UMass Dartmouth

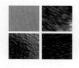

PEDIATRIC REHABILITATION NURSING

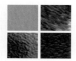

PEDIATRIC REHABILITATION NURSING

Patricia A. Edwards, EdD, RN, CNAA
Nursing Director
The Shriver Center University Affiliated Program
Waltham, Massachusetts
Rehabilitation Nursing Consultant, Private Practice
Rockport, Massachusetts

Dalice L. Hertzberg, MSN, RN, CRRN
Colorado University Affiliated Program
Instructor
University of Colorado School of Medicine
University of Colorado Health Sciences Center
Denver, Colorado

Susanne R. Hays, MS, RN, CRRN, CCM
Advanced Practice Nurse
Pediatric Rehabilitation and Developmental Disabilities, Private Practice
Albuquerque, New Mexico

Nancy M. Youngblood, PhD, CRNP
Assistant Professor and Coordinator
Nurse Practitioner Programs
LaSalle University School of Nursing
Philadelphia, Pennsylvania

W.B. SAUNDERS COMPANY
A Division of Harcourt Brace & Company
Philadelphia   London   Toronto   Montreal   Sydney   Tokyo

W.B. SAUNDERS COMPANY
A Division of Harcourt Brace & Company

The Curtis Center
Independence Square West
Philadelphia, Pennsylvania 19106

Library of Congress Cataloging-in-Publication Data

Pediatric rehabilitation nursing / Patricia A. Edwards . . . [et al.].—1st ed.

p.   cm.

ISBN 0–7216–5425–8

1. Pediatric nursing.   2. Rehabilitation nursing.   I. Edwards, Patricia A. (Patricia Ann).   [DNLM: 1. Rehabilitation Nursing.   2. Pediatric Nursing.
3. Rehabilitation—in infancy & childhood.   WY 150.5 P371 1999]

RJ245.P437   1999

610.73′62—dc21

DNLM/DLC   98–5825

PEDIATRIC REHABILITATION NURSING   ISBN 0–7216–5425–8

Printed in the United States of America.

Last digit is the print number: 9   8   7   6   5   4   3   2   1

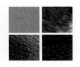 # Contributors

Mary G. Boland, MSN, RN, FAAN
François Xavier Bagnoud Professor of
    Community Pediatric Nursing
School of Nursing
University of Medicine and Dentistry of
    New Jersey
Newark, New Jersey

Michael Comeau, MS, RN
Faculty, Massachusetts Bay Community
    College
Framingham
Clinical Nurse Specialist, Pediatrics
Dana-Farber Cancer Institute
Boston, Massachusetts

Lynn Czarniecki, MSN, RN, C, CNS-C
Advanced Practice Nurse
François Xavier Bagnoud Center
School of Nursing
University of Medicine and Dentistry
    of New Jersey
Newark, New Jersey

Janet Duncan, RN, BSN, CPON
Staff III, Oncology Program
Children's Hospital
Boston, Massachusetts

Cynthia H. Himes, RN, CRRN
Nursing Supervisor
Children's Seashore House
Philadelphia, Pennsylvania

Kathleen Ryan Kuntz, MSN, RN, CRRN, CLCP, Cm
Clinical Preceptor, University of
    Pennsylvania School of Nursing
Clinical Instructor, Thomas Jefferson
    University School of Nursing
Core Faculty, Children's Seashore House
Philadelphia
President, Rehab Advantage
Jamison, Pennsylvania

Deb Ryan Michalak, RN, BSN
Director of Nursing
Misericordia Home South
Chicago, Illinois

Teresa A. Savage, PhD, RN
Adjunct Assistant Professor, Maternal Child
    Nursing
Post-doctoral Research Fellow, Primary
    Health Care/Social Ethics
College of Nursing, University of Illinois at
    Chicago
Clinical Nurse Specialist, Pediatric
    Neurology, Rush Presbyterian-St. Luke's
    Medical Center
Chicago, Illinois

Preface

Pediatric rehabilitation nursing has evolved over the past 25 years from the separate practices of pediatrics and rehabilitation into a true specialty practice committed to the care of children and adolescents with disabilities and chronic conditions and to their families. No nursing textbook until now addressed this new specialty.

Pediatric Rehabilitation Nursing brings together a unique body of knowledge specific to the care of children and adolescents with disabilities and chronic conditions and to their families. It was conceived as a method of filling a need we discovered in our discussions with colleagues and in our search for a single source that provided both theoretical information and guidance, as well as information about the child's growth and development and the impact of pediatric rehabilitation nursing care on the family.

This book provides an important reference for nurses in a multitude of practice settings. It is based on a combination of core values and beliefs about the worth of the individual. A continuum of care—from hospital to home and community—is presented with emphasis on rehabilitation management in the least restricted environment necessary to maximize the potential of the child, adolescent, and family.

As mentioned, the purpose of this book is to provide a reference for pediatric rehabilitation nurses that combines clinical guidance, information on growth and development, and consideration for the families of children with special health care needs. It is written also for those who care for and about children and adolescents with disabilities and chronic conditions and for their families. *Pediatric Rehabilitation Nursing* is designed to support the clinical practice of the registered nurse who works with children in a pediatric rehabilitation setting or with children who have rehabilitation needs and problems. It can also be used as a course textbook by nursing students in graduate courses in pediatrics, rehabilitation, ambulatory care, community health, and family health. This text can act as a supplement in undergraduate upper division courses in which content on children with special health and developmental needs is required. We also believe that this text is appropriate for practicing nurses in a variety of settings—inpatient, outpatient, community, and long-term care—especially new graduates in rehabilitation settings.

The book has four sections that provide a comprehensive resource for the practicing nurse and essential information for nursing students and new graduates. Part I begins with chapters that introduce the reader to pediatric rehabilitation nursing and its standards of practice, ethics, legislation and public policy, principles, and community-based care and models. Part II focuses on health promotion and management; physical and psychosocial health care patterns and nursing diagnoses; family-centered care; and growth and development and the home, school, and community environments. Part III integrates information on specific nursing care relevant to given disorders. The design of each chapter includes information on the disorder, particularly etiology and incidence, clinical aspects, functional limitations, diagnoses, therapeutic management, impact on the family, and application of the nursing process. Part IV addresses further dimensions in pediatric rehabilitation nursing. Chapters include content related to research, advanced nursing practice, outcome, and program evaluation and future directions—including health care reform, community integration, technology, genetic research, alternative therapies, and aging with a disability.

PAE
DLH
SRH
NMY

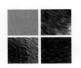

Acknowledgments

A book of this scope is not possible without the encouragement and assistance of many people—family members, contributors, professional colleagues, and friends—as well as the support provided by the collegial relationship among the four authors. The authors wish to extend special thanks to our families for their patience and support in the process of creating this book—to Bill, Jon, and Beth Edwards; Howard Hertzberg; Francis and Jeannette Hays; Joellen Hollingsworth; Carolyn Hoffman; and Benjamin and Erinn Hart.

We also thank the colleagues and friends who supported our original concept; provided information, resources, and assistance; reviewed chapters; and offered encouragement throughout the project, especially members of the ARN Pediatric Special Interest Group, staff at the Children's Specialized Hospital, faculty and staff at the Colorado University's Affiliated Program, particularly Cordelia Robinson, PhD, RN, FAAN, Randi Hagerman, MD, Ann Grady, MS, OT, Renee Charlifue-Smith, MA, and Tracy Price Johnson; Marilyn Krajicek, EdD, of the University of Colorado School of Nursing; and Amy Bodkin, MS, PT, of the University of Colorado School of Physical Therapy, as well as Judith Walker, Judy Taylor, and Judy Ducharme for technical assistance and support.

Finally, we want to acknowledge all of the children, adolescents, and families who have had a tremendous impact on our knowledge and learning over the years and who have increased our sensitivity to their special needs and problems.

NOTICE

Nursing is an ever-changing field. Standard safety precautions must be followed, but as new research and clinical experience broaden our knowledge, changes in treatment and drug therapy become necessary or appropriate. Readers are advised to check the product information currently provided by the manufacturer of each drug to be administered to verify the recommended dose, the method and duration of administration, and the contraindications. It is the responsibility of the treating physician, relying on experience and knowledge of the patient, to determine the dosages and the best treatment for the patient. Neither the publisher nor the editor assumes any responsibility for any injury and/or damage to persons or property.

THE PUBLISHER

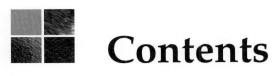

Contents

Part I

Perspectives on Pediatric Rehabilitation Nursing Practice

Chapter 1

Introduction to Pediatric Rehabilitation Nursing

Dalice Hertzberg and *Patricia A. Edwards*

The practice of pediatric rehabilitation nursing has evolved over the past 20 years from a mere combination of pediatrics and rehabilitation into a true specialty committed to the care of children with disabilities or other chronic conditions and their families. Nurses in this field, in a collaborative relationship with the interdisciplinary team, provide a continuum of care so that children can become contributing members of society and function at their maximum potential. Pediatric rehabilitation nursing is described by the Association of Rehabilitation Nurses (ARN) as:

> ... both specialized and diverse—a combination clearly reflected in the populations the specialty serves. Infants, children and adolescents with a variety of disabling conditions receive specialized care from pediatric rehabilitation nurses in settings ranging from hospital to home, from clinic to school. Physical, emotional, social, cultural, educational, developmental and spiritual dimensions are all considered in a holistic approach to care. The unique qualities of each child are cherished and fostered. (ARN, 1992)

Table 1–1 shows some of the roles of the pediatric rehabilitation nurse.

This chapter introduces the terms and definitions commonly used in pediatric rehabilitation, the historical evolution of pediatric rehabilitation, the clients served by pediatric rehabilitation providers, the settings in which pediatric rehabilitation is practiced, and the concepts, assumptions, and values that form the base of pediatric rehabilitation nursing practice.

TERMS

Many terms are used to describe the situation of a child with a disability or other chronic condition. To establish a common frame of reference and avoid the confusion that results when a term is used without clear definition, the following terms are defined: child, family and family-centered care, habilitation and rehabilitation, health care services (including primary, secondary, and tertiary interventions), disability and handicap, chronic condition, and children with special health care needs.

Child

The focus of care, the child, refers to neonates, infants, toddlers, school-aged children, and adolescents. Instead of using varying terms throughout the book, we choose to refer to all age groups from birth through 21 years of age as children. The terms child and children are used throughout the text for consistency and brevity.

Family and Family-Centered Care

"Family" refers to:

> the basic unit of society having as its nucleus one or more persons consistently serving in the care giving role for the child. This role may be filled by a parent, foster parent, guardian, brother or sister, ... (New England SERVE, 1989, p. 76)

"Family-centered care" is a philosophy of care that recognizes the pivotal role of the

3

Table 1–1   ROLES OF THE PEDIATRIC REHABILITATION NURSE

Advocate

Functions as a child and family advocate
Facilitates the child and family's transition from hospital to home and community
Promotes community and governmental knowledge of pediatric rehabilitation issues

Coordinator

Works as a valued member of the health care team
Brings together the expertise of health professionals and integrates that knowledge into the comprehensive continuum of care
Facilitates the design and implementation of the family's individual plan of care

Leader

Demonstrates leadership through clinical expertise and delegates responsibilities to other members of the team
Acts as an agent of change
Consults with other health professionals

Teacher

Shares knowledge and skills
Offers counseling and support to families about the special needs of their children and adolescents with disabilities
Teaches other individuals (both in the healthcare field and in the community) about the special aspects of children's and adolescent's rehabilitation needs

Team Member

Works as part of an innovative and creative unit
Collaborates in the development of new service delivery models that best meet the needs of young clients and their families

Primary Care Provider

Implements nursing care based on a sound knowledge base, scientific principles, and a documented therapeutic plan

Reprinted with permission of the Association of Rehabilitation Nurses (ARN) from *Pediatric rehabilitation nursing: role description*. Skokie, IL: ARN. Copyright 1992. Association of Rehabilitation Nurses, 4700 W. Lake Avenue, Glenview, IL 60025-1485.

family in the lives of children with disabilities or other chronic conditions. It is a philosophy that strives to support families in their natural caregiving roles by building on their unique strengths as individuals and parents. This perspective promotes normal patterns of living at home and in the community and views families and professionals as equals in a part-

nership committed to excellence at all levels of health care. The ability and willingness of nurses and health care providers to share knowledge and control of health resources with families, empowering them to act as advocates for themselves and their children, is an integral part of family-centered care. Key elements of family-centered care are found in Table 1–2 and are discussed further in Chapter 9.

Rehabilitation and Habilitation

Because pediatric rehabilitation includes the management of children with both acquired and developmental disabilities, the words "habilitation" and "rehabilitation" can be used to differentiate the approaches between the two types of disability. These terms are described as follows:

> Habilitation includes all the activities and interactions that enable an individual with a disability to develop new abilities to achieve his or her maximum potential, whereas rehabilitation is the relearning of previous skills, which often requires an adjustment to altered functional abilities and altered lifestyle. (Burkett, 1989, p. 239)

The primary difference between rehabilitation of children and rehabilitation of adults is the developmental potential of the child. The child or adolescent may receive an injury resulting in disability at any age, with very different consequences for his or her future depending on the age and developmental level at which the trauma occurred. Children who are born with genetic disorders, who are premature, or whose fetal development is affected by maternal disease, injury, or substance abuse require services focused on habilitation rather than rehabilitation.

Whereas rehabilitation refers to the relearning of skills or behaviors lost as a result of disease or injury, habilitation refers to the process of acquiring skills and behaviors by an individual whose development has been affected by disease or other disabling conditions since birth or very early childhood. This process includes procedures and interventions designed to help the individual achieve greater mental, physical, and social development. Children and adults who are diagnosed with a developmental disability often receive habilitative services. Habilitation often can be even more challenging than rehabilitation, because the child must achieve developmental tasks for the first time while hampered by the disability or chronic health condition.

Table 1-2   THE KEY ELEMENTS OF FAMILY-CENTERED CARE

Incorporating into policy and practice the recognition that the *family is the constant* in a child's life, while the service systems and support personnel within those systems fluctuate.

Facilitating *family/professional collaboration* at all levels of hospital, home, and community care: care of an individual child; program development, implementation, evaluation, and evolution; and policy formation.

Exchanging complete and unbiased information between families and professionals in a supportive manner at all times.

Incorporating into policy and practice the recognition and *honoring of cultural diversity*, strengths, and individuality within and across all families, including *ethnic, racial, spiritual, social, economic, educational, and geographic diversity.*

Recognizing and respecting *different methods of coping* and implementing comprehensive policies and programs that provide *developmental, educational, emotional, environmental, and financial supports* to meet the diverse needs of families.

Encouraging and facilitating *family-to-family support* and networking.

Ensuring that *hospital, home, and community service and support systems* for children needing specialized health and developmental care and their families are *flexible, accessible, and comprehensive* in responding to diverse family-identified needs.

Appreciating families as families and children as children, recognizing that they possess a wide range of strengths, concerns, emotions, and aspirations beyond their need for specialized health and developmental services and support.

Reproduced with permission of the Association for the Care of Children's Health, 7910 Woodmont Ave., Suite 300, Bethesda, Maryland, 20814. From Shelton, T., & Stepanek, J. (1994). *Family-centered care for children needing specialized health and developmental services.*

Children With Special Health Care Needs

The phrase "children with special health care needs" describes a heterogeneous group of children who have a need for ongoing specialized health services in addition to well child care. The definition includes children from birth to 21 years of age who have any of a broad spectrum of disabilities or chronic conditions diagnosed at any time during the pre-natal period or childhood. Such chronic conditions may require adaptations for daily functioning, periodic or prolonged hospitalizations, or special services in the home, school, or community setting. Examples of the types of disabilities and conditions these children have include cerebral palsy, human immunodeficiency virus (HIV) infection, diabetes, myelodysplasia, or cystic fibrosis (New England SERVE, 1989).

Health Care Services

"Health care services" refers to practice in primary, secondary, and tertiary settings. Primary level intervention includes well child care, preventive measures, routine screening, health promotion, and health education. Secondary level intervention consists of treatments or strategies to limit the effects of disabilities and prevent complications. Tertiary level intervention targets optimal function and improved outcome and is brought about by methods such as corrective surgery and educational and self-care interventions focused on developing lifelong coping and adaptation skills. These services may be delivered in inpatient, ambulatory, and community-based settings, including tertiary care centers, hospitals, specialty clinics, neighborhood health centers, and the home.

Disability and Handicap

There is an appropriate distinction between the terms "disability" and "handicap." Disability is an established variation with potential functional significance. Disability is defined by the Americans With Disabilities Act (ADA) as "the inability to perform key life functions" (Watson, 1990). The World Health Organization (WHO), in an effort to describe the effects of disability in a global context, has devised a system called The Consequences of Disease and Injury, which includes the concepts of disease, impairment, and disability. The term handicap represents the degree of limitation or hindrance produced by the disability at the environmental or societal level (WHO, 1980).

The term "developmental disability" is popularly used to refer to children with congenital conditions that cause disability, as well as to individuals who are mentally retarded. Legally, for the purpose of provision of services that are mandated by the federal government and provided by states, the definition of a developmental disability found in the Rehabilitation Comprehensive Services and Developmental Disabilities Amendments of 1978 (Public Law 95–602) is as follows:

A severe, chronic disability of a person which: (A) is attributable to a mental or physical impairment or a combination of mental and physical impairments; (B) is manifested before the person attains the age twenty-two; (C) is likely to continue indefinitely; (D) results in substantial functional limitations in three or more of the following areas of major life activity: (i) self-care, (ii) receptive and expressive language, (iii) learning, (iv) mobility, (v) self-direction, (vi) capacity for independent living, and (vii) economic sufficiency; and (E) reflects the person's need for a combination and sequence of special interdisciplinary, or generic care, treatment, or other services which are of lifelong or extended duration and are individually planned and coordinated.

The subsequent Developmental Disabilities Act of 1984 (Public Law 98–527) retains the same elements contained in this definition.

Chronic Condition

The term "chronic condition" refers to any long-term condition that interferes with daily functioning. It has one or more of the following characteristics: "It is permanent; leaves residual disability; is caused by a non-pathological alteration; requires special training for rehabilitation; is expected to require a long period of supervision, observation or care" (Hymovich & Hagopian, 1992, p. 19).

HISTORICAL PERSPECTIVE

Although the specialty of pediatric rehabilitation nursing is relatively new, the interest in and commitment to services for children with disability or chronic illness dates back well over 100 years. For instance, in 1829, Dr. Samuel Gridley Howe opened the New England Asylum for the Blind and began a program for two blind students. In the last two decades of the nineteenth century, a number of

other institutions were founded to meet the needs of children. One developed from a "fresh air" summer home into an accredited hospital dedicated to the unique needs of children with physical disabilities and respiratory ailments. Others began as a special place to help underprivileged children from the slums and operated as a respite summer program for children, or a fresh air camp. Table 1–3 provides a specific timeline of rehabilitation institutions, and Figures 1–1 through 1–4 show a series of pictures of the various activities in these institutions.

Near the end of the nineteenth century, greater attention was focused on the education and training of children with physical disabilities. Many cities and states established special schools for these children, and some of the beginning endeavors in the area we

Table 1–3 PEDIATRIC REHABILITATION EVOLUTION

Pre-1880

1829	School for Blind Students—New England Asylum for the Blind

1880–1900

1872	Summer convalescent facility for children needing long-term care—Children's Seashore House
1883	Fresh air summer home—Hospital for Sick Children
1889	The Cleveland Rehabilitation Center
1891	Country place for slum children—Children's Country Home (now Children's Specialized Hospital)
1892	Summer respite program for crippled children—Teaching and Visiting Guild for Crippled Children (now Blythedale Children's Hospital)
1893	The Boston Industrial School for Crippled and Deformed
1895	Children's fresh air camp (now Health Hill Hospital)
1895	Fresh air sanitarium (now LaRabida Children's Hospital)
1898	Home for incurables (now Newington Children's Hospital)

Early 20th Century

1902	Home for crippled children (now The Rehabilitation Institue—Pittsburgh)
1922	Happy Hills Convalescent Center (now Mt. Washington Pediatric Hospital)
1930	Elizabethtown Hospital and Rehabilitation Center
1937	Children's Rehabilitation Institute (now the Kennedy Institute—Baltimore)

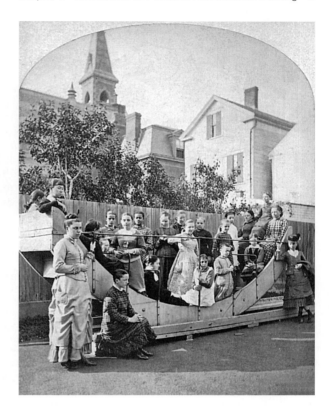

Figure 1–1   Institute for the Blind, South Boston, 1871. (Courtesy of Perkins School for the Blind, Watertown, MA.)

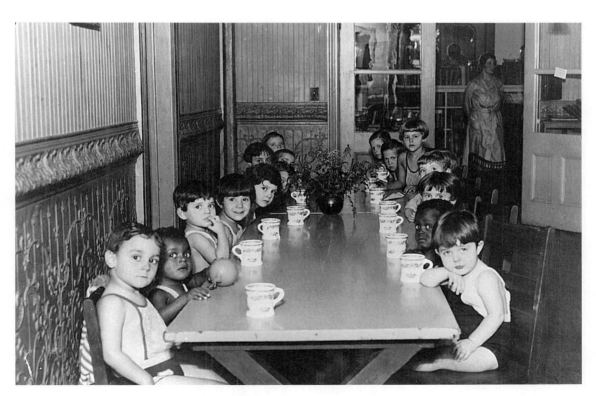

Figure 1–2   Children's Country Home, Westfield, New Jersey, 1920s. (Courtesy of Children's Specialized Hospital, Mountainside, NJ.)

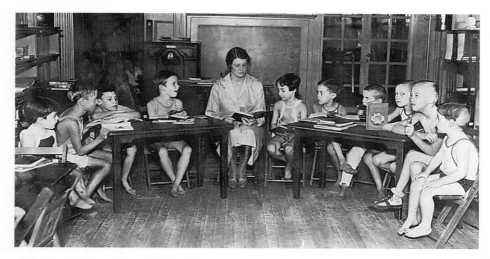

Figure 1–3 Children's Country Home, Westfield, New Jersey. (Courtesy of Children's Specialized Hospital, Mountainside, NJ.)

now call rehabilitation were made by private individuals or groups in one specialized area, such as blindness or orthopedic problems.

During the first decade of the twentieth century, society began to focus on the needs of individuals with disabilities by providing a therapeutic environment for the treatment of specific disabilities while beginning to address individuals' educational and vocational needs. This was especially important for children who need to have a separate environment that supports their specific developmental, educational, and family needs as well as treat their specific condition.

World War I had a tremendous impact on the American practice of physical medicine. A special hospital for physical reconstruction was designed to treat wounded soldiers and others requiring rehabilitation, and the need for providing educational and vocational rehabilitation that would restore a sense of meaning to their lives was recognized. In Europe, the first spinal centers incorporated the concepts of aseptic technique and functional education.

In the following two decades, attempts were made to define and implement the role of therapists, to define rehabilitation as a

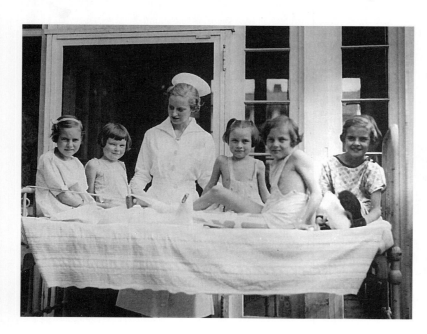

Figure 1–4 Children's Country Home, Westfield, New Jersey. (Courtesy of Children's Specialized Hospital, Mountainside, NJ.)

process that helped a disabled person become capable of engaging in a remunerative occupation, to provide rehabilitation services beyond the needs of the military and outside hospital walls, and to encourage the use of simple physical therapy modalities by all physicians. The impact of polio and the development of spinal cord injury centers stimulated many advances in rehabilitation, such as development of the iron lung, positive-pressure ventilation, pneumobelts, wrist-driven hand splints, and prototypes for other mobility devices.

In the latter part of the twentieth century, the pediatric rehabilitation facilities that "began as summer homes or chronic facilities, evolved and changed to meet the needs of the times and advances in medical technology" (Edwards, 1992, p. 192). Some examples of these changes include pediatric rehabilitation hospitals that are consolidating with acute pediatric services; establishing a long-term care unit; opening a satellite pediatric rehabilitation inpatient unit; operating as an academic center; and offering day school programs. Additionally:

> They are important facilities for rehabilitation, as children need to have separate therapeutic environments that support their developmental, educational and family needs as well as their specific condition. These facilities are continuing to evolve in purpose, scope and mission, and they are changing to serve children with a variety of disabling conditions (Edwards, 1992, p. 192).

PEDIATRIC REHABILITATION POPULATION

Death rates in infancy and childhood have declined markedly during the twentieth century, most noticeably in the case of infections as a cause of death. Most of the deadly childhood diseases prevalent in the early part of the century have been controlled by the development of effective vaccines and implementation of public health standards that are among the best in the world. In addition, advances in pre-natal diagnosis and preventive interventions for a number of birth defects, such as neural tube defects (e.g., spina bifida, anencephaly) have also served to decrease the incidence of these conditions (Centers for Disease Control and Prevention [CDC], 1995b).

Despite these advances, a number of health problems have increased in frequency. Injuries, whether accidental or intentional (e.g.,

child abuse, homicide), are now the third leading cause of death in the United States (Baker, O'Neill, & Karpf, 1992). For children aged 1 to 4 years, 45% of all health problems are caused by injuries, compared with 12% of health problems caused by congenital anomalies. For children 5 to 15 years of age, the percentage of health problems caused by injury increases to 56% (Baker, O'Neill, & Karpf, 1992).

Violence is a major cause of death and disability among children and youths in the United States. In 1992, more than 5000 children were killed by guns—one child every 98 minutes (Children's Defense Fund, 1995). Thousands more survived injuries incurred from guns, with sequelae ranging from soft tissue to brain and spinal cord injuries.

As the number of births to adolescent mothers rise, so do the number of premature and low-birth-weight infants. More babies are born at very low birth weights and earlier in gestation and are surviving, putting them at greater risk for chronic conditions and disability. Increasing rates of poverty in the United States contribute to poor pre-natal and ongoing health care, and maternal substance abuse results in infants born with congenital conditions and affected by cocaine and alcohol. Increases in homelessness and substandard living conditions lead to more health, developmental, and nutritional problems in children (Children's Defense Fund, 1995).

The *National Health Interview Survey* found that the rate of limitation of activity, a method of measuring the effect of disability on the individual, has doubled since 1960, as has the proportion of children who are identified as having a major limitation of activity (National Center for Health Statistics, 1993). Data from the Survey of Income and Program Participation for 1991–1992 (National Center for Health Statistics, 1993) indicate that of the estimated 48.9 million people who have a disability, 3.8 million are 17 years of age or younger. For children younger than 3 years of age, the prevalence of disability is 2.2%; for children from 3 to 5 years of age, the prevalence of disability is 5.2%; for children aged 6 to 14 years, the prevalence of disability is 6.3%; and for adolescents 15 to 17 years of age, the prevalence is 9.3%. In all age groups, more males are disabled than females, with the gender-specific difference being greatest in the 6- to 14-year-old age group.

The impact of disabilities is disproportionately greater in children than in adults in the United States. Disabilities that begin during childhood account for about one third of the years of disability in the total U.S. population, including both children and adults. The increasing percentage of disability in children with age most likely reflects the greater ease of identification of functional deficits by schools and health care providers as a child's performance becomes more complex and more readily measured by objective means. Despite the use of these methods, the prevalence of disability in children is still very likely underestimated (CDC, 1995a).

Pediatric rehabilitation involves children with chronic conditions affecting the neurologic and musculoskeletal systems as well as those conditions significantly affecting child development. Trauma is a primary cause of disabling conditions in children, with head injury alone accounting for approximately 200,000 hospital admissions yearly (Molnar & Perrins, 1992). Trauma may result from falls, automobile and other accidents, child abuse, and violence (e.g., shootings). Head injury is the leading cause of death in children, youths, and young adults; half of all mortality is due to trauma in children younger than 15 years of age. Of this group, head injuries cause half of trauma deaths. Of children who survive head injury, about 10 in 100,000 experience severe brain injury, with disabilities ranging from persistent vegetative state to learning and adjustment problems (Fletcher, Ewing-Cobbs, Francis, & Levin, 1995). Head and spinal cord injuries are the most disabling forms of trauma in children and youths.

A second important cause of disability in children is prematurity and low birth weight. Children who are born earlier than 30 weeks of gestation are at greater risk for some form of disability or chronic condition than infants born at term. These conditions range from learning disabilities, which occur in 6.5% of all children (National Center for Health Statistics, 1993), to cerebral palsy, which occurs in 2 in 100 births (Molnar, 1992). Another significant cause of disability in children is congenital or genetic conditions. These conditions include the mid-line deficits such as cleft palate and myelomeningocele, syndromes resulting from TORCH infections of the mother, muscular dystrophies, and other genetic and teratogenic causes. Birth defects occur in an estimated 150,000 babies born each year (Sever, 1993). Birth defects, which may be categorized as congenital anomalies, cause approximately one out of every five infant deaths (National Center for Health Statistics, 1993).

Table 1–4 MOST COMMON DIAGNOSTIC CLASSIFICATIONS

Diagnosis	Respondents	Percentage of Facilities
Traumatic brain injury	84	73
Spinal cord injury	63	55
Cerebral palsy	52	45
Spina bifida	28	24
Bronchopulmonary dysplasia	20	17
Cerebrovascular accident	18	16
Burns	14	12
Orthopedic problems	34	30
Neurologic problems	32	28

Edwards, P. (1995). Pediatric Special Interest Group survey results. *ARN News*, 11(1), 4.

In 1994 the Pediatric Special Interest Group of the Association of Rehabilitation Nurses conducted a survey of its members (Edwards, 1995). One section of the questionnaire asked for a list of the five most frequently encountered diagnoses. Table 1–4 shows the most common classifications. Some of the diagnoses, such as orthopedic and neurologic problems, were grouped for reporting purposes. Other less common diagnoses identified included behavior problems, muscular dystrophy, developmental disabilities, anoxia, failure to thrive, and Guillain-Barré syndrome.

The numbers of children and families requiring pediatric rehabilitation services are increasing as a result of advances in medical care and technology. This includes areas such as emergency care, intensive care and neonatal intensive care, and home and community care. As a result of these advances, children are surviving previously fatal conditions to return to their homes, schools, and communities with disabilities, dependent on life-sustaining medical equipment, and requiring an intensity of care and services that was unheard of only 10 years ago. Pediatric rehabilitation services are required to enable these children to reach the stage at which they can rejoin their community, and for their families to learn the skills they need to provide the necessary care for the child.

WHERE DOES PEDIATRIC REHABILITATION TAKE PLACE?

The variety of services and service sites described represent a continuum of services that are available to every child with a disability or chronic condition. The type and intensity of services that are accessed by the family is determined by the nature and severity of the child's condition, the family's insurance, their geographic location (urban or rural), and the availability of specialty pediatric rehabilitation services in the area.

A pediatric rehabilitation facility promotes the rehabilitation of children with disabling conditions through an integrated program of medical, nursing, therapy, psychological, social, and vocational evaluation and treatment. During the course of the program, a major portion of evaluation and treatment is furnished within the facility. The facility and its operations may be connected with a hospital or may be free-standing. All health-related services are prescribed by or under the general supervision of physicians specializing in rehabilitation medicine or developmental pediatrics. More recently, physicians interested in pediatric rehabilitation pursue residencies in both physiatry and pediatrics and then become board certified to practice in both specialties.

Rehabilitation facilities for children serve a specific client population from birth to 21 years of age who have lost function or ability because of an injury, congenital condition, or disease. With the help of an interdisciplinary team of health care providers specializing in pediatric rehabilitation and the care and support of the child's family, a child can develop or recover the skills necessary to resume the activities of everyday life. The facility may provide additional developmental, educational, family, or social services as warranted by the needs of the child and family.

Rehabilitation services for children fall within the continuum of health care. According to Perrins (1988), 85% of what individuals who have a chronic illness need is based on their needs as a human being, whereas 15% of their needs come from the risks or threats to health presented by a specific disease condition. Acute care rehabilitation services take place after an injury or surgical procedure, as soon as the child's condition is stabilized. Acute care rehabilitation services are delivered in the inpatient setting in either a free-standing rehabilitation center or a rehabilitation unit in a hospital. Ideally, rehabilitation in the form of therapeutic exercises, proper positioning, and family counseling may be initiated as soon as several days following the injury. Children with congenital or developmental disabilities or with conditions acquired through a past trauma may be candidates for corrective surgical interventions; for example, dorsal rhizotomy for relief of spasticity stemming from cerebral palsy. In such cases, the rehabilitation team is generally involved in the decision to do the surgery, along with the child and family, and may initiate therapeutic interventions as early as the first day following the surgery.

Sub-acute rehabilitation services are provided for children who require inpatient treatment but not at the initial intensity required just after an injury. Sub-acute services for adults are delivered in long-term care settings such as skilled nursing facility units, nursing homes, or various types of day treatment centers. Sub-acute services for children are more often delivered in day treatment programs, allowing the child to go home to his or her family at night and on weekends, or in specialized residential settings.

Outpatient rehabilitation services account for the majority of services used by children with disabilities and their families. Many children with congenital or developmental disabilities may never require hospitalization but receive the most benefit from therapeutic interventions delivered in serial appointments with therapists and nurses, as well as periodic evaluation by a rehabilitation physician. Visits to the rehabilitation clinic for periodic check-ups may occur yearly or more or less frequently, depending on the age of the child, the severity of symptoms, and the effects of the disabling condition. The family's funding source for health care and their proximity to the outpatient clinic is also a major determinant of frequency and scheduling of services.

Community-based services are delivered in the natural environments of the child—the home, the school or day care, or early intervention center. These services are delivered by nurses, therapists, psychologists, social workers, and special education teachers on a periodic basis, as prescribed by the physician and the child's individual education plan (IEP) or individualized family service plan (IFSP). Within the school system, the IEP and IFSP are plans that are formulated by the family and community service providers to meet the child's educational and related service needs.

Current concerns about the deleterious effect of prolonged institutional care on development and advocacy on the part of parents who want to care for their children at home has resulted in the exploration of alternatives to normalize the environment of the child with a disability to the greatest extent possible. Technologic advances are among the factors that have made home care and community care a viable alternative for the great majority of children with severe disabilities and chronic conditions. The development of portable ventilators, home dialysis, and home cardiorespiratory monitors are examples of technology that make home and community management possible.

School systems also provide services for children with disabilities. The Individuals With Disabilities Education Act of 1993 (IDEA; Public Law 102–119), mandates the provision of related services that are necessary for a child with a disability or chronic condition to benefit from public education. IDEA instructs states to provide a free, public education to all children from 3 through 21 years of age, regardless of disability, in the least restrictive environment (i.e., the most typical and usual environment possible). Part H of IDEA provides for early intervention services for children from birth through 3 years of age, and part B provides for preschool services for children with disabilities.

In addition, philosophical developments, such as those reflected in legislation such as IDEA and ADA, have resulted in more opportunities for children with disabilities to participate in the daily activities of their nondisabled peers in schools, communities, and recreational activities. These philosophical changes on the part of health and human service providers have largely been brought about by the efforts and influence of parents collaborating with professionals who seek equality of opportunity for children regardless of their disability.

Although the IDEA legislation was the culmination of many years of political action on the part of families, educators, and health care providers, it has not met with universal approval from school districts and the general public. Inadequate funding, lack of availability of supportive services and training for teachers, and philosophical differences have jeopardized IDEA. The law is up for re-authorization by Congress, and it is unclear whether or not it will survive in its present form. Additional information about legislative issues is presented in Chapter 4.

Services facilitating the transition of children from one delivery setting to the next are crucial to the child's attainment of appropriate age-related roles. Children with disabilities experience transitions many times during their lifetimes, moving from hospital to home, from pre-school to grade school, from grade or middle school to high school, and from high school to college, a vocational setting, or independent living. Specific skills—academic, social, and physical—are required for the child to be successful in a new grade, with new friends and new expectations of his or her abilities.

One of the most crucial of these skill sets are vocational skills. Vocational skills encompass not just the physical or cognitive ability to perform a specific job, but the judgment, social skills, and self-discipline necessary to hold down a job, be on time, get along with other employees and managers, and take direction and criticism. Performance of meaningful employment may involve not only physical adaptations to the workplace but specific training for the adolescent or young adult with a disability in critical social and emotional skills.

In addition to academic-related transitions, there are health-related transitions. During adolescence, most children learn the self-help skills that allow them to appropriately seek health and medical care when they are ill as well as the skills that maintain health. Children with disabilities must master these skills as well as others; the complexity of their medical condition requires greater skills in self-care, judgment, and motivation in seeking medical assistance when needed.

Transition also occurs in the type of health care provider from whom the individual seeks care. Typically, children with disabilities receive well child care from a pediatrician or pediatric nurse practitioner, or occasionally from a family practice physician. Specialty health care services are provided by pediatric specialists, such as pediatric neurologists, pediatric orthopedic surgeons, pediatric physiatrists, clinical nurse specialists, and nurse practitioners. As the child becomes an adult, his or her health care needs change and should appropriately be provided by adult health practitioners, such as internists for primary care, general practice urologists, and other adult specialists. Failing to undergo this transition may present a significant problem, because pediatric providers are not always able to provide safe, appropriate adult health care. Young adults with disabilities may go totally without health care or receive inconsistent preventive care or minor acute illness care. This can jeopardize overall health, reduce opportunities for early detection of problems and preventive services, and jeopardize the continuity of care to which they are entitled.

Although the great majority of children with disabilities remain with their biologic family, situations exist in which the biologic family is unable to provide a safe environment for the child or is unable to provide the specialized care that the child needs. In these situations, out-of-home or residential care may be an option. In most cases of out-of-home care, county or facility social services or child welfare workers are involved with the child and family. Social services involvement may be sought by the family or ordered by the court. In most states, a permanency plan is required for children with disabilities in out-of-home settings; this plan must work to ensure the best interests of the child and help to meet the child's needs for care and nurturing during the growing years. Placements range from medical foster homes and adoptions to private or state-run group homes and institutions.

CONCEPTS AND ASSUMPTIONS

Pediatric rehabilitation nursing care is based on a set of primary concepts and assumptions that help to provide the philosophical basis for services and direct the focus of care. These assumptions describe the major differences between the rehabilitation of adults and the rehabilitation of children. Children with disabilities all receive some level of habilitative care. Because of the developmental process, children are always developing and maturing. Whereas rehabilitation services can help restore skills lost after injury or disease, habilitation takes place as the child continues to mature, both physiologically and psychologically.

"Developmental theory is a cornerstone of pediatric rehabilitation nursing" (ARN, 1992). The disruption of life experiences that occurs with injury, disease, or congenital condition puts the child's growth and development in all domains in jeopardy. A comprehensive understanding of the developmental stages and the interaction of the disability or condition with physiologic and socio-emotional developmental tasks is crucial to providing appropriate pediatric rehabilitation nursing care.

"Pediatric rehabilitation nurses recognize the importance of family involvement in the young person's development and are advocates for children and their families. The young client and his or her family form the core of the rehabilitation team" (ARN, 1992). Children are totally dependent on their family for nurturing, love, and care as they grow and develop. When this process is interrupted by injury or disease, the family becomes even more important to the child. In pediatric rehabilitation nursing, the child and family cannot be separated, and the family unit as a whole is the recipient of services. The child's physical and emotional development depends on the family's ability to tend to the child's needs. Whereas an adult with a disability may learn how to train, hire, and fire personal attendants, a child will simply not survive without their family or a family substitute. Even those children who end up in foster care frequently develop significant problems in relating to others due to a lack of initial bonding and inconsistency of caregivers. These problems significantly affect the child's ability to learn and to function as a productive, happy adult.

Another aspect of pediatric rehabilitation that differs from that of adults is the complexity of the long-term outlook for services and care. For adults, rehabilitation services, in seeking to restore lost function, need be concerned only with the developmental consequences of adulthood. Rehabilitation of children, however, must take into account not just how the child might best function at the age when the injury occurred, but how that disability and its treatment will impact his or her future development and achievement of adult abilities, roles, and relationships. For example, a 5-year-old child had a head injury that has affected his memory. Whereas the physical effects of the injury may be treated by ankle braces and physical therapy, the inability to remember new information has far-reaching implications for school, work, and relationships that will last throughout his life span.

More specifically, children differ from adults physiologically, and these differences have tremendous implications for rehabilitative care. Immaturity of systems and vital organs leads to differences in fluid maintenance, homeostatic control mechanisms, and vulnerability to infection and disease. Treatment of fractures and choice and dosage of medications will also be different. Airway management, emergency procedures and equipment, and size and replacement schedule of assistive devices and durable medical goods such as wheelchairs and braces are also affected. Differences in developmental level affect treatment goals, teaching methods, approaches to the child and family, safety considerations, and expectations with regard to independence. These differences are addressed in more detail in Chapter 7.

Assumptions about the nature of care and where it is delivered are: education for pediatric nursing must be oriented to family-centered, community-based, and coordinated care that is sensitive and responsive to the beliefs, practices, and strengths of the specific cultural group; and much of the care of children with acute or chronic illness or disability will be shifted from the hospital to community settings, including homes, schools, day care centers, and primary care clinics.

CORE VALUES IN PEDIATRIC REHABILITATION NURSING

At the center of nursing practice are the core values and beliefs that guide the care that nurses give and the services they provide. Options for more independent and productive life have been greatly expanded as a result of the enactment of legislation based on an affirmation of values such as inclusion for all persons in the community and a focus on supporting abilities instead of trying to "fix" disabilities. The Individuals With Disabilities Education Act (IDEA), the Rehabilitation Act Amendments of 1992, the Americans With Disabilities Act (ADA), and the Technology-Related Assistance for Individuals with Disabilities Act (Tech Act) all reflect values of family–provider partnerships and equal opportunity for people with disabilities to achieve independence and productivity in the mainstream of society. These legislative actions promote the right of all people to be part of the naturally occurring activities of society, along with a variety of supports that can make these opportunities become reality. These policies provide critical components for extending the rehabilitation process into the community.

Increasing costs of health care are expected to significantly affect delivery of rehabilitation services. Health policy-makers are redefining health to include a sense of well-being and achievement of each individual's full potential, which may be modified by illness, disability, or environmental hazards (U.S. Public Health Service, 1990). This expansion of the traditional definition of health and illness and the medical model approach to health care is supportive of changes presently occurring in rehabilitation services to children. Shapiro (1993) noted that historically the medical model of disability measured independence by how far one could walk after an illness or how far one could bend his or her legs after an accident. In contrast, independence can now be redefined as the control a person with disabilities has over his or her life. Independence can effectively be measured not only by the tasks one can perform but by the quality of one's life lived with family and friends within the greater community.

This book is based on a combination of core values that support belief in the worth of the individual and validate the potential for growth, self-actualization, and happiness that each child possesses, despite disability or circumstance. These core values are:

1. Each individual, child or adult, has an intrinsic worth and value to themselves, their families, and society.
2. Each child has the right to grow and develop with peers, disabled and non-disabled, in play groups, child care programs, schools, work environments, and recreation facilities. Each child has the right to inclusion in health care services, school, work, and community.
3. Each child is regarded as an integral part of his or her family, making the family the center of services in pediatric rehabilitation.
4. Families have the right to choose and maintain control of health, rehabilitation, and educational services for their child through shared decision making with the interdisciplinary health care team. Parents are entitled to clearly worded, accurate, timely, and non-biased information from health and rehabilitation providers to enable them to make the best choices based on their knowledge of their child and their family. Each child has a right to be informed about his or her care and to be part of the care-planning process according to his or her developmental level.
5. The family has the right to equal access to health care services that assist their child to attain his or her greatest potential.
6. Children and adolescents with disabilities and their families are entitled to the same legal and ethical rights as any other child and family.

In addition to these values, services for children with disabilities and their families must meet specific criteria to best meet the needs of this diverse, varied population. Based on the experiences of pediatric rehabilitation nurses and on the testimony of families, individuals with disabilities, and other pediatric and rehabilitation specialists, the following standards were adapted from the values adopted by the New England SERVE Regional Task Force on Quality Assurance (New England SERVE, 1989). These should be used as guidelines for best practices for pediatric rehabilitation nursing care and services.

Community-Based

Competent services are available at a local level or as close to the child and family's home as possible. In many cases, specialty pediatric rehabilitation centers are located in regional centers far from the child and family's home, often in a different state. In these cases, every effort must be made to link and collaborate with service providers in the home community and to effect as early a discharge from the hospital as possible to facilitate the child and family's return to the community.

Comprehensive

A broad range of health, educational, social, and related services are included in care. In each setting—inpatient, outpatient, home, school, and community—nurses are an integral component of the care and services provided.

Continuous

Care is maintained without interruption, regardless of changes in the child's service providers, site of services, or method of payment. Continuity of care is crucial to maintaining and improving gains in health, development, and independence.

Coordinated

A comprehensive system of assessment, planning, intervention, and evaluation should be in place to form a cohesive approach to each therapeutic issue. This system encompasses not only the child's inpatient stay but also outpatient, school, and community services.

Collaborative

Rehabilitation services are delivered in collaboration with the family. The parents of the child with a disability, and later the young person himself or herself, work in partnership with nurses and other members of the rehabilitation team.

Developmentally Oriented

Care based on the child's functional level as well as his or her chronological age provides the most effective approach to rehabilitative and habilitative services.

Documented

All aspects of care and services are recorded in a system that is accessible to family, other providers, and evaluators of health care. Families have a legal right to any and all information contained in their child's medical record and should be able to review the chart at any time.

Efficacious

Care is based on scientific evidence and practices and is focused on achieving anticipated outcomes in health and functional status.

Family-Centered

Care and service providers recognize and respect the role of families in the lives of children. Families should receive support in their natural caregiving roles, which promotes adaptive patterns of living and ensures family collaboration and choice in services provided to the child.

Individualized

Care and services reflect the unique physical, developmental, emotional, social, educational, and cultural needs of the child within the context of the family.

Inclusive

An important component of health care and services is a system for advocacy that ensures full participation of the child and family in society.

Interdisciplinary

Because of the complexity of health, educational, and social issues involved in the lives of children with disabilities and their families, interdisciplinary services provide the most effective method of meeting the child's and family's needs. The interdisciplinary team is composed of providers from three or more disciplines who work collaboratively with each other and the family to provide effective health and rehabilitative services.

Culturally Appropriate

Care is non-discriminatory and respects the race, ethnicity, primary language, religion, gender, sexual orientation, marital status, medical condition, and economic status of the family.

Safety

Care is free from unnecessary risk by ensuring use of adequate facilities, procedures, equipment, and well-trained staff. It is crucial for facilities that are not familiar with pediatric care to obtain the proper size and type of equipment, especially emergency equipment, when caring for children with rehabilitation needs. It is equally important for pediatric facilities that maintain a very low number of children with disabilities to maintain familiarity with rehabilitation and disability-related care (New England SERVE, 1989).

INFLUENCES OF ATTITUDES AND BELIEFS ON PEDIATRIC REHABILITATION NURSING CARE

Individuals who are valued tend to select experiences that contribute to their growth and development and that of others (King, 1984). Pediatric rehabilitation nurses must be committed to facilitating the growth and development of children and families in all possible ways. An understanding of values, attitudes, and beliefs and the resulting clinical choices nurses make is crucial to quality pediatric rehabilitation nursing care. Values, beliefs, and attitudes arise from experience and are determined by an individual's upbringing, cultural heritage, professional beliefs, and environment and are developed and refined over time.

A value is defined as a learned goal or standard that influences choices and helps to guide both groups and individuals toward meaning in their lives. Holding a value involves an active process of choosing and prioritizing beliefs and acting on them (King, 1984). Values are always positive or negative attributes. Behaviors are indicators of values.

A belief is the acceptance of a position or statement about a subject, an individual, or a group. Beliefs are not inherently positive or negative, but they may influence attitudes, which are positive or negative. For example, if an individual believes that computers are an important communication tool, that belief does not necessarily cause them to feel strongly for or against using computers (Morgan & King, 1971).

Attitudes are influenced not only by family but also by peers, information received, and educational experiences. Attitudes are the tendency to respond either favorably or unfavorably to a person, object, group, or situation. Attitudes tend to be based on categorization of individuals or groups according to similarities or differences. Although this strategy may sometimes be useful in generalizing about people encountered in everyday activities, it may also lead to discrimination. Because attitudes are learned, they may be changed (Morgan & King, 1971).

The words individuals use when referring to themselves or others are powerful tools in delineating identity (Zola, 1993). The power of naming or labeling a person or a group of people goes far beyond the contemporary trend of "political correctness." For example, the term "handicapped" brings to mind a person who is less able than others to perform a job or meet basic needs. It has a negative connotation and may stigmatize the individual (i.e., brand them as being different). Often people perceive those who are stigmatized to be inferior, less capable, or less competent. Using language such as "cripple" or "spastic" to refer to a person with a disability reinforces these negative, dependent qualities and defines that individual as inadequate to self and others.

In addition, the generalization that results from these practices tends to define the individual according to only one of his or her many characteristics. When one hears the words "disabled person," the characteristic of disability is first and is the defining characteristic of the person. When one uses the words "person with a disability," the person is put first, and the disability becomes another characteristic, like having blond hair or brown eyes. The term "handicap" is used appropriately to refer to a barrier to full participation in society, such as an architectural barrier or an attitudinal barrier (WHO, 1980). A person is not referred to as "having a handicap" but as experiencing a handicap placed on them by society, for example, the employer who does not believe a person is competent because he uses a wheelchair or the child care provider who refuses services to a family because their child has cerebral palsy (Blaska, 1993).

The words used to refer to children with disabilities and their families reflect nurses' values and attitudes. Just as the terminology used to refer to members of racial or ethnic groups is respectful of cultural differences, so the terms used to refer to people with disabilities show respect for individual health or functional differences. One way of showing this respect for people with disabilities is by using people-first language. By describing someone as "a child with cerebral palsy" instead of a "CP child," a "spastic," or a "victim of cerebral palsy," one puts the person first and the disability second and focuses on the ability rather than the disability.

Parents of children with disabilities often feel strongly about how health care providers refer to their child. Phrases such as "the CP kid" label and stigmatize the child and make it more difficult for care providers to see beyond the disability to the child. Children with disabilities are more similar to other children than they are different, and they need the same things as any other child—love, caring, a nurturing home, and opportunities for learning, play, and fun. It is most appropriate when working with families to ask how they prefer to speak about their child when referring to the disability or chronic condition. Families may have different preferences and ask that you use terms such as "physically challenged," "exceptional," or "differently abled." Table 1–5 lists other acceptable terminology that puts people first.

These values and attitudes affect behavior toward families and their children. Value-free professional behavior is a myth (King, 1984). Assessment, planning, and evaluation and the daily interventions used to support the child's development and restoration of function are all colored by the set of learned responses and judgments that make up attitudes. Failure to examine one's own values and attitudes may lead to a loss of potential alternative actions when making decisions about patient care. Whether nurses listen to parents concerns with empathy or impatience, support parents' decision making over that of the rehabilitation team, or offer or withhold hope to families who seek information about their child's condition are determined by ingrained values, attitudes, and assumptions.

Parents, older children and youths, and adults with disabilities report that the attitude nurses exhibit toward them helps to determine the level of collaboration and the relationship that develops with the rehabilitation team. Attitudes such as devaluing parents'

Table 1–5 PEOPLE-FIRST TERMINOLOGY

Use	Avoid
Person with a disability or who has a disability, people with disabilities or who have disabilities	The disabled, the handicapped, invalid, cripple, deformed, victim, defective
People without disabilities, typical person, non-disabled people (less preferred)	Normal, healthy, able-bodied
Wheelchair user, uses a wheelchair	Wheelchair-bound, confined to a wheelchair
Congenital disability, birth anomaly	Birth defect, affliction, deformity
Has cerebral palsy, has spina bifida, person with a developmental disability, person with quadriplegia	Victim of cerebral palsy, stroke victim, cerebral palsied, spastic, para, quad
Has had polio, experienced polio, has a disability as a result of polio	Suffers from polio, is afflicted with polio, post-polios
People who have mental retardation, person with mental retardation	The mentally retarded, mentally deficient, retardate, retard, feeble-minded person, idiot
Person with Down syndrome	The Down kid, mongoloid
Person who has epilepsy, people with seizure disorders, seizure, epileptic episode or event	The epileptic, epileptics, fits, epileptic fits
People who have a mental illness, person with a mental or emotional disorder	The mentally ill, crazy, psycho, mental case
Person with a speech or communication disability	Tongue-tied, dumb
People who are blind or visually impaired, person who is deaf or hearing impaired	The blind, the deaf, the hard of hearing, deaf-mute, deaf and dumb

Adapted from *Talking about disability: a guide to using appropriate language*. Nashville, TN: The Coalition for Tennesseans with Disabilities.

opinions and what they have to say, labeling parents who question health care providers as "pushy parents," and preventing questions from being answered; providers who have a patronizing or paternalistic (or maternalistic) attitude toward parents and do not give them the full information about their child's condition; or attitudes that devalue the family's cultural or economic status all work to set up adversarial relationships that seriously affect the quality and efficacy of care offered and received.

Most frequently, nurses fail to examine their behavior or attitudes toward clients unless an incident occurs to challenge their beliefs. Such an incident, for example, encountering a paternalistic or patronizing attitude from health care providers directed toward oneself or a family, can stimulate reflection about one's own attitudes toward children with disabilities and their families (Leff & Walizer, 1994).

Attitudes, like behavior, can be changed in the same way they are constructed—by experiences, by information, and by peer influence. Examination of one's own attitudes toward children with disabilities and their families is crucial in providing care based on quality standards. Group exercises, using methods such as role play, problem-based learning tutorials, case study discussion of value-laden situations, and listing and prioritizing personal values can help to clarify attitudes and values and how they affect nursing care.

Another way of assessing attitudes toward families and children with disabilities is to read about or listen to parents, teens, or adults with disabilities talk about their own experiences with the health care system and how these experiences affected their self-esteem and their attitudes toward health care and rehabilitative services. Talking about past encounters with nurses and other rehabilitation providers, including what was helpful to families and what was not, and doing some collaborative problem solving can positively affect attitudes toward parents and children as well as strengthen collaborative partnerships between health providers and families.

SUMMARY

Pediatric rehabilitation nurses in their roles as leaders, advocates, and educators can have a very positive influence on the lives of children with disabilities and chronic conditions and their families. By facilitating transitions from hospital to home and community and offering counseling and support to families, they can provide assistance in meeting identified needs. By designing an individualized plan of care that incorporates the values and beliefs mentioned previously, they can positively influence the quality of the child's life and interactions with family and friends within the greater community.

REFERENCES

Association of Rehabilitation Nurses. (1992). *Pediatric rehabilitation nursing: role description*. Skokie, IL: ARN.

Baker, S., O'Neill, B., & Karpf, R. (Eds.). (1992). *The injury fact book* (2nd ed.). New York: Oxford University Press.

Blaska, J. (1993). The power of language—speak and write using "person first." In M. Nagler (Ed.). *Perspectives on disability*. Palo Alto, CA: Health Markets Research.

Burkett, K. (1989). Trends in pediatric rehabilitation. *Nursing Clinics of North America*, 24(1), 239–255.

Centers for Disease Control and Prevention. (1995a). Disabilities among children aged >17 years—United States, 1991–92. *Morbidity and Mortality Weekly Report*, 44(3), 609–612.

Centers for Disease Control and Prevention. (1995b). Surveillance for anencephaly and spina bifida and the impact of prenatal diagnosis—United States, 1985–1994. *Morbidity and Mortality Weekly Report*, 44(4), 1–13.

Children's Defense Fund. (1995). *The state of America's children yearbook*. Washington DC: Children's Defense Fund.

Edwards, P. (1992). The evolution of rehabilitation facilities for children. *Rehabilitation Nursing*, 17(4), 191–192, 195.

Edwards, P. (1995). *Pediatric Special Interest Group survey results*. ARN News, 11(1), 4–5.

Fletcher, J., Ewing-Cobbs, L., Francis, D., & Levin, H. (1995). Variability in outcomes after traumatic brain injury in children: a developmental perspective. In S. Broman & M. Michel (Eds.). *Traumatic brain injury in children*. New York: Oxford University Press.

Hymovich, D., & Hagopian, G. (1992). *Chronic illness in children and adults: a psychosocial approach*. Philadelphia WB Saunders.

King, E. (1984). *Affective education in nursing*. Rockville, MD: Aspen Systems Corp.

Leff, P., & Walizer, E. (1994). *Building the healing partnership: parents, professionals, and children with chronic illnesses and disabilities*. Cambridge, MA: Brookline.

Molnar, G. (1992). Cerebral palsy. In G. Molnar (Ed.). *Pediatric rehabilitation*. Baltimore: Williams & Wilkins.

Molnar, G., & Perrins, J. (1992). Head injury. In G. Molnar (Ed.). *Pediatric rehabilitation*. Baltimore: Williams & Wilkins.

Morgan, C., & King, R. (1971). *Introduction to psychology.* New York: McGraw-Hill.

National Center for Health Statistics. (1993). *1988 National health interview survey, child health supplement (NHISCH), advance data from vital and health statistics,* Number 190; cited in Ficke, R. (1992). *Digest of data on persons with disability.* Washington, DC: National Institute on Disability and Rehabilitation Research, U.S. Department of Education.

New England SERVE. (1989). *Enhancing quality: standards and indicators of quality care for children with special health care needs.* Boston: New England SERVE.

Perrins, J. (1988). Presentation at Rochester University Affiliated Program 20th Anniversary Conference, Rochester, NY.

Sever, L. (1993). Birth defects and their causes: the importance of surveillance. *Childhood Cancer Research Institute,* Dec/Jan, 7–11.

Shapiro, J. (1993). *No pity.* New York: N.Y. Times Books, Random House.

U.S. Public Health Service. (1990). *Healthy people 2000. National health promotion and disease prevention objectives.* U.S. Department of Health and Human Services, DHHS PUB. No. (PHS) 91-50213. Washington, DC: U.S. Government Printing Office.

Watson, D. (1990). The Americans With Disabilities Act: more rights for people with disabilities. *Rehabilitation Nursing,* 15(6), 325–328.

World Health Organization. (1980). *International classification of impairments, disabilities and handicaps: a manual of classification.* Geneva, Switzerland: World Health Organization.

Zola, I. (1993). Self, identity and the naming question: reflections on the language of disability. In M. Nagler (Ed.). *Perspectives on disability.* Palo Alto, CA: Health Markets Research.

ADDITIONAL RESOURCES

Johnson, B., Jeppson, E., & Redburn, L. (1992). *Caring for children and families: guidelines for hospitals.* Bethesda, MD: Association for the Care of Children's Health.

Selekman, J. (1991). Pediatric rehabilitation: from concepts to practice. *Pediatric Nursing,* 17(1), 11–14, 33.

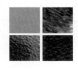

Chapter 2

Standards of Professional Nursing Practice and Quality Care

Patricia A. Edwards

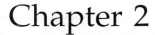

Nursing as a profession is accountable for the unique service that it provides to the public and is responsible for regulating the actions of its members. This begins with a formalized definition of nursing and the scope of its practice and includes a description of the practice base and its development; the system for nursing education; the structure of nursing service delivery; and the mechanisms for quality review, such as standards of practice.

This chapter answers the question, "What are standards and why do we need them?" The American Nurses Association (ANA) definition of nursing and scope of nursing practice is introduced, and standards for nursing practice in the areas of rehabilitation, including pediatric rehabilitation, related specialty practice, and school health nursing are explained. Additionally, standards for both professional education and quality care in nursing are discussed. An understanding of the standards that govern nursing practice is essential in the planning and implementing of care and the evaluation of pre-determined outcomes.

WHAT ARE STANDARDS?

Standards are pre-established criteria that identify the required components for achieving excellence in nursing practice. They provide specific quality indicators that can be measured and monitored. Criteria that determine how each standard is measured must be identified in advance so they can be applied to actual practice. These include the judgments, skills, and competencies required to provide care. Standards should be research based and derived from current knowledge and proven practice but reviewed and changed as health care and nursing practice are transformed.

Three types of standards have been identified and developed: structure, process, and outcome. Structure standards provide an overall framework for reviewing the organization and its policies, resources, and rules of conduct. Process standards detail how care is to be given, and outcome standards describe what responses should be expected at the completion of care and treatment. Standards also define the expected service outcomes for individuals with disabilities and the expected performance levels for both health care providers and the organization to achieve outcomes. Process standards are the organizational norms that describe how the providers or programs perform to produce quality outcomes. Outcome statements specify the expected outcomes of the supports and services.

Standards express values derived from evolving knowledge, new perceptions and interests, power shifts in health care environments, and increasing sensitivity to multiple stimuli on the part of individuals and systems. There has been a shift toward more comfortable health care environments, flexibility in non-clinical routines, and encouragement of client participation in care planning and seeking preventive care. Examples of trends in standards terminology are presented in Table 2–1 (Williamson, 1992).

SOURCES OF STANDARDS

Standards can be generated in a variety of ways and by different groups. Health care

Table 2-1 EXAMPLES OF TRENDS IN STANDARDS

From	To	Examples
Environmental Care		
Utilitarian	Comfortable	Carpets, easy chairs, curtains
Clinical	Domestic	Pictures, plants, smaller spaces
Harsh	Gentle	Low lights and noise, attention to wall color
Lack of privacy	Privacy	Single rooms, bathrooms
Creating dependence	Supporting independence	Aids to mobility and communication, easy access
Non-clinical Routines		
Rigid	Flexible	Choice of bedtime, feeding schedule
Imposed	Negotiable	Choice of day/time for admission or procedure
Batch	Individual	Choice from menu, individual appointment
Closed	Open	Unrestricted visiting, parent with child
Practitioner-Patient Interaction and Communication		
Impersonal	Personal	Continuity of care, same practitioner
Autocratic	Consultative relationships	Participate in care planning, informed choice
Inducing dependency	Supporting autonomy	Information, explanation, values and status recognized
Clinical Care		
Care in institution	Care at home	Pediatric, dying
Inpatients	Day patients	Surgery, diagnostic tests
Long inpatient stays	Shorter stays	Post-operative
Severe physiologic stress	Less severe	Quicker return to normal
High psychological stress	Lower stress	Information, support, continuity
Higher risk	Lower risk	Careful protocols, non-invasive procedures
Curative care	Preventive care	Screening, counseling, early detection

From Williamson, C. (1992). *Whose standards? Consumer and professional standards in health care* (pp. 123–124). Philadelphia: Open University Press. Reproduced with permission. All rights reserved.

professionals examining various aspects of their own work activities or professionals and academics in other disciplines can promulgate standards. The experience and observations of consumers, working collaboratively with professionals, can lead to the development of systems and practice standards that reflect the dynamic interplay of ideas, feelings, and interests.

Health care standards are based on government regulations and guidelines and established by organizations such as the Joint Commission on Accreditation of Healthcare Organizations (JCAHO), the Commission on

Accreditation of Rehabilitation Facilities (CARF), and consumer groups. These health care accrediting bodies have developed various methods to identify levels of quality for patient care processes and outcomes. JCAHO has provided quality assurance monitoring and evaluation standards that assist health care organizations in evaluating how efficiently and effectively they carry out governance, managerial, clinical, and support processes in providing high-quality care to their clients. The JCAHO survey and accreditation decision-making process is for reassessing the methods incorporated into the day-to-day operations that most affect patient outcomes. CARF was founded in 1966 to establish guidelines for rehabilitation services. CARF standards for program evaluation measure the efficiency and effectiveness of the system and patient satisfaction.

Standards specific to nursing care are established by governmental agencies, health care organizations such as JCAHO, and nursing organizations such as the American Nurses Association and the Association of Rehabilitation Nurses (ARN). According to the ANA, standards of nursing practice describe an expected level of performance ". . . by which the quality of nursing practice can be judged" (ANA, 1991). Included in the ANA document *Standards of Clinical Nursing Practice* are standards of care and standards of professional performance (ANA, 1991). These standards have been expanded by the ARN and other nursing groups to include the scope of specialty nursing practice and components specifically related to the various fields of nursing practice.

NURSING'S SOCIAL POLICY STATEMENT

In 1995, the ANA Congress of Nursing Practice revised the nursing profession's social policy statement, which represents the profession's commitment to the people it serves. The document contains descriptions of nursing's knowledge base, the scope of practice, and the profession's regulatory activities (ANA, 1995).

In the previous document, nursing was defined as "the diagnosis and treatment of human responses to actual or potential health problems" (ANA, 1980). The revised document acknowledges the following features of contemporary nursing practice:

- Attention to the full range of human experi-

ences and responses to health and illness without restriction to a problem-focused orientation
- Integration of objective data with knowledge gained from an understanding of the patient or group's subjective experience
- Application of scientific knowledge to the processes of diagnosis and treatment
- Provision of a caring relationship that facilitates health and healing (ANA, 1995, p. 6)

Nurses in both basic and advanced practice are involved in the provision of nursing care. Within each of these levels, nurses demonstrate competence along a continuum and may choose to specialize in one particular nursing area. Those practicing at the basic level are graduates of approved nursing programs who have qualified for Registered Nurse (RN) licensure. If they focus on a specialty area of practice, their additional knowledge and expertise may be recognized through certification. Advanced practice nurses have specialized or concentrated in one field of nursing and acquired additional practice knowledge and skills through study at the master's or doctorate level. This level is characterized by integration of theoretical, practical, and research-based knowledge, as well as expansion of clinical practice skills. Certification is attained at the completion of graduate study.

SCOPE OF REHABILITATION NURSING PRACTICE

Specialty organizations also delineate the practice scope for nurses who have chosen to focus in one area. The Association of Rehabilitation Nurses collaborated with the ANA in 1988 to devise a general description of the aims, beliefs, roles, and functions that are part of rehabilitation nursing practice. In 1994, ARN revised the general description of the parameters of this specialized area of practice. In that document, the specialty practice area of rehabilitation is described as "The diagnosis and treatment of human responses of individuals and groups to actual and potential health problems relative to altered functional ability and lifestyle" (ARN, 1994, p. 3). Specialized practice characteristics include knowledge and clinical skills to deal with the impact of chronic illness and disability on clients, families, and the community. Also included is a description of the responsibilities of rehabilitation nursing practitioners in providing a competent level of professional nurs-

Table 2–2 STANDARDS OF REHABILITATION NURSING PRACTICE

Standards of Care	Standards of Professional Performance
Assessment	Quality of care
Diagnosis	Performance appraisal
Outcome identification	Education
Planning	Collegiality
Implementation	Ethics
Evaluation	Collaboration
	Research
	Resource utilization

ing care and practice. As shown in Table 2–2, these responsibilities consist of both standards of care and standards of professional performance.

Standards of care are designed to assist the rehabilitation nurse in the integration of nursing process into client-centered actions. Additional responsibilities such as maintaining a safe environment, providing culturally relevant care, teaching self-care activities, and planning for care continuity are inherent in these standards. Standards of professional performance include activities related to behavior in the professional role. These expectations of the rehabilitation nurse should be viewed in light of his or her position, education, and practice setting.

Two levels of rehabilitation nursing practice are also described: generalist practice and advanced practice. All professional nurses involved in the field of rehabilitation should possess basic knowledge of rehabilitation technologies and therapies and the clinical skills that enable them to perform specific activities. Advanced practice requires an advanced degree in nursing, preferably with a rehabilitation nursing concentration; focuses on interdisciplinary collaboration; and includes leadership, clinical practice, consultation, education, and research (ARN, 1994).

Building on the ARN (1994) document, a new set of standards was developed for nurses in advanced practice. In the *Scope and Standards of Advanced Clinical Practice in Rehabilitation Nursing* (ARN, 1996), advanced practice is defined, and the education, settings, roles, and other parameters for practice are described. Within the standard of care on implementation, five specific interventions are listed: health promotion, health maintenance, and health teaching; case management/coordination of care; referral; consultation; and prescriptive authority and treatment. In the standard of professional performance, the following areas are new emphases: self-evaluation, leadership, the interdisciplinary process, and research.

PEDIATRIC REHABILITATION NURSING PRACTICE

The pediatric rehabilitation nurse uses these clinical and professional practice standards in interactions with children, adolescents, and families and provides interventions consistent with the total rehabilitation program. Because children differ from adults in many ways, the pediatric rehabilitation nurse must possess additional knowledge and skills to meet the needs of this population. The following are specific components of pediatric rehabilitation nursing practice:

- Using appropriate theory and content
- Maintaining professional practice standards
- Approaching crises systematically
- Collaborating with all members of the team in the plan of care
- Participating in research
- Pursuing professional development
- Providing health education (ARN, 1992)

The pediatric rehabilitation nurse uses appropriate theory and specialized content as the basis for clinical decision making in the application of the nursing process. Specific theories and bodies of knowledge used are growth and development, learning, family and group dynamics, communication, and leadership. Because the pediatric rehabilitation nurse must assist children and their families in dealing with predictable developmental crises and the impact of these events, the nurse must possess the theoretical knowledge and clinical skills to intervene in promoting health and development. Collaboration with other professionals, the child, and the family is essential in assessing, planning, implementing, and evaluating an individual plan of care. Knowledge of the scope of practice of fellow members of the rehabilitation team ensures a plan that is comprehensive, coordinated, designed to meet identified needs, and geared toward promoting optimum well-being. Specific components of pediatric rehabilitation nursing practice are found in the Appendix.

Within a specific health care setting, the standards may be used to address specific diagnoses, problems, or patient populations. One example is a standard developed at a rehabilitation hospital with a pediatric unit, for *Care of the Child and Family* (Nursing Standards Committee, 1994). It specifically states that the pediatric rehabilitation nurse provides a comprehensive, coordinated approach to the care of the child and family and recognizes the importance of family involvement in all aspects of care. The components of the standard include developmental tasks, problems and needs, and interventions, and these are presented in detail for each age group from neonate through adolescent. A standardized nursing care plan developed from the standard addresses the nursing diagnosis of Altered Growth and Development. This care plan format provides a method of documentation for goal attainment, interventions, and progress toward discharge outcomes. A quality assurance monitor relevant to the standard and care plan provides a means of evaluation, and the results are used in additional educational programming for staff and revisions and modifications of the standard and the care plan.

SPECIALTY PRACTICE STANDARDS

The Individuals with Disabilities Education Act of 1990 (IDEA) reinforced the need for the development of standards for nurses providing early intervention services. As defined by the law, nursing services include:

> . . . a) the assessment of health status for the purpose of providing nursing care including the identification of patterns of human response in actual or potential health problems; b) provision of nursing care to prevent health problems, restore or improve functioning and promote optimum health and development; and c) administration of medications, treatments and regimens prescribed by a licensed physician (U.S. Department of Education, 1989).

In 1993 the *National Standards of Nursing Practice for Early Intervention Services* (Consensus Committee, 1993) were developed to enable nursing implementation of Part H of IDEA (1990) and also to provide a guide for further standard development in specific settings. The ANA (1991) standards previously mentioned were used as an organizing framework for these standards, which are applicable to both general and advanced practice and include structure criteria that focus on the environment and its resources. The document includes complementary definitions, functions within an interdisciplinary, collaborative framework, and reflects the current state of knowledge in the field.

Another group of standards that govern nursing practice are those for the *Care of Children and Adolescents with Special Health and Developmental Needs* (Consensus Committee, 1994), which were designed to broaden the scope of the *National Standards of Nursing Practice for Early Intervention* (Consensus Committee, 1993) to include children with special health and developmental needs. These standards are also organized using the ANA (1991) framework and include the components of care and professional performance. Within these standards is the recommendation that nurses consult appropriate specialty practice guidelines and care plans that identify the current state of practice and knowledge. Also included is a general structure standard that identifies the need for adequate resources and an institutional commitment to quality care and evaluation to ensure effective service delivery. These standards can be used to inform many constituencies, including policy makers, about what constitutes quality care; provide guides for developing evaluation methodologies and reimbursement mechanisms; and characterize the components of individual practice and systems of care.

STANDARDS FOR NURSING EDUCATION

Historically, nursing has made strong efforts to develop and expand its educational standards, and the accreditation process is essential to these endeavors. The National League for Nursing (NLN), in its accreditation process, has developed and improved the standards for nursing education and places emphasis on the total nursing education program and its compliance with pre-determined criteria. It is the belief of the NLN that "... specialized accreditation provides for the maintenance and enhancement of educational quality, provides a basic assurance of program improvement and contributes to the improvement of nursing practice" (NLN, 1990, p. 2).

Another set of standards for education specifically addresses pre-licensure and early professional education for the nursing of children and their families. This includes degree-related education for students in programs preparing the RNs' as well as the new graduates' education early in their professional careers. These are stated as 11 goals that should be implemented across all nursing educational settings. These goals are based on the following assumptions, which are in accord with the concepts, assumptions, and core values discussed in Chapter 1. The education must be:

> ... 1) oriented to family-centered, community-based and coordinated care that is sensitive and responsive to the beliefs, practices and strengths of cultural groups; and 2) much of the care of children with an acute or chronic illness or disability will be shifted from the hospital to community settings, including homes, schools, day care centers and primary care clinics (Pridham, 1994, p. i).

The 11 goals reflect concepts of primary concern for pediatric rehabilitation nurses working with children and their families and fall into three categories: child, family, and societal factors; clinical problems or areas, and care delivery (Table 2–3).

STANDARDS FOR SCHOOL HEALTH NURSING

The specialty of school nursing also applied the *Standards of Clinical Nursing Practice* (ANA, 1991) in the development of a document that identifies specialty standards of practice for the school nurse. Ten specialty standards of school nursing practice encompass the role and scope of practice in contemporary school nursing, which is a complex and diverse practice that involves three frequently overlapping roles: generalist clinician, primary caregiver, and manager.

The nurse in the role of the generalist clinician delivers health services and education to school children and families. The primary care role involves the provision of health services with the school as the setting for care delivery. Much of the everyday practice of school nurses is in the management role: case management, management of health education programs and screening, and supervision of other personnel and services.

The standards of school nursing practice are divided into six role concepts (Proctor et al., 1993):

- Provider of client care, which includes clinical knowledge, nursing process, and dealing with clients with special health care needs
- Communicator
- Planner and coordinator of client care, which includes program management, collaboration within the school system, and collaboration with community systems
- Client teacher, which includes health education
- Investigator which includes participation in research
- Professional development within the discipline of nursing

As the school nurse role has expanded to meet the needs of a more diverse client population, the collaborative model for delivery of services within the school setting has also expanded to a larger community that extends beyond the immediate school population. These standards of school nursing practice provide a common framework for development and evaluation of service delivery systems, quality assessment, and development and use of information and reimbursement systems, as well as shared policies and procedures for the multiple specialties practicing in schools or school-linked collaborative programs.

STANDARDS OF QUALITY CARE

In Chapter 1, a critical set of values and assumptions are presented that form the base for the development of standards of quality care that can assist all members of the health care team to assess the quality of the present service systems. These values and assumptions are inherent in the document *Enhancing Quality: Standards and Indicators of Quality Care for Children with Special Health Care Needs*, produced by the New England SERVE regional task force on quality assurance (Epstein et al., 1989). Resources, activities, and collaborative roles are described in these standards, useful definitions of the inherent concepts are provided, and a framework of organization that focuses on differing levels within the health care system is presented.

These standards can be used in the following ways:

- As an educational tool to define components of quality care
- As a guide in selecting caregivers or sites and identifying parents' rights and responsibilities on the team
- As a basis for developing educational or training programs for families and professionals and as a catalyst for discussion of shared concerns
- As a tool for agencies in conducting self-surveys to assess care delivery and develop quality improvement systems

Table 2–3   GOALS FOR PRE-LICENSURE AND EARLY PROFESSIONAL EDUCATION FOR THE NURSING OF CHILDREN AND THEIR FAMILIES

Child, Family, and Societal Factors

The nurse will integrate knowledge of the unique anatomic structures, physiologic processes, and psychologic processes of children from birth through adolescence in assessments and in plans, interventions, and evaluation of care.

The nurse will use opportunities to influence positively the health behavior of children and families.

The nurse will provide supportive care for children and families experiencing separation, loss and/or bereavement.

The nurse will use knowledge of how the economic, social, and political environment influences the child's health and the family's care of the child to: (a) make assessments, plan strategies, and implement approaches to care of the child that are in accord with the family's economic and social situation and available resources; and (b) work with others in the community to make and implement plans for the healthcare needs of children.

Clinical Problems or Areas

The nurse will provide and promote safety in order to prevent injury and support the development of the child.

The nurse will make assessments, plan strategies of care, and intervene in ways that promote the growth and development of the child with a chronic condition or disability, support the child's and family's management of care, and promote a healthy lifestyle.

When providing care to children with acute illness or injuries and their families, the nurse will make assessments, plan strategies of care, and intervene in ways that promote growth and development of the child and support the child's and family's management of care.

Care Delivery

The nurse will use the family-centered approach to: (1) assess needs, plan, implement interventions, and evaluate outcomes relevant to the health care needs of children in partnership with children and their families; (2) work with other health care providers and the family to promote coordinated service delivery; and (3) advocate for family-centered care of children. The nurse will participate in developing and working within service delivery systems to support practice that is consistent with principles of a family-centered approach.

The nurse will acknowledge and integrate into health care the beliefs, practices and values of cultural groups defined by geography, race, ethnicity, religion, or socioeconomic status.

The nurse will communicate effectively with child and family and others who participate in the care and education of the child and family.

The nurse will respond to an ethical, moral, or legal dilemma concerning the child's health in ways that promote the development of families and children, assist them in making decisions, and support them in implementing the decisions.

From Pridham, K. (1994). *Standards and guidelines for pre-licensure and early professional education for the nursing care of children and their families* (pp. 10–12). Washington, D.C.: Maternal and Child Health Bureau, U.S. Department of Health and Human Services.

These standards are organized into five sections. The first section focuses on the individualized services received by the child and family; the second adds the characteristics of the team of professionals delivering the services; the third includes health care agency responsibilities; the fourth addresses the role of the state health department in promoting quality; and the fifth expands beyond the agency to community and societal supports. Table 2–4 lists desired outcomes that reflect the values and philosophies that are the core of these standards.

PROFESSIONAL REGULATION

Every state has its own Nurse Practice Act that defines the limits within which each nurse is expected to care for clients and pro-

Table 2–4   DESIRED OUTCOMES FOR ENHANCING QUALITY

The Child

Grows and develops toward independent adulthood; develops a positive self-image; is knowledgeable about his/her illness or disability; develops ways of managing the impact of his/her illness or disability; and gives feedback that he/she is satisfied with the care received.

The Family

Is knowledgeable about the child's condition, prognosis, treatment plan, and available resources; feels comfortable in caring for the child's special health care needs; effectively uses a range of resources to meet the needs of the child and other family members; maintains social integrity; maintains financial integrity; and gives feedback indicating satisfaction with the availability of resources, the process used in the delivery of care, and their involvement in decision making.

The Health Care Professional or Team

Delivers care resulting in health status outcomes consistent with optimal expectations for children with special health care needs; maintains a high level of education and training; responds to the needs of families as defined by families; coordinates care with others delivering services to children; and derives professional satisfaction and growth in delivering care to children and families.

The State Health Department

Provides leadership in the development of the health care system; utilizes standards of care to promote quality; establishes a health data and information system; guides the allocation of public resources to meet the special health care needs of children; initiates statewide efforts in the primary and secondary prevention of chronic illnesses and disabling conditions; and collaborates with public and private agencies and providers on behalf of children with special health care needs.

The Community

Values all children; integrates children with special health care needs into all aspects of community life; recognizes that its life is enriched by the integration of children with special health care needs; supports and engages in broad advocacy efforts by agencies, parents and professionals; provides a coordinated system of care responsive to children with special health care needs; and supports services to children with special health care needs through public and private funding.

From Epstein, S., Taylor, A., Halberg, A., Gardner, J., Walker, D. & Crocker, A. (1989). *Enhancing quality: standards and indicators of quality care for children with special health care needs* (pp. 69–71). Boston: New England SERVE Regional Task Force on Quality Assurance.

vides a framework within which practice can be evaluated. These specific acts are designed to protect the public by delineating the legal scope of nursing practice. The nursing license is an indication to the public that the nurse has the minimum qualifications for safe nursing practice. In some instances, legal parameters of nursing practice may also be defined by federal laws, such as those that dictate Medicare standards. Individual professional licensure is a protective mechanism legislated by the public to ensure the basic and minimum competencies of the professional nurse. Beyond that, society allows the nursing profession the right and responsibility for regulating its own practice.

The professional obligations of the nurse to safeguard clients are grounded in the ethical norms of the profession, the *Standards of Clinical Nursing Practice* (ANA, 1991), and state nurse practice acts. Nurses must be aware of the policies and procedures within their individual practice settings, the state nurse practice act, and state and federal regulations governing the settings in which they work. This is especially important in the area of delegation, in which the pediatric rehabilitation nurse entrusts the performance of nursing tasks to assistive personnel. Although the performance of the task is delegated in selected situations, the nurse maintains accountability for the total nursing care provided to the child. Three things must occur for delegation to take place: the authority for delegation must be in the state Nurse Practice Act; the nurse must document an assessment to show appropriateness of the delegated activity; and the nurse is obligated to determine the assistant's competence to perform the task and must supervise its performance.

CREDENTIALING/CERTIFICATION

Unlike state licensure, certification is a voluntary credentialing activity that serves to acknowledge and validate the expertise of the nursing professional and demonstrate adherence to a set of recognized practice standards. An individual who has attained a specific certification level possesses the appropriate knowledge, clinical competence, and experience to provide services based on sound practice principles. Certification of rehabilitation professionals plays a role in ensuring quality outcomes for clients.

Certification in specific nursing areas is awarded through activities of a number of non-governmental agencies: the American Nurses Credentialing Center (ANCC), the ARN, and the Commissions for Insurance Rehabilitation and Rehabilitation Counselor. Generally, certification requires education in the particular specialty area, a minimum number of years of clinical practice, letters of reference, and a written examination. The certifying organization establishes the number of years for which certification is valid and the process for its renewal, usually through continuing education, clinical practice, or retaking the examination. The ARN, as the professional organization for pediatric rehabilitation nurses, is responsible for the credentialing procedure and certifies generalists who have concentrated their practice in rehabilitation. On successful completion of the certification process, the nurse is entitled to the designation Certified Rehabilitation Registered Nurse (CRRN).

With the publication of the new standards for advanced practice in rehabilitation nursing, a core curriculum was developed as a resource for nurses. This publication (Johnson, 1997) outlines the body of knowledge of rehabilitation advanced practice. It focuses on four areas: core knowledge of the theory and practice of advanced practice nursing, principles of advanced direct practice, application and conduct of research as well as program evaluation and outcomes, and advocacy and health care policy. Additionally, a second certification program was implemented to recognize advanced practice nurses in the specialty of rehabilitation. To be eligible for the examination, the nurse must have a master's degree or doctorate in nursing, current RN license, and current CRRN credential. After the successful completion of the certification process, the nurse is entitled to use the designation Certified Rehabilitation Registered Nurse–Advanced (CRRN-A).

OUTCOME AND PROCESS MONITORING

Standards are written to apply to a broad population. When applying the standards, the needs of each individual must be considered, and plans to meet their needs must be developed and implemented. There is also an obligation to show that the programs work and deliver the promised end result. This can be accomplished through program evaluation documenting the benefits to clients. It is important to show that the outcomes result from the program or service. Many programs use efficiency and effectiveness measures to quantify and qualify rehabilitation outcomes. The process used to deliver rehabilitative care is as important as the client outcome and end result. Program evaluation and quality assurance methods allow the rehabilitation institution and program to monitor quality efficiently and effectively.

One of the standards of care for rehabilitation nursing practice is Outcome Identification. This standard states that "the rehabilitation nurse identifies expected outcomes individualized to the client" (ARN, 1994, p. 10). These outcomes are derived from the identified nursing diagnoses, are formulated with the input of the client and others involved in care and treatment, and are realistic and attainable in relation to client capabilities and available resources. The standard of care labeled Evaluation specifies the nurse's activities and involvement in evaluating the client's progress toward attainment of the identified outcomes. These are integral components of the nursing process.

Standards have also been set to provide the health care team with a method of assessing the quality of existing service systems. From these standards, statements of anticipated outcomes have been developed to summarize desired outcomes for the child and family, the health care providers and agencies, and the community.

SUMMARY

Standards of clinical nursing practice must reflect changes in organizational and community practices, and those responsible for their development must remain responsive to the impact of changes on children with disabilities or chronic conditions and their families. Understanding trends makes it possible to predict what will be the next development for specific practice issues so that standards can be revised accordingly. It is anticipated that the number of standards in health care will increase over time as new issues are identified. The pediatric rehabilitation nurse is accountable for the quality of the service he or she delivers and must be oriented toward the development of action plans leading to individualized outcomes.

REFERENCES

American Nurses Association. (1980). *Nursing: a social policy statement*. Kansas City, MO: American Nurses Association.

American Nurses Association. (1991). *Standards of clinical nursing practice*. Washington, D.C.: American Nurses Association.

American Nurses Association. (1995). *Nursing's social policy statement*. Washington, D.C.: American Nurses Association.

Association of Rehabilitation Nurses. (1992). *Pediatric rehabilitation nursing role description*. Skokie, IL: Association of Rehabilitation Nurses.

Association of Rehabilitation Nurses. (1994). *Standards and scope of rehabilitation nursing practice*. Skokie, IL: Association of Rehabilitation Nurses.

Association of Rehabilitation Nurses Advanced Practice Task Force. (1996). *Scope and standards of advanced clinical practice in rehabilitation nursing*. Glenview, IL: Association of Rehabilitation Nurses.

Consensus Committee. (1993). *National standards of nursing practice for early intervention services*. Lexington, KY: University of Kentucky College of Nursing.

Consensus Committee. (1994). *Standards of nursing practice for the care of children and adolescents with special health and developmental needs*. Lexington, KY: University of Kentucky College of Nursing.

Epstein, S., Taylor, A., Halberg, A., Gardner, J., Walker, D., & Crocker, A. (1989). *Enhancing quality: standards and indicators of quality care for children with special health care needs*. Boston: New England SERVE Regional Task Force on Quality Assurance.

Individuals With Disabilities Education Act of 1990, Pub. L. No. 101-476.

Johnson, K. (Ed.). (1997). *Advanced practice nursing in rehabilitation: a core curriculum*. Glenview, IL: Association of Rehabilitation Nurses.

National League for Nursing, Division of Education and Accreditation. (1990). *Policies and procedures for accreditation for programs in nursing education* (6th edition). New York: NLN.

Nursing Standards Committee. (1994). *Care of the Child and Family*. Boston: Spaulding Rehabilitation Hospital.

Pridham, K. (1994). *Standards and guidelines for prelicensure and early professional education for the nursing care of children and their families*. Washington, D.C.: Maternal and Child Health Bureau, U.S. Department of Health and Human Services.

Proctor, S., Lordi, S., & Zaiger, D. (1993). *School nursing practice: roles and standards*. Scarborough, ME: National Association of School Nurses, Inc.

U.S. Department of Education. (1989, June 22). *Early intervention programs for infants and toddlers with handicaps: final regulations. Federal Register, 54, 119.*

Williamson, C. (1992). *Whose standards? Consumer and professional standards in health care*. Philadelphia: Open University Press.

ADDITIONAL RESOURCES

England, B., Glass, R., & Patterson, C. (1989). *Quality rehabilitation: results-oriented patient care*. Chicago: American Hospital Publishing Inc.

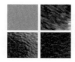

Chapter 3

Community-Based Health Care Delivery Systems

Patricia A. Edwards

Children with disabilities or chronic conditions and their families are particularly vulnerable to the effects of myriad problems stemming from the interaction of environment and physiology. Though the health care system has made tremendous technologic breakthroughs in many areas of treatment, serious issues remain regarding the best approach to the delivery of the care needed to protect children's health and well-being. In Chapter 1 it was stated that care needs to shift to a family-centered, community-based system that links providers with the home and the larger environment in a continuum of services. The pediatric rehabilitation nurse, in the pivotal roles of advocate and collaborator, can be the key to facilitating the transition of the child and family from inpatient service to home and promoting awareness of the need for community-based services.

This chapter describes community-based service delivery systems, including the types of services provided, how these services are organized, where they are located, and who delivers the care. Criteria for quality services and the organizational factors that affect these systems are discussed, and the projected delivery systems of the future are described.

COMMUNITY-BASED SYSTEM

Community-based service systems are defined by Gittler (1988) as "an organized network of integrated and coordinated services delivered at the local level" (p. 1). These services are necessary to decrease fragmentation of care and to provide a range of services that are timely, consistent, available, accessible, and cost-effective. Community-based service systems promote normal patterns of growth and development for children, who deserve to live with their families in their own communities.

Such a comprehensive delivery system has several advantages. It ensures a wide distribution of service centers geographically within the community, making services readily available to those families without transportation; it avoids duplication and promotes coordination of services by health, education, and social service providers; it allows for a truly multidisciplinary team concept in the delivery of services; and it responds to the special needs of various cultural groups found in the community as well as tailors services to the individual needs of a particular family.

Barriers to providing comprehensive, quality health care to children and families include financial constraints; complexity of agencies and systems designed to provide services; lack of knowledge about the value of early intervention, how to access services, which resources are appropriate, and how to attain eligibility; and philosophical differences regarding the delivery of services (i.e., institution versus inclusion versus segregated programs). In many instances, the "system" is a fragmented approach with confusing eligibility requirements and shrinking resources, or the services are available but not truly accessible.

As mentioned in Chapter 1, a move toward home care for children with disabilities or chronic conditions is underway. This trend suggests the importance of integration into the larger community as well. For families, this involves the complicated activities and daily anxieties of maintaining their child at home with strangers, nurses, home health aides, therapists, and other caregivers as continual and changing visitors. For community-based personnel, extensive planning, creativity, and preparation are necessary for successful integration of the child into programs and activities. In many instances, extensive training of personnel must take place to enable children with disabilities or chronic conditions to successfully participate in school, community, and other programs without detriment to their health status. Community-based providers need to be aware of strategies to enhance the child's growth and development and provide family support, as well as have an understanding and appreciation of their role as a visitor in the home when providing care to the child.

The development of an appropriate delivery system requires an understanding of the multiple facets of the community system. The elements of a community system are "... the family's neighborhood, health, recreational, educational, social and political institutions" (Hymovich & Hagopian, 1992, p. 73), and these all have an effect on its functioning. As a method to help the pediatric rehabilitation nurse understand the impact of the community on the child and family, a community assessment is a useful tool. Knowledge gained from this in-depth look at the child's environment can give the nurse valuable insight while assisting the family in ensuring access to services and advocating for changes to increase service availability.

The community assessment should provide information to assist the pediatric rehabilitation nurse in understanding the central core of the community, its people, and the available resources. Identifying community health needs and patterns of use is also essential. In assessing community strengths and deficits, the nurse should assess the following areas:

- The values and beliefs of the people, including both demographics and a historical perspective
- The physical environment, including condition of structures in the community and their accessibility, climate, resources, boundaries, and community problems
- Local health and social service agencies, including scope, accessibility, demographics of users, and availability of resources
- The economic subsystem and financial and labor force characteristics
- Safety services (e.g., police, fire, emergency), environmental factors (e.g., sanitation, water), and transportation, both public and private
- The political structure, especially influential individuals and politically active groups
- Formal and informal communication sources
- Community educational facilities, including school enrollment, funding, and available services
- Types of recreation, such as play areas and barrier-free facilities

One method of assessment, The Community Oriented Needs Assessment (CONA) model, was developed to enhance communication between service providers and the community. In this model, data are collected from three sources: demographic profiles, key informants, and individual consumer interviews. There are a number of advantages with this model, including involvement and education of consumers. Its primary goal is to establish a database of information that can be used in planning to meet community needs (Neuber, 1980).

Once a basic understanding of the community is developed, the service delivery system can be assessed to determine what activities must be undertaken to make the concept of community-based, coordinated care a reality. The essential elements of a service system are presented in Table 3–1. With these elements in mind, the community-based health care delivery system should make services available for all types of children and their families in or near their home communities. The design should be flexible and family-centered, and should include primary, secondary, and tertiary health services as well as other specialized programs.

This system should be resource-based as opposed to service-based; this requires a change in perspective on the part of care providers. There are three critical differences in the systems. Resource-based practices lead to:

1. The development of community-based systems and the use of local individuals and organizations to provide services. This can increase access and flexibility and provide a more comprehensive, permanent program.
2. Community resources that are expandable

Table 3–1   ELEMENTS OF THE SERVICE SYSTEM

The service delivery system should serve a broad population of children who have health problems requiring something beyond routine and basic care. This includes children with disabilities and handicapping conditions, chronic illnesses and conditions, health-related educational problems, and health-related behavior problems, as well as children at risk for disabilities, chronic conditions, and health-related educational and behavioral problems and their families.

The service delivery system should make available and accessible for both children and their families comprehensive services that include primary level basic care, secondary level specialized care, and tertiary level highly specialized care provided by a combination of community-based physicians and clinics, other health care providers, regional medical centers and clinics, and tertiary medical centers and clinics. Other needed services and programs include early intervention services, educational services, vocational services, mental health services, social services, recreational and arts programs, and family support services such as parent-to-parent support and respite care.

The service delivery system should be community based. To the extent possible, needed services should be provided to children and their families in or near their home communities. The relevant geographic area for the purpose of developing a service delivery system will vary widely between states and within states.

The service delivery system should provide services that are coordinated. Multiple services from different providers should be delivered in a complementary and consistent manner. The system should also provide services in a timely manner and in the proper sequence.

The service delivery system should provide services that are family centered. The fact that the family is the constant in the child's life while the service system and personnel within the system fluctuate should be recognized, and family–professional collaboration at all levels should be facilitated. Unbiased and complete information about the child's care should be shared with families on an ongoing basis in an appropriate and supportive manner. Programs and policies that are comprehensive and provide emotional and financial support to meet the needs of families should be implemented. Family strengths and individuality should be recognized, and different methods of coping should be respected. The developmental needs of infants, children, and adolescents and their families should be recognized and incorporated into the system, and parent-to-parent support should be encouraged and facilitated. The design of the system should be flexible, accessible, and responsive to family needs.

Adapted from *A national goal: building service delivery systems for children with special health care needs and their families.* (1988). Rockville, MD: National MCH Resource Center.

and flexible, allowing families access to a number of agencies and providers consistent with their needs and priorities.

3. Broader supports that are part of larger systems that link families and facilitate informal networks which can include a multitude of individuals and organizations.

SERVICE COMPONENTS

Family-centered care, a fundamental part of the system, is defined in Chapter 1, and its key elements are outlined in Table 1–2. Family-centered care is part of a system that responds to the needs of children and their families rather than requiring them to adapt to the system. This type of care supports and assists families in their role as primary care-givers, is responsive to needs of families as defined by families, and recognizes and respects the role of the family as decision-maker, teacher, and advocate. Family members are equal partners in collaborative relationships with professionals, participate in decision making, and guide practices. This true partnership is one in which family members and health care professionals share information as integral members of the team and are of mutual benefit to each other.

A model articulated by Dunst and colleagues (1988), termed the enablement model, is aimed at promoting independence and growth. Those seeking assistance are viewed as capable and responsible, and it is the role of the professional to create opportunities for resources and skills to be acquired. Implicit in this model is the assumption that "those providing help or assistance acknowledge the strengths of those seeking help, and that help-givers assist families in seeing, developing and using their capabilities" (Shelton & Stepanek, 1994, p. 16).

Family-centered services must be comprehensive, accessible, flexible, and part of community-based systems. Family support services should be based on the changing needs of families and include physical and environmental needs (e.g., food, clothing, medical and dental care); economic, social, cultural, and recreational needs; adult and child education and child care needs; employment, vocational, and transportation needs; and emotional and communication needs. Education and training in care of the child, respite care, homemaker assistance, parent support, individual or group therapy, and self-help groups are some of the services that are needed. Assistance with obtaining resources, housing, and financial counseling and determining financial eligibility for aid are also included. Efforts are focused on the development of resources that will continue over time and can be used by others in the community or culture.

A checklist developed by the Institute for Family-Centered Care (1994) contains elements that should be used to evaluate the incorporation of family expertise in policy decisions and program development at all levels of care—hospital, home, and community. Some items on the checklist relate to recognizing family members' expertise and financially compensating them for it, including them as educators and on committees, and publicly acknowledging their contributions.

Comprehensive care requires a range of services with varying degrees of intensity that are available and accessible. Preventive, early identification, diagnostic, and treatment services, as well as habilitation and rehabilitation, are all parts of the system. Linkages between large medical centers providing tertiary care and community health professionals providing primary and secondary care are established. Large medical centers, where children with special health care needs receive high-quality, specialized care, are an important component in the system. This tertiary level of service must continue to be centralized but have strong linkages with community professionals providing secondary level care.

Efforts should also focus on identifying primary care needs and providing for these within the home and community. Early identification and intervention services, as well as educational and vocational services, should be a component of the community-based service system. Mental health services, family support services, and access to social services

are also essential. Recreational services, art programs, and other leisure activities enrich lives and improve functioning.

Collaboration between community-based service providers must be truly integrated and coordinated. Three important areas for collaboration are planning through a structured process to determine total system needs and priorities; actual delivery of services with a common intake process and sharing of basic information; and identifying funding sources. A collaborative partnership must be integrated into the decision-making process at all levels of health and developmental care. "While the goal of family/professional collaboration is becoming more of a reality in some hospital-based settings, it is essential that the same goal be extended into home-based and community-based care as well" (Shelton & Stepanek, 1994, p. 18). The concept of service coordination was included in the Individuals with Disabilities Education Act of 1990 (IDEA, Part E) as an approach to providing interdisciplinary services to children. One professional providing services to the family assumes the role of service coordinator, which includes coordinating the process of assessment; participating in Individual Family Service Plan (IFSP) development; identifying appropriate services with the family and assisting with access; monitoring service provision; facilitating transitions; and advocating for the family in the hospital setting.

CASE MANAGEMENT AND MANAGED CARE

Case management, a critical service for children with disabilities or chronic conditions, is a systematic organization of resources whose components include assessment, development and implementation of a service plan, and evaluation of outcomes. It should be family-centered and community-based through the use of networks of integrated services at the local level.

Several models of case management developed as a result of the requirement in Part H of the 1986 amendment to the Education for All Handicapped Children Act. One is described as "a coordinative function that includes activities designed to assist and enable an eligible child and the child's family to obtain appropriate early intervention services" (Davis & Steele, 1991, p. 15). These models might include a parent–professional partnership, an involved agency as the case manager, one professional who is currently providing services as case manager, or a combination of persons as case manager.

In many instances, it is nurses and pediatric rehabilitation nurses in particular who function in this important role in a partnership with the child and family. Nurses receive specific education in several necessary skills of case management: assessment, care planning, evaluation, leadership, service delivery, and quality assurance. They have knowledge about appropriate documentation practices and the ability to communicate with other providers and translate information for all team members.

A number of specific activities are part of the case manager's role: periodic developmental assessment and evaluations; development and update of the IFSP; evaluating services provided; and identifying, coordinating, and monitoring resources. The nurse is also uniquely qualified to assist other health professionals in collaborating with the family to make decisions about provision of services and to provide and manage comprehensive, family-centered, community-based care.

One specific approach, developed as part of a demonstration project of the Handicapped Children's Early Education Program (HCEEP), was called "Project Continuity." The project's goal was "to articulate a care coordination approach that would be family-centered and provide a bridge between the health care, education and social service systems for medically fragile infants and toddlers" (Jackson, Finkler, & Robinson, 1992, p. 224). Over the course of the project, the term "case management" evolved into "care coordination" to more appropriately reflect the provision of services for the child and family. The model that developed provides for comprehensive services during hospitalization, assistance in transition to home, and follow-up in the community. Coordination activities occur at both the individual and team levels.

Functions at the individual level might include:

- Coordinating assessments and the IFSP process
- Facilitating team communication and problem resolution
- Monitoring plan implementation and recommending modifications
- Assisting the family in securing services and participating as team members and advocates
- Participating at the system level in identifying and developing needed services

Functions at the team level might include:

- Ensuring that assessment occurs and the IFSP is developed and implemented
- Identifying resources and strengths in the community
- Ensuring regular evaluation of the IFSP

Managed care is now at the forefront of plans at both the state and national levels to reform health care systems and the delivery of care. It has been defined as a series of strategies to manage the quality and cost-effective delivery of health care through the appropriate use of resources. Although the managed care plan has the potential to result in better access and care, the focus must be on comprehensive service systems that promote healthy social, emotional, and physical growth, especially for children with disabilities or chronic conditions and their families. Included in this focus should be health promotion and disease prevention services that are integrated and family-centered and provided at locations where they are easily accessed (e.g., home, day care, school), as well as specialty and support services. There must be adequate funding methodologies in place for the services, as well as ongoing evaluative mechanisms to ensure that managed care arrangements appropriately serve children and families.

The following considerations should be given special attention. Financing methodologies should ensure funding for public health functions; public accountability for the assessment of the quality of care and monitoring of health outcomes should be an expectation; and strategies for developing adequate and appropriate services in the community must be in place. "Adequate and collaborative planning that addresses ongoing structural problems in the health care delivery system must occur in effecting the complex change-over to managed care" (Hess, 1993, p. 24).

A clinical model was developed by the Medicaid Working Group (1992) to help selected programs develop new care models and reimbursement mechanisms to improve the delivery of services. There are six components of clinical management in this model, and four of these, called the Core Components, are critical to the role described in the model. These components are primary care, urgent care, assessment and care planning, and coordination of services. The two optional components, case finding and intake and ongoing service development, can be implemented according to the characteristics of the organization. The nurse practitioner is the identified health care provider uniquely suited to this role of Primary Care/Clinical Manager. "Combining primary care responsibilities with the more traditional case management . . . can extend clinical decision-making into the home. Home-based care safely and effectively reduces the use of costly acute care services" (Medicaid Working Group, 1992, p. 11).

PARTNERSHIPS IN HEALTH CARE DELIVERY

Changes in the federal legislation for programs serving children with disabilities or chronic conditions have produced various system development efforts. To assist personnel in developing systems that are coordinated, family-centered, and culturally sensitive, the Maternal and Child Health Bureau (MCHB) developed the following definition of primary care:

> Primary care for children and adolescents is personal health care delivered in the context of family, culture and community whose range of services meets all but the most uncommon health needs of the individuals being served (MCHB, 1994, p. 1).

Additionally, it is the "integration of services that promote and preserve health, prevent disease, injury and dysfunction, and provide a regular source of care for acute and chronic illnesses and disabilities" (MCHB, 1994, p. 1). Primary care is the usual point of entry into the larger health care system, and the providers of primary care serve as coordinators of health and human services. The provider of primary care shares an ongoing responsibility for health care with the family and incorporates community needs and resources into clinical practice.

The characteristics of primary care are:

It serves as the child and family's "first contact" with the health care system and guides the child and family to the most appropriate resources.

It provides coordination of services and mechanisms for transfer of information.

It supports the right of the family to participate in the assessment and provision of care.

"First contact" care means that the primary care provider serves as the usual point of entry into the system when a medical or health-related need arises, guiding children and families to the most appropriate source of care. The primary care provider is continuous over time, not only in the case of illness but also for the provision of preventive services. "Coordinated care is the linking of health care events and services so that the patient receives appropriate care for all his/her health problems, physical as well as mental" (Johansen, Starfield, & Harlow, 1994, p. 5).

The primary care provider transfers information and links treatment plans through continuity of information systems and provides a comprehensive array of health services tailored to the needs of the individuals being served. Other elements of primary care that were discussed in Chapter 1 include community-oriented care; family-centered care; accessible, culturally competent care; and developmentally appropriate, accountable care. Primary care is important to children with disabilities or chronic conditions to maintain wellness, enhance growth and development, provide a basis for specialty/rehabilitation services, and treat minor acute illness before it becomes severe.

Primary health care for children with disabilities or chronic conditions can be provided through systems and services using nurses in advanced practice such as pediatric nurse practitioners, clinical nurse specialists, and pediatric rehabilitation nurses. One model, called "Partners in Caring" (Weis & Sharpton, 1993), is a state-wide primary care initiative in Wisconsin. A pediatric nurse practitioner, working in collaborative practice with community health nurses, provides health education, preventive health services, case finding, referrals, and anticipatory guidance. A close working relationship is also maintained with the family's primary care provider.

In San Diego, another program called REACH (Rural Efforts to Assist Children at Home) encompasses the provision of primary care and case management in the home using pediatric nurse practitioners. The four dimensions of practice as part of the program are management of well child care, management of chronic illness, management of minor pediatric illnesses, and case management. The program is designed to provide more comprehensive care and decrease fragmentation of care, as well as to increase the child and family's compliance with prescribed medications, diets, and instructions. In addition, REACH can increase school attendance, decrease or prevent emergency department visits, and encourage more appropriate use of resources (Martinez, Schreiber, & Hartman, 1991).

The emergence of comprehensive school health services for adolescents and school-based clinics has also provided a model for nursing involvement. Typically, these services are staffed by a team that includes a nurse practitioner and provides primary health care services, diagnosis and treatment of minor injuries, medications, immunizations, laboratory tests, referrals, counseling, and educational services. Although this type of program remains controversial because it shifts even more responsibility, that of health care, to the already overburdened educational system, it nonetheless remains an effective method of reaching school-aged children and adolescents. According to Palfrey (1994), ". . . the major benefits of such programs are their accessibility, acceptability, comprehensiveness and efficacy" (p. 72).

At present, there is tremendous variability in school-based services as a result of inconsistencies in planning, funding, staffing, and commitment. Despite these variations, four basic components are found in most schools: screenings (e.g., physical examination, sports physicals, periodic height and weight checks, immunization monitoring, vision and hearing testing), infectious disease policies, emergency procedures, and a curriculum aimed toward health promotion. Areas of concern regarding school-based clinics are related to the sensitive issues of reproductive health services, lack of coordination among clinics, inadequate financial support, and inability to provide 24-hour accessibility (Palfrey, 1994).

INDIVIDUALIZED SERVICE QUALITY

Services and systems are changing rapidly and will continue to do so in the years to come. As a result, it is of utmost importance that the quality of these services be evaluated, and service quality, in terms of how it might look from the child's point of view, must be considered. From the child's perspective, a good service would:

Value me as a unique individual—let me be me

Let me build genuine relationships—really care about me

Meet my needs—both ordinary and special

Involve my family in my care and in any decisions about me

Recognize me as a child first, with a disability second

Let me influence the way I live—give me real choices

Enable me to learn and change and grow

Be flexible and responsive and accessible—adapt to me when appropriate and gently encourage me to change when necessary (Marchant, 1992, p. 494)

To use these statements in designing care and to create specific quality indicators, consider the following when deciding what a good service should be like.

- Is the service or system built around the individual needs of children and families?
- Are families involved in planning and delivering care?
- Are families enabled through a strong, caring relationship that is guiding and supporting them rather than doing things for them?
- Does the service meet both specialized and ordinary needs, and is it flexible and user friendly?
- Does the design of the service recognize the child first while still meeting his or her special needs?
- Does the system empower the child and family and help all members learn useful skills and grow?

The key features of an effective organization in relation to these criteria are: it must have clear aims and an explicit value base, and it must provide good staff support for cultivating commitment and enabling caring. "A service that cares for and values its staff is far more likely to enable them to be able to really care for and value the children they serve" (Marchant, 1992, p. 505).

FUTURE DELIVERY SYSTEMS

In the late 1980s, the concept of functional supports was proposed as an alternative to the services continuum, putting people into community programs. This concept emphasized "the creation of a network of formal and informal supports that a person with a disability needs to meet his or her day-to-day demands" (Karan & Greenspan, 1995, p. 10). The key to this perspective is to view the community as the place where everyone has a right to live and work, and strive toward resolving barriers that inhibit participation as well as provide support to children with disabilities or chronic conditions and their families. This must also be accompanied by real social connections and the development of links to the community.

In the future, the values that are a part of

this community membership paradigm will shift the reality of practice closer to the goal of full inclusion for children with disabilities or chronic conditions and their families. Heightened interest in natural supports as a way to maximize the quality of the lives of children and families holds the promise of enhancing personal growth and satisfaction. Natural supports are defined as:

> . . . resources and strategies that promote the interests and causes of an individual with or without disabilities, that enable him or her to access resources, information, and relationships inherent within integrated work and living environments, and that result in the person's enhanced independence, productivity, community integration, and satisfaction (Karan & Greenspan, 1995, p. 210).

Strategies and resources that might be used to enhance natural supports are behavioral support, health assistance, in-home living assistance, community access and use, befriending, employee assistance, and financial planning. Four sources of support might include:

- The competency of the individual to make choices
- Family, friends, and coworkers
- Assistive devices and job and living accommodations
- Currently available rehabilitative services

The term "natural supports" came from the vocational literature and refers to the use of community resources and other resources from typical daily life to assist an individual with a disability to have a successful job in the community. More recently, the term has been used to refer to the non–service system resources that families of children with disabilities or chronic conditions may draw from to help them meet their own needs and those of the child. Examples of sources of natural supports for children and families include church congregations or other religious fellowship groups, neighbors, friends, family or extended family members, children's play groups, and private or public services provided to the general public that are not focused on providing disability-related services. Examples of this last category include recreation centers, child care centers or homes, housekeepers or cleaning services, nanny or au pair services, and educational or recreational camps.

System resources such as those provided by the social service system, health care system, and vocational system are used primarily to support the individual or family in their efforts to enhance personal choice, contribute to the community through each person's unique gifts and strengths, and build relationships with neighbors or neighborhood groups. Natural supports are those already available in the community.

The language of natural supports is derived from the value that all individuals and families are members of the community, that is, the language of inclusion. Natural supports and full community inclusion go together. They are supports that are natural to the place, time, delivery, and person and are not necessarily related to the disability service system. The language used to describe the situation deviates from "institutional" or health care language and refers to the needs and situations common to all people. For example, people with disabilities live with roommates rather than staff or providers; they bathe themselves, clean their homes, or do their laundry rather than perform activities of daily living or learn programs; friends come to visit rather than volunteers; and people have fun rather than participate in outings.

Changes will need to be made in federal policy and regulations as the roles of professionals and families shift to encompass concepts such as "power sharing" and parent activism. The education of nurses and the delivery of nursing services will need to be explored to support the shift of practice from the helping model to one based on empowerment. Pediatric rehabilitation nurses will benefit from an examination of their professional attitudes and practices as they seek to involve children and families in their own health management. Additional training and education in some areas will be warranted, and nursing research is needed to generate information on changes in health care and evaluate the focus of service delivery.

SUMMARY

Service delivery systems for children with disabilities or chronic conditions and their families must be available at the local level. There are a number of models for these systems that vary from state to state, but the system should be an expansion of collaborative arrangements between clinical services. The service delivery system must have a generic orientation and the ability to serve a broad population and offer a range of different types of services (*A national goal*, 1988).

Delivery of these services in or near the home communities facilitates the promotion of normal patterns of living and a focus on the family as equal partners in the care of children.

REFERENCES

Amendment to the Education for All Handicapped Children Act of 1986. Pub. L. No. 99-457.

A national goal: building service delivery systems for children with special health care needs and their families. (1988). Rockville, MD: National Maternal and Child Health Resource Center.

Davis, B., & Steele, S. (1991). Case management for young children with special health care needs. *Pediatric Nursing*, 17(1), 15–19.

Dunst, C., Trivette, C., & Deal, A. (1988). *Enabling and empowering families: principles and guidelines for practice.* Cambridge, MA: Brookline Books.

Gittler, J. (1988). *Community-based service systems for children with special health care needs and their families.* Iowa City: National MCH Resource Center.

Hess, C. (1993). *Managed care for women, children, adolescents and their families: a discussion paper with recommendations for assuring improved health outcomes and roles for state MCH programs.* Washington, D.C.: The Association of Maternal and Child Health Programs.

Hymovich, D., & Hagopian, G. (1992). *Chronic illness in children and adults: a psychosocial approach.* Philadelphia: WB Saunders Co.

Individuals With Disabilities Education Act of 1990, Pub. L. No. 101-476.

Institute for Family-Centered Care. (1994). Checklist: incorporating family expertise in policy and program development. *Advances in Family-Centered Care*, 1(1), 10.

Jackson, B., Finkler, D., & Robinson, C. (1992). A case management system for infants with chronic illnesses and developmental disabilities. *Child Health Care*, 21(4), 224–232.

Johansen, A., Starfield, B., & Harlow, J. (1994). *Analysis of the concept of primary care for children and adolescents: a policy research brief.* Baltimore, MD: The Johns Hopkins University Child and Adolescent Health Policy Center.

Karan, O., & Greenspan, S. (Eds.) (1995). *Community rehabilitation services for people with disabilities.* Boston: Butterworth-Heinemann.

Marchant, R. (1992). Caring for children with special needs. In McCarthy, G. (Ed.) *Physical disability in childhood: an interdisciplinary approach to management.* New York: Churchill Livingstone, pp. 493–506.

Martinez, N., Schreiber, M., & Hartman, E. (1991). Pediatric nurse practitioners: primary care providers and case managers for chronically ill children at home. *Journal of Pediatric Health Care*, 5(6), 291–298.

Maternal and Child Health Bureau. (1994). *Primary care for children and adolescents: definition and attributes.* Rockville, MD: Health Resources and Services Administration, Public Health Services, U.S. Department of Health and Human Services.

Medicaid Working Group. (1992). *Nurse practitioners as clinical managers.* Boston: Boston University School of Public Health.

Neuber, K. (1980). *Needs assessment: a model for community planning.* Beverly Hills, CA: Sage Publications.

Palfrey, J. (1994). *Community child health: an action plan for today.* Westport, CT: Praeger.

Shelton, T., & Stepanek, J. (1994). *Family-centered care for children needing specialized health and developmental services*, (3rd ed.). Bethesda, MD: Association for the Care of Children's Health.

Weis, D., & Sharpton, S. (1993). Partners in caring: a state-funded primary care initiative for children. *Journal of Pediatric Health Care*, 7(1), 31–36.

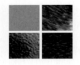

Chapter 4

Legislation and Public Policy

Patricia A. Edwards

■

Children, especially those with disabilities or other chronic conditions, are a very vulnerable part of this country's population. They have no power or voice because they cannot vote and need advocates who are willing and able to influence and shape important health policies. Pediatric rehabilitation nurses, who interact continually with families, health care professionals, and the community, are in a position to provide a strong voice in shaping health policies for children and their families. This chapter provides a historical perspective on rehabilitation legislation in general, as well as more recently enacted laws (Watson, 1990), especially the Americans with Disabilities Act (1990). Specific legislation for services for children are described, with special emphasis on the education acts. Current issues surrounding universal access and coverage, the balanced budget amendment's threat to the medical safety net, and the elimination of entitlements and other health care reform efforts also are described. The advocacy role, an integral part of the pediatric rehabilitation nurse's practice, and the role of parents in speaking out for the needs of their children are examined. Suggestions are made for increased involvement in public policy decision making at the state and federal levels.

HISTORICAL PERSPECTIVE ON REHABILITATION LEGISLATION

The beginning of a congressional interest in rehabilitation came with the passage of the National Defense Act (1916). This Act provided for vocational training for soldiers,

through instruction and study, that would enable them to perform more efficiently while in the military and be better equipped for a job in civilian life. This act was followed in 1917 by the establishment of a vocational education program under the Smith-Hughes Act. It provided grants to the states for vocational education on a matching basis and established a federal board with responsibility for veterans' vocational rehabilitation.

The Soldier Rehabilitation Act of 1918 expanded the role of this board to provide vocational rehabilitation for disabled veterans. This was the basis for the Vocational Rehabilitation Act in 1920, which provided funds for "vocational guidance, training, occupational adjustment, prostheses and placement services" (Bitter, 1979, p. 16.) Four subsequent amendments were made to this law.

The 1943 amendments to the *Vocational Rehabilitation Act* broadened financial provisions, defined vocational rehabilitation more comprehensively, and extended services to the mentally handicapped. Amendments in 1954 reshaped the role of the federal government in the rehabilitation program and established a working relationship between the public and private sectors. Significant features of this amendment were the provision of training grants for nurses and other rehabilitation professionals, as well as grants to remodel or expand facilities. With the 1965 amendments, the federal cost share of rehabilitation was enlarged to 75% and benefits were extended. Construction assistance for building rehabilitation centers was authorized, and extended client evaluation was allowed to determine whether the rehabilitative services would help the individual be more employable. Amendments in 1967 and 1968 provided services for migratory workers, eliminated state residency requirements, established the National Center for Deaf-Blind Youths and Adults, expanded services to family members, and provided for other programs and services such as vocational evaluation and work adjustment (Bitter, 1979).

In 1935, the vocational rehabilitation program was continued and strengthened by the Social Security Act, the first permanent base for the vocational rehabilitation program. This act provided for increased grants and support and continuous authorization. The 1936 Randolph-Sheppard Act authorized the licensing of vending stands in federal buildings to be operated by qualified blind persons and set a precedent for similar arrangements at the state level.

These major historic trends were interrelated. The availability of services moved from exclusion to inclusion; entitlement of services moved from charity to right; and location of services moved into educational settings. Overall, the trend was from segregated, isolated services to more integrated programs, academic integration with special education classes in regular schools, and social integration and legal access to services through compulsory education laws (Bersani & Nerney, 1988).

RECENT REHABILITATION LEGISLATION

Rehabilitation Act

The Vocational Rehabilitation Act, as amended in 1968, was replaced by the Rehabilitation Act (PL 93-112) in 1973. By bringing the needs of severely disabled individuals to the forefront of the rehabilitation mission, it began a new era. This act actually represented a compromise between two branches of the government. The legislation was originally intended to provide for rehabilitation services regardless of whether the recipient could be expected to obtain or return to gainful employment. The act's purpose was to develop and implement rehabilitation programs for individuals with disabilities that would maximize employability, independence, and integration into the workplace and the community. It emphasized service for individuals with the most severe disabilities, and required that a written, individualized program be

provided for every client. Title V, Section 504, entitled "Nondiscrimination Under Federal Grants and Programs," provided that qualified individuals may not be excluded from benefits, programs, or activities receiving federal assistance. It was further strengthened by the subsequent section, which specified that the Civil Rights Act of 1964 could be applied to individuals discriminated against in employment on the basis of their disability.

The Vocational Rehabilitation Act also established the Rehabilitation Services Administration and provided funding for projects with industry programs, centers for independent living, and the Architectural and Transportation Barriers Compliance Board. This board was empowered to make recommendations regarding accessibility in the areas of transportation, in compliance with the 1968 Architectural Barriers Act (PL 90-480), which mandated access to federal buildings for people with disabilities. Section 504 of the 1973 Vocational Rehabilitation Act incorporated redefined standards for accessibility. The Rehabilitation Act was amended in 1974 and again in 1978 to continue appropriations, strengthen programs for the blind, and change the definition of developmental disabilities. It provided grants to states to fund vocational rehabilitation services, including evaluation, diagnosis, training, and employment placement, and independent living centers in certain areas of the country on a demonstration basis. In 1984 an amendment extended the provisions of the 1973 Vocational Rehabilitation Act, a 1986 amendment placed emphasis on needs of Native Americans and technology development, and a 1992 amendment emphasized "people-first" language (Fifield & Fifield, 1995).

1980s Rehabilitation Legislation

The 1980s were an important time for rehabilitation legislation; during this decade, seven acts pertaining to the needs of people with disabilities became law. These laws can be classified in three categories: benefits, services, and access. Benefits legislation was designed to make it both desirable and possible for disabled individuals to contribute as members of society through certain financially related benefits that were provided or extended. Service legislation pertained to rehabilitation services provided directly to disabled individuals, and to the overall policies that govern the manner in which society treats individuals with disabilities. Access

Table 4-1   REHABILITATION LEGISLATION, 1980–1986

Year	Legislation	Provisions
1980	Education Amendments (PL 96-374)	Provides centers, services, personnel, training, and research related to educational needs of children with disabilities.
1980	Social Security Disability Amendments (PL 96-265)	Extends trial work periods for the disabled, enabling them to retain social security benefits. Places gainfully employed disabled in a special benefits category for needed services.
1982	Surface Transportation Assistance Act (PL 97-424)	Encourages removal of architectural barriers in transportation industry.
1983	Education of Handicapped Act (PL 98-199)	Ensures access to educational opportunities for children with disabilities.
1984	Vocational Educational Act (PL 98-524)	Requires states to provide funds for individuals with disabilities to have access to available vocational educational opportunities.
1984	Rehabilitation Amendments (PL 98-221)	Modifies definition of severely disabled and places lower age limit at 16 years. Extends provisions of 1973 Rehabilitation Act.
1986	Rehabilitation Amendments (PL 99-506)	Emphasizes rehabilitation needs of Native Americans with disabilities. Provides funding for rehabilitation engineering to develop technologically current devices for individuals with disabilities. Decreases federal share of the basic state rehabilitation program. Expands influence of the National Council on the Handicapped.

Watson, P. (1988). Rehabilitation legislation of the 1980s: implications for nurses as health care providers. *Rehabilitation Nursing*, 13(3), 137.

legislation was intended to enable individuals with disabilities to move about freely and to participate fully in all societal activities. Table 4–1 cites each of the seven pieces of legislation and their provisions. These laws were important for three reasons. They signified the status of the rehabilitation mission in the United States, predicted future directions for legislation, and suggested ways in which nurses could influence the future of legislation (Watson, 1988). Three pieces of legislation directly affected educational services and ensured access to educational opportunities for children and adolescents with disabilities.

Technology-Related Assistance for Individuals With Disabilities

The Technology-Related Assistance for Individuals with Disabilities Act of 1988 (PL 100-407) expanded the availability of services and

recognized the importance of assistive technology in the lives of children with disabilities. This act broadly defined assistive technology as items that add to the individual's functional ability and provided impetus for states to assess needs for types of services. In 1994, an amendment (PL 103-218) strengthened and expanded the original act and required states to:

- have policies regarding access and funding for assistive technology (AT) services
- implement strategies to overcome barriers to access for underrepresented groups
- coordinate state agency activities
- assist individuals with disabilities to access funding for and procurement of AT devices
- provide outreach to increase access for rural populations
- place emphasis on delivery of services to children (Arizona Technology Access Program, 1996).

Americans With Disabilities Act

At the beginning of the 1990s, another milestone occurred with the passage of the Americans with Disabilities Act (ADA, PL 101-336). As shown in Table 4–2, this act had four components that addressed access in the areas of employment, services, accommodations, and telecommunications. It also included a new, simpler definition of disability.

> Disability: The term disability means, with respect to an individual (A) a physical or mental impairment that substantially limits one or more of the major life activities of such an individual; (B) a record of such an impairment; or (C) being regarded as having such an impairment. (ADA, 1990)

Individuals with recorded impairment or regarded as having an impairment were included in this definition. This piece of legisla-

Table 4–2 AMERICANS WITH DISABILITIES ACT OF 1990

Title I: Employment

Employers cannot discriminate against a qualified disabled job applicant or employee in any manner related to employment and benefits.
Employers must make their existing facilities accessible and usable by individuals with disabilities
Accommodations in all aspects of job attainment and performance are required in order to place individuals on an equal plane with the nondisabled.

Title II: Public Services

Qualified disabled individuals must have access to all services and programs provided by state or local governments.
Public rail transportation must be made accessible to disabled individuals and supplemented with a paratransit system.

Title III: Public Accommodations and Services Operated by Private Entities

Virtually every entity open to the public must now be made accessible to the disabled.
A study is to be conducted concerning accessibility of over-the-road transportation

Title IV: Telecommunications Relay Services

Telephone companies are required to furnish telecommunications devices to enable hearing and speech impaired individuals to communicate by wire or radio.

Watson, P. (1990). The Americans With Disabilities Act: more rights for people with disabilities. *Rehabilitation Nursing*, 15(6), 326.

tion was the first to place compliance responsibilities and costs on the private sector and will probably influence future legislative efforts significantly. Various provisions were directly or indirectly applicable to families with children with disabilities. For example, parents were protected from discrimination with respect to employment hiring practices based on their status as parents of a child with a disability, and parents were protected from being denied health insurance because of their child's condition. Additionally, parents of children with disabilities could expect increased availability of accessible transportation services and greater access to structures in their communities related to education, shopping, and recreation. The ADA also prohibited denial of child care services solely on the basis of a child's disability. This provision increased the availability of child care for families of children with disabilities or other chronic conditions.

The ADA was an impressive piece of legislation that led to substantial increases in societal mobility for people with disabilities; however, issues such as the following remained to be addressed:

1. Eligibility requirements need to be modified, because employment potential remains a criterion for receiving the available services.
2. Medical and other assistance benefits need to be reviewed so that people with disabilities do not lose benefits while in the process of becoming independent economically.
3. Legislators and the public need to be assisted in realizing that increasing the level of function for individuals with disabilities can be cost-effective for the whole country (Watson, 1990).

LEGISLATION FOR SERVICES FOR CHILDREN

The twentieth century saw the beginning of increased societal concern for maternal and child health, and in 1909 President Theodore Roosevelt held the First White House Conference on Children. The treatment of children in orphanages and work settings and their physical and emotional health was discussed, and a decade later, the second conference examined children's well-being and health during the depression.

The first piece of legislation specific to the area of maternal-child health was the Sheppard-Towner Act of 1921. Small amounts of money were given to states that participated in establishing prenatal clinics for poor women under the provisions of this act. The passage in 1935 of the Social Security Act provided grants to states to promote, improve, and develop maternal-child health services, including services to crippled children. Title V established the Crippled Children's Service (CCS). Matching funds were provided by states to establish programs such as Child Welfare Services and Aid to Families with Dependent Children (AFDC). Title V of the Social Security Act has been amended a number of times to reflect current concerns for maternal and child health. In 1985 PL 99-272 changed the name of the CCS to the Program for Children with Special Health Care Needs (CSHCN). State CSHCN programs serve a variety of functions, including support of services through reimbursement procedures similar to those of Medicaid, direct provision of services, mechanisms to coordinate care, and methods for disseminating effective treatments and new service delivery arrangements. Some agencies offer educational programs to health care professionals and the general public about issues related to children with special health care needs. Many states are closely involved in planning new health care initiatives.

In 1965 Title XIX of the Social Security Act established Medicaid, which provided additional funds for health services for children, and Title XX provided for day care for needy families. The Early Periodic Screening, Diagnosis and Treatment Program (EPSDT) and the Women, Infants and Children (WIC) supplemental food program were also developed under Medicaid. EPSDT provides comprehensive services for children from birth to age 21 years, including screening, diagnosis, treatment for identified conditions, and follow-up (Velsor-Friedrich & Frager, 1990).

In 1964 the Economic Opportunity Act, Title V, created Head Start, which continues to provide comprehensive, early childhood development services and programs. Grants were awarded directly to local public schools and agencies as well as private organizations. Each program must include education, health and social services, and parent involvement. At least 10% of the children must be identified as having a disability. The Human Services Reauthorization Act, Title I (1986), is the current reauthorization for these services. The 1997 appropriation was $3.577 billion dollars (U.S.), with approximately 800,000 children

enrolled. The 1994 Head Start Reauthorization Act established a program called Early Head Start to serve families with infants and toddlers. Table 4–3 provides an outline of recent legislative initiatives for children.

Developmental Disabilities Act

The Developmental Disabilities Act of 1970 (PL 91-517) was advocacy legislation whose purpose was to address service gaps to better meet the needs of persons with disabilities. This act established councils with consumer membership in each state to plan for and monitor disability services and programs. The Developmental Disabilities Assistance and Bill of Rights Act of 1975 (PL 94-103) amended the previous act by authorizing developmental disability programs and providing grants to states to fund services and special projects. Additional amendments in 1978 (PL 95-602) changed the definition of developmental disabilities, and the 1984 amendment (PL 98-527) provided a more functional approach to the definition. Other provisions of the original act and amendments include requirements for state planning councils, state plans to address unmet needs of individuals with developmental disabilities, the establishment of a system to advocate for and protect rights, and the development of university-affiliated facilities to implement training programs for individuals in the developmental disabilities field (Bersani & Nerney, 1988). The 1987 amendment (PL 100-146) required that studies be conducted to determine consumer satisfaction with services and program effectiveness (Fifield & Fifield, 1995).

Education of the Handicapped Act

The 1970 Education of the Handicapped Act (PL 91-230) defined handicapped children and was the first recognition of a separate category for people with learning disabilities. Within the U.S. Office of Education, this act also created a Bureau for the Education and Training of the Handicapped and made funds available for projects affecting handicapped students (Bersani & Nerney, 1988). The 1975 Education For All Handicapped Children Act (PL 94-142) was a series of amendments to the 1970 Education of the Handicapped Act and was of great significance for children with disabilities or other chronic conditions. This act and its amendments provided for a free, appropriate public education for each handicapped child, with full protection for

Table 4–3 LEGISLATION FOR CHILDREN'S SERVICES

Year	Legislation	Provisions
1970	Developmental Disabilities Act (PL 91-517)	Addresses service gaps; plans for and monitors disability programs.
1970	Education of the Handicapped Act	Defines handicapped children and makes funds available for them.
1975	Developmental Disabilities and Bill of Rights Act (PL 94-103)	Provides funds for developmental disabilities programs and special projects. Amendments in 1978 changed the definition of developmental disabilities and in 1984 provided a more functional approach. The 1987 amendment requires studies of program effectiveness and customer satisfaction.
1975	Education for All Handicapped Children Act (PL 94-142)	Series of amendments to the 1970 act require provision of educational and support services for all children older than age 3 years, including Individual Education Plans. Amendment in 1984 expanded services.
1981	Omnibus Reconciliation Act (OBRA)	Creates MCH Block grants. Consolidates programs and adds Sudden Infant Death Syndrome, lead-based poisoning prevention, and hemophilia treatment. Amendment in 1990 broadened state mandates and emphasized the development of community-based systems.
1986	Early Intervention Amendments (PL 99-457) to Education for All Handicapped Children Act	Mandates education and services for 3- to 5-year-old children with a developmental disability in the least restrictive environment. Creates or expands early intervention services for children from birth to 3 years of age under Part H of the statute.
1990	Individuals with Disabilities Education Act (IDEA; PL 101-476)	Amendment changed the name of the act and added transition, assistive technology, rehabilitation counseling, and social work to the services that may be provided. Amendment in 1991 emphasized people-first language.

the procedural rights of children receiving special educational services and their parents. It mandated special education and support services to be provided in the least restrictive environment for children older than 3 years of age, Individualized Education Plans (IEP), and due process for questions of eligibility or extent of services offered. The priorities of this act were to seek out those children not currently receiving an education and to serve them and the most severely disabled persons (Bersani & Nerney, 1988).

The 1975 Education for All Handicapped

Children Act was amended in 1984 (PL 98-199) and again in 1986 (PL 99-457). At that time a new discretionary program to help each state plan, design, and implement a comprehensive, multidisciplinary program of early intervention services for infants, toddlers, and families was established. Early Intervention added Part H, which mandates education and related services in the least restrictive environments for 3- to 5-year-old children with developmental disabilities. Part H also creates or expands early intervention services for children from birth through 2 years of age. The key components of the birth to 2-year-old section specified under PL 99-457 are:

- inclusion of outreach case finding in a "Child Find" effort
- provision of comprehensive evaluation, assessment, and diagnostic services
- development of a plan of services for the child and family (IFSP)
- flexibility of service delivery models and services in a variety of settings
- listing of qualified providers available for those making staffing arrangements
- funding through Medicaid, third-party insurance, and state and local moneys
- family-centered delivery of services that is integrated and community-based and supports families in their caregiving roles
- case management or care coordination with the assignment of specific professionals
- administrative aspects and leadership through designation of a "lead" agency in the state assisted by an Interagency Coordinating Council

There are three major components of the professional's role in implementing PL 99-457:

1. "Child Find," which provides for screening, identification of community resources, and determination of eligibility for services
2. Assessment through interdisciplinary evaluation, including assessment of medical needs, monitoring of health needs, and parent and professional education
3. Development and implementation of the IFSP in collaboration with other professionals and the family; provision of services, follow-through, and family support

Roles and functions of identified service providers include:

Nurse: responsible for medical well-being, which may involve preventive measures and treatment of medical disorders

Physical Therapist: focuses on gross motor development and is responsible for the child's positioning, handling and movement

Occupational Therapist: responsible for the child's sensory development and integration, with an emphasis on sensory information processing

Speech/Language Pathologist and Audiologist: responsible for development of communicative abilities, oral-motor facilitation, feeding therapy, and development of preverbal communication

Social Worker: provides a link between program and family and has knowledge of the family's dynamics, information about siblings, and an understanding of family stresses

Infant Special Educator: responsible for educational programming and assessment, child and family advocacy, and referral to other services

Psychologist: responsible for psychological assessment, counseling of child and family, and consultation regarding behavior and development

Nutritionist: provides guidance to ensure optimal nutrition and proper diet and treats dietary problems (Widerstrom, Mowder, & Sandall, 1991)

Individuals With Disabilities Education Act

A 1990 amendment (PL 101-476) to the Individuals with Disabilities Act changed the name to Individuals with Disabilities Education Act (IDEA) and added transition, assistive technology, rehabilitation counseling, and social work to the services provided. The scope was expanded to include other areas of disability, traumatic brain injury, autism, attention deficit disorder, and serious emotional disturbance. The 1990 amendment included updates, results of program evaluations, and appropriations for funding, and recommends recruitment of staff from ethnic minority groups so the needs of children with limited proficiency in English are addressed. In a 1991 amendment, people-first language was emphasized and funding increases outlined, including specific instructions concerning Native American infants and children living on reservations.

At present, Part H of IDEA is a federally mandated but state-administered program. States receive some funding from the federal government and some funding from state appropriations. Because of the difficulties in levels of funding and the resources available in communities, the extent and frequency of early intervention services may vary. Although Part H is a federal mandate, states differ in the amount and type of services they offer to eligible children and families. The extent and type of services offered by the state is determined by the Part H lead agency, named by the Governor of each state, which administers early intervention services in that state. The lead agency is not always the Department of Education; it may also be the Department of Health, Department of Human

Services, or a Developmental Disabilities state agency.

School systems also provide services for children with disabilities. IDEA (PL 101-476) mandates the provision of related services that are necessary for a child to benefit from public education. IDEA instructs states to provide a free, public education in the least restrictive environment (i.e., the most typical and usual environment possible) to all children from 3 through 21 years of age, regardless of disability. Part H of IDEA provides for early intervention services for children from birth through 3 years of age administered by the identified lead agency, and Part B of IDEA provides for pre-school services administered through the local school districts. The issue of exactly what setting constitutes the least restrictive environment is often debated. Current educational philosophy suggests that full inclusion of all children, regardless of disability, in the same classroom with their non-disabled peers is the attainable ideal. Many leaders in education and special education believe that it is the intent of IDEA to promote inclusive services whenever possible.

However, the realities of differing educational philosophy, scarce funding and resources, inadequate training and support for teachers in the skills and knowledge needed to teach children with differing needs in one classroom, and the often significant challenges created by including children with severe behavioral problems or children who require complex medical support often lead to segregated classrooms or even separate schools. Although many parents are willing to fight for their child's right to attend school with non-disabled peers, other parents fear for their child's vulnerability in a regular classroom and prefer a segregated setting where specialized services are more easily available and their child is not exposed to the risk of teasing or demeaning behavior from peers.

Related services may include one or more services provided by or paid for by the school district in which the child resides. These services include special education, psychology, social work and counseling, speech and language therapy, audiology services, physical therapy, occupational therapy, nursing, and transportation services. Medical care is not included. Testing to determine whether or not the child qualifies for these services on the basis of developmental delay, disability, or learning or psychological disabilities is also provided to families at no cost through the

Child Find system. Each child aged 3 through 21 years who qualifies receives an Individual Education Plan (IEP) on a yearly basis to plan for and monitor services. Only those services identified in the IEP are provided through the school district. Young children who qualify for services through Part H of IDEA receive an Individualized Family Service Plan (IFSP) that provides for family support as well as intervention services for the child. These services are provided on an intermittent basis and are often supplemented by families who receive private therapies paid for out-of-pocket or by insurance. Frequently, the related services the child receives through the school district fail to meet the child's complete therapy needs because they are limited to the child's ability to learn and participate in the school environment.

Omnibus Budget Reconciliation Act

The Omnibus Budget Reconciliation Act (OBRA) in 1981 created Maternal and Child Health Services block grants and consolidated programs. The 1990 Omnibus Budget Reconciliation Act (PL 101-239) amendments to Title V altered the program's mission, broadened the mandate of state programs, gave a more generic orientation to the definition of children to be served, emphasized the development of community-based systems, and described how minimum standards must be established for community-based services. This amendment required states to spend 30% of the funds from the Maternal and Child Health Services block grant on children with special health care needs and to improve the service system for these children and their families by promoting family-centered, community-based, coordinated care. This significantly altered the service system for these children and created changes in how care was provided, monitored, and reimbursed.

Personal Responsibility and Work Opportunity Reconciliation Act

The Personal Responsibility and Work Opportunity Reconciliation Act of 1996 (PL 104-193) decreased support for many programs serving children and families, including Aid to Families with Dependent Children (AFDC), the JOBS program (a work and training program for welfare recipients), and Emergency Assistance to Families with Children, and replaced them with the provision of flat (fixed-amount) block grants of federal funds given to states called Temporary Assistance for Needy Families (TANF). This act eliminated provision of child care help and the special "At Risk" category, cut the food stamp program, and reduced nutrition aid through the Child and Adult Care Food program. It also redefined disability in childhood by "limiting Supplemental Security Income (SSI) to children who meet a set of official conditions called the 'medical listings'." This caused a large number of children to be denied SSI, and many also lost Medicaid (Children's Defense Fund, 1996, p. 5).

HEALTH CARE REFORM: NURSING IMPLICATIONS

The number of individuals in society who are accurately characterized as severely disabled can be expected to increase over the next 20 years. Individuals will spend shorter periods of time in inpatient settings and will be discharged to the community in early stages of rehabilitation. The resultant burdens and responsibilities on families is likely to increase. This trend will be accompanied by increased demands for long-term care facilities to house individuals who cannot be maintained in the home for various reasons. A greater number of youths with severe disabilities will have reached a stage in life when society expects gainful employment and independent community living. There will be many disabled individuals who will be alive because of technological advances but will require lifelong rehabilitation services.

Initiatives like the Contract with America would have altered the very structure of the federal government's response to children's needs, severely restricting the nation's ability to produce healthy, well-educated, well-cared-for children far into the future. More than 500,000 children with disabilities face possible denial of help under the SSI program. Congress has had numerous opportunities to improve the delivery of services to children and families in a number of program areas by consolidating selected federal programs that are not entitlements. Thoughtful consolidation of programs with similar goals and purposes in such areas as child care, job training, and child abuse prevention and treatment could improve the quality of services and increase program accountability while reducing administrative complexity and duplication of effort.

In 1993 the American Health Security Act was proposed, to offer a set of critical reforms and a beginning solution to the health care financing and delivery crisis that confronts children with special health care needs and their families. It promised access to a federally guaranteed, specified package of primary, preventive, and acute health care services and prescription drugs regardless of health status, income, family employment, or ability to pay. It offered critical reforms of the health insurance system and provided an initial step toward building an adequate system of home- and community-based long-term care for children with chronic health conditions. However, the legislation was never enacted, and many proponents continue the effort to make health care reform a reality.

What is needed is available, affordable health insurance; access to primary and specialty care; insurance coverage that is continuous and portable with prohibition of pre-existing conditions and waiting periods; elimination of annual or lifetime caps; setting of caps for out-of-pocket expenses; accessible information for families; and simple enrollment procedures.

Jameson and Wehr (1995) recommend health care reform that addresses the special needs and concerns of children to provide access to services. Current health coverage is inadequate because insurers do not recognize the difference between the needs of children and adults. To protect the interests of children, a pediatric standard of care should be created "to evaluate the appropriate type and scope of health services for children" (Jameson & Wehr, 1995, p. 2). Included in this standard would be basic health services for children that would foster the goal of healthy development and "guarantee that health services of particular value to children are not compromised by a plan's cost management efforts" (Jameson & Wehr, 1995, p. 3).

PUBLIC POLICY INVOLVEMENT/ ADVOCACY ROLE

One of the roles of the pediatric rehabilitation nurse as stated in the Association of Rehabilitation Nurses role description (1992) is that of advocate. This role includes:

- functioning as a child and family advocate
- facilitating the entire family's transition from hospital to home and community
- promoting community and governmental knowledge of pediatric rehabilitation issues

Nurses from many practice settings, including rehabilitation, community health, academia, developmental, and acute care, have much to contribute to the provision of care for children with disabilities or other chronic conditions. Care coordination can be easily incorporated into the nursing process and the implementation of services for families. Nurses are especially suited to identifying and meeting the needs of families with children, with or without risk factors, because they provide education and support for practices that facilitate the child's developmental potential (Hansen, Holaday, & Miles, 1990).

Nurses can impact on public policy decisions and provide valuable input on today's major health care issues. When an important issue is being addressed by legislators at the state or federal level, nurses should call or write their senator or representative and share their viewpoints and opinions. This is especially important for children's issues, because children do not have a strong voice or representation in the political arena. The nurse does not need to be an expert on the health care issue, but it is important that the nurse states his or her position clearly when calling or writing. The American Nurses Association has developed a *Legislative Action Handbook* (Nurses Strategic Action Team, 1993) to assist nurses in making their voices heard.

Nurses speaking on behalf of the rehabilitation needs of individuals and families, using clinical examples and anecdotal evidence along with documented research findings, have the power to dramatically affect the character of legislation put forth by the U.S. House of Representatives and Senate. State legislatures can also be informed of specific community child care needs. For example, welfare reform has shifted the AFDC program to the states through block grants, and nurse advocates need to urge their state government to invest at least the same amount of money in new programs as their present funding for AFDC.

Nurses need to have skills in many areas and an extensive knowledge base to perform their various roles. Expertise in pediatric rehabilitation nursing must be blended with continuing education regarding regulations, legislation, and strategies for affecting public policy to allow for articulation and collaboration in the political arena. Nurses as advocates for children with disabilities and their families can reflect current concerns: the cost and quality of care and access to all levels of health care services for the greatest number of people. When nurses understand proposals such as health care reform they can combine this understanding with their nursing knowledge and experience to explain the impact of legislation. Nurses must be politically astute

so that they know how to present the situation in the most effective way possible. Pediatric rehabilitation nurses can also be effective consultants to state agencies in the development of standards for health and safety.

Parents and other family members need to become more sophisticated in their understanding of the impact of legislation and the health care system from which they must seek services. "Knowledgeable families will insist on being supported, not served, in settings that include everyone . . ." and become increasingly influential in the political and legislative areas that affect them and their children (Shoultz & Smith, 1995, p. 183). It is critical for nurses, parents and other family members to maintain awareness of how political candidates plan to provide support for children. Candidates should be asked their position on cuts in federal support for basic services, provision of health care for every child, and other initiatives to improve children's lives.

SUMMARY

Progress is made when clinical gains, policy reform, and favorable legislation all occur at the same time. For the rest of the century, activity will probably focus more on the use of legislation and litigation to make existing rights into realities and threats will come from budget cuts and Supreme Court decisions (Bersani & Nerney, 1988). Monetary provisions in the past have decreased the federal share of the costs of the basic state rehabilitation program from 80% to 75%. Among the states, there are varying commitments to the concepts of rehabilitation and special education and varying financial resources to support the programs. The characteristics of rehabilitation legislative action at the state and federal level will be governed to a large degree by the ideologies of the prevailing political party at any given time.

Numerous suggestions have been made for improving care and preventing health problems in childhood. As we look to the future, specific actions must be taken to represent children's needs and invest in their health and well-being. Pediatric rehabilitation nurses at all levels of practice can provide a strong body of representation to influence child health policy and make a difference in the quality of children's lives. Collaboration with families, consumers, and other service providers is imperative to make systems accessible and well coordinated and to ensure that these systems foster the child's developmental progress.

Many politicians campaign that children are their priority, so nurses need to remind them that equal opportunity must begin with our youngest children. Report after report demonstrates that preventive investments in our most vulnerable children can save lives and millions of dollars. Investment in child health and education benefits all of society by contributing to our country's health, security, and economic competitiveness.

REFERENCES

Americans With Disabilities Act of 1990. Pub. L. No. 101-336.

Arizona Technology Access Program. (1996). *The technology-related assistance for Individuals with Disabilities Act.* Institute for Human Development, Northern Arizona University [On-line]. Available: www.nau.edu/ihd/techfact.html

Association of Rehabilitation Nurses Pediatric Special Interest Group. (1992). *Pediatric rehabilitation nursing role description*, Skokie, IL: Association of Rehabilitation Nurses.

Bersani, H., & Nerney, T. (1988). *Legal and legislative initiatives in disability.* In V. VanHassell, P. Strain, & M. Hersen (Ed.), *Handbook of developmental and physical disabilities* (Chap. 11). New York: Pergammon Press.

Bitter, J. (1979). *Introduction to rehabilitation.* St. Louis: C.V. Mosby.

Children's Defense Fund. (1996). *Summary of new welfare law* [On-line]. Available: www.tmn.com/cdf/welfarelaw.html

Fifield, B., & Fifield, M. (1995). *The influence of legislation on services to people with disabilities.* In O. Karan & S. Greenspan (Eds.). *Community rehabilitation services for people with disabilities* (Chap. 3). Boston: Butterworth-Heinemann.

Hansen, S., Holaday, B., & Miles, M. (1990). The role of pediatric nurses in a federal program for infants and young children with handicaps. *Journal of Pediatric Nursing*, 5(4), 246–251.

Jameson, E., & Wehr, E. (1995). *Drafting national health care reform legislation to protect the health interests of children* [On-line]. Abstract from Pediatric Standard. Available: nncf.unl.edu/health.pedstand.html

Nurses Strategic Action Team. (1993). *Legislative action handbook.* Washington, DC: American Nurses Association.

Shoultz, B., & Smith, P. (1995). *Shifting roles of parents and families.* In O. Karan & S. Greenspan (Eds.). *Community rehabilitation services for people with disabilities* (Chap. 8). Boston: Butterworth-Heinemann.

Velsor-Friedrich, B., & Frager, B. (1990). The federal government and child health. *Journal of Pediatric Nursing*, 5(1), 56–58.

Watson, P. (1988). Rehabilitation legislation of the 1980s: implications for nurses as health care providers. *Rehabilitation Nursing*, 13(3), 136–141.

Watson, P. (1990). The Americans with Disabilities Act: more rights for people with disabilities. *Rehabilitation Nursing*, 15(6), 325–328.

Widerstrom, A., Mowder, B., & Sandall, S. (1991). *At-risk and handicapped newborns and infants: development, assessment and intervention.* Englewood Cliffs, NJ: Prentice Hall.

ADDITIONAL RESOURCES

Children's Defense Fund. (1995). *The state of America's children yearbook.* Washington, DC: Children's Defense Fund.

Cohen, H. (199_). Services for young children with disabilities: new directions and emerging issues. *Physical Medicine and Rehabilitation*, 5(2), 427–441.

Craven, G., & Gleason, C. (1995). Public policy and rehabilitation nursing. In S. Hoeman (Ed.). *Rehabilitation nursing: process and application*, 2nd Ed. (Chap. 5). Boston: CV Mosby.

Frager, B. (1990). A national child care crisis: action for the 90s. *Journal of Pediatric Nursing*, 5(3), 229–231.

Ireys, H., & Nelson, R. (1992). New federal policy for children with special health care needs. *Pediatrics*, 90(3), 321–327.

Karan, O., & Greenspan, S. (Eds.). (1995). *Community rehabilitation services for people with disabilities.* Boston: Butterworth-Heinemann.

National Center for Education in Maternal Child Health. (1993). *Children with special health needs.* Arlington, VA: National Center for Education in Maternal Child Health.

New England SERVE Regional Task Force on Health Care Financing. (1994). *Assessing the adequacy of health care reform proposals: an analysis of the American Health Security Act of 1993.* Boston: New England SERVE Regional Task Force on Health Care Financing.

Parette, H., & VanBiervliet, A. (1991). Rehabilitation assistive technology issues for infants and young children with disabilities: a preliminary examination. *Journal of Rehabilitation*, July/Aug/Sept, 27–36.

Phillips, W., & Spotts, M. (1994). Medicolegal issues in the US. In S. Campbell (Ed.). *Physical Therapy for Children* (Chap. 33). Philadelphia: WB Saunders.

CASE STUDY—Oral Testimony Before the State Legislature Health Care Committee

Good morning Chairman McDonough, Chairman Montigny, and members of the Health Care Committee. I am Patricia A. Edwards, the Secretary of the Board of Directors of the Massachusetts Nurses Association. I have a Masters degree in Parent-Child Health Nursing and extensive experience in pediatrics and rehabilitation services for children with special health care needs. Today, I am specifically addressing the issue of expansion of state-funded coverage for the 160,000 uninsured children in Massachusetts. First, some background information.

From a health perspective, the years between birth and 5 are critical. This is a time of rapid physiologic change. Optimal neurologic and musculoskeletal growth is crucial to the development of cognitive, psychomotor, and speech and language skills. The first 2 years also mark the identification of many minor, or perhaps a few major, health problems. For children with diagnosed health problems, the pre-school years also represent a time when surgery, special equipment, and therapies may be needed to eliminate a medical problem or reduce its later impact.

A key assumption in pediatric care is that unless optimal levels of wellness are promoted, a child's potential to function may be adversely affected. Although children who have a handicapping condition or are chronically ill may not be sick in the common use of the term, the nature and extent of their disabilities puts them at higher risk for recurrent illnesses and unwarranted secondary disabilities.

However, in this area we face a paradox. Tremendous advances in technology during the past decades have made possible the prevention and remediation of disabilities. At the same time, funds for services have become less available, particularly for low-income families.

Now I would like to make a few comments relating specifically to the health care reform bill under discussion. I agree with those who sense that the signs are favorable for meaningful health care financing reform this year and believe that a priority must be availability of health insurance for children and families, along with access to community-based, comprehensive services. A system of coordinated care is needed that is more responsive to the needs of families as well as more cost-effective and efficient. First, the expansion of funding for children's health should be included as an integral part of the bill and not be solely contingent on passing a tax increase. The benefits of the Children's Medical Security Plan (CMSP) include services for children from only 1 month to 12 years of age and cover only regular visits. It must be expanded to include prevention and hospitalization, and the age limit must be increased to 21 years. Second, the drug subsidy program should also include children and individuals with disabilities and not just the elderly. CMSP covers only a minimum of prescription medical payments. Third, because there are no provisions in the bill for health care coverage for family members, many children will remain uninsured and have only limited access to services if the previously mentioned changes do not take place in CMSP. Improving access to care and the quality of life for children and their families needs to be a priority, and employers should be required to include family coverage with pediatric preventive care and health supervision services in their health benefits packages.

The provisions of this bill are a good beginning to solving the problem of access to insurance but are only a "baby" step toward what should be the ultimate goal—universal access to health care for all. Many groups and individuals articulate the growing realization that child health providers and educators serve a common constituency. This awareness has led to a reexamination of the relationship between health and education, and recent reports of national commissions call explicitly for better health and education coordination.

In closing I pose this question. "How visible and important are children in our state?" In recent years, children's issues have found their way into the political rhetoric, but rarely as serious, central, or dominant themes. The National Commission on Children ends its child-focused document *Beyond Rhetoric* with the following:

> The National Commission on Children calls on all Americans to work together to change the conditions that jeopardize the health and well-being of so many of our young citizens and threaten our future as an economic power, a democratic nation, and a caring society. Our failure to act now will only defer to the next generation the rising social, moral and financial costs of our neglect. Investing in children is no longer a luxury, but a national imperative.

Here in Massachusetts we must make a commitment to a child-oriented agenda as part of our program of health care reform. Thank you.

■■■

REFERENCES

Children's Defense Fund (1995). *The state of America's children yearbook*. Washington, DC: Children's Defense Fund.

Palfrey, J. (1994). *Community child health: an action plan for today*. Westport, CT: Praeger.

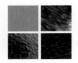

Chapter 5

Financing Health Care

Patricia A. Edwards

For many of us, the system for financing health care in this country is just not working. Health care costs are rising, benefits through our insurance plans are shrinking, and a significant percentage of the population have no health insurance coverage at all. It has been predicted that many millions of Americans will be without health insurance by the year 2000, and others who may be lucky enough to have some health insurance will find their coverage inadequate and unable to meet their family's needs. Families whose children have serious ongoing health needs are disproportionately represented in both of these groups.

Proposals for changing the delivery of health care in the United States and its financial implications are being discussed in many forums at a variety of levels. Articles in professional journals and the popular press, as well as television media coverage, cite that health care spending has risen dramatically, as has the number of uninsured Americans. "A significant policy debate has begun on how to reform health care financing so that rising costs can be contained and health care coverage provided to the Americans currently without health insurance" (New England SERVE, 1991, p. 1). Children with disabilities or other chronic conditions are a significant group in this debate. They require specialized health and related services and have health care needs that are broader and deeper than those of the population as a whole. These children require a system of financing that covers a range of services and benefits and supports coordination of services and quality assurance efforts. An increasingly large number of families, characterized as the "working poor," have incomes too high to qualify for Medicaid or the entitlement programs, yet are unable to afford health insurance due to cost or lack of availability through the workplace. Numerous proposals have been presented at both the federal and state levels but, to date, only minimal changes have been made in financing structures.

The system for delivery of health care services to children is threatened by major reductions in the rate of growth of funding under federal initiatives to balance the budget. Overall, children are a large percentage of the Medicaid recipients in the country, but they account for only a small percentage of the dollars spent. The concept of block grants poses a further threat to access, and there will be ongoing competition for limited dollars on the state level. When block grants are established, minimum federal standards for children's services should be included as a requirement for the receipt of block grant funds, and access issues should be closely monitored in the transition to such an approach.

Because children with disabilities or other chronic conditions are heavy users of the health care system, their families spend a great deal of time trying to understand and decide how to pay for their care. This often includes using a complicated mix of private health insurers and public programs. Getting general information or specific questions answered can be a long, drawn-out, and confusing process. As the cost of health care increases, benefits and eligibility may be subject to change. In addition, a job shift for a parent can result in a change in health insurance benefits, a change in health care providers, or even the loss of insurance. In addition to placing demands on schools, community programs, and health care institutions, this group of children and their families are often required to forego basic health services, make sizable out-of-pocket payments, or both. Because of pre-existing conditions, these children may be excluded from the family's insurance coverage and may be more likely to be dependent on public programs for their care and services.

This chapter describes the various financing methods in place to cover health care services, the economic issues related to preventive services, what an "ideal" system should be like, how to assist families in assessing their financial status and securing necessary funding for their child, and what the future may hold in the way of health care reform.

FINANCING METHODS

Health care for children with disabilities or other chronic conditions is primarily financed by the following methods: private insurance, public programs, philanthropic sources, and family funds. This may be through a single payor or a combination of methods, depending on family income, place of residence, the child's condition, and the benefits package provided by an employer (Table 5–1). The availability of voluntary organizations and the family's ability to advocate for the child's rights also have a significant impact on funding for various services and other needs (O'Grady, 1992). Knowledgeable pediatric rehabilitation nurses can assist the family in obtaining information about funding sources and advocate for their right to access health care benefits and services.

Private Insurance

The world of private health insurance is a complex and confusing one that has changed dramatically in recent years and will continue to change as more emphasis is placed on cost containment efforts and less funding is available from other sources. "The proportion of health care costs paid by private insurance has represented between 30 and 40 percent of all national expenditures" (McCarthy & Minnis, 1994, p. 1161). Companies that provide private insurance are under state regula-

Table 5–1   PRIVATE AND PUBLIC SOURCES FOR HEALTH CARE

Private Insurance

- Commercial insurance companies
- Blue Cross Hospital and Blue Shield Physician Service Plans ("The Blues")
- Employer self-insurance
- Health Maintenance Organizations (HMOs)
- Preferred Provider Organizations (PPOs)

Public Programs

- Medicaid (Federal and State)
- Federal Employees Health Benefits Program (FEHBP)
- Civilian Health and Medical Program of the Uniformed Services (CHAMPUS)
- Native American Services Program
- Other federal, state, and local programs

Other Private Sources

- Hospital non-patient revenues
- Philanthropy
- Consumer out-of-pocket

---

tions that require the provision of certain benefits. To exempt themselves from these mandates, many employers have chosen to become self-insured and provide medical coverage for their employees.

There are different ways to buy insurance and different types of insurance to buy. Both of these issues have an impact on what the insurance is likely to cover and cost. Most people purchase health insurance through their employer and are part of a group plan. This type of plan represents the best coverage for the least cost because risks are spread over a group. Some people buy individual plans directly from an insurance company or through an insurance agent and pay the entire premium. Private insurance varies with the benefits and cost-sharing requirements written into the policy, and features that can affect coverage include lifetime maximums (i.e., the maximum amount of dollars for all medical care per insured person), stop-loss provisions (i.e., an insured annual limit on out-of-pocket expenditures), and covered or limited services (e.g., equipment, therapies, home nursing care). The coverage may include increased cost-sharing requirements with employee deductibles and co-payments, and the insurer may have case management programs in place to assist with access to services and monitor utilization.

The main source of coverage for children

with disabilities or other chronic conditions is private insurance, whose purpose is to provide pooled protection against the risk of unexpected medical and financial demands (Votroubek, 1990). With traditional plans, the insurance company covers some percentage of the cost of service with a co-payment, and there may also be annual deductibles. Whether this type of plan is the best choice for a family depends on their particular needs and the specifics of the plan. Although traditional plans allow the widest choice of providers, both primary and specialty care, as well as of hospitals or clinics, out-of-pocket costs may be higher. These health insurance policies may contain combinations of the following: major medical insurance, hospital/medical insurance, prescription drug coverage, disability income protection, dental expense insurance, and long-term care insurance.

Fee-for-service plans pay after the service is provided, and prepayment plans provide services for regular, fixed payments. "The problems faced by families who depend on fee-for-service health insurance to finance care for a child with a chronic condition are evident in looking at the exclusion and limitations of these policies. The insurer usually does not pay for pre-existing conditions. Thus if a family was not adequately covered before the child acquired the chronic condition, a fee-for-service plan often will not cover the medical expenses related to the chronic condition" (O'Grady, 1992, p. 46). Other exclusions include payments for preventive health care, rehabilitation services, and devices such as hearing aids and eye glasses. Additionally, coverage for non-medical health needs such as special education, transportation, and home renovations are generally excluded.

Managed Care

Pre-paid health plans are both the insurer and the health care provider. These are systems that integrate the delivery and financing of health care services, such as health maintenance organizations (HMOs), self-contained and preferred provider organizations (PPOs), and networks of providers that contract to deliver health care to a group or individuals for a pre-set fee. In this type of plan, the choice of provider may be restricted, but there are fewer out-of-pocket costs. There is usually good coverage for primary or preventive care, but these plans may be more restrictive of specialty services.

A wide variety of insurance arrangements are available as a result of the evolution of "managed care." This "encompasses a variety of innovations in both the delivery and financing of health care that are intended to eliminate unnecessary and inappropriate health care and reduce costs" (McCarthy & Minnis, 1994, p. 1183). Managed care is an organized system of coverage that includes the integration of facilities, services, and products. Health maintenance organizations (HMOs) are perhaps the best known examples of managed care systems.

"HMOs provide a pre-defined, comprehensive set of health services to a voluntarily enrolled population within a specified geographical area" (McCarthy & Minnis, 1994, p. 1186). They focus on the primary care practitioner as the main provider for the child and family and are more likely to offer preventive services. A variety of models evolved in response to the needs of the consumers, including:

- group model (single, multispecialty medical group)
- network model (two or more independent medical groups)
- staff model (own staff of physicians)
- independent physician association (IPA) model (loose organization of independent physicians)
- mixed or open-ended plan

After joining an HMO, the family must select a primary care physician who authorizes care by any other physician or hospital within the plan. However, if a child with a disability or chronic condition requires a health care professional with special expertise, this type of health coverage may not be adequate for the child if such a provider is not available in the HMO. Services that may be excluded include long-term care, therapies lasting longer than 60 days, prosthetics, and durable medical equipment. "Advantages of the pre-paid plan for the family are the coverage of primary care and access to a different mix of services that may include pediatric nurse practitioners and clinicians, and nutrition and social services with expertise in various problems of living with a chronic condition" (O'Grady, 1992, p. 47).

Managed care, specifically HMOs, presents some problems for families of children with disabilities or other chronic conditions, but they also offer advantages over traditional insurance coverage. "HMOs are less likely to have exclusions for pre-existing conditions and are more likely to protect families against out-of-pocket costs. HMOs are also more likely to cover ancillary therapies, home health care, outpatient mental health services and medical case management" (Hoyt, 1995, p. 1). Problems may arise, however, when families are restricted from seeing specialists and limited to shorter rehabilitation stays that decrease the time available for children and families to cope with problems and learn how to manage their care. "Often inpatient stays are approved on a week-to-week basis, leaving both the family and the rehabilitation staff uncertain about long range treatment and discharge planning" (Cole, 1996, p. 1).

Public Programs

Medicaid

"Medicaid is a federal- and state-funded program administered by the individual states in the form of public assistance programs for low income groups, families with dependent children, the elderly poor and the disabled" (McCarthy & Minnis, 1994, p. 1194). Benefits and eligibility requirements vary from state to state. Much of the original intent of Medicaid has changed as Congress has taken actions to add new services and criteria through the Budget Reconciliation Acts. Each state can choose which services it will fund, but there are some that are mandatory. These include inpatient services, outpatient clinics, laboratory tests and x-rays, certain skilled nursing care facilities, physician's office visits, and intermittent home health visits by a nurse. However, states may impose limits on the duration and scope of the services. Since the early 1980s, as a result of attention given the situation of a child named Katie Beckett, states have obtained waivers to design programs that offer special services and expand services provided in the home and community. "Some services allowed through waiver programs include private duty nursing at the child's home, case management services, experimental medications, transportation services, respite care, rehabilitation services, speech, hearing and language disorder therapy and certain preventive services" (Kaufman, 1991a, p. 281).

Civilian Health and Medical Program of the Uniformed Services

Medical treatment is available at any Department of Defense facility for active military personnel and their dependents under the Civilian Health and Medical Program of the Uniformed Services (CHAMPUS). "CHAMPUS is a program of medical benefits provided by civilian health professionals for military families who are unable to use government facilities because of distance, overcrowding or unavailability of appropriate medical treatment. It resembles a traditional health insurance plan in that beneficiaries must pay a deductible, may have out of pocket costs and may also be limited to a preferred provider panel of physicians" (O'Grady, 1992, p. 48). Children with disabilities or other chronic conditions may be eligible for services in one of two ways: the home health benefit or the Program For The Handicapped (PFTH). The home health benefit provides "skilled nursing care, primarily as an intermittent visit, physician visits, durable medical equipment, oxygen, parenteral and enteral nutrition, physical therapy, disposable medical supplies, and medications" (Kaufman, 1991b, p. 380). These services are limited, and children requiring custodial care are not eligible. The PFTH program provides for dependents who are mentally retarded or severely physically handicapped. "These services include diagnostic tests, rehabilitation, durable medical equipment, disposable supplies, transportation and in-home nursing care" (Kaufman, 1991b, p. 380). Prior approval is required, a $1000 per month limit is imposed, and only those children not eligible for other public programs or institutionalization can receive the services. Children who require custodial care are not eligible (Kaufman, 1991b).

Native American Services Program

The Native American Services Program is a federal program that ensures the availability of comprehensive health care and services to Native American Indians and Inuits. These services include hospital and ambulatory care, preventive and rehabilitative services, and community and environmental health programs.

Federal Employees Health Benefits Program

The Federal Employees Health Benefits Program (FEHBP) is the largest employer-sponsored health care program and provides health insurance coverage for federal government employees and their dependents. It offers three types of plans:

Government-wide plan: service benefit plan under National Blue Cross and Blue Shield Association
Employee/union organization plan: member employees or annuitants
Comprehensive medical plans: contracted health care in designated locations

Other Programs

Other programs include the following:

The Developmental Disabilities Program, which does not provide funds directly to families but supports services such as home nursing care and respite care (Kaufman, 1991b).

The Early and Periodic Screening Diagnosis and Treatment Program (EPSDT) is "intended to enable Medicaid-eligible children to receive basic screening in order to identify actual or potential health problems including mental and physical developmental concerns. It is also intended to fund diagnostic and/or treatment services for health problems that are identified during the screening process. Additional mandates to EPSDT include vision, dental, hearing and developmental assessments" (Kaufman, 1991a, p. 281).

The Supplemental Security Income Program (SSI) provides an important access to essential health services for lower-income, disabled Americans, both children and adults, who would not otherwise qualify for assistance. In 37 states, individuals eligible for SSI who do not otherwise qualify for Medicaid can do so through a provision that links the two programs (Perrin & Stein, 1991). "When SSI is applied for on behalf of a child, the income and resources of the child's parents, as well as the child's disability, are considered when determining eligibility" (Kaufman, 1991b, p. 381).

Children's Medical Services–State Programs, first established in 1936 as Title V (Crippled Children's Services) of the Social Security Act, have undergone major changes, culminating in a consolidation of all the programs into the state programs for Children with Special Health Care Needs (CSHCN). This revision eliminated most federal treatment requirements for categorical illnesses and specific services and gave the states greater discretion in the provision of services (Kaufman, 1991a).

Other Private Sources

Even with coverage from a private health plan and public programs, a family may be left with uncovered expenses. They should be assisted in identifying special discretionary funds available through hospitals or health care centers in the local community, and some communities have access to private endowments with which to help families in this situation. Hospitals and health care providers may be willing to negotiate reduced payment. Voluntary agencies or social organizations may also assist. These agencies require a full description of medical needs and how the problem affects the whole family.

Consumer out-of-pocket expenses vary among the services needed and provided, with more than half being used for medications. In 1990, 4% of the total expenditures for health care came from private sources such as philanthropy and non-patient revenues. Pediatric rehabilitation nurses must "be aware of the services available in your state, what is covered and what is not, what are the barriers to receiving needed care, and how to help those who need resources access them" (Kaufman, 1991b, p. 381).

FUNDING FOR ASSISTIVE TECHNOLOGY

Finding funding is the most significant problem faced by families and children who need assistive technology. A 1992 study found that many of the purchases were made by the family members with no assistance from other sources because of equipment denials by third-party payors. The two main reasons that equipment was denied were that the item was not a medical necessity or it was not a covered expense. The Technology Related Assistance for Individuals with Disabilities Act of 1988, described in Chapter 4, provided grants to the states to increase the availability of assistive technology (AT), conduct needs assessments, develop innovative programs, manage public awareness and provision of information, and identify policies that promote the availability of AT. This program has been limited in its impact because it has not been adequately funded (O'Day & Corcoran, 1994). The 1994 amendment has, however, expanded and strengthened the original act and placed emphasis on delivery of services to children.

Medicaid, when it was enacted, included a provision for rehabilitation and other services to assist families and individuals attain or retain independence or self-care. This provision has been used on behalf of individuals with disabilities to gain access to assistive technology. In Medicaid regulations, the definitions of physical and occupational therapy and services for individuals with speech, hearing, and language disorders contain the statements that they include necessary supplies and equipment. "This is the minimal standard for the service so if a PT prescribes supplies or equipment to promote independence or self-care it is used to prove necessity. The equipment and services are all available to children under Medicaid as a result of major changes in the law in 1989 which mandated a national standard for children" (Bergman, 1994, p. 28).

FAMILY-CENTERED FINANCING

Nurses working in a setting with children with disabilities or other chronic conditions must help families and caregivers anticipate potential financial problems so they can take measures to address or avoid these problems. It should be a priority for the nurse to assess the funding sources available and assist the child and family in gaining access to services.

The nurse should begin with an identification of the child's needs–what they are now and what they will be in the future. A specific diagnosis for the child's health problem or disability can be a very important element in getting payment for services or access to a public program. Discuss with the family the best words to use in describing the child's problem. Determine the benefits available at present and explore others that could be applied for if the child and family meet eligibility requirements. If the family is considering enrolling in a managed care plan or HMO, The National Health Council and the National Patient Empowerment Council suggest asking the following questions (Cole, 1996):

- Can the primary care practitioner be a specialist knowledgeable about the child's condition?
- Can a physician outside the plan be consulted? Is there an additional fee for that service or for a second opinion?
- What hospitals might be used and what services are provided?
- Are medically necessary services, including home-based rehabilitation, durable medical equipment, and prescription medications, provided?

Are there co-pays and deductibles or a lifetime maximum per-person coverage?

When making referrals, choose appropriate agencies and resources and document the needs. Describe the medical necessity of the service or equipment using language that is meaningful to the payor and personalize the request with pictures showing the child and family using the equipment. Explain how the service or equipment will prevent more costly medical needs, and seek support from other health care providers who can help support and document the need. In your role as advocate, take steps to influence decision-makers.

Use a friendly style, be persistent, and follow the prior approval system when you know it is required. Be prepared to negotiate, and try to clarify who will pay for what services and resources. Private plans and public programs may deny an application for benefits, so be prepared to try and change decisions in favor of the child and family. Seek clarification, ask for the explanation in writing, and always be ready to resubmit. If you use the appeals process, ask for their appeals policy and for assistance in filing an appeal.

Education, training, and support must be provided to families, especially when the decisions are complicated and technical. The financing system should pay for services that allow families to determine priorities for care and function effectively as primary decision-makers. Having contact with other families of children with disabilities or other chronic conditions can offer much needed support. These families should be encouraged to support each other, share concrete ideas, and speak up for reform. A unified parent and professional voice about the serious inadequacies in the present health care financing system can influence the reforms. Families must be prepared to check benefits thoroughly when negotiating new insurance or changing employment.

It is also very important that parents consider the potential impact of the child's situation on their work and finances and find sources of financial support. They may need assistance in finding child care services and arranging schedules so that they do not need to miss work for extended periods or quit their jobs. Financing from multiple sources needs to be coordinated to increase efficiency, prevent duplication, and ensure that the child and family receive maximum access to services and resources. Always ask for specific cost of supplies, equipment, or services, and regularly assess the effectiveness of services to take advantage of changing technology and new therapies.

IDEAL SYSTEM

In 1990 a regional task force was established in New England to assess existing health care financing systems for children with disabilities or other chronic conditions and examine new proposals for reform. After a year-long study, the task force defined 14 criteria for consideration and grouped them under five main headings: Access, Benefits, Quality, Family Participation, and Cost Containment. In a publication titled *Ensuring Access* (New England SERVE, 1991), each criteria is defined, followed by a list of indicators in a question format. This document is intended for use in:

- assessing state and federal financing proposals
- education regarding family-centered financing system components
- evaluating health financing systems

Access

The first criterion under Access is *universal coverage*. This must include access to health care that is adequate and affordable and includes both primary and specialty care. The statement "access to health care is maintained regardless of changes in child's age, health status, family income, employment status, geographic location, or change in health insurance" (New England SERVE, 1991, p. 5) provides a standard for universal coverage programs.

The second criterion, *provider and service availability*, means affordable and timely access to appropriate specialists, especially for those in under-served areas. Mandates and incentives must be in place for acceptance of public and third-party payor reimbursement.

The third criterion specifies *consumer choice* of providers and facilities. This is especially critical because of the need for specialized services and the maintenance of relationships that contribute to continuity of care.

The fourth criterion is *family coverage*. This should include children with disabilities or other chronic conditions and provide a financing system for the family as a unit. All children within the family are included in both routine and specialized services regardless of pre-existing conditions and family structure.

Benefits

Criteria under Benefits include prevention, comprehensive benefits, community-based care, and coordinated care. *Prevention services* such as screening and family education are included in the financing system. The family has access to preventive services such as immunization, health promotion services such as parenting skills, and injury prevention services such as auto restraints and safety locks through the financing system.

Comprehensive benefits are provided through a full range of health and health-related services, including:

- adequate primary and specialty medical and surgical services
- specialized nursing and support services
- mental health services
- assistive technologies
- nutritional counseling and services
- specialized dietary products
- home health care
- hospice
- care coordination
- long-term occupational and physical therapy
- long-term speech, language, and hearing services
- adaptive equipment
- medications (New England SERVE, 1991, p. 12)

Families should also be able to access support and specialized services such as respite care and housing adaptation.

Services are provided in *community-based* settings as close to home as possible toward the goal of community integration. Community-based providers are encouraged to obtain the appropriate training to serve families of children with disabilities or chronic conditions. Financing is available for services such as nursing, physical therapy, occupational therapy, and speech therapy, both in the home and in other settings such as schools, day care centers, and outpatient facilities.

Care coordination occurs with communication among multiple providers and cooperation in planning for the needs of children with chronic health conditions. Care for children is paid for by various financing methods.

Quality, Family Participation, and Cost Containment

Quality assurance, the indicator under the criterion Quality, occurs when mechanisms are built into the system that maximize best practices and eliminate utilization problems.

The criterion Family Participation includes indicators that reflect the family role in *decision making* and *resource allocation*. The family is recognized and supported as the primary caregiver and decision-maker, especially in developing the plan of care.

Cost Containment, the fifth criterion, includes the provision of *flexible benefits* that are *coordinated* and the concept of *administrative efficiency*. The financing system should pay for services that are efficient, effective, and coordinated and that avoid duplication.

THE ECONOMICS OF PREVENTION

The health care financing system in the United States has evolved with a bias toward financing acute illnesses despite the demonstrated effectiveness of preventive services. Although the beneficial effects of prevention are well documented, costs are unclear as the impact of prevention on health has preceded determining the economic impact.

> Understanding how financial resources are, and should be, used in preventive health care involves consideration of one of three models: investment, insurance or consumption. In the investment model of prevention, today's cost is weighed against the financial consequences of tomorrow's event. The insurance model stipulates that spending in the present will avoid a potential adverse outcome in the future. The consumption model considers prevention as an expenditure providing benefits today (for example, a sense of well-being from physical activity). Considering prevention as a good to be consumed today places the emphasis on active prevention; individuals spending the time, energy and money to change behavior, with the possibility of an immediate payoff (Simmons, 1993, p. 3).

Given the importance of prevention in maintaining the health of children with disabilities or other chronic conditions, it is critical for pediatric rehabilitation nurses to articulate the needs of this group to ensure the delivery of effective preventive health care. In the report *Nursing's Agenda for Health Care Reform* (ANA, 1991), a broad-based strategy for restructuring the health care system was outlined, and this report can be incorporated into a program specific to the needs of these children and their families. "The report calls for a federally defined standard package of essential health care services, including preventive services. Also emphasized is the development of provider-client relationships,

directed at prevention activities, that will ultimately improve health outcomes in a cost-effective manner" (Simmons, 1993, p. 7). How specifically can the pediatric rehabilitation nurse address these issues for children and families? The following are some specific suggestions:

Begin by influencing the consumer to raise awareness of prevention and its value.

Provide testimony to governmental bodies and develop position statements on prevention issues.

Lobby for equitable reimbursement for preventive health care.

Participate on a team that collects or analyzes cost-effectiveness data.

REFORM STRATEGIES AND FUTURE NEEDS

In the past few years there has been tremendous activity in the area of health care reform, but it has not resulted in major restructuring or change. Two areas that did receive attention dealt with reform of the welfare system and portability of insurance, and both have a major impact on families with a child with a disability or other chronic condition.

Under the new welfare reform law, states receive a "capped" block grant, which is the equivalent of prior years' payments for AFDC benefits, Aid to Families with Dependent Children (AFDC) administration, Emergency Assistance, and JOBS (the work and training program for welfare recipients). "Additional, small sums are appropriated for several purposes, including supplemental grants to states that have high rates of population growth and that have low amounts of federal welfare spending per poor person; bonuses to 'high performing' states; bonuses to states that demonstrate a net decrease in out-of-wedlock births; and loans at market interest rates to states" (Children's Defense Fund, 1996, p. 1). Provisions of the welfare bill agreed to by the U.S. House and Senate include:

1. AFDC is replaced with block grants to states, which would run their own programs and set eligibility requirements and benefit levels
2. Restrictions on children's eligibility for SSI disability benefits are tightened
3. Students are eligible for school lunch programs as long as they are eligible for free public education.

Legislation was passed guaranteeing the right of an individual to change employers without losing coverage, protecting the currently insured and restricting limitations due to pre-existing conditions. The portability provisions in the bill include group insurance portability, availability of individual insurance as well as group coverage, required enrollment, prohibitions of exclusions based on health, and guaranteed renewability. The bill also introduced the concept of a program of tax-deferred medical savings accounts that allow individuals to shelter income to pay routine medical bills.

As the discussions about health care reform continue, pediatric rehabilitation nurses must continue to be knowledgeable, involved participants at all levels and in a variety of settings. As advocates for quality care and access, nurses must provide input on definition and scope of services and on implementation strategies for families and children with disabilities or other chronic conditions.

Some areas that have been considered and will continue to be explored are managed competition and a single-payor system. General recommendations for reform include:

- mandatory health care coverage for all
- wide diversity of insurers in a competitive market
- stronger consumer incentives to shop for care
- sharing of financial risk associated with decisions regarding utilization
- risk-adjustment process focusing on providing quality services at a low premium (McCarthy & Minnis, 1994)

The challenge is to provide high-quality care through a more equitable and efficient process of health care delivery and financing.

SUMMARY

"Public and private programs for financing care for children with chronic conditions are complex and ever changing. They are marked by inadequacies and inequalities among counties within a state and among states" (O'Grady, 1992, p. 58). Providers must be knowledgeable about how the family is paying for care and about referral options. Assistance in purchasing appropriate insurance or gaining access to public programs requires persistence but is crucial to implementing the plan of care and meeting the child's needs.

The process of finding funding for the health care of a child with a disability or other chronic illness is complicated and at times very frustrating for the family. The pediatric rehabilitation nurse must help the family clearly articulate what is needed, fully investigate all possible benefits through private coverage plans and public programs, enlist allies when support is needed, and finally, by sheer perseverance, find the necessary financing for the needs of the child.

REFERENCES

American Nurses Association (1991). *Nursing's Agenda for Health Care Reform: Executive Summary.* Kansas City, MO.

Bergman, A. (1994). Funding for assistive technologies. *Rehabilitation Management,* June/July, 26–31.

Children's Defense Fund. (1996). *Summary of new welfare law* [On-line]. Available: tmn.com/cdf/welfarelaw.html

Cole, N. (1996) Facing the realities of managed care and HMOs. *Spinal Cord Injury Update,* UW Rehabilitation Medicine [On-line]. Available: weber.u.washington.edu/rehab/sci/6–1/hmo.html

Hoyt, D. (1995). What families need to know about managed care. *Iowa Child Health Specialty Clinics Report,* 10(1), 1–2.

Kaufman, J. (1991a). An overview of public sector financing for pediatric home care, part I. *Pediatric Nursing,* 17(3), 280–282.

Kaufman, J. (1991b). An overview of public sector financing for pediatric home care, part II. *Pediatric Nursing,* 17(4), 380–381.

McCarthy, T., & Minnis, J. (1994). The health care system in the U.S. In Hoffmeyer, U., & McCarthy, T. (Eds.). *Financing health care,* Vol. 2, pp. 1147–1293. Boston: Kluwer Academic Publishers.

New England SERVE. (1991). *Ensuring access: family-centered health care financing systems for children with special health care needs.* Boston: New England SERVE.

O'Day, B., & Corcoran, P. (1994). Assistive technology: problems and policy alternatives. *Archives of Physical Medicine and Rehabilitation,* 75(10), 1165–1169.

O'Grady, R. (1992). Financing health care for children with chronic conditions. In Jackson, P., & Versey, J. (Eds.). *Primary care of the child with a chronic condition,* pp. 45–60. St. Louis: CV Mosby.

Perrin, J., & Stein, R. (1991). Reinterpreting disability: changes in SSI for children. *Pediatrics,* 88(5), 1047–1051.

Simmons, S. (1993). The economics of prevention. In American Nurses Association (Ed.). *Prevention across the life span: healthy people for the 21st century* (Chap. 1). Washington, DC: ANA Council of Community Health Nursing, American Nurses Publishing.

Votroubek, W. (1990). Financing pediatric home care. In McCoy, P., & Votroubek, W. (Eds.). *Pediatric home care* (Chap. 3). Rockville, MD: Aspen.

ADDITIONAL RESOURCES

Children's Defense Fund. (1995). *The state of America's children yearbook*. Washington, DC: Children's Defense Fund.

Fox, H., Wicks, L., & Newacheck, P. (1993). State Medicaid health maintenance organization policies and special needs children. *Health Care Financing Review*, 15(1), 25–37.

National Leadership Coalition for Health Care Reform. (1993). *Excellent health care for all Americans at a reasonable cost*. Washington, DC: National Leadership Coalition.

Neff, J., & Anderson, G. (1995). *Protecting children with chronic illness in a competitive marketplace*. *JAMA*, 274(23), 1866–1869.

Newacheck, P., & McManus, M. (1988). Financing health care for disabled children. *Pediatrics*, 81(3), 385–394.

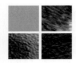

Chapter 6

Ethical, Legal, and Moral Issues in Pediatric Rehabilitation

Teresa A. Savage and *Deb Ryan Michalak*

FAMILY-CENTERED APPROACH IN ETHICAL DECISION MAKING

Whether a child is in a hospital, rehabilitation facility, community setting, nursing home, or home, the parents have the moral and legal responsibility for all decision making for their child. In instances in which the parents no longer have legal custody, the parents are often informed of, if not included, in the major health care decisions for their child. The goals for the child's care and treatment are planned with the family. The family's resources and coping ability are primary considerations in identifying the rehabilitation setting, the goals of rehabilitation, and the family's ability to meet the child's needs. Difficult and complex questions surround the care and treatment of a child in rehabilitation. Should life-sustaining treatment be given if needed, or should only comfort care be given? If the child survives severe trauma and will have profound disabilities and the parents do not want the child to live, are their wishes to withhold or withdraw treatment respected? Discussion of ethical decision making by the parents for their child is addressed later in this chapter.

In most cases, the goal is to get the child home. Some children require such intense nursing care that their families cannot provide that care at home or do not have the resources to have nursing care in the home. In balancing the needs of the child with the needs of the family, decisions are made regarding the best location for the child to live. Many factors enter into the decision—the needs of the child, the resources of the family (both emotional and financial), the values and culture of the community in which they live, and the needs of the child's parents and siblings. Ethics plays a huge part in deciding whether or not to bring the child home. The values of the family need to be clarified. The parents must weigh the needs of the child with their ability to provide what the child needs. Nurses and other professionals can assist the family in making decisions. Parents need accurate information and the health care team's prognostications, and they need to be able to discuss their feelings in a non-judgmental atmosphere. Parents should participate in the acquisition of information regarding community services for their child and should investigate those services. Weekend passes permitting the child to be at home for short periods on a trial basis allows the parents to try out care methods. Even if parents do manage at home for a period of time, the child's needs or the family's situation may change so that out-of-home placement once again is considered.

There is an assumption that the best place for a child is at home with parents, yet not all families can manage the care of a child with disabilities. The attitude of the health care team should be one of facilitation and support of the decision that the parents deem best for the child and family. Feelings of parents may vacillate between hopelessness and joy. Chronic sorrow, as first described by Olshansky (1962), can be misinterpreted by the health care team as depression or detachment. The health care team may question the parents' ability to care for the child at home. Perceived pressures from the parents' community or cultural background can make the parents feel responsible for their child's predicament and may obscure an honest appraisal of their caregiving abilities. The cause of the child's condition, whether accidental, congenital, or unknown, may leave parents with feelings of guilt that they could have or should have prevented the child's problem. Callahan (1988, p. 326) acknowledges a "minimal decency" expectation that parents will care for their ill children, but unending, self-sacrificing care should not be expected. Society does not at present have supports for those caregivers, who primarily are women. The burden of caregiving can outweigh the moral obligation for families to provide care at home. Callahan's argument is based on ethical principles of autonomy and nonmaleficence. He uses principles to support his argument, but also includes consideration of context, relationships, and self-sacrifice. Those factors are elements in the ethic of care, a perspective of ethical decision making described by Gilligan (1982). Ethical principles and the ethic of care are discussed further later in the chapter.

Ethical Principles

There are four primary ethical principles that guide moral behavior: autonomy, beneficence, justice, and nonmaleficence. Other principles, such as fidelity, veracity, and truth-telling, have their foundation in one or more of the primary ethical principles.

Autonomy

Autonomy is having the freedom to make choices. Underlying this principle is a respect for persons that must be present for one truly to be autonomous. There are moral and legal aspects of autonomy.

Autonomy reflects the person's will to choose a particular course of action. Some philosophers have proposed that a person's will is guided by reason; others suggest that will is guided by desires and emotions. For many people, reason, desires, and emotions enter into their decisions. What makes the decision autonomous, however, is the freedom that person has in making a choice. Coercion, whether positive, in terms of incentives, or negative, in terms of punishment, invalidates autonomy. In the health care arena, coercion takes the form of paternalism.

Paternalism occurs when others believe they know what is best for the patient. In the past, patients were not always told their diagnosis in the paternalistic belief that they did not need to know and that it could be upsetting and thereby counterproductive to their recovery. In this situation the patient lacks critical information and is unable to make an autonomous decision.

Another threat to autonomy is the determination of competence. The concept of competence has a moral and a legal side. The moral side is again embedded in paternalism. It is appropriate, both morally and legally, to be paternalistic in terms of children. Because children usually lack the wisdom and experience to make certain decisions, parents are expected to make decisions for them that are in the child's best interests. This standard for decision making is the best interests standard. If a patient is unconscious, a surrogate is expected to make decisions that the patient would make if able to communicate. This standard is referred to as the substituted judgment standard. Competence, defined as the capacity to make a specific decision at a specific point in time (Buchanan & Brock, 1990, pp. 18–19), is determined both physiologically, psychologically, and legally. Most institutions have policies for the determination of competency for the purposes of giving informed consent. States have laws and standards that specify how competence is determined for individuals with cognitive deficits living in the community.

The law recognizes a person as being autonomous to make decisions when they have reached a certain age, usually 18 years, and have not been declared incompetent to make decisions about person or property. Children are presumed to be incompetent to give informed consent and are not autonomous in decision making unless they have been declared mature minors. A minor child, under the age of 18 years in most states, cannot give consent for health care with certain exceptions defined in state laws. Such exceptions usually pertain to obtaining contraceptives, counseling and treatment for substance abuse, or treatment for psychiatric conditions. In all other conditions, a parent or legal guardian has the authority to give or refuse consent for health care decisions. If the parents' decision does not seem to be in the best interests of the child, however, the health care team may challenge the decision. For example, a child with hemorrhagic shock from trauma needs a blood transfusion, and the parents, who are Jehovah's Witnesses, refuse to consent to the blood transfusion. Even though it is clear that the child will die without the transfusion, the parents' religious beliefs prohibit the acceptance of a blood transfusion. The health care team faces a conflict between respecting the parents' religious tradition and preserving the life of the child. In most instances, the health care team, usually the attending physician, will take medical custody for the purposes of consenting to the life-saving blood transfusion. The law supports these actions of the health care team in putting preservation of the child's life over respect for the parents' religious beliefs. In other cases, it is not clear cut as to what is in the best interests of the patient.

The autonomy of the child is exercised by the parents or legal guardian. Open, honest communication between health care providers and parents facilitates decision making for the child. Parental autonomy, however, is not absolute. As child advocates, if the health care team believes that the parents are not making decisions in the child's best interests, it may be necessary as a last resort to take medical custody of the child. Buchanan and Brock (1990) make a distinction that parental authority should not be abrogated if the parents' decision fails to maximize the child's well-being. Only in those instances in which the child would risk serious harm is custody sought. Occasionally when the state is involved, a guardian is appointed to advocate for the child's interests apart from the parents' interests. This route is sometimes used when parents disagree about what is in the child's best interests.

Beneficence

Beneficence means "to do good." Health care providers were probably motivated by beneficence when they chose health care as their profession. The challenge of beneficence is determining what is "good" in a specific situation. As with the child in the previous example who was hemorrhaging and whose parents refused to consent to a blood transfusion, giving blood was seen as a good by the health care team but not by the parents. Rehabilitation goals of restoring function, preventing further complications, and assisting the child and family to adapt reflect the ethical underpinning of beneficence.

Justice

The principle of justice is often seen in its broad context of macroallocation. Macroallo-cation is the allocation of resources at a systems level (e.g., funding of public health, hospitals, grants, or projects for the health of a community). Microallocation involves the decisions about an individual (e.g., decisions to admit to a hospital, the use of home health nursing, or the use of a specific technology such as a ventilator, parenteral nutrition, or motorized wheelchair). The fair distribution of the benefits and burdens of society is one definition of distributive justice. An example of distributive justice outside the health care arena is taxation. The tax burden is distributed among citizens according to tax law. In exchange for taxes, citizens receive the benefits of public services such as education, police and fire protection, libraries, and many other services on a local, state, and federal level. An example of distributive justice in health care is the allocation of organs for donation. The United Network for Organ Sharing (UNOS) has a system for ranking patient need and distributing available organs in a prioritized fashion. The appropriate use of resources is an issue of justice. Criteria for admission to intensive care or rehabilitation units reflect the institution's or the rehabilitation unit director's views of what is fair and just. With the increase in health care financing through managed care companies, the determination of eligibility for benefits under the specified coverage is an issue of justice. Decision making is limited by the options available under the patient's insurance plan. With children, however, the situation is again different than with competent adults. A competent, underinsured adult can decide to forgo a therapy, such as a coronary artery bypass graft procedure, that would deplete all of the person's financial resources. Treatment decisions with children are more complicated. A child may not be discharged from the hospital on a ventilator because the parents do not have insurance or are underinsured. Even a stellar insurance plan with a million dollar maximum can be depleted by a catastrophic illness or injury.

In the past, cost has not been a factor in ethical decision making at the bedside, except when competent adult patients entered it into their decision making. Decisions about treatment were to be made based on the best interests of the patient. To factor in the patient's ability to pay would be to risk discriminating against the poor. From 1987 to 1990, the state of Oregon developed a program in which treatment for certain conditions was prioritized and funded by public dollars.

Through a lengthy and elaborate process, a list of treatments and diagnoses was generated. All treatments and diagnoses above a certain number were funded; those that fell below were not funded. Immunizations for children were funded; intensive care for a pre-term infant weighing 500 g was not funded. The implementation of the program was challenged by the Bush administration, which wanted to ensure the program was in compliance with the newly passed federal law, the Americans With Disabilities Act. However, within the increase of managed care plans in many states, both public and private insurance plans are reducing the number of conditions covered and the cap on spending per condition.

The financial aspect of the justice issue in ethical decision making has received a great deal of attention. The question of whether or not a certain course of action is "right" or "fair" or "just" must still be addressed apart from the question of who will pay. Although it may be more expedient to look at only the options available to parents, instead of offering them options they cannot obtain, that may be a disservice to them. Changes in the law have occurred after parents wanted options seemingly not available to them, such as organ transplantation, school inclusion, or home care vs. institutional placement. In these instances, the parents have chosen what they believe is the right decision for their child.

Ethical Approaches Supporting Justice Decisions

Various ethical theories support justice decisions. As in the state of Oregon, to fund the more efficacious treatments (appendectomy vs. ICU for a 500-g pre-term infant) is a utilitarian approach. Utilitarianism supports the choice that would bring about the greatest amount of benefit to the greatest number of persons. In this approach, there is a minority who will not benefit from the utilitarian choice. Another ethical theory is deontology. In deontology, an act is judged as inherently good or bad apart from the consequences of the act. A deontologic approach might be one of denying funding for all abortions in the reasoning that abortion is terminating life and a deontologist may believe that it is always wrong to terminate another person's life. There would be no exceptions in instances of rape, incest, genetic abnormality, or to save the life of the mother.

The decision to allocate resources can be based on the evaluation of the consequences of a given course of action or on the act itself. Saving the life of an infant born early and weighing 500 g could be seen as a good act because preserving life is a good, but if the child is likely to be profoundly impaired, the consequences of the act of implementing life-sustaining treatment in intensive care may not be a good. This is a particularly difficult decision to make because the long-term outcomes of very-low-birth-weight infants are not completely clear. The ethical principle of justice focuses on the balance of benefits and burdens of an action or decision. The benefits and burden to the child, to the family, to the community, and to society at large are part of the justice issue.

Non-maleficence

The ethical principle of nonmaleficence is summed up in the Latin phrase, "primum non nocere," translated as "above all, do no harm." Health care providers have a duty to prevent harm from occurring in the course of a child's care. Again, as in the determination of what is good, there is also debate over what is harm. There are many short term harms in health care—brief pain or discomfort associated with an injection of an antibiotic or pain associated with a surgical procedure. In weighing the benefit of the antibiotic or the surgical procedure against the burden of the fleeting pain of the injection or the post-operative pain and discomfort during recovery, one determines whether or not the benefit outweighs the burden. Other benefit–burden analyses are more difficult.

In pediatric rehabilitation, every treatment decision is analyzed regarding its relative benefit or burden to the patient. For example, a child with quadriplegic cerebral palsy has bilaterally dislocated hips. Surgery could correct the dislocations. The child is unable to sit unsupported and does not appear to be uncomfortable. To put the child through surgery might be more of a harm than a benefit if the surgery would not improve function or relieve a painful condition or could result in surgical complications.

The discussion about what is a harm gets more complicated when it is argued that a child's continued existence constitutes a harm to the child and family. Setting aside the interests of the family for a moment, the child's existence is examined. Harm should be viewed as unrelievable pain and suffering. It is impossible to know the pain and suffering another person is experiencing and whether or not the pain and suffering is unbearable. The interpretation of pain and suffering of a child is often enmeshed in the pain and suffering of the caregiver. Concern for the child's future in terms of the level of care the child will require and the increasing physical demands on the caregiver as the child grows into an adult enters into the decision-making process. For some children, rehabilitation restores their functioning and assists the child and family in adapting to whatever changes have occurred. For others, the illness or injury is so extensive that development is stunted at a very young level. Growth will occur, but the child will not develop beyond a very cognitively limited level. In those cases, the quality of life of these children is assumed to be poor. To maintain a level of wellness and function achieved after rehabilitation, a great deal of resources, such as nursing care, therapies, acute medical care, adaptive equipment, and daily personal attendance, are needed. If there is little hope for improvement in function, how much resources should be invested? Should maintenance therapy be given but life-sustaining therapies withheld? Since the child cannot tell the caregiver what is preferred, the parents are the ones who face these decisions.

To make decisions, the parents must be fully informed of the diagnoses, prognosis, and treatment and non-treatment options. Prognosis cannot always be made with certainty, and the uncertainty adds to the complexity of decision making.

ETHIC OF CARE

Kohlberg (1976) described the stages of moral development, in which a person uses increasingly sophisticated reasoning in making decisions. The higher stages of reasoning involve applying ethical principles to determine the right decision. Kohlberg's research had only male subjects, so it should not be generalized to both men and women. A student of Kohlberg's, Carol Gilligan (1982), investigated how women decided to have an abortion. She found that these women did not apply ethical principles in abstraction. They considered the context of the situation, and made decisions that would preserve their relationships and relieve burdens. The perspective that Gilligan described has been coined the "ethic of care" approach to decision making; Kohlberg's application of ethical principles is the "justice"

perspective. In resolving ethical problems, both perspectives are used.

Decision-Making Strategies

There are many ethical decision-making models in the nursing and ethics literature (Aroskar, 1980; Bunting & Webb, 1988; Curtin, 1978; Silva, 1990; Thompson & Thompson, 1985; Jonsen, Siegler, & Winslade, 1992). These models follow a linear, step-wise process of gathering data, sorting the options, evaluating consequences of the options, and arriving at a decision.

Nurses make ethical decisions in the judgments and actions they take in the course of providing nursing care. They quickly gather and analyze the data at hand and the options, make and implement their plan, and evaluate their actions.

Nurses are also involved in ethical decision making in patient care. They provide information to parents and help them clarify their values. Helping the parents identify resources, deal with their feelings, and find and use supports in their community are all ways in which nurses influence ethical decision making of parents.

Ethical problems in the clinical arena are often embedded in clinical, social, and interpersonal issues. Ethical decision-making models assist in sorting the questions and identifying the ethical aspects of the questions. The Savage Model for Facilitating Ethical Decision Making (Table 6–1) is one such ethical decision-making model, used to illustrate the decision-making process in the following case.

CASE STUDY

"Billy" is a 9-year-old with spina bifida who was burned in a fire in his home. His 4-year-old brother died in the fire. He has two living siblings—Joey, a 6-year-old brother with spina bifida and a 2-year-old sister. He had an older sister who also had spina bifida and died of complications. Both Billy and his 6-year-old brother have lived in several foster homes for most of their lives since being removed from their parents' home for neglect. The parents separated after that, and Billy's mother has been working toward getting the boys back. She was awarded custody 4 months earlier.

When the fire broke out, Billy's mother

Table 6–1 SAVAGE MODEL FOR FACILITATING ETHICAL DECISION MAKING

1. Gather facts of the case and understandings of those parties involved.
2. Identify the questions and goals.
3. Organize a meeting with key players—parents, physicians, nurses, social workers, therapists, and others who might assist in the decision making.
   a. Pose questions, clarify information, set goals.
   b. Explore options and their consequences and ethical ramifications.
   c. Make plan for future management of case.
4. Provide information, referrals, education, and emotional support to family.
5. Participate in implementation of decision, if appropriate.
6. Review the process, evaluate your role, and revise process as needed.

was not home. She said she had gone next door for a little while and returned home when she heard the sirens. Billy and Joey were taken to separate burn centers. The 4-year-old sibling was pronounced dead at the scene, and the 2-year-old sibling was unharmed. Joey was discharged after 2 weeks. Billy remained in the hospital for 8 weeks and was transferred to a rehabilitation facility. His mother wants to take him home after rehabilitation, but the child welfare agency has removed all the children from her custody. Billy was ambulatory without assistance prior to the fire but will not walk now. He does not want to go back with his mother, but he also does not want to be separated from his brother, who wants to go back to his mother. The child welfare agency is asking the rehabilitation team to advise them on Billy's needs and their assessment of the mother's ability to meet his needs.

Application of the Savage Model for Facilitating Ethical Decision Making

1. Gather facts of the case and understandings of those parties involved.
What were the circumstances resulting in the children being removed from the parents initially? What happened the evening of the fire? What was Billy's functional level prior to the fire?
Prior to the fire, Billy walked and ran without assistance but needed help with

urinary catheterization. At this point, he states he cannot walk and refuses to try. The mother visits regularly and, in discussion with the social worker, said that her two boys were removed from the home when their older sister died from sepsis after a wound on her foot became infected and her mother did not give her antibiotics as prescribed. The child welfare agency investigated and believed that the boys were not being catheterized. The mother admitted that she should have given her daughter the antibiotics and should have been catheterizing the boys, but she was young and did not know any better. She says she loves her children and wants them all together. She still sees her ex-husband and hopes for a reconciliation, although he blames her for their eldest child's death. Regarding the fire, she went next door to return something she had borrowed from her neighbors and stayed a while to talk. The children had gone to bed. When she heard sirens, she rushed home. The firefighters were there and there was nothing she could do by that time. Since then her neighbors have taken her in and she has received gifts of clothing and toys for the children.

2. Identify the questions and goals.
What does the child welfare agency say about what happened and the possibility of the mother getting custody of the children? What is the father's position regarding custody of the children? The goal is for the boys to be discharged to a safe environment where they will receive appropriate care. Another goal is for the oldest boy to return to his pre-fire functional level.

The Ethical Question: What Is in the Best Interests of the Children—Being Discharged to Their Mother or Not?

The mother was reported to the child welfare agency by her daughter's treating physician, who had prescribed the antibiotics and hospitalized the daughter when she returned to the clinic in a septic state. The child welfare agency investigated and determined that the boys were not receiving appropriate care. They were not being catheterized regularly although the mother had been taught and supplies were being delivered to the home. The agency made a contract with the mother that specified what she would need to do to regain custody of her two children. When she met those criteria, her boys were returned to her under agency supervision. The agency now questions the wisdom of that decision, and has stated to the mother that since a death resulted from her negligence, they will seek a court order to sever parental rights. The father has made phone contact with the rehabilitation facility but has not visited and has not sought custody. He does not provide any financial assistance to the family.

3. *Organize the meeting with key players—parents, physicians, nurses, social workers, therapists, and others who might assist in the decision making.*

A meeting was organized by the primary nurse and attended by the attending physician, the primary nurse, the physical therapist, the social worker, the child welfare worker, the ethics consultant, the clinical nurse specialist from the spina bifida clinic who observed the boys prior to the fire, and the school nurse from Billy's school. Both parents were invited; the mother arrived 30 minutes after the meeting began. The father did not attend or call.

a. Pose questions, clarify information, and set goals.

Are the parents able to meet the children's needs? (Each person shares their assessment of the boys, what their needs are at this time, and what they project their needs will be in the future.) It was learned that Billy had been walking and even running without any adaptive devices prior to the fire. He was taught clean intermittent catheterization and performed it under supervision both at home and at school. The child welfare worker related that the foster home the boy had been in prior to returning to their mother was no longer available, and it would likely take several weeks to find another home for special needs children. The child welfare worker stated that the agency would not approve of the children returning to the mother's custody, and the father will not accept custody. No other relative can be located to accept the children, so continued hospitalization until a foster home can be found is their recommendation. The mother stated her desire to get her children back and said that God had punished her for being out of the house the night of the fire by taking one of her children. She does not think she should be punished any further by having the rest of her children taken from her. The attending physician stated that

the decision about where the children go is not intended to punish her but to do what is in the children's best interests. They must be in a home where they can receive safe and appropriate care and supervision. If the children are not returned to her at this time, that does not preclude her ever regaining custody. The mother wept.

Goals:

- Get Billy back to pre-fire functional level.
- Promote independence in self-care activities.
- Keep the boys together.
- Find appropriate foster home for the boys.
- Continue counseling to help the boys cope with these events.
- Recommend continued counseling and other assistance for the mother in her quest for reuniting the family.
- Allow supervised visits by the mother.

b. Explore options and consequences of the options.

Option 1. The boys are discharged to their mother.

Consequences: With continued supervision and support, the boys may thrive, although they have been removed from the mother's care for neglect and the deaths of two siblings have been attributed to their mother's neglect. The team believes the risk to the children is greater than the benefit of reuniting the family. Although Joey wants to return to his mother, Billy does not, and the mother has not demonstrated that she will provide the needed care or exercise the best judgment for the children's welfare. Billy told the primary nurse that he loves his mother, but that she did not take care of them and frequently left them home alone.

Option 2: The boys are discharged to the same foster home.

Consequences: With careful screening, education, and supervision, the boys should receive appropriate care. Through continued work with their mother, the family may eventually be reunited. The boys will be together. It may take weeks before one home for both boys is found.

Option 3: The boys are discharged to separate foster homes.

Consequences: Although their physical care needs would be met, both boys expressed fear of being separated. The rehabilitation team prefers keeping the boys in their facility until one home is found for both of them, but the utilization review department will not approve of continued hospitalization because their therapies can continue on an outpatient basis.

Option 4: Discharge the boys to a residential facility or nursing home.

Consequence: This option was not deemed the most appropriate and least restrictive environment for the boys. It would allow the boys to stay together.

Option 5: Keep the boys in the rehabilitation facility until one foster home for both of them is found.

Consequence: The utilization review department indicates that both boys have exhausted their inpatient coverage. Their rehabilitation can continue on an outpatient basis. There is a waiting list for admission into the facility.

The team continued to discuss the merits and drawbacks of each option. The ethics consultant asked questions to elicit their thoughts on what option would be in the children's best interests. On the spectrum from "ethically prohibited" to "ethically obligated," all the options fell between, in the "ethically permissible" category, although the child welfare worker believed the option of discharging the children to their mother was "ethically prohibited."*

   c. Make plan for future management of care.
   The child welfare worker will attempt to locate one foster home for both children. The social worker will assist in finding a family. Since the boys are ready for discharge, the child welfare worker will place them in separate homes until one home is found. The team stated their strong preference that the boys be kept together.
   The child welfare worker will arrange for regular visits between the mother and children and will discuss the feasibility of another contract toward the mother regaining custody, although the chances seem slim at this time.

4. *Provide support to family in terms of information, referrals, and education. Provide emotional support through sensitivity to and respect for their feelings.*

Several members of the rehabilitation team will work with the foster parents so they can learn how to care for the children and negotiate the health care system. They will also work with the mother so she may stay abreast of their care needs. Referrals were made to community providers (therapists, nurses, educators), and they were able to see Billy before his discharge.

5. *Participate in implementation of decision, if appropriate.*
   The children will be discharged when the foster parents have demonstrated their understanding of the care the children need and can perform procedures such as clean intermittent catheterization.

6. *Review the process, evaluate your role, and revise process as needed.*
   At the regular team meetings, the team will review the process of facilitating the decision regarding what is in the children's best interests. The ethics consultant offers a written analysis for the team to review. The decision-maker in this case was the child welfare worker, who depended primarily on the information and recommendations of the rehabilitation team. The child welfare worker communicated with her supervisor, who had the legal authority to make health care decisions for Billy.

Each team member must review their own role in this case and think about what they would do differently, if anything. The people at the conference may not have reached a consensus about what was in the children's best interests, but the process allowed for positions to be heard and options to be explored. Although the mother no longer had custody of her children, she was informed, asked for her input, and could interact with the team members.

Additionally, each team member can work through their professional organizations to effect a change that would impact cases like Billy and Joey's. Such efforts might include community education about fire prevention, increased need for specialized foster care, need for greater and longer supervision of children released to parental custody, need for preconception education about the multifactorial etiology of spina bifida, and the need for parenting classes and support groups for parents of children with chronic illness or disability.

---

*Ethically prohibited ←—Ethically permissible—→ Ethically obligatory
Option 1 Options 2, 3, 4, 5

ETHICS COMMITTEE

In 1982 fewer than 2% of hospitals had an ethics committee (Ross, 1986). Ethics committees had been recommended in the 1976 New Jersey Supreme Court opinion of the Karen Ann Quinlan case. Quinlan was a young woman who had experienced apnea and cardiac arrest for unknown reasons and was resuscitated. She remained in a persistent vegetative state and her parents sought permission to disconnect her ventilator. In the New Jersey Supreme Court opinion, Judge Karen Teel granted the parents permission to have the ventilator disconnected, but also urged hospitals to form prognosis committees as a measure to keep cases like Quinlan's out of the courts. Prognosis committees would be composed of physicians who would render their opinions on the patient's prognosis (Ross, 1986).

By the end of 1983, ethics committees had flourished in response to the case known as Baby Doe. Baby Doe was an infant with Down syndrome who died when his parents decided to forgo life-sustaining surgery to repair a tracheoesophageal fistula. The Reagan administration invoked the Baby Doe regulations that threatened the loss of federal funding to any facility that discriminated against the handicapped. The regulations were struck down as being imposed arbitrarily and capriciously. The federal government instructed states to amend their child abuse and neglect acts to ensure that infants receive appropriate medical treatment. The courts encouraged the proliferation of ethics committees in hopes that they would keep cases out of the courts. By the end of 1983, more than one half of U.S. hospitals had ethics committees.

Ethics committees have three purposes: to educate, to develop policy, and to review and deliberate cases. The manner in which cases are referred to the ethics committee varies from institution to institution, as does their composition. The purpose of committee deliberations is to provide ethical reflection on the options in a given situation. The ethical analysis from the committee's deliberations are shared with the health care team in the form of a formal consultation note on the chart or may be communicated to the attending physician verbally. There are pros and cons to ethics committees, as outlined in Table 6–2.

As a member of an ethics committee, the nurse can contribute as a clinician, as a manager, and as a patient advocate. As a *clinician*, the nurse can ask probing questions that may not occur to a non-clinician member. Nurses often have insight into family dynamics because they usually have spent a greater amount of time with the patient and family than other health care professionals. Although the nurse's interpretation of the family dynamics does not take the place of working with the family directly, their positions and values are represented during ethical deliberation by the committee.

As a *manager*, the nurse understands the intricacies of the implementation of various options being deliberated. Because not all nursing staff members can attend the ethics committee meeting, the nurse on the committee can serve as a liaison for sharing pertinent information from the committee's deliberations and recommendations.

As a *patient advocate*, the nurse directly involved with the patient may be invited as an ad hoc member to participate in committee deliberations or may be asked to share his or her perspective in the data-gathering phase of the deliberation process. The nurse, as do all others involved with the patient, attempts to decide what is in the patient's best interests. Particularly in pediatrics, it is difficult to know what is in the patient's best interests when the patient is either unable to commu-

Table 6–2 ETHICS COMMITTEE PROS AND CONS

Pros	Cons
Multidisciplinary perspectives	"Groupthink" (dominant members' opinions prevail)
Forum for communication	Intrusive in physician-patient relationship
Anticipatory discussion of potential conflicts	Potential for bureaucratic inefficiency
Clinical focus	Rubberstamp of physician's opinion
Objective, detached deliberation	Potential for disenfranchising interested parties not
Policy development	appointed to the committee
Promotion of awareness of ethical issues	

nicate or is considered too immature cognitively or emotionally to participate in decisions. If the nurse believes that the best interests of the patient are not being served by the recommended course of action, then there is an obligation to present that point of view. In a family-centered approach, the nurse acts as an advocate for the family unit, but there are situations where the nurse may see a conflict between the family's interests and patient's interests. In those instances, the nurse should examine his or her own personal feelings about the situation and share the biases uncovered from this introspection. The committee benefits from the nurse's point of view and rationale.

For example, a 10-year-old child named Michael survived multiple gunshot wounds and has been in a rehabilitation center for 3 months. Bullets severed his spinal cord and damaged both kidneys, necessitating dialysis. The mother has not visited during the hospitalization despite saying many times that she would be in "tomorrow," neither has she followed through on arrangements for post-discharge care. The utilization review department requires medical certification for continued rehabilitation treatment and is pressuring the attending physician to discharge the patient. The mother, when reached by telephone by the nurse, admitted that she has a substance abuse problem. She has three other children who live with her mother, who has visited Michael but does not believe that she can take care of him in her home. The nurse appreciates the enormous responsibilities that the mother now faces, but has concerns that Michael's needs may go unmet in this family. The mother refuses to permit Michael to go to a foster home or residential facility. The nurse, as an advocate for the patient's needs over the mother's needs, refers Michael's case to the ethics committee.

Nurses can benefit from the presence of an accessible ethics committee. Because of the prolonged contact with patients, nurses learn of conflict or disagreement with the plan of care. Nurses may not agree that a particular course of action is in the child's best interests. If the usual methods for resolving the issue do not succeed, the ethics committee is a resource for the nurse. The Joint Commission on Accreditation for Healthcare Organization (JCAHO, 1995) mandated that there be a mechanism for nurses in resolving ethical issues. Ethics committees are one way for hospitals to meet that mandate.

The nurse's role on the ethics committee, like that of other committee members, is to participate in educational activities, develop policies, and participate in case deliberation. Education of fellow committee members on pediatric rehabilitation philosophy is especially important. Nurses are the primary persons on the health care team to educate families and assess a family's abilities to manage a situation. These experiences are valuable in case deliberation.

Nurses also are the primary persons who recognize the need for policies to address certain clinical issues. In the past, nurses would be given verbal orders to withhold resuscitation, yet without a written order, would feel compelled to resuscitate if the patient arrested. Nurses began to insist that policies regarding resuscitation be written and followed so the plan of care would be clearly delineated for the entire health care team.

ETHICAL, LEGAL, AND MORAL ISSUES IN PRACTICE

Severely Ill Newborns

Infants experiencing complications at birth, such as prematurity, meconium aspiration, or congenital defects, pose ethical problems in the delivery room. In most instances, the infant is resuscitated and transferred to a neonatal intensive care unit (NICU). The myriad of decisions made during the neonatal period are not discussed in this chapter; what is relevant is that many children who experience problems as newborns develop chronic illness or disabilities. At the point of discharge, the diagnosis is usually known; a chromosomal anomaly such as trisomy 18, post-birth asphyxia, post-meningitis, prematurity, or multiple congenital anomalies sometimes warrant further hospitalization, but not in an intensive care nursery. NICU graduates requiring habilitation may also need sophisticated health care. Pre-term infants who need supplemental oxygen, infants with neurologically depressed sucking abilities, infants who had meningitis, or infants with multiple interventions such as tracheostomy, gastrostomy, ileostomy, and ventriculoperitoneal shunt might be transferred to a unit or facility for stabilization and transition to home, foster home, or residential facility.

Diagnosis and Prognosis

Although the child has survived trauma or multi-system physiologic problems, one cannot always predict the extent of impairment a child will experience or the developmental level a child may reach. In some cases, however, it is most unlikely that the child will recover or that development will be unaffected. Those cases include certain chromosomal abnormalities, extensive structural defects of the brain such as hydranencephaly or holoprosencephaly, and insults to the brain such as bleeding that extends into the parenchyma or profound asphyxia at birth.

Once a diagnosis and prognosis has been made, the parents are counseled regarding the projected future needs of the child. Drotar and colleagues (1975) described the stages some parents pass through when learning of their child's problems. Upon receiving the disturbing news, parents may work through periods of shock and disbelief, denial, anger, and bargaining. Some parents eventually reach acceptance, whereas others may never fully accept their child's diagnosis and prognosis. Olshansky (1962) described a "chronic sorrow" that parents may experience. The grief that the parents felt on learning the bad news is once again acutely felt when triggered by an event, such as failure to reach a developmental milestone. Chronic sorrow can also be triggered by events such as sending birth announcements, celebrating the child's first birthday, or when the child enters kindergarten but is unable to walk independently.

Decisions that are made during this early period in the child's life may reflect the parents' optimistic desire that the child will surpass expectations and function at a much higher level than anticipated. Aggressive treatment of conditions, a search for a cure, and a rejection of any actions that signify acceptance of the diagnosis and prognosis characterize their behaviors. During this time, the parents may switch physicians, try a new medical center or find a new interdisciplinary team, or resort to unorthodox treatments. Other families react to the diagnosis with sadness but are able to accept the changed child and incorporate the child back into the family.

Collaborative Decision Making

Thorne and Robinson (1989) identified phases in the relationship between patients and health care providers. Blindly trusting that the health care provider can find the answers to their problems, patients (and in this case, parents) have a "naive trust." At some point in the relationship, the health care providers

"fall from grace," and the parents are disenchanted. Over time, the parents develop a "guarded alliance" with their child's health care provider in which they learn how to work with the health care provider and may even move to a collaborative partnership with the health care provider.

For young children with disabilities, early intervention services are available. Therapies to inhibit primitive reflexes and normalize tone, sensory stimulation, oral-motor facilitation to improve oral feedings, and vestibular stimulation can be provided as appropriate. Parents work with nurses and therapists to learn to read their child's cues. Parents also work toward adapting to the special needs of their child. This work includes integrating the child into the family, coping with the loss of the "perfect" baby, and learning to negotiate health care and educational systems to secure services.

Part of the work of parenting is to decide what interventions are in the child's best interests. Parents have voiced concerns about the suffering they perceive their child could be experiencing, especially those children with respiratory difficulties, gastroesophageal reflux, seizures, or spasticity. Procedures such as tracheostomy, gastrostomy, tendon release, or multi-drug medication regimens seem ordinary to pediatric rehabilitation professionals but may be seen as extraordinary by some parents. In an acute care setting, these interventions are proposed almost reflexively when a "fixable" problem is present. The long-term impact of the intervention, however, needs to be examined in more depth.

Decision Making in Acute Care Setting vs. Long-Term Setting

Children are admitted to an acute care setting after a trauma or life-threatening illness for a level of health care they cannot receive at home or in other health care facilities. The assumption is that all available technology will be used to save the child's life. Tertiary care medical centers, which have the most sophisticated, state-of-the-art medical and nursing care, exist to reduce morbidity and mortality. They usually are affiliated with universities and have an additional mission to advance knowledge. When a child presents with a medically remediable problem, the inclination is to provide the intervention to remedy the problem. For example, the problem may be that a child with traumatic brain injury is experiencing respiratory distress. Relieving the respiratory distress through tracheostomy and mechanical ventilation can be achieved in an efficient, matter-of-fact manner at an acute care facility. The functional level of the child will not be improved by the respiratory rescue, although it may prevent further damage from hypoxia should the child survive without transfer to an acute care facility.

The dilemma arises when the child is transferred to a rehabilitation or chronic care facility but the parent, guardian, or other caregiver does not wish aggressive treatment to be given. The child may be transferred because the options of treatment are limited, yet the decision to accept the most aggressive treatment may not have been made prior to transfer. Some facilities, such as nursing homes, child care centers, or schools, may feel legally compelled to transfer the child to an emergency department or pediatric intensive care unit when they do not have the technology or expertise to treat a life-threatening condition. The health care providers in the acute care facility are perplexed when consent has been given for transfer yet is being withheld for treatment.

In long-term care facilities options are limited because technology intentionally is limited so as not to duplicate services offered by the acute care facility and because the cost would be prohibitive. Just as acute care facilities may have a "Do Not Resuscitate" policy, long-term care facilities may have a "Do Not Transfer" policy as well. Episodes are treated to the limit of the available technology, and transfer to an emergency department or summoning of emergency medical personnel is not done. Some long-term care facilities prefer to transfer the child to a facility where treatment, if chosen, is available rather than preclude that option for the child. The finality of the decision to forgo treatment influences the caregivers in the long-term care facility to ensure that the parents have the option of treatment and can make an informed decision to forgo treatment. Acute care facilities, however, often function as though the decision to accept treatment is made on transfer. Confusion and questions of appropriate use of resources are generated at this time.

Once the child is transferred, the potential benefits of the intervention should be weighed against the burdens. Some philosophers have considered prolonging the life of severely developmentally impaired children as the "injury of continued existence" (Engelhardt, 1975) or have argued that life itself is a harm to the child (Kahn, 1994). Parents worry about the pain the child may suffer if the problem is not relieved, the pain the child will suffer undergoing the procedure, and the benefit to be gained. Although there may be little or no improvement in functional abilities that the intervention can offer, the intervention may provide comfort or may make the physical care of the child easier and safer to give. For example, the child may have significant gastroesophageal reflux that is both painful for the child and dangerous in terms of aspiration. A Nissen fundoplication and placement of a gastrostomy involves anesthesia, a surgical incision, a stab wound, IV fluids, a temporary nasogastric tube, and a period of recovery. The child will be at reduced risk of a life-threatening aspiration and should not experience any further esophagitis from reflux. Although relief from pain and reduced risk of aspiration may be seen as adequate reasons for putting the child through the discomfort of the procedure, one might argue that death by aspiration would be a natural demise for a disabled child and to remedy the reflux would be to interfere with "nature." Some proponents of this position, however, conveniently identify unwanted interventions as "unnatural" and other interventions such as immunizations or anticonvulsants as standard medical care.

Best interest decisions in the long-term care facility are rarely easy to make. Decisions made about the simplest intervention become complex when applied to the profoundly impaired infant, child, or adult. For example, a 12-year-old child with spastic quadriplegic cerebral palsy, mental retardation, and dysphagia with a history of feeding problems begins to exhibit respiratory problems associated with mealtimes. Initially mild in character, the respiratory events develop into manifestations of aspiration. The intervention seems direct—the child will need nutritional support, partially or wholly, via tube. The question of best interest, however, is a much more difficult challenge. Questions posed may include: Is this the end of the child's "natural" ability to survive? Will tube feeding prolong life? Will there be complications related to tube feedings? Will more interventions be necessary? If tube feeding is not pursued what will happen? Will the child die of pneumonia? Will the child die of starvation? Do tube feedings hurt? What is more uncomfortable—tube feedings or the inability to eat? Should the child be given a tracheostomy? Once started, where does the intervention lead?

In an acute care setting, where diagnostic tests and interventions are readily available, a moral imperative—"because it can be done, therefore it should be done"—has been re-oriented to "because the child needs it, it must be done unless there is an overriding reason to withhold it." In long-term care settings, the act of seeking specialist consultation or transferring to another facility increases the "burden" of the intervention. For families in rural areas with few resources, travel and expense may also significantly increase their burden. The analysis again returns to the focus of identifying what is in the child's best interests. In our experience, the caregivers in the acute care setting have a tendency to support those interventions that would prolong the child's life. Occasionally, there are those health care professionals who see a life-threatening condition as a "window of opportunity" for the child to die and would see the child's death as a blessing. Still others may argue that to invest further resources in an impaired child is an inappropriate allocation of resources.

Family Decisions to Withhold or Withdraw Treatment

In the past, infants and children with neurologic impairment characterized by profound cognitive and motor disability did not survive or succumbed to a variety of conditions incompatible with long-term survival. Survival in the neurologically disabled child has been extended with medical intervention, nursing care, and therapeutics but still is often limited to late childhood or adolescence (Crichton, Mackinnon, & White, 1995; Eyman, Grossman, Chaney, & Call, 1993). When an infant or child is diagnosed with a disorder that offers no hope of improvement or cure, life expectancy is frequently discussed. The parent is told that the child will live "a few years" or a "short time." Dialogue regarding treatment and resuscitation may take place at the time of diagnosis and prognosis, but decisions to limit treatment or withhold resuscitation are rarely made at the time of the initial illness or injury.

Wishing to end their child's perceived suffering but not yet ready to forgo all treatment, the parents may decide not to pursue hospital-based treatment but rather treat the child's acute episodes within the home or in a health care facility. Limitations set by these environments allow the parent to let go of the dream that the child will return to the pre-morbid state.

To facilitate understanding and promote consistency in care, a care conference may be held. At the conference, a plan is developed that outlines the goals of interventions: namely, routine care as the child can tolerate—school, therapies, and elimination of non-beneficial interventions.

The nurse can assist the family in making decisions by providing them with accurate, clear information, or assisting them in accessing the information, and listening to the family's questions and concerns. The role of the nurse working with the family at this time can be very difficult. The nurse may identify with the family's grief. The nurse may have "bonded" with the child and see the parents as distant and uninvolved. As a facilitator for decision making and as a child advocate, the nurse can influence the parents by listening to their issues, assisting them in getting all the information they need to make their decision, helping to identify resources for the family that would have a bearing on the decision, and letting them know when a decision needs to be made.

Chronically Ill Children

Although life-threatening episodes can occur in children with disabilities or chronic conditions, the bulk of interactions families have with the health care system is the office visit, the occasional "tune-up" in the form of a brief hospital stay, or admission for corrective surgery. Children with conditions such as cystic fibrosis, arthritis, cerebral palsy, myelomeningocele, prematurity, and sickle cell disease often require close medical management and occasional hospitalization for tests, surgeries, complications of the condition, and rehabilitation. Children who have been successfully treated for cancer and have some sequelae either from the cancer or from the treatment are included in this category. Prior to a procedure and in anticipation of untoward outcomes, parents need to be advised of the resuscitation policy in the institution. The impetus for this comes from the Patient Self-Determination Act (Omnibus Budget Reconciliation Act, 1990), a federal law applying to all facilities that receive federal funds. The law stipulates that patients must be asked whether or not they have an advanced directive, and if not, if they want information about it. The law does not apply to children, because children are not considered autonomous to make advance directives. However, the attitude that resuscitation status must be discussed and clearly communicated on admission persists. For a small subset of children who the health care team suspect may experience a life-threatening event during hospitalization, the health care team may pursue the discussion with the parents to better understand their views. At face value, this effort to have clear communication is admirable. The effect on the families, however, is not always reassuring. Anecdotally, parents have described discomfort having multiple caregivers raise the issue of their child's demise and their involvement in that event. They have resisted efforts to sign any document that gives their consent in allowing their child to die. Despite the policy's intent to prevent harm, the parents feel as though the issue is "rammed down their throats" and that they are made a party to their child's death. If parents resist efforts to clarify resuscitation status, they risk being labeled "in denial." If they choose a course that the health care team does not agree with, their motives and competence are challenged. The person on the health care team designated to discuss this issue with the parents must make a detailed note in the chart so that the parents are not bombarded by many people in this regard. Should the health care team suspect that the child's best interests are not being served by the parents' decision, the health care team should consult the institution's ethics committee or ethics consultant.

Older Children Participating in Treatment Decisions

The law recognizes a minor's right to make decisions under four conditions: the "child" reaches the age of majority, the "child" is emancipated through marriage or military service, "child" is declared a mature minor through a court proceeding, or the parents have not fulfilled their parental child care responsibilities (state statutes may vary). Short of these conditions, the parents or legal guardian have decision-making authority, although some states permit adolescents to obtain health care services such as birth control, treatment for substance abuse, psychiatric conditions, and pregnancy without parental consent. There are instances of children who seem fairly sophisticated in understanding their medical condition and prognosis. Health care providers sometimes get caught between the child seeking truthful information and the

parents' admonition not to tell the child the truth. In a protective gesture, the parents wish to shield the child from information that they believe would be distressing to the child or that they, the parents, may not be able to discuss with the child. For example, the parents may insist that the child not be told that the upcoming surgery is for amputation of a leg. The surgery is a necessary curative or palliative measure for osteogenic sarcoma. The parents may believe that the child would resist the surgery, even if it meant death. Most nurses find the scenario of keeping the child uninformed as horrifying. Evaluation of the child's ability to reason and deal with bad news can be conducted by appropriate professionals such as a psychologist, social worker, or psychiatric clinical nurse specialist. Counseling sessions with the parents to advise them of the health care team's strong opposition to deceiving the child and the plan for assisting the parents in communicating with their child is shared.

Respect for children is seen in actions to inform them of what is about to happen to them, answer their questions, and seek their cooperation. Their developmental level, intellectual abilities, method of communication, and parental wishes influence the way information is communicated to them. Because the parents have the decision-making authority, the child's consent to a treatment is not legally required. Most of the time, discussions occur outside of the child's presence and the child is then informed of the decision. In some families, the parents discuss options with the child to seek the child's preferences, or the parents may ask the health care team to share all information in the child's presence. Different communication styles, cultural beliefs, and child-rearing practices influence the parents' view of how much or how little to include the child in the decision-making process. Children with chronic conditions acquire a medical sophistication beyond their years. Their experience with their illness gives them a perspective no one else has, so their views should carry a great deal of weight in decisions.

For example, a 16-year-old boy with Duchenne muscular dystrophy should be consulted about whether or not he wants mechanical ventilation to treat pneumonia. If the teenager has the ability to understand the options and to weigh the consequences, risks, and benefits of the options and makes a choice that is consistent with his stated beliefs and desires, his decision should be honored.

A developmental assessment can be done to learn if he has the capacity to participate in decisions of this gravity prior to asking for him to make a decision. A dilemma occurs when the child is offered a choice and then his choice is rejected when he disagrees with his parents or the health care team. Similarly, a dilemma arises when the health care team supports the child's preferences when they are in conflict with the parents' preferences.

As child advocates, the health care team may work with the parents to persuade them to honor their child's wishes, although this may tread the thin line between "educating" them and "coercing" them. In extreme cases, the health care team may seek court involvement to emancipate the minor for the purposes of consenting to or refusing medical treatment.

A patient in rehabilitation may experience depression and could be considered "appropriately depressed." A 15-year-old boy who suffered a severed spinal cord from a gunshot wound may be "appropriately depressed" about his loss of function and its impact on his future. He might refuse treatment and state that he wishes he were dead. As with adults, an attempt should be made to discern whether or not this behavior represents a clinical depression, a transient response to the patient's current condition, or a persistent and repeated request.

The health care system has been reluctant to withhold or withdraw treatment in children. Prior to the changes in attitudes surrounding Baby Doe, parents and physicians privately made decisions to withhold or withdraw treatment (Duff & Campbell, 1973). The concern that children with disabilities would be discriminated against has evolved into a difficult process in which they become "prisoners of technology." Situations arise in which children will express their wishes that they no longer be given life-sustaining treatment. Every effort must be made to give the child's request serious consideration. Although this consideration seems inconsistent with rehabilitation philosophy, there are those exceptional cases in which continued existence is an overwhelming burden to the child. Respect for the child's wishes, in addition to insurmountable evidence favoring non-treatment, tips the balance of burden over benefit of treatment. The Health Care Surrogate Act of Illinois of 1991 provides one example of a law outlining the choosing of surrogate decision-makers and the types of choices they can make (Table 6–3).

Table 6–3 HEALTH CARE SURROGATE ACT (ILLINOIS)*

A surrogate can be identified for the purposes of refusing life-sustaining treatment for a child. The child must meet one of the qualifying conditions: (1) be in an irreversible vegetative state, (2) be terminally ill, or (3) have an incurable, irreversible condition. A hierarchic list of possible surrogates includes legal guardian, parents, grandparents, other adult relatives, and close friends. The attending physician speaks with the potential surrogates and identifies the surrogate for the purposes of refusing a life-sustaining treatment. Occasionally, the child is in the custody of the state; in this case, the legal guardian is the surrogate. In other situations, the parents may be very young (13 or 14 years of age) but are emancipated minors and have the legal right to make the decision, but the grandmother is the primary caregiver. The physician, after meeting with both the mother and grandmother, may identify the grandmother as the surrogate decision-maker for this decision. The surrogate can only refuse life-sustaining treatment. If consent for treatment is sought, the parent retains legal authority to consent or refuse.

*1991. Pub. Act 87–749.

Justice Issues in Allocation of Resources

Decisions to allocate health care resources are no longer being made by patients and their health care providers. Public and private insurance companies have engaged intermediaries to manage benefits to reduce costs. In rehabilitative care, insurance companies may limit coverage for a stay that is less than what the rehabilitation team has recommended. Insurance coverage varies in paying for assistance in the home once parents take their child home. Children with disabilities often require the attention of multiple pediatric subspecialists, but their access to specialists is contingent on referral from their primary care provider. Pediatricians who are not accustomed to caring for children with disabilities may not provide the necessary education to the family to prevent complications or to make appropriate referrals in a timely fashion to effectively treat the complications. Ideally, a managed care environment promotes wellness and rehabilitation through coordination of care. This approach saves costs over the long term by detecting problems early and reducing complications.

Justice issues in the allocation of health care resources can be divided into two areas:

microallocation, or those decisions made about a particular patient, and macroallocation, or those decisions about distribution of resources to all of society. Managed care is an intersection of macroallocation and microallocation. Health care expenditures for one individual have an effect on all other individuals in that particular plan. Rehabilitation nursing has a stake in both microallocation and macroallocation.

Microallocation Issues

The initial ethical issue in microallocation is the decision by the acute care practitioner, usually the physician, to refer the patient for rehabilitation. Although outcomes can be improved with early transfer to a rehabilitation facility (Edwards, 1987), the initial decision to refer for evaluation does not rest with the rehabilitation staff.

The decision to refer may be affected by the acute care physician's knowledge about rehabilitation but also may rest on the family's ability to pay. Many facilities limit the number of patients on public assistance, or the patient's own insurance company may not approve of the transfer if a less expensive option, such as home care with outpatient therapies, is feasible. The patient's insurance plan may have a lifetime limit on rehabilitation services, and the parents may opt to save the benefit for a later time. If the child is being considered for transfer to a rehabilitation service and the parents do not have insurance to cover the costs, is it ethically appropriate to tell them of services they cannot access? Children have often remained in the acute care facility, where multidisciplinary services are provided but not as intensively as in a rehabilitation unit. Payors, however, are limiting coverage in these cases, and parents and physicians are notified that they will be responsible for the hospital bill after a certain date if their child remains in the hospital.

Best interests and parental consent (except in instances previously discussed) also dictate the allocation of resources at the bedside. In the past decade, however, as insurance coverage reimbursements have been capped, the length of inpatient and rehabilitation stays and the number of outpatient and therapy visits have been reduced. Families have had to absorb more of the cost for physician visits, deductibles for hospitalizations, outpatient and therapy visits, and purchasing durable medical equipment. Every use of resources is being scrutinized by either the payor (or its designee) or the parents. For example, a child with an intractable seizure disorder is hospitalized after sustaining a fall at the onset of a seizure. The charge nurse implements the unit's "seizure precaution" protocol and orders a suction machine and the appropriate-sized airway at the bedside and padded side rails. The mother asks what the charge is for having the suction machine at the bedside. No one immediately knows, but after a few phone calls, the charge nurse learns that it is over $300 per day. The mother states that she has never had to suction her son during a seizure and produces a spiral notebook documenting every seizure he has had over the past two years. The charge nurse realizes that protocols are meant as guidelines and should be modified as the patient's condition warrants, but she finds that the patient, a 10-year-old who functions cognitively at the level of a 4- or 5-year-old, drools excessively, and she is concerned that he may need suctioning. The safety net of having the suction machine at the bedside does not seem unreasonable, although the cost does seem excessive to her. The mother understands the nurse's discomfort, but assures her that she knows her son and also knows that she will have to bear a larger portion of the hospital bill because of the suction machine charge. The two compromise by having a suction machine available at all times on the unit (the unit budget bears the cost of this) and, in the event of a seizure, the nurses will use their judgment regarding the need for suctioning.

Other ethical issues are not that readily resolved. Caps on in-home nursing care hours have strained the financial, physical, and emotional limits of families. Cultural and societal expectations that the family must always provide for its members' health and welfare are no longer realistic. The changing social landscape of non-traditional nuclear families, frequent relocation of families for jobs, more mothers in the workplace, and more single-parent households has left many parents without family or community support. Much of the work of child-rearing and caring for sick or disabled family members traditionally falls to female members of the family. The expectation used to be that if the mother was working, she would quit her job to care for a sick or disabled child. For single mothers, the workload of a full-time job (to secure health care benefits for herself and children) and nursing care of her child was overwhelming. The only resolution many could find was to accept public assistance that included medical coverage, but they had to be financially destitute or they would have "spend-downs," a fixed monthly amount they must pay to qualify for public assistance.

In these circumstances, every expenditure is justified and costs are contained. The concern is that not only are unnecessary expenditures reduced, but necessary expenditures are also reduced. The payor is quick to deny payment for services that are not efficacious or health-related. In pediatric rehabilitation, services that improve function and positively impact self-worth may not be seen as medically indicated. A communication device for a brain-injured child may be viewed as an educational need or a "toy" by an insurance company. Likewise, a request for in-home respite care may be seen as paying for a family's babysitter, and the family is advised to use relatives, neighbors, or religious group members as babysitters. These microallocation decisions are derived from the same attitude affecting the macroallocation issues, but there is an inconsistency in the societal message. Much work is needed in educating payors and lobbying for expanded coverage.

Macroallocation Issues

Society, through the Baby Doe case, sent a strong message that a child's life is to be saved and preserved regardless of that child's quality of life. Cost was not to enter into this decision-making process, and costs of more than $1 million for the hospitalization of one premature infant were not uncommon. Not much has changed since the Baby Doe incident in 1982.

Once the child is discharged from the hospital, services are difficult to obtain. Some states have programs to assist families in the costs of re-hospitalization or subspecialty office visits, but eligibility requirements according to the child's diagnosis and the family's income must be met. Educational programs vary from state to state. Public Law 94-142, the Education for All Handicapped Children Act (later retitled the Individuals With Disabilities Act), ensures that states are mandated to have free and least-restrictive education for children 3 to 21 years of age, but the types of services available vary among school districts within the state. Early intervention programs, also known as 0–3 programs, provide services at no cost or for a nominal charge, but there are long waiting lists in some areas, or parents are expected to

drive more than 50 miles one way three times per week to get services at the center.

The societal mandate that ostensibly values life does not extend beyond the medical facility. Government administrations have moved to reduce public support of programs and encourage private enterprise to absorb the costs. In other countries, such as England and Sweden, a cradle-to-grave commitment to provide medical, educational, and other related services is made once a child's life is rescued and disability is discovered. Two movements in the United States have been headed on a collision course: the movement to contain health care costs and the rights movement for the disabled. This clash of movements is best represented by the Oregon Health Care Plan. In 1989, Oregon legislators passed laws that would provide health care coverage for nearly one-half million uninsured Oregonians. This uninsured group consisted of the poor, the working poor, and those who were denied coverage because of pre-existing conditions. Employers were mandated to offer health care coverage to their employees or pay a tax to the state for providing coverage. The state's plan listed benefits in a prioritized order to be covered by the plan. A cut-off point indicated benefits that would not be covered, such as intensive care for 23-week-gestation pre-term infants or liver transplants for alcoholics with cirrhosis. The rankings were derived from a "mathematical cost-utility formula" that rendered a net value of providing the benefit (White, 1992, p. 13). The Medicaid waiver was not approved because there were concerns that the plan may not adhere to the protections afforded the disabled in the Americans With Disabilities Act (ADA). In 1993, the Clinton administration issued a conditional waiver after Oregon made substantial revisions in their plan which increased both benefits and costs but retained prioritized benefits. The implementation of the plan began to occur in 1994, but its viability remains questionable (Campbell, 1993). The effects of health care reform on children with disabilities and chronic conditions and their families are discussed at length in Chapter 5.

Caplan, Callahan, and Haas (1987) acknowledged that society has not wrestled with the ethical questions in resource allocation in rehabilitation because those in need of rehabilitation are often not valued by society. The elderly, the disabled, and the chronically ill lack the attributes of vigor and vitality that society values. Budget-wrangling in Congress has been characterized as pitting the needs of children against the desire to balance the budget and provide tax cuts. Children who are disabled and chronically ill risk disenfranchisement by a society that questions their usefulness in that society. The utilitarian viewpoint forces child advocates to appeal to a sense of community in caring for the most vulnerable in society. "The provision of care and social support for persons with chronic illness by temporarily well and able-bodied citizens reflects an acknowledgment of the links that join the sick and the well, the young and the old in a community of common humanness and vulnerability" (Jennings, Callahan, & Caplan, 1988, p. 15).

One other societal trend in macroallocation issues is blaming the victim. Society values independence and industriousness in its members. It also values personal responsibility, although the increasingly litigious nature of society seems to belie this. This is represented in attitudes toward irresponsible behavior, such as riding a motorcycle without a helmet, not wearing seatbelts, diving in the shallow end of a pool, driving while intoxicated, having unprotected sex, smoking, or drinking alcohol to excess. When disease or disability is attributed to lifestyle, society is critical of the behavior and resentful of the use of resources for that person. Society may forgive the lack of judgment of a child or adolescent while blaming the parents for the lack of supervision or control over the situation resulting in the injury or illness. This societal attitude is reflected in the public's unwillingness to support programs and funding for services for persons with disabilities and integrate them back into society. The need for the Americans With Disabilities Act reflects society's reluctance to accept people with disabilities. Rehabilitation professionals have an ethical obligation to educate the public and lobby for and with persons with disabilities on their behalf.

The Nurse's Role in Bioethics

As professionals, nurses have a code of ethics to guide their professional behavior (American Nurses Association, 1985). Using the Code for Nurses to clarify obligations is a beginning point for the nurse in analyzing a situation. In an effort to update the Code, a task force appointed by the American Nurses Association (ANA) Board of Directors spent 2 years revising the provisions and interpretive statements contained therein. The revised code is slated for debate in the ANA House of Delegates in June 1998.

In pediatric rehabilitation, the nurse advocates for patients, families, and the profession. In the intimate relationships between nurse and patient, the nurse must keep professional boundaries to remain therapeutic. In pediatrics, it is easy to feel strong emotions of affection and protection for the patients. Deep friendships can develop between parents and nurses. These relationships can be facilitating or counterproductive. The professional role of the nurse is to be empathetic and supportive but to avoid relationships that foster dependence or cloud the nurse's judgment. Socialization of the novice nurse into the professional role can prepare the nurse for the therapeutic nurse-patient-family relationship (Savage & Conrad, 1992).

In developing the relationship with the family, the pediatric rehabilitation nurse rarely starts with a clean slate. The parents have had experience with nurses in an acute care facility, and this can affect the relationship in the new facility or with providers in the community. Thorne and Robinson (1989) have described three stages experienced by patients with chronic illness and their families. Although their study was conducted primarily with adults (77 patients aged 2 to 16 years), experienced pediatric rehabilitation nurses may recognize the behavior of their patients' families in the researchers' description of the three stages. The first stage is naive trust, in which the family has certain expectations of the health care providers as being all-knowing and altruistic. When the health care providers fall from this pedestal, the family experiences the second stage: disenchantment. The family's trust is shattered, and they realize that the health care provider is not all-knowing. Thorne (1993) details the frustration and doubt the families feel during this stage. Eventually, the families regain a new trust in which they feel empowerment in a "guarded alliance" with the health care providers. Parents often view the nurse as their ally in negotiating the health care system and are well-served by the nurse who teaches the parents how they themselves can negotiate the health care, social service, and educational systems. Likewise, nurses often learn a great deal from parents on how to manage the needs of children with disabilities in the community.

Alternative Medicine

Alternative medicine, or complementary medicine, is increasing in popularity among families of children with disabilities and chronic conditions. Parents may seek alternative therapies when mainstream medicine either has nothing else to offer, has failed to deliver the expected results, or has unacceptable risks or side effects. In one study, one in three Americans had used an adjunct to conventional treatments, most commonly for chronic conditions (Eisenberg, Kessler, & Foster, 1993). Variously called "alternative," "complementary," or "unorthodox medicine," these preventative practices and interventions are drawn from outside mainstream medical practice in the United States and are generally held in low regard by the scientific community because of a lack of reproducible scientific research supporting their efficacy. At present in the United States, practitioners of these therapies are often not licensed and lack the level of regulation applied to medical doctors. The level of acceptance of alternative medicine by medical doctors ranges from outright hostility to tolerance to use of alternative as well as mainstream methods. Interest in alternative medicine and health care is evidenced by the formation of The Office of Alternative Medicine by the National Institutes of Health (Toran, 1996). The terms alternative and complementary are used interchangeably throughout this section.

The purpose of this section is not to explore the pros and cons of alternative medicine but to examine the ethical issues nurses may face in working with families who seek information about or use alternative therapies. However, a brief description of the purpose and use of forms of alternative therapies commonly used by parents of children with disabilities and chronic conditions is provided to aid readers who lack experience in this area.

Alternative or complementary medicine emphasizes the achievement and maintenance of health using an integrated, holistic approach to diet, lifestyle, and environment and drawing on various philosophies. Most alternative health practices are based on four principles. The first principle is the healing power of nature, which uses "natural" methods and substances to enhance the power of the body and the mind to heal itself. Natural substances are those that occur in nature, are not man-made, and are held by alternative health practitioners to be non-toxic. The second principle is to do no harm. The third principle is to identify and treat the cause of the problem and not just eliminate the symptom. The fourth principle is that the

physician or practitioner is viewed as a teacher, and that patients are active participants in their treatment. Practitioners of alternative health care perceive mainstream medicine as primarily disease-focused; fragmented into specialties that fail to recognize the whole person, especially the interrelationship of mind and body; and dependent on medications and treatments that can be as harmful as the disease itself (Burton Goldberg Group, 1993; Marti & Hime, 1995; Toran, 1996).

Examples of alternative medicine include homeopathy, hydrotherapy, chiropractic, prayer, Doman-Delacato or patterning, biofeedback, meditation, therapeutic touch, acupuncture, Yoga, herbalism, vitamin therapy, massage, Christian Science, dietary therapy, chelation therapy, craniosacral therapy, environmental medicine, and bodywork. This is by no means an exhaustive list but includes many of the therapies often consulted by families for children with disabilities or chronic conditions.

Wardwell (1994, p. 1061) described alternative medicine as a "residual definition" because it is composed of practices outside of "orthodox" medicine. The mainstream form of medicine practiced in this country by physicians is referred to variously as "mainstream," "orthodox," "Western," or "allopathy." All of these terms refer to methods and techniques that are based on reproducible scientific research and performed by licensed and certified practitioners meeting national standards of practice. For the purposes of this section, this type of medicine is referred to as mainstream medicine.

Alternative Therapies

In most states, the law assumes that a minor child (a child younger than 18 years of age) is incompetent to make medical decisions. The law also presumes that the parent is competent and will make decisions in the child's best interests. If the parent's or parents' ability to make decisions is in doubt or if the decision seems irrational to the health care providers, the parental decision may be challenged. Decisions regarding customary medical treatment can be very difficult, but when parents have been given the facts and the advice of their child's health care providers, the law supports their decision. For example, when the parents of Baby Doe decided to forgo life-saving surgery, they had been given advice from both a pediatrician who favored surgery and the mother's obstetrician, who advised against surgery. The Indiana Supreme Court affirmed the parents' right to make the decision to forgo treatment when they had been given opposing medical opinions from reputable physicians. The exceptions in which parental decision making is usurped are when the treatment is clearly efficacious and the life of the child is threatened without treatment, and when the parents choose alternative treatment not accepted by standard mainstream medical care.

The most common instance of parents rejecting clearly effective treatment is when parents who are Jehovah's Witnesses refuse to consent for blood transfusions for their child. With the concern for blood-borne pathogens, Jehovah's Witnesses opposition to blood transfusion does not seem that inappropriate, but blood transfusions have been a low-risk, life-saving procedure for decades. The prohibition against blood transfusions for Jehovah's Witnesses is based on their beliefs; when those beliefs are not shared by the attending physicians and other health care providers, the balance of benefits over risks tips in favor of giving the blood. There have been other public examples of parental decision making being challenged. Parents who decided to forgo customary treatment for their child's leukemia in favor of laetrile therapy were ordered by a Massachusetts court to submit their child for chemotherapy (Weir, 1989, pp. 115–116). The court based its decision on the fact that the laetrile therapy was not accepted medical treatment. Laetrile was not (and is not) accepted medical treatment, nor was it legally available in the United States. Laetrile had potentially fatal side effects, and the parents had stopped standard medical treatment. The standard medical treatment was not without toxic side effects and did not guarantee cure, but through a rigorous scientific process, it was determined to be the state-of-the-art treatment for leukemia.

Whenever the parents refuse the suggested plan of treatment or non-treatment, the decision-making process bears review. Every case varies, but case precedents often set the standard for decisions in a given jurisdiction. The nurse needs to ascertain the relevant case law for each particular issue. Because the applicable laws vary from state to state, the discussion here remains general. In efficacious, accepted treatment, when the child's life is at stake, the courts favor treatment. In the Messenger case, a father who was also a physician removed his 780-g pre-term infant from a ventilator when his request to forgo the ventilator was not heeded. The infant died, and the father was charged with involuntary manslaughter (Peabody & Martin, 1996). When the benefit of accepted treatment is ambiguous or uncertain, the parents' wishes are respected. When the attending physician believes that treatment would be futile, the parents' wishes are respected, unless the provider is morally opposed to providing treatment. At that point, the provider may transfer the care of the child to another provider who does not have the moral opposition, or the provider may seek court intervention in withholding or withdrawing treatment. Court decisions to withhold treatment deemed futile by the health care providers have not always supported the physician's position. The court supported one husband's request to continue the ventilator for his elderly wife who was in a persistent vegetative state (Helen Wanglie case), and another court supported a mother's request that the ventilator be continued for her child with anencephaly (Baby K) (Bernat, 1994).

Although parents are given much freedom in child-rearing practices, they do not have absolute autonomy. Immunizations (with medical exceptions or exceptions for religious or personal beliefs), school attendance (with home school or medical exceptions), car seats, alcohol and tobacco restrictions, disciplinary methods, baby-selling, and child labor all reflect changes in societal attitude toward children and the relationship between child and parent. Children used to be treated as property of their parents. Even quiet decision making between parents and physician to withhold or withdraw treatment came under scrutiny with Baby Doe. There is an assumption that parents are the best persons to make decisions for their children, but that assumption is arguable. Parents do not solely determine what is in their child's best interests. When parents make alternative choices, their decisions are not challenged unless there is the possibility of harm to the child. The harm may be from forgoing standard treatment or from trying an alternative treatment.

When parents seek information on alternative therapies, nurses can direct them to local libraries. Information may be available through health science center libraries, but families may not be able to easily access these libraries. Nurses can facilitate obtaining information without endorsing or condemning the specific practice. Such resources include the American Holistic Medical Association and the American Holistic Nursing Association. Additionally, states may have specific licensed practitioners such as chiropractors, massage therapists, or acupuncturists. Critical to informed consent is the educational process. It behooves the health care team to review the material given to the parents. The principle of autonomy is respected by the informed consent process; the principle of nonmaleficence is exercised by advising the parents of the potential harms of attempting a specific unorthodox treatment or forgoing orthodox treatment in favor of a probably harmless but potentially worthless therapy.

Some nursing programs have integrated alternative therapies into their educational and research programs. The Center for Human Caring at the University of Colorado School of Nursing has a program devoted to "complementary modalities" (Cleaveland & Biester, 1995, p. 122). Nurses may feel ambivalent about supporting mainstream medicine and discouraging alternative medicine, which is the posture most institutions would expect nurses to adopt. Most institutions such as hospitals and rehabilitation facilities are strongly influenced by mainstream medicine, if not totally controlled by physicians. Apart from the debate on the efficacy of alternative medicine, nurses have devoted more attention and research to family adaptation and coping, and realize that hope is a powerful factor in both recovery and adaptation. To limit parents' access to information or to thwart their efforts in seeking alternative therapies when the risk of harm to the child is low may threaten the relationship between the parents and the rehabilitation team. Instead, the rehabilitation team might design a trial of the alternative therapy that would respect the parents' choices, limit the possibility of harm to the child, and perhaps demonstrate a benefit. The benefit can be measured in terms of family functioning, reduced parental stress, or through more traditional outcomes.

REFERENCES

American Nurses Association. (1985). *Code for nurses with interpretive statements.* Kansas City, MO: American Nurses Association.

Aroskar, M. A. (1980). Anatomy of an ethical dilemma: the theory. *American Journal of Nursing,* 80(4), 658–60.

Bernat, J. L. (1994). *Ethical issues in neurology.* Boston: Butterworth-Heinemann.

Buchanan, A. E., & Brock, D. W. (1990). *Deciding for others: the ethics of surrogate decision-making.* New York: Cambridge University Press.

Bunting, S. M., & Webb, A. A. (1988). An ethical model for decision-making. *Nurse Practitioner,* 13(12), 30–34.

Burton Goldberg Group. (1993). *Alternative medicine: the definitive guide.* Puyallup, WA: Future Medicine Publishing Inc.

Callahan, D. (1988). Families as caregivers: the limits of morality. *Archives in Physical Medicine and Rehabilitation* 69, 323–328.

Campbell, C. S (1993). Gridlock on the Oregon trail. *Hastings Center Report,* 23(4), 6–7.

Caplan, A. L., Callahan, D., & Haas, J. (1987). Ethical and policy issues in rehabilitation medicine. *Hastings Center Report,* 18(1), S1–20.

Cleaveland, M J., & Biester, D. J. (1995). Alternative and complementary therapies: considerations for nursing practice. *Journal of Pediatric Nursing,* 10(2), 121–2.

Crichton, J. U, Mackinnon, M., & White, C. P. (1995). The life-expectancy of persons with cerebral palsy. *Developmental Medicine and Child Neurology,* 37, 567–576.

Curtin, L. L. (1978). A proposed model for critical ethical analysis. *Nursing Forum,* 17(1), 12-7.

Drotar, D., Baskiewicz, A., Irvin, N., Kennell, J., & Klaus, M. (1975). The adaptation of parents to the birth of an infant with a congenital malformation: a hypothetical model. *Pediatrics,* 56(5), 710–7.

Duff, R. S., & Campbell, A. G. M. (1973). Moral and ethical dilemmas in the special-care nursery. *New England Journal of Medicine,* 289(17), 890–894.

Education for All Handicapped Children Act of 1975. Pub. L. No. 94-142.

Edwards, P. A. (1987). Rehabilitation outcomes in children with brain injury. *Rehabilitation Nursing,* 12(3), 125–127.

Eisenberg, D., Kessler, R., & Foster, C. (1993). Unconventional medicine in the United States: prevalence, costs and patterns of use. *New England Journal of Medicine,* 328, 246–52.

Engelhardt, H. T. (1975). Ethical issues in aiding the death of young children. In M. Kohl (Ed.). *Beneficent euthanasia* (pp. 180–192). Buffalo, NY: Prometheus Books.

Eyman, R. K., Grossman, H. J., Chaney, R. H., & Call, T. L. (1993). Survival of profoundly disabled people with severe mental retardation. *American Journal of Diseases in Children,* 147, 329–336.

Gilligan, C. (1982). *A different voice.* Cambridge, MA: Harvard University Press.

Health Care Surrogate Act of Illinois of 1991. Pub. Act 87-749.

Jennings, B., Callahan, D., & Caplan, A. L. (1988). Ethical challenges of chronic illness. *Hastings Center Report* 18(1), S1–16.

Joint Commission on Accreditation of Healthcare Organizations. (1995). *Accreditation manual for hospitals.* Chicago: Joint Commission on Accreditation of Healthcare Organizations.

Jonsen, A. R., Siegler, M., & Winslade, W. J (1992). *Clinical ethics: a practical approach to ethical decisions in clinical medicine* (3rd ed.). New York: McGraw-Hill.

Kahn, J. P. (1994). Genetics and the problem of harm. In J. F. Monagle & D. C. Thomasma (Eds.). *Health care ethics: critical issues* (pp. 12–23). Gaithersburg, MD: Aspen.

Kohlberg, L. (1976). Moral stages and moralization: the cognitive-developmental approach. In T. Lickona (Ed.). *Moral development and behavior: theory, research and social issues*. New York: Holt, Rinehart, and Winston.

Marti, J., & Hime, A. (1995). *The alternative health and medicine encyclopedia*. New York: Gale Research Inc.

Olshansky, S. (1962). Chronic sorrow: a response to having a mentally defective child. *Social Casework*, 43, 190–193.

Omnibus Budget Reconciliation Act of 1990, Pub. L. No. 101–508. §§ 4206, 4751 (Nov. 5, 1990).

Peabody, J. L., & Martin, F. I. (1996). From how small is too small to how much is too much. *Clinics in Perinatology*, 23(3), 473–487.

Ross, J. W. (1986). *Handbook of hospital ethics committees*. Chicago: American Hospital Association.

Savage, T. A., & Conrad, B. A. (1992). Vulnerability as a consequence of the neonatal nurse-infant relationship. *Journal of Perinatal and Neonatal Nursing*, 6(3), 64–75.

Silva, M. C. (1990). *Ethical decision making in nursing administration*. Norwalk, CT: Appleton & Lange.

Thompson, J. E., & Thompson, H.O. (1985). *Bioethical decision-making for nurses*. Norwalk, CT: Appleton-Century-Crofts.

Thorne, S. E. (1993). *Negotiating health care: the social context of chronic illness*. Newbury Park, CA: Sage.

Thorne, S. E., & Robinson, C. A. (1989). Guarded alliance: health care relationships in chronic illness. *Image: Journal of Nursing Scholarship*, 21(3), 153–157.

Toran, M. (1996). Alternatives in the mainstream. *Case Manager*, 7(4), 55–63.

Wardwell, W. I. (1994). Alternative medicine in the United States. *Social Science Medicine*, 38(8), 1061–8.

Weir, R. F. (1989). *Abating treatment with critically ill patients: ethical and legal limits to the medical prolongation of life*. New York: Oxford University Press.

White, J. H. (1992). The Oregon plan's impact on the future of healthcare reform. *Health Progress*, 73(100), 12–14.

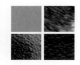

Chapter 7

Principles of Pediatric Rehabilitation Nursing

Dalice L. Hertzberg

As a relatively new sub-specialty of the practice of rehabilitation nursing, many of the underlying principles of care and service for pediatric rehabilitation clients are drawn from both general rehabilitation and developmental pediatrics. Concepts of growth and development are an integral part of pediatric rehabilitation nursing. This chapter provides a framework within which to better understand and influence the internal and external factors affecting the child with a disability and his or her family.

FRAMEWORK FOR UNDERSTANDING THE INTER-RELATIONSHIP OF HEALTH, DISABILITY, AND SOCIETY

Disability occurs as a part of the continuum of health and illness and strongly influences quality of life. Disability arises as the consequence of a disease, a congenital or genetic condition, or some type of impairment of health or physical function.

International Classification of Impairments, Disabilities and Handicaps Model

The International Classification of Impairments, Disabilities and Handicaps (ICIDH) was originally developed and published in 1980 by the World Health Organization (WHO) to describe and classify the consequences of disease in the context of health experience (Badley, 1995; WHO, 1980). A taxonomy such as the ICIDH offers a framework within which to understand the driving forces of disability—physiologic, social, and envi-

ronmental—and to develop interventions that can affect the individual with a disability in the areas of prevention, prevention of secondary conditions, health maintenance, health promotion, and quality of life.

The ICIDH framework describes three planes on which the consequences of disease are played out: impairment, disability, and handicap.

Impairment

The first plane, impairment, is concerned with the effects at the level of the body—a part of the body that does not operate in the expected manner, dysfunction or malfunction of an organ, or an absent body part. Examples of dysfunction at the first plane include an amputated limb, a diabetic pancreas, myelomeningocele, and arthritic joint stiffness.

Disability

The second plane, disability, operates at the level of the individual and his or her performance of activities. Examples of dysfunction at the second plane are difficulty walking due to an amputated leg, the need for daily insulin injections by a person with diabetes, lower extremity paralysis from spina bifida, and mobility limitations from stiff joints in a person with arthritis.

Handicap

The third plane, handicap, is concerned with the consequences of the impairment and disability at the social level. For example, an individual with a leg amputation might not experience handicap on a social level unless his or her amputation results in a societal disadvantage—that is, the gap between society's expectations of an individual and the individual's ability to meet those expectations. Examples of a disadvantage on this plane might be job discrimination or physical disfigurement that leads to few social contacts and relationships. Similarly, persons with diabetes may experience handicap as a result of disability if frequent illness and hospitalization prevent them from qualifying for health insurance. The child with myelomeningocele who is unable to participate in intramural sports with peers may be disadvantaged socially and thus encounter a social handicap as a result of the disability.

In the context of the ICIDH framework, the term handicap refers to the situation in which the ability to sustain a survival role (WHO, 1980) is affected by an impairment or a disability. Survival roles are dimensions of experience in which competence is expected. They are derived from Maslow's hierarchy of needs (Maslow, 1970) and include such typical life activities as physical independence and self-care; mobility; expected life occupations or activities such as attending school, working, parenting, or recreation; participation and maintenance of social relationships; and economic self-sufficiency (Badley, 1995; WHO, 1980). Typical life activities are circumscribed by the individual's age, gender, social and cultural factors, and environment. Therefore, what constitutes a handicap in a white, middle-class suburb might vary significantly from a condition that causes a handicap in rural New Mexico or in the low-income housing projects of New York City. The relations among impairment, disability, and handicap in the ICIDH framework are represented in Figure 7–1.

The term "handicap" is used here to refer to the interaction between societal role expectations and the altered roles experienced by individuals with disabilities, and not to describe an individual. Thus, the individual is not handicapped but rather experiences handicap due to the barriers and limitations imposed by his or her community and society. In some ways, the concept of handicap in the ICIDH framework is closely related to the concept of discrimination in the Americans With Disabilities Act in that it is based on disadvantage. Disadvantage occurs when the individual is unable to conform to societal norms. The Americans With Disabilities Act prohibits discrimination on the basis of disadvantage due to disability. Despite this clarification, in present day use, the term handicap is not well accepted as proper or "people-first" terminology, and in this country the term has negative connotations, as discussed in Chapter 1. Use of the term "handicap" represents an important objection to the ICIDH framework.

Although at first glance the ICIDH framework appears to be constructed in a primarily linear fashion, the nature of disability is dynamic, varying with changes in the internal and external environments of the individual. Correspondingly, the designation of a person's disability also may fluctuate using this framework. The ICIDH has been criticized for primarily representing adults and not satisfactorily capturing the interaction of development and the influence of family on the child with a disability. Subsequently, other conceptual models based on the ICIDH framework have been developed to expand on the environmental and social influences on the individual and describe outcomes in terms of functional limitations or societal expectations as opposed to handicap. The ICIDH framework is presently undergoing massive revision and expansion by an international team sponsored by WHO. The new version will more fully represent the continuum of disease conditions, disability, health, and quality of life with regard to individuals of all ages and national origins.

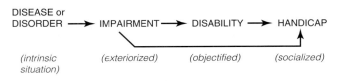

Figure 7–1   Graphic representation of the consequences of disease. (Adapted from the *International Classification of Impairments, Disabilities, and Handicaps: A Manual of Classification Related to the Consequences of Disease.* Geneva: World Health Organization, 1980, p. 30.)

Conceptual Model of Disablement in Childhood

Another model derived from the ICIDH framework posits the domains of impairment, functional limitation, disability, and social role performance, which takes the place of handicap in the ICIDH terminology (Coster & Haley, 1992). This Conceptual Model of Disablement in Childhood meshes the disablement framework, described previously, with three additional constructs: a developmental framework, representing developmental states and experiences; a contextual framework, representing the setting, environment, conditions of the desired task, and presence or absence of social support; and measurement constructs that include mastery of discrete functional skills, performance of

functional activities, and performance of social, family, and personal roles. The goal of this model is to encompass societal expectations of the child with age-appropriate behavior and achievement of specific motor tasks, with the modifiers of environmental influences and caregiver assistance. The outcome, social role performance, is viewed in context of the desired social, family, and personal roles. A functional evaluation tool, the Pediatric Evaluation of Disability Inventory (PEDI; Coster & Haley, 1992), was derived from this model and is used extensively in pediatric rehabilitation. A representation of the model is included in Figure 7–2.

Another extension of the model of disablement in childhood was suggested by Patrick, Richardson, Starks, and Rose (1994). This construct was developed to illustrate the pro-

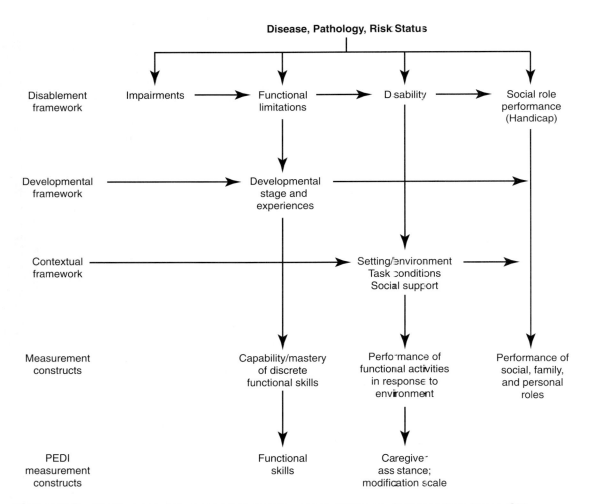

Figure 7–2   Working conceptual model of disablement in childhood. (Adapted from Haley, SM (1992). Motor assessment tools for infants and young children: A focus on disability assessment. In H. Forrsberg (Ed.). *Treatment of Children with Movement Disorders: Theory and Practice*. Basel, Switzerland: Karger Publishers. Reproduced with permission of S. Karger AG, Basel.)

cess of primary prevention and health promotion in people with disabilities, particularly those with conditions that occur early in life (e.g., cerebral palsy, spina bifida), and to show the opportunities for intervention at all levels. This construct, the Framework for Promoting the Health of People with Disabilities, describes the environment of people with disabilities and its influences on five planes that represent the individual's life: the total environment, the life course and events, the disabling process, opportunity, and quality of life. Potential interactions between the environment and the individual on these five planes provide different opportunities for intervention and prevention. This model assumes that disability is not a linear process and that it does not proceed in a predictable manner. The Framework for Promoting the Health of People with Disabilities is shown in Figure 7–3.

One of the strengths of the Framework for Promoting the Health of People with Disabilities is in its inclusion of the potentials for different interventions and opportunities that may slow, stop, or reverse the process of disablement. The disablement process may be affected by efforts to restore function, to prevent the development of secondary conditions that may either worsen existing conditions or lead to new problems; or interventions that may reduce the disadvantage experienced by the individual's lack of opportunity to participate in the community. A significant advantage of this model over others is that it encompasses changes and experiences that occur across the life span. Although the term "interventions" implies a passive role for the child with a disability, outcomes and effects may be brought about by the child, the family, and members of the community, as well as professionals (Patrick, Richardson, Starks, & Rose, 1994).

These models present interdisciplinary frameworks that can be used to assess, plan, implement, and evaluate interventions and services. They provide methods with which to measure change in function while taking into account the evolving skills and competencies of the developing child and influences of the family, caregivers, and the environment. The models described in this section also provide frameworks for applied research on pediatric rehabilitation interventions that are applicable across disciplines. Greater consideration and use of these models by the pediatric rehabilitation nurse is crucial to a greater understanding and application of the concepts of impairment, disability, and social role performance within the rehabilitation community.

Basic Concepts

Rehabilitation and habilitation of children is irrevocably enmeshed with the process and outcomes of growth and development. Whether a child is born with a malfunction of organ or limb or receives an injury resulting in damage to the maturing brain or musculoskeletal system, the trajectory of future abilities is determined in large part by growth, development, and maturation.

As stated in Chapter 1, the term "habilitation" refers to the development of new skills and abilities in the presence of major organ impairment, most commonly impairment of the neurologic or musculoskeletal system. "Rehabilitation" describes the process of relearning skills and behaviors after an injury or illness.

Ideally, the process of rehabilitation is characterized by a comprehensive, high-quality, coordinated, integrated system (Albrecht, 1992). Whatever the comprehensiveness and quality of the process, rehabilitation is a primary force shaping the lives of children with disabilities and their families. Unfortunately, families seeking rehabilitation services for their children are often confronted by a maze of bureaucracies, denial or refusal of insurance benefits, and often prohibitively high-cost services. The rehabilitation process is described in *The Specialty Practice of Rehabilitation Nursing, A Core Curriculum* (1993) as "a planned and orderly sequence of individualized services designed to meet the unique needs of each disabled person" (Rehabilitation Nursing Foundation, 1993, p. 4).

Key components of this process for children with disabilities and their families include

- the collaborative interaction of an interdisciplinary health care team
- the understanding by all team members, including the child and family, that the unique contribution of each discipline to the total rehabilitation outcome is an integral part of a holistic model of service
- accountability on the part of each member of the team for enhancing the interventions and goals of other members of the rehabilitation team
- use of a problem-solving approach focused on long- and short-term outcomes

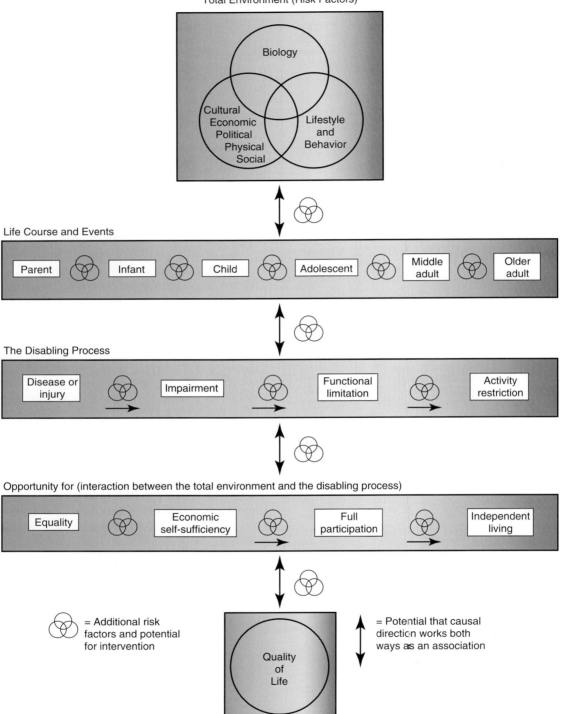

Figure 7–3 Framework for promoting the health of people with disabilities. (Adapted from Patrick, D., Richardson, M., Starks, H., & Rose, M. (1994). A framework for promoting the health of people with disabilities. In D. Lollor (Ed.). *Preventing Secondary Conditions Associated with Spina Bifida or Cerebral Palsy: Proceedings and Recommendations of a Symposium.* Washington, DC: Spina Bifida Assocation. Reprinted with permission.)

- recognition of the unique impact of the disability for the child and family

The pediatric rehabilitation process is occurring more frequently in out-patient and community settings, as well as in acute care settings and rehabilitation centers, as discussed in Chapter 1.

The process of pediatric rehabilitation nursing includes:

- assessment and evaluation of the child's condition and of the family's coping and expectations, including a developmentally-appropriate functional assessment
- identification of family and team concerns
- formulation of short-term and long-term goals and determination of desired outcomes
- development of a treatment plan
- implementation of the treatment plan
- evaluation of the treatment plan, comparing projected goals and outcomes with the child's actual achievement of skills and knowledge, involving a functional assessment tool
- ongoing revision of goals, outcomes, and the treatment plan, if necessary

This process takes place in full collaboration with the family and with the child if he or she is developmentally able.

Function

Key to understanding the process of development in the presence of disability is the concept of function. Function is often defined as the usual and characteristic action of an object. Cech and Martin (1995) describe function as "the natural required, or expected activity of a person or thing" (p. 4).

When used in the context of human activity, function may refer to the action of an organ or body part or to the activity of the individual as a whole. The term refers to the overall ability of the individual to perform purposeful activities required for survival or required by society. These basic functions include mobility, specific movement, and strength of different muscle groups; sensory abilities, such as hearing, seeing, physical sensation, and communicating; and cognitive abilities, including problem-solving ability, learning, emotions, mental state, affect, and behavior (Verbrugge & Jette, 1993).

In the practice of rehabilitation, the term "function" frequently is used to describe the individual's ability to interact with the environment to meet the individual's physical, social, or psychological needs. Function is often used interchangeably with performance (Hens, 1989). In children, the definition of function becomes even more complex, taking into account the constant changes in ability and potential brought about by development and maturation. Additionally, when considering function in children, one must take into account the effect of the caregiver on the child's overall functional status, because true independence does not begin to occur until adolescence.

The term "functional status" is used to describe the child's ability to walk, perform self-care, interact with others in a meaningful way, and learn new information and apply it to everyday life and work. A child's function represents not just the child's capability and developmental achievement at a specific age, but the receptivity of and barriers present in the environment that help or hinder the child's efforts. The definition of functional status in a child is dependent on the child's age at the time of diagnosis or trauma and his or her pre-morbid developmental level.

Functional limitations are restrictions in functions due to disease, impairment, or injury (Verbrugge & Jette, 1993). The child's surrounding environment, whether home, school, community, or workplace, can modify the effect of functional limitations, either increasing or decreasing them. The demands of the environment can be modified in a number of ways to reduce the impact of functional limitations. Demands may be reduced by use of activity accommodations, environmental modifications, social support, assistive devices, and changes in time requirements and frequency of demands (Verbrugge & Jette, 1993). For example, a 10-year-old girl with cerebral palsy walks with ankle-foot orthoses (AFO braces) and a walker. She is skilled at using her communication device, a Dynavox (Sentient Systems Technology, Inc., Pittsburgh, PA), with which she can choose letters and words to compose a computer-spoken statement or a visual readout. She does her homework on an adapted computer, and maintains a "B" average. Because she moves more slowly than her classmates, she is allowed extra time to travel between classrooms at school. She participates in adapted physical education and is learning how to be the assistant coach for the girls' soccer team. She gets along well with the other children and has satisfying friendships.

This child has significant functional limitations in mobility, speech and language, and fine and gross motor abilities. Despite her disability and the potential limits presented to her functional status, she has a supportive family and teacher, and the school has made the accommodations necessary to help her succeed. Additionally, the other children in her class accept her for her sunny personality and good sense of humor, and are able to see past her braces, walker, and communication device to the real person. This situation exemplifies the effects that societal expectations, social support, and environmental influences can have on functional limitations.

OUTCOMES IN PEDIATRIC REHABILITATION NURSING

The Changing Definition of Outcomes

An outcome is the end product of a process. In rehabilitation practice, an outcome is a projected goal regarding changes in the functional status of an individual. These changes or improvements in function are based on the quantity and quality of interventions; the individual's diagnosis and intrinsic factors such as personality and motivation; risk of complications; and the designated time span to attain the goal, in terms of days, weeks, months, or years. Outcomes are measures of functional performance at the level of disability (Johnston, Wilkerson, & Maney, 1993). Outcome terminology is also used to refer to quality assurance outcomes, which may pertain to additional factors in rehabilitation and other fields, such as cost, length of stay or service, program evaluation, efficacy of services, educational services or programs, and number of clients served. Outcomes are frequently used to measure functional gains as a result of rehabilitation team and rehabilitation nursing interventions. Outcome statements reflect the expectation of how the individual should look, feel, or act as a result of the rehabilitation interventions and are more comprehensive than goals. Outcome criteria are specific, clear statements describing the expected result, against which actual outcomes are measured. At this time, there are few functional outcome criteria that pertain to pediatric rehabilitation nursing.

The definition of desirable outcomes for children is changing. As rehabilitation moves more and more into the community, interventions are provided in community settings such as homes, schools, child care centers, and recreational programs. On site, inclusive services take place in the natural environments of children and are increasingly integrated into their daily activities instead of being provided in isolated clinics or centers. This more holistic model of services has evolved along with the philosophy of community inclusion for children and adults with disabilities to shift the language of outcomes toward that of overall quality of life and life satisfaction. Independence begins to take on an enhanced meaning, focusing not only on the tasks the child can perform but on the quality of life for that child at home, at school, and in the community. Independence is now more likely to be defined as the control the individual with a disability has over his or her own life, or the degrees of control the child with a disability and his or her family have over their lives (Shapiro, 1993). Outcomes that are based on integration of interventions into daily activities allow the family a greater role in determining desirable, meaningful outcomes.

The determination of functional outcomes is not a static process but a dynamic one, and it is a process that occurs in close collaboration with the child's family and the interdisciplinary team of rehabilitation service providers. Just as the child's development and maturation present a changing panorama of possibilities, the outcomes of rehabilitation services must reflect this outlook. The process described requires an ongoing system of assessment and evaluation to best provide the most effective and meaningful interventions to maximize the child's developmental and human potential.

Quality of Life

The concept of quality of life is a key factor in determining the outcomes of pediatric rehabilitation services. Quality of life has been described in many different ways: as personal well-being (Pope & Tarlov, 1991; Marge, 1994); as "physical, care-related, psychological, social and economic factors that bear on a person's self esteem" (Miller, Steele, & Morse, 1994, p. 89); and as "an individual's perception of their position in life in the context of the culture and value systems in which they lie and in relation to their goals, expectations, standards and concerns" (The WHOQOL Group, 1995, p. 1405), among others. Most of the definitions agree that quality of life is subjective, is based on the individual's or the family's perceptions; and includes factors in addition to health status and health care services. Quality of life for children or adults with disabilities shares the same features as that for people without disabilities.

Campbell's (1977) definition of quality of life describes satisfaction with 10 domains of life, in addition to absence of perceived stress. The 10 domains of life are: health, work, marriage, housing, community, standard of living, social relationships, creative expression, education, and future prospects for growth and development. Children with disabilities, due to personal and societal factors interacting with the effects of the disability, often experience difficulty in attaining satisfaction within these 10 domains. Unstable health, difficulties with communication and learning, and altered physical appearance often interfere with societal expectations and result in social isolation, reduced access to education, limited opportunities for making friends and working, and curtailed future prospects for emotional and creative growth. These aspects of well-being are measured both by the perception of the individual and family and by the perception of the society in which the child and family live.

The second part of Campbell's definition of quality of life is absence of perceived stress. Although some stress is necessary to promote optimum performance, too much stress can lead to physical and psychological ills. The subjective assessment that life is generally easy, that needs are met without undue expenditure of time and money, and that life proceeds at a comfortable pace and is not rushed hardly seems to apply to the busy lives of most families today. However, the perception of stress encompasses in large part comparison of one's own situation against that of others. Large or frequent hospital bills, frequent time spent away from work for a child's medical or therapy appointments, and the ever-increasing limitations of insurance coverage for services deemed essential by parents and health and rehabilitation providers all contribute to ongoing stress and reduce quality of life for families of children with disabilities.

One study (Goode, 1990) surveyed adults with disabilities and service providers about the principles of quality of life and found the following:

The same factors and relationships are as important to people with disabilities as people without disabilities.

Quality of life is experienced when basic needs are being met and when the opportunity to pursue and achieve goals is present.

The meaning of quality of life in major life settings is validated by a wide variety of people with disabilities, their families, and service providers.

An individual's quality of life is interrelated with that of other people in the environment.

Quality of life reflects cultural heritage.

Presence of a high quality of life for children with disabilities and their families is dependent on the ability of the child and family to meet both basic and higher level needs and the availability and accessibility of adequate resources. Nurses and other members of the rehabilitation team practicing in the range of settings that offer habilitation and rehabilitation services have a unique opportunity to improve quality of life for children with disabilities and their families.

Factors Influencing Outcomes in Pediatric Rehabilitation

The complex and continual interaction between bio-psycho-social factors and environmental factors determines long-term and short-term outcomes in pediatric rehabilitation and habilitation. The process of growth and development is one of the most crucial factors influencing short-term and long-term functional outcomes. Michaud (1995) identified five factors associated with pediatric brain injury outcomes: pre-injury factors, injury-related factors, acute management factors, factors in the post-rehabilitation environment, and developmental factors. For the purposes of this chapter, those factors are further broken down and expanded to include age; growth, development, and maturation; severity, extent, and location of injury; health status, nutrition, and intrinsic biologic factors; psychosocial factors; environmental factors; and family influences.

Age

The age of the child is a significant defining factor for size, biologic capacity of all body systems, and expectations of abilities, behavior, and lifestyle. Although all children do not grow, develop, and mature at exactly the same rate and time, they all follow the same developmental sequence. The child's size influences the risk for and response to injury. Infants are more vulnerable to cervical spine and spinal cord injury because of the elasticity of ligaments around the cervical spine and poor head control (Allen & Ferguson, 1985). Children who weigh less than 18.14 kg (40 lb) are more vulnerable to injury in an automobile because of their weight and size and require specialized restraint systems such as car seats. Premature infants and neonates are more vulnerable to the effects of excess or inadequate oxygen as a result of the immaturity of their central nervous systems (CNS) and the tiny, delicate blood vessels in their brains.

The developmental expectations of parents, teachers, rehabilitation specialists, and other health care providers are based on the age of the child. Adults compare their expectations with the child's performance to determine whether or not the child is behaving appropriately and has achieved the designated developmental milestones at the prescribed time. These age-related expectations form the basis for functional goals during the rehabilitation process. As the child ages, constant adaptation to the demands of environment and of developmental expectations must occur for the child to remain developmentally appropriate, or "on track" for age.

Children who have a disability, whether acquired or congenital, are either delayed in their achievement of developmental tasks or fail to achieve them as a result of lags in maturation and difficulties in adapting to new experiences caused by the underlying condition. In some cases, neurologic impairment appears to increase as children who were born prematurely and diagnosed as having mild, moderate, or severe insult grow and develop (Gilfoyle, Grady, & Moore, 1990). As the child gets older and developmental demands and expectations become more complex, the child with a disability falls further and further behind. In essence, the gap between performance and expectations widens with increasing age. For example, the child who was born with spina bifida, which affects mobility, CNS function, bowel and bladder function, musculoskeletal function, and cognitive abilities, is able to "keep up" fairly well with developmental expectations, supported by assistive devices such as braces or a wheelchair, until he or she reaches middle school age. Then, as the requirements for functional ability, school performance, and social skills increase, the child with spina bifida, who lacks physical maturation, the ability to explore the environment fully, and the cognitive ability to process complicated information,

fails to adapt to the ever-changing environment and expectations and loses more and more ground developmentally. Development of functional goals takes into account not only the child's chronologic age but also the child's actual performance of tasks and developmental achievements, whether or not they are appropriate for age.

The child's age at the initiation of habilitation or rehabilitation services significantly affects the outcomes of those services. For children born with a congenital condition or who acquire a disabling condition early in life, the key to their success in late childhood, adolescence, and adulthood lies in early identification of delays and disability and early and consistent intervention by the family and health care providers (Guralnick, 1993; Russell & Free, 1994). Children who experience trauma, disease, or a congenital condition and do not receive rehabilitation or habilitation services soon after the onset of the condition may develop complications that significantly affect their developmental and functional potential. Physical changes that occur as a result of the condition, such as spasticity, bowel and bladder dysfunction, and motor deficits, if untreated, may progress to joint contractures; chronic constipation and stretching of the walls of the colon; incontinence, reflux, and bladder or kidney infection and damage; and loss of independent mobility. As the child grows older and gains in size and weight, complications may progress more rapidly, especially during growth spurts. Some examples of changes with rapid growth include tightness in tendons such as hamstrings or heel cords, which do not grow as quickly as the long bones do during growth spurts; changes in bladder function that typically occur between 1 and 3 years of age and may result in increased bladder and sphincter tone leading to inadequate emptying or reflux; and changes in size and weight that require frequent, often yearly, checks for assistive devices or prostheses that are outgrown and causing pressure. Maintaining an understanding of these age-related changes is critical to effective rehabilitation nursing care.

Children with neurologically based disabilities are influenced by age and development-related reflex patterns. In children with early brain injury or cerebral palsy, persistence of primitive reflexes, most of which usually disappear by 6 months to 1 year of age, are a major interference with the achievement of functional skills. Development of postural reflexes, which allow the child to remain upright and balanced and generally appear as primitive reflexes are extinguished, is frequently delayed.

Growth, Development, and Maturation

The period of the child's development, and the tasks to be achieved during that developmental period, greatly influence rehabilitation outcomes. For example, a young child who loses motor abilities at a time when physical exploration of the environment is crucial to learning will be at a greater risk for developmental difficulties than a child who loses motor abilities at a later age, when physical exploration of the environment is less of a factor in learning. Conversely, an adolescent boy who experiences a spinal cord injury and loses function is more at risk for emotional problems related to body image and sexuality than a 2-year-old child with a spinal cord injury.

Pre-existing developmental delays in a child who is injured may further jeopardize outcomes. The juxtaposition of prior difficulties with learning or motor development adds to the complexity of the problem and may alter expectations of the child's ability to reach an age-appropriate developmental level following rehabilitation. A good example of this situation is the 5-year-old boy who was born at 34 weeks gestation to a 17-year-old mother who admitted to using crack during her pregnancy. The child's motor development was not delayed, but instead progressed faster than that of most other children of the same age. Speech and language abilities were delayed, and the mother had difficulty finding a preschool that would accept him due to his impulsive and aggressive behavior. He was hit by a car when he ran into the street after getting off the school bus, resulting in a severe head injury, a fractured right femur, and multiple abrasions. Following acute rehabilitation, he continued to have significant difficulties with behavior and attention and required one-to-one supervision both during school and at home. The pre-existing developmental and behavioral difficulties continued to affect the child's performance and learning potential and added to the functional deficits experienced after the injury.

"Plasticity" of the immature brain is the term used to describe the apparently greater propensity for adaptation of the CNS of young children. Because neurons are still forming, growing, and developing, it is believed that some types of damage to the brain may be overcome by the process of development. Developmental factors such as axonal growth and development of myelinization may account for this greater capacity for adaptation in young children, as well as greater ease of development of reciprocal pathways to take the place of those that have been damaged (Cech & Martin, 1995). Recent evidence suggests that CNS plasticity now appears to be evident in adults as well (Gans, 1993). All of these neurophysical factors combine to influence the ability of the child to respond and benefit from rehabilitative interventions. Early intervention programs for children from birth to 3 years of age are designed to take advantage of these physiologic processes.

Other physiologic characteristics of the developing organism predispose children to a greater degree of "moldability" than adults. Bone growth and increases in osteogenesis result in more rapid healing after fracture, as well as easier correction of bony deformities such as clubfoot, which may be treated solely with splinting. Inhibitive casting of extremities in children with brain injury reduces the response of persistent primitive reflexes and can improve gait and coordination.

When a young child experiences injury to the CNS, the processes of neurodevelopment offer an advantage with regard to restoring lost function. However, as stated previously, the earlier in life the injury occurs, the more learning needs to take place before the child can achieve adult or near-adult development and function. If those CNS functions that are needed to learn, store, and retrieve new experiences are lost or significantly affected by the injury, the child's long-term outcomes will be poorer despite the inherent plasticity of the developing brain.

The theory of critical periods of development postulates that each developmental phase or domain has a critical period for achievement of developmental milestones. Prior to the critical period, body systems are not yet mature enough to enable the child to achieve the task. After the critical period has passed, if the developmental task has not been achieved, it will become either more difficult to achieve or the full functional potential of the task will not be achieved. This theory is discussed in more detail in Chapter 10. Rehabilitation interventions should be timed to take advantage of these critical periods in development whenever possible.

As children grow and develop, they increase and improve their abilities to perform functional tasks by adapting to their environment and cataloguing, integrating, and storing feedback from new experiences. Children who acquire a disabling condition later in childhood benefit from established skills, coping mechanisms, knowledge, relationships, and support systems already established, as well as the adaptation skills that come with a longer duration of life experience (Gilfoyle, Grady, & Moore, 1990). Although injury or disease may result in permanent losses in one or more functional areas, re-learning previously mastered skills may be somewhat easier than learning new skills with an altered physical and cognitive capacity. For example, the child who receives a head injury at 16 years of age already has a large repertoire of skills, information, and tried-and-true coping abilities. The 16-year-old must re-learn those skills and information, but due to his age and level of development, these abilities and capabilities are more established than in a child who is 2 years old. In many ways, the 16-year-old is more like an adult, since the majority of developmental tasks have been achieved. The 2-year-old child with a head injury has developed some skills in interacting with the environment but is extremely limited in life experience and still has many skills and a great amount of information to process and store before adulthood is reached. This young child is at a much greater disadvantage, having so much to learn and so many skills to develop in addition to recovering from a serious injury. The typical pattern of disability that occurs with head trauma (e.g., memory, processing of information, storage of information, and motor deficits) makes the process of attaining the functional skills needed to succeed in adulthood much more difficult and complicated. The younger the child is when the disability occurs, the longer the rehabilitation process will continue to take into account changes in function as a result of development. The components of memory, integration, and organization of information are crucial for learning. The less time the child has had to learn before the disabling event, the more information and skills still remain to be learned so that the child can function successfully in society. The child who experiences cognitive deficits at an early age is at great disadvantage as a result of altered memory, integration, and organization. With an altered cognitive ability, especially one of memory, learning is much more difficult to achieve, and the lack or delay of learning knowledge and functional skills

causes the greatest deficits for young children. In premature infants, the degree of risk of disability remains difficult to predict.

Another factor that is key to developmental progression is mobility and the ability to explore the environment. Infants and young children learn through experience, and movement is crucial to that process. In addition to the requirement for movement to develop strength and coordination, the initiation of purposeful movement requires both intent (i.e., a goal, such as bringing a toy to mouth), developmentally programmed behaviors (e.g., turning to suck, development of protective responses), and repeated experience. The interval from infancy through pre-school is a critical period for motor development. Rehabilitation interventions for young children with motor disabilities are focused on facilitating the child's mobility.

Both acute and ongoing rehabilitation services must take into account the amount and degree of change the child will undergo during continued growth and developmental periods. Interventions that take into account the child's level of development at the time of the injury must not stop at that point, but should continue to evolve to incorporate changes in growth and acquisition of developmental skills. Skill acquisition is often delayed or even prevented by injury, and interventions are designed to support the child's acquisition of developmentally appropriate skills as much as possible. An important part of rehabilitation interventions for children is providing adaptive equipment that will temporarily or permanently take the place of lost functions, such as communication devices, hearing aids, prostheses, and mobility and positioning devices.

Severity, Extent, and Location of Injury

Injury to the CNS is the most damaging type because of its effect on motor, sensory, and cognitive functions. Initial improvement results from reduction of swelling in brain or spinal cord tissue or removal of an impinging object such as a bone splinter. Some restoration of function may occur for months or even years after the initial injury. Although research is extensive in this area, there is as yet no definitive method to restore or re-grow damaged CNS cells, and there is no evidence that CNS tissue can heal itself (Farel & Hooper, 1995). What restoration occurs is thought to depend on development of reciprocal nerve pathways to take over the work of the damaged nerves or re-learning the performance of skills in different ways using different behavioral strategies (Farel & Hooper, 1995).

Severity, extent, and physical location of the condition or injury substantially affects the habilitation or rehabilitation process and interacts with other factors such as the child's age and level of development. A premature infant with large areas of porencephalic cysts in the brain has a poorer outcome than an infant with a grade I intraventricular bleed in the motor cortex (Allen, 1991), suggesting that the size of the affected area of the brain has a direct effect on outcome. Severity in children with head injury is measured by depth of coma, duration of impaired consciousness, and length of post-traumatic amnesia and is considered the major factor in outcome (Fletcher, Ewing-Cobbs, Francis, & Levin, 1995; Michaud, 1995). The presence of associated injuries to other organ systems, such as chest injury, is also a predictor of outcome in terms of survival in pediatric head injury (Michaud, Rivara, Grady, & Reay, 1992). In children with myelomeningocele, the level of the spinal cord dysfunction influences both short-term and long-term functional outcomes. Dysfunction at vertebral level L4-5 suggests the potential for more independence in mobility and self-care skills than in the child with a high thoracic myelomeningocele (Badell, 1992).

Health Status, Nutrition, and Intrinsic Biologic Factors

In addition to development, a child's state of health influences his or her ability to participate in and benefit from habilitation and rehabilitation. Health and development are intertwined—threats to the child's health, such as serious infections, are also threats to the child's development and growth. The adequacy of the child's immune system affects not only the ability to resist infection after an injury or diagnosis of a disabling condition, but can influence acquisition of a disabling condition. The child who is immunosuppressed, whether due to medications (e.g., chemotherapy for cancer), disease (e.g., HIV/AIDS), or an undiagnosed cause, is more vulnerable to infections from relatively benign sources. Cytomegalovirus, a minor flu-like condition in most people, causes serious infection in children with AIDS. Other infections that cause disabling conditions include meningitis and encephalitis, Guillain-Barré syndrome, and transverse myelitis.

The child's state of nutrition is also an important factor in rehabilitation (Molnar & Kellerman, 1992). Children with cerebral palsy may be unable to take in enough nutrients by mouth to meet the energy needs of their brain and body; this seriously hampers their rate of development and puts them at significant risk for infection, skin breakdown, and delayed growth. Burns and severe multiple trauma place tremendous metabolic and nutritional demands on the body. Supplemental nutrition and frequent analysis of the adequacy of nutritional factors is necessary to maintain life in the short term and to facilitate rehabilitation in the long term.

Other intrinsic biologic factors that influence outcomes in the child with a disability include presence or absence of other complicating medical conditions; genetic make-up, which includes inherited vulnerabilities and strengths as well as genetic disorders; the child's unique trajectory of growth; and the child's psychological and emotional make-up (Molnar & Kellerman, 1992), including his or her degree of resilience (Russell & Free, 1994; Morse, 1994). The term "dual diagnosis" is used to refer to an individual with a disability who also is diagnosed with a psychiatric condition or substance abuse. The presence of either diagnosis significantly complicates the rehabilitation process. Children who have a psychiatric condition as well as a physical disability must receive interventions that address both conditions as well as the interplay between the conditions. In the developmental disabilities literature, the term "diagnostic overshadowing" is used to refer to children and adults with developmental disabilities and concurrent psychopathology (White, Nichols, Cook, Spengler, Walker, & Look, 1995). Adolescents with a pre-existing history of substance abuse, perhaps even contributing to the disability, tend to have poorer outcomes with regard to self-care and independence and may experience a reduced quality of life (Hoeman, 1996). Another term, "multiple disability," is used to refer to children who have more than one major disabling condition. Children who are deaf and blind, who have both spinal cord and head injury, or who have multiple functional deficits due to genetic causes, teratogenic causes, or pre-natal infection, require creative and flexible comprehensive interdisciplinary rehabilitation services to meet their developmental needs.

Just as with any other child, the child who is born with a disabling condition or acquires a disability through trauma may have other unrelated medical conditions that require close supervision by a medical specialist. Conditions such as asthma, juvenile diabetes, cardiac disease, renal disease, or cancer require modification of interventions and often slow the child's progress through rehabilitation. Outcomes are formulated to include significant factors related to the child's medical condition as well as the disability. The child with diabetes must re-learn the self-care activities required for the diabetes as well as adapt to the functional deficits caused by the disability. Frequently a pediatric medical specialist such as an endocrinologist or cardiologist becomes a member of the rehabilitation team. Families who were accustomed to assisting the child in managing a medical condition, such as asthma, may become overwhelmed by the increased care needs of a spinal cord injury and may have more difficulty providing the child with the necessary support.

The genetic inheritance of the child determines his or her ability to adapt to the environment, potential life-span, and frequency and occurrence of disease, infections, and malignancies. Genetic make-up also determines the parameters within which a child's development unfolds. Factors such as the child's height, the age at which the child walks, and the child's intellectual development are influenced by the genes, chromosomes, and DNA sequences provided by the child's parents. As stated by Wright (1995), "Each person's individual genetic pattern forms the outside framework on which all aspects of health and illness interact" (p. 1114). The Human Genome Project, a long-term, international study to identify and map all of the genes in the human body, has located the specific genes, chromosomes, and sites on the chromosomes that are responsible for a number of genetic conditions that affect health. Even in the absence of a diagnosed genetic disorder, the child's genetic pattern interacts with environmental influences and other factors that affect the outcomes of the rehabilitation process.

Psychosocial Factors

Each child and family brings to the rehabilitation process a unique combination of personal characteristics, culture, coping mechanisms, and adaptation skills which will modify the short-term and long-term outcomes for the child. Although adults must adjust and adapt to their acquired disability only once, albeit for a long period during and after rehabilitation, children must re-adjust to the changes brought about by disability many times as their bodies and abilities change with development. Each developmental phase brings changes in expectations, physical size and abilities, functional skills, and social interactions. The typical transitions of childhood, such as moving up in school, changing friends and schoolmates as schools are changed, dating, formation of an independent identity, vocational planning, and entering the employment market, are made more demanding and stressful for the child as a result of the disability.

The presence or absence of several key psychosocial factors will in large part determine the success of the child and family in adapting and coping with the ongoing life changes in the presence of disability. All of the psychosocial factors discussed in this section interact to influence coping and adjustment in the child and family and therefore affect rehabilitation outcomes. More detailed information about psychosocial factors and coping in pediatric rehabilitation nursing can be found in Chapter 13.

The culture of the child and family and the degree of assimilation into the dominant or majority culture are key factors in adaptation and adjustment to disability. The term "culture" is used here not just to describe a particular nationality or ethnic heritage and beliefs, but also to describe the unique cultural blend that is special to each individual family. The use of the word "culture" in this way is based on the assumption that each family has their own individual culture, composed of ethnicity, life experiences, the methods used to communicate and solve problems in the family, and the child and family's beliefs about health, illness, roles of family members, and life goals. The family's culture will strongly influence their reactions to the disability, the changes that the child has experienced and will experience, and the efforts of the rehabilitation team. Depending on their culture, the family may perceive one aspect of the child's disability to have more or less importance to them, and focus more on or ignore that area during rehabilitation. Examples are families that value intellectual ability over mobility, and families that value the child's appearance, or visibility of the disability, over its functional effects.

Another cultural factor that influences the

rehabilitation process is the value the child and family place on independence (Hertzberg, 1993). The dominant belief systems in the United States value personal independence over almost anything else, as does the rehabilitation and health care service system. Many families and older children do not value independence as highly, but rather see themselves as part of a community, which exists primarily to provide support and meaning to the lives of its members. In this case, interdependence is the strongest value, with the expectation that family members, extended family, friends, and other members of the community will all work together to support each other. Often, differences between the cultural and health values of rehabilitation team members and the child and family can produce serious conflicts and misunderstandings that can jeopardize the effectiveness of the rehabilitation process. More information on family issues and cultural issues is provided in Chapter 9.

The concept of resilience applies both to children and families, and helps to determine their ability to successfully adapt to changes. Resilience is generally described as the ability to rebound and recover from stressful events, physical and emotional trauma, and adverse circumstances. Individuals and families who exhibit resilience are able to quickly recover strength, good spirits, and a positive attitude, which enables them to resume their lives in a normal way after physical or social setbacks. Resilience was first studied after World War II, when it was found that some concentration camp survivors were more able to cope with their experiences of suffering and loss than others, and were more successful with work, relationships, and families. The characteristic of resilience in children with disabilities and their families allows them to better cope with the often discouraging and frustrating experiences that accompany disability in this country. Experiences such as multiple losses, financial problems, repeated setbacks in health and development, fragmented health care, and the multiple challenges posed by changes in insurance coverage and managed care present children and families with almost unceasing stressors. Resilience is often seen in those children who grew up with adverse circumstances, such as poverty, an abusive family, or a disabling condition, and went on to become productive, happy members of their communities. The Center for Children with Chronic Illness and Disability has published a list of family strengths that are supportive of resilience that includes factors such as family size, attitudes, resources, relationships, modes of communication, beliefs, and the presence of additional stressors (Morse, 1994).

A concept that is closely related to resilience is that of locus of control. Individuals who exhibit an internal locus of control believe that they have control over life events and are able to influence outcomes. In contrast, external locus of control is based on the belief that external forces determine life events, and the individual has little ability to affect or change themselves or these events. Locus of control does not represent the single determining factor in a child or a family's ability to cope with or adjust to disability, but it is an important aspect that interacts with other psychosocial factors that influence coping. The child and family's locus of control influences the family's approach to the rehabilitation process and helps to determine whether they respond in a more passive manner, allowing others to lead in decision-making and implementation of the rehabilitation plan, or whether they "take charge," actively seeking information and participating as active members of the rehabilitation team. Often, nurses and other members of the rehabilitation team may make value judgments about which characteristic is more desirable and may favor an active, involved family over one that is less actively involved. This approach can bring about conflicts between the family and the rest of the rehabilitation team and can jeopardize a collaborative working relationship and rehabilitation outcomes. Although most of the research in this area has been done with adults, these concepts have occasionally been examined in children (Hoeman, 1996).

Environmental Factors

A crucially important factor that influences the child's habilitative or rehabilitative success, as well as development, is the environment. Environment is described as the conditions, circumstances, and influences surrounding and affecting the development of an organism. "Milieu" is the term used to describe the cultural and social environment. An optimal environment is one that promotes the most favorable potential for the attainment of desired outcomes.

Betz, Hunsberger, and Wright (1994) describe seven components of the social milieu and physical environment to portray the range of forces that influence a child's development and modify his or her outcome. Due to their importance as factors influencing rehabilitation, family and culture are also addressed later in this chapter and discussed in greater detail in Chapter 9.

The first component of the social milieu is culture and lifestyle. Culture describes the cultural and ethnic characteristics of the primary caregivers. Lifestyle refers to the family structure; that is, the relationship and configuration of family members and other caregivers within the home.

Family environment is the second component. Family interactions, parenting skills, roles and relationships of family members, birth order of children, and family size compose the family environment. The family environment is the most important influence on the young child and can make a major difference in both short-term and long-term outcomes for the child with a disability. Just as the child is influenced by the environment, so is the family. External and internal stressors such as finances, health and illness, role changes, work stresses, relational difficulties, social and cultural factors, and family relationships all shape the ability of the family to respond to the needs of its children.

The school milieu, which is the third component, encompasses influences of skill training, cultural transmission, and self-actualization that occur during the child's educational career from pre-school through high school. School is second only to the family in providing socialization and learning opportunities to the child. Increasingly, schools also provide health and rehabilitative care for children with disabilities or chronic conditions and are a key factor in discharge plans and long-term supportive services.

The characteristics of the world outside the home make up the neighborhood, the fourth component of the child's environment. This aspect of the environment is also often referred to as the community. Many neighborhoods today are no longer safe places for children and present even greater risks for children with disabilities. Increasing violence, traffic patterns, and the availability of illegal drugs all increase risk factors for children. Rural neighborhoods differ from urban neighborhoods with regard to availability of support and resources, safety risks, size, and diversity.

Socio-economic status is the fifth component of the social milieu. This term refers to the family income level. Families who are at or below the poverty line tend to have higher death rates, higher rates of disability, higher infant mortality, a greater incidence of accidents, less educational attainment, and are less likely to have private health insurance (Children's Defense Fund, 1995).

Mass media is the sixth component of the child's environment. Television is the major source of information about the world for most children, as well as a primary socializing tool. Violence and sex in television programs influence children's behavior, as well as their moral and ethical development. Television viewing takes the place of more active pursuits and interferes with family communication and problem solving. Children with disabilities often use television as their main source of entertainment and recreation.

The seventh component, the physical environment, is made up of the pre-natal environment and the external environment. The prenatal environment is the initial basis for child development. Maternal nutritional deficits, malpositioning of the fetus in the uterus, maternal metabolic and endocrine imbalances, teratogens ranging from radiation exposure to substance abuse, Rh incompatibility, and maternal infections set the stage for the neonate's initial attributes as well as for later development. The external physical environment, including safety factors, cleanliness, exposure to lead, contaminated food or water, weather, and presence or absence of pollution, affects the child's activity level, risk factors for illness or injury, and recreational options. Both the pre-natal environment and the external physical environment contribute factors that can either complicate or facilitate development and the habilitation or rehabilitation process.

Family

The family is the first, most crucial influence on the child, and can "make or break" the rehabilitation process. The love, direction, and support they give the child during the early developmental years determines in large part the characteristics of the adult. Family members direct and nurture the child based on their ability to provide food, shelter, and health care; respond in a timely manner to the child's basic physical and emotional needs; and provide a stimulating and safe environment for the child to explore and learn. The initial bonding of the child and family at the child's birth sets the stage for the establishment of trust and the later ability to relate to other human beings in fulfilling, reciprocal relationships. In addition to their genetic contributions, the family forms the basis for transmission of culture, including values, beliefs, spirituality, and world view. The developing child's behavior, life decisions, outlook, and ability to cope and adapt successfully to stressors and life events are primarily shaped by family influences. The skills and behaviors the child learns from the family in the first few years of life will determine his or her future success in interacting within the greater community and the world. Just as these crucial skills and behaviors affect the child's ability to function in the community, they also color the child's ability to use the input and information provided by nurses, therapists, educators, and other rehabilitation team members. Research suggests that in early intervention services for children at risk for or having disabilities, family support services are among the most effective interventions in producing desired developmental outcomes in both the short and long term (Guralnick, 1993). The scope of family issues that may relate to and result from the presence of a child with a disability is more thoroughly explored in Chapter 9.

Quality and Quantity of Intervention

The final factor is the efficacy of rehabilitation interventions and the skills and knowledge of the rehabilitation team. Although it is not clear whether or not rehabilitative or habilitative interventions actually accelerate the repair of damaged CNS tissue, it appears that the adaptive skills gained by the child and family increase function and improve coping. Despite their widespread use in practice, research has yet to demonstrate that pediatric rehabilitation medicine interventions actually produce the desired outcomes (Michaud, 1995). Despite the paucity of research-based foundations, rehabilitative and habilitative practice focuses on promoting appropriate skills by providing a developmental environment in which the child can receive the most benefit, based on past experience, clinical practice, and adaptation of interventions from developmental pediatrics and adult rehabilitation. Interventions may target the child directly, such as during physical, occupational, or speech therapy sessions, or may focus on the family, teaching them to provide the therapeutic environment once the child is discharged home.

Rehabilitation interventions are focused on retraining for lost skills, prevention of secondary disability and complications; and training in developing compensatory strategies (Michaud, 1995). Prevention of secondary disability is particularly important for children because of the inter-relationship of growth and development. Interventions must take into account the effects of changes in height, weight, and maturation over time. Activity levels may change both from improvement in the underlying condition and as a result of developmental and age-related causes. Whereas adults in rehabilitation can change quickly with regard to functional skills and repair of damaged tissues, children have the added aspects of developmental progression and maturation to take into consideration. Braces or assistive devices that take an extended period to fabricate or obtain may not fit when they are finally delivered due to the child's growth. Leg braces, canes, walkers, or wheelchairs must be evaluated at least once a year and sometimes more frequently if the child experiences a growth spurt. Rehabilitative or habilitative interventions do not stop when the child is discharged but must continue many years, often through early adulthood, via frequent and periodic evaluations of functioning, health, and developmental progress. Interventions, especially those for infants and younger children, are designed to use play to promote development and the achievement of functional goals. Risk of secondary conditions increases with age and maturation, just as the types of potential secondary disabilities change with age. When formulating goals and outcomes and planning interventions, nurses and other rehabilitation team members must draw on their knowledge of development, the ways that the specific disability affects and is affected by the development, and the child's personality, environment, functional skills, and needs.

The amount and timing of rehabilitation and habilitation interventions is also important. Emergency management and acute rehabilitation management of injury significantly affects outcomes. Surgical evacuation of subdural hematoma and timely management of CNS swelling and intracranial pressure are good examples of well-timed interventions. Accurate assessment skills and early detection of physiologic changes in the acute post-injury period are essential to pediatric rehabilitation nursing. In the neonatal period, prompt diagnosis of the disabling condition is crucial, as is prenatal diagnosis for genetic conditions.

In the past, the "more is better" approach often resulted in children receiving intensive therapies several times a day or two to three times weekly in outpatient programs. For children with developmental disabilities or those receiving outpatient therapy, the amount of time spent in therapy took up the majority of their and the families' time and energy and left little opportunity for other family activities, recreation, school, or play. Typical life activities were put aside for therapeutic interventions focused on functional goals, with less attention paid to the importance of friends and daily activities. Presently, the focus of interventions is changing, with more emphasis on services provided in typical, inclusive settings such as schools, child care centers, and homes. Restrictions in the availability of funding for pediatric rehabilitation services across the spectrum of settings have also influenced the frequency and timing of rehabilitation and habilitation interventions provided by hospital-based centers and community service providers.

Early intervention services promote development in infants and young children who are at risk for delays or disability. To be successful, early intervention services must be coordinated, comprehensive, community-based, and family centered. According to the Individuals With Disabilities Education Act (IDEA), children from birth through 3 years of age are most likely to benefit from therapeutic interventions aimed at preventing disability or reducing the severity of disabling conditions. Therapeutic services that fall within the scope of early intervention include:

- newborn screening and developmental screening of young children
- identification of congenital conditions
- early detection of sensory impairments
- identification of children who are at increased risk for developmental delay due to environmental factors
- therapeutic intervention for all identified delays and risk factors, particularly for premature and low birth weight infants
- provision of family support services (Bennett, 1984).

Provision of early intervention services is based on the following assumptions:

All development is influenced by early experience.

Each child's development is the product of the complex and crucial interaction of genetic, biologic, and environmental factors.

Sensitive or critical periods exist for the development of specific skills that correspond with rapid and maximal CNS growth and development that occur in the first 3 years of life, such as speech, fine and gross motor strength and coordination, and cognition.

Gaps or delays in development tend to increase over time; that is, the older and more mature a child becomes, the greater the developmental delay appears when compared with peers.

Early sensory deprivation from visual or hearing deficits results in loss of many functional skills and significantly interferes with the ability to learn (Bennett, 1984).

There are many factors that influence outcome in pediatric rehabilitation nursing that are both common to the majority of children in rehabilitation and unique to individuals. The pediatric rehabilitation nurse takes into account the range of influences on the child with a disability and his or her family when designing interventions and formulating outcomes for both acute and long-term rehabilitation services.

REHABILITATION NURSING CARE: KEY DIFFERENCES BETWEEN CHILDREN AND ADULTS

Understanding the unique interactions of aspects of growth, development, and maturation, with common areas of functional intervention addressed in rehabilitation, is critical to the competent performance of pediatric rehabilitation nursing. Discussion of the key differences between adults and children can assist with this understanding (Table 7–1).

Children are not just little adults. Because of the influences of growth, development, and maturation; differences in timing of services; goals of services and interventions; frequency of follow-up appointments; and availability of caregivers; rehabilitation team members require additional knowledge and skills to competently provide care. As stated in Chapter 1, disabling conditions in children may be either congenital (i.e., a condition identified at birth) or acquired (i.e., conditions resulting from trauma or disease). Gans (1993) identified three temporal patterns of conditions commonly seen in pediatric rehabilitation. The conditions can be categorized as transient, static, or progressive. Transient conditions occur, are treated or run their course, and gener-

Text continued on page 105

Table 7-1   PHYSIOLOGIC DIFFERENCES BETWEEN CHILDREN AND ADULTS

Physiologic Characteristics	Implications for Care
Cardiac Function	
Congenital heart defects ranging from mild (patent ductus arteriosus) to severe (tetralogy of Fallot) may affect cardiac function and result in pulmonary hypertension, congestive heart failure, and the child's ability to eat, grow, and develop.	Review the medical record, and question parents as to the presence of underlying cardiac conditions. When designing interventions, allow for more time to eat, frequent rest periods, and increased monitoring of response to activity.
In infants, the heart is located higher in the chest, because the diaphragm is higher and the rib cage is shorter. The apical impulse is located at the 5th intercostal space in infants and at the 4th or 5th intercostal space in older children. The thin chest wall allows for easier auscultation of chest sounds.	Assessment of cardiac function must take into account the differences in anatomic location of cardiac landmarks. Physiologic murmurs are common.
Normal heart rates are higher in infants than in older children and adults, and blood pressure is lower in infancy.	Charts indicating age-normed heart rates and blood pressure measurements should be used. Blood pressure cuffs should be chosen for the arm and leg size and age of the child. For arm cuffs, the bladder should be two thirds the length of the upper arm; for the lower extremity, the bladder should be two thirds the length of the thigh.
Respiratory System	
Diaphragmatic abdominal breathing predominates in the neonatal period through 5 years of age.	Dressings, braces, casts, or splints that restrict abdominal movement will restrict breathing. Be aware that signs of respiratory distress are different in young children.
Respiratory rate in children is increased, especially in infants; irregular rate of breathing is the norm in very young children.	Use charts listing normal rates for age, and be aware of normal variations in respiratory rate.
A very supple chest wall leads to retractions (pulling in of the skin around the sub-sternal area, supra-clavicular area, and ribs) with respiratory distress; circumoral cyanosis is a late sign of respiratory distress.	Be aware of the different signs of respiratory distress in young children. Remove clothing to observe chest for respiratory effort; pulse oximetry is a reliable indicator of poor oxygenation in children.
Children exhibit greater oxygen consumption and increased heat loss, resulting in an increased metabolic rate.	Oxygen flow rate will vary based on age, size, and condition; children exhibit respiratory distress much more rapidly than adults. An increased metabolic rate may result in even more increases in oxygen consumption.
Infants are obligate nose breathers for the first 3 weeks of life and have a large tongue. The larynx is placed 2 to 3 vertebrae higher than in the adult.	Anything that causes nasal obstruction (nasogastric tube feedings, nasal congestion, bedding) will compromise oxygenation and breathing.
Mucous membranes are extremely vascular in children, who have more soft tissue and less cartilage.	Results in an increased susceptibility to trauma and disease. Airways are more likely to collapse with tracheal injury due to intubation or tracheostomy.

Table continued on following page

Table 7–1 PHYSIOLOGIC DIFFERENCES BETWEEN CHILDREN AND ADULTS *Continued*

Physiologic Characteristics	Implications for Care
Respiratory System *Continued*	
Airways in children are much smaller than those in adults, creating four times the air resistance as that in adults.	Children are more vulnerable to injury to the airways with invasive procedures such as tracheostomy and suctioning. There is an increased risk of respiratory infection and of obstruction with edema, further compromising the airway. Hospitals, clinics, emergency departments, emergency medical systems, schools, or other community agencies must keep appropriately sized emergency equipment on hand.
Fluid and Electrolyte Balance	
The young child has a high ratio of body surface area to body volume.	Fluid loss progresses rapidly in young children and most rapidly in infants. Young children with diarrhea, high fever, or vomiting must be monitored closely for signs of dehydration such as dry mucous membranes, "tenting" of skin, infrequent urination, inability to produce tears, and severe lethargy leading to coma.
Infants are unable to concentrate urine until 3 months of age.	Specific gravities are low, and urine tends to be dilute. There is an increased risk of dehydration and metabolic imbalance.
Young children are unable to process large quantities of fluid at a time.	Younger children are at a greater risk for fluid volume excess when receiving intravenous fluids. Fluid and electrolyte losses must be made up carefully by following standard guidelines for pediatric fluid maintenance and rehydration.
Immune System	
Young children, especially infants, have a diminished mucosal resistance to organisms. Near-adult levels of resistance are reached by 2 to 5 years of age.	Disease is easily transmitted through mucous membranes by mouthing of toys and other objects. Young children have an average of 7 to 10 respiratory infections per year.
Neonates and infants have an immature immune system.	Severe infections develop rapidly in young children. Symptoms such as a fever of 100°F–101°F and lethargy in infants younger than 4 months are likely to suggest a severe infection such as meningitis or sepsis.
Increased lymphatic tissue in the growing child results in a relatively pronounced response to infection.	Enlarged lymph nodes are a common finding in children, even several weeks after an infection. Children with immune system deficits may have chronically enlarged lymph nodes.
Laboratory values vary with age as well as with gender, and differ among neonates and infants, older children and adolescents, and adults. Young children tend to respond to infection with an increased neutrophil count, greater than that seen in older children and adults.	Laboratory value charts for children should be consulted when attempting to determine normal values.
Hematologic System	
Normal hemoglobin and hematocrit vary with age and gender, as do all types of blood cells. Young children tend to show an increased neutrophil count with increased numbers of immature neutrophils with infection.	Knowledge of normal blood counts for age and variation with disease is critical. Charts that are normed for age and gender should be used.

Table 7–1   PHYSIOLOGIC DIFFERENCES BETWEEN CHILDREN AND ADULTS *Continued*

Physiologic Characteristics	Implications for Care
Hematologic System *Continued*	
Rapid growth in early childhood results in an increased risk of iron deficiency anemia due to the immature hematopoietic system.	Yearly monitoring of hemoglobin and hematocrit in young children is necessary; adequate nutrition includes iron-rich or iron-enriched foods.
Gastrointestinal System	
Infants are predisposed to increased gastric motility, decreased gastric emptying, and gastroesophageal reflux.	Infant feeding practices reflect these physiologic characteristics. These factors should be considered when supplementing diets with nasogastric or gastrostomy feedings to prevent side effects such as aspiration from reflux, regurgitation, and diarrhea.
The infant's metabolic rate is higher than that in older children and adults.	The metabolic rate increases even more with illness or injury and may result in the need for supplemental tube feedings or parenteral nutrition.
Infants have a decreased gag reflex.	Nasogastric tube insertion is somewhat easier; orogastric tubes are used frequently in premature and term infants. Choking may be a greater risk with rapid oral feeds.
Infants younger than 1 year old have increased permeability of the intestines.	This factor is theorized to be the basis for the infant's greater susceptibility to allergic gastrointestinal problems.
The young child's rectal and intestinal mucosa is thin and easily traumatized.	Use dietary interventions first when treating constipation. If enemas or suppositories are necessary, slow, careful administration of enema solutions and suppositories is indicated.
In infants and young children, feeding is associated with oral gratification and meeting emotional and social needs as well as growth and development.	Conditions or procedures that interfere with the feeding process between mother and infant disrupt the infant's and family's well being and may affect attachment and development.
The immature liver is less able to detoxify substances.	Medication dosages and frequencies require careful monitoring and calculation of the appropriate dosage by weight or body surface area. Children receive lower doses of medications and may require longer intervals between dosing. Long-term medications must be changed with changes in growth.
Neurologic System	
Due to the immaturity of the neurologic system, involving changes in the numbers of axons, dendrites, production of neurotransmitters, and myelination, neurologic status in young children may change quickly, and changes may be difficult to detect.	Young children are not able to communicate as easily as older children, making detection of changes in neurologic function more difficult. Often, the only early signs of neurologic deterioration are lethargy, irritability, or anorexia.
In infants, sutures are not fused and fontanels are open, with the anterior fontanel closing at around 10 to 12 months and the posterior fontanel closing at about 3 to 4 months of age.	Increased intracranial pressure may be detected in young children by the presence of a bulging fontanel and increased head size. Nystagmus and lethargy may also be seen with increased intracranial pressure.
Developmental differences in the ability to communicate make it more difficult to assess changes in level of consciousness following injury.	To assess coma in children, use age-normed scales such as the Glasgow Coma Scale for Verbal Response in Infants or the Rancho Los Amigos Pediatric Coma Scale.

Table continued on following page

Table 7-1 PHYSIOLOGIC DIFFERENCES BETWEEN CHILDREN AND ADULTS *Continued*

Physiologic Characteristics	Implications for Care
Neurologic System *Continued*	
Brain wave patterns become more organized and rhythmic, increasing in frequency and decreasing in amplitude.	Electroencephalogram readings that are normal for young children may suggest abnormalities in adolescents.
The immature neurologic system is more vulnerable to trauma.	Thirty percent of all seizure disorders begin before 4 years of age. Infants between 6 weeks and 3 years of age are more likely to experience febrile seizures.
The terminus of the spinal cord changes in vertebral level from infancy to adulthood. In newborns, the cord terminates at L3, and in adults at L1-2.	Tethering of the cord may result in neurologic degeneration due to growth in children with dysfunction of the spinal cord.
Musculoskeletal System	
Children's bones contain more cartilage, are more porous, and contain an active growth area (the epiphyseal growth plate).	Due to increased cartilage, fractures in children may be more difficult to detect. Additionally, fractures across the growth plate are more difficult to detect due to its appearance on x-ray films. Due to the presence of the growth plate and the ongoing process of growth, bones tend to remodel quickly after fracture, and some angulation may self-correct. However, rotational deformities are less likely to correct on their own. Fractures through the growth plate may result in angulation of the bone or injury to the growth plate itself, resulting in cessation of growth in that area. Long bones, since they are more porous, tend to absorb more energy before breaking and are more likely to bow than fracture.
The periosteum is thicker and more richly supplied with blood in children.	Greenstick fractures are more common. Fractures heal more quickly due to the rich blood supply.
Ligaments are more lax in the spine.	Spinal cord injuries may occur without bony malformation on x-ray films. Hyperflexion of the neck in infants, which may occur with cardiopulmonary resuscitation, can cause spinal cord injury.
Soft tissues surrounding joints are more elastic.	Sprains and dislocations are unusual with normal activity.

Data from Cusson, R. (1994). Altered digestive function. In C. Betz, M. Hunsberger, & S. Wright (Eds.). *Family-centered nursing care of children* (2nd ed.). Philadelphia: WB Saunders; Daberkow-Carson, E., & Smith, P. (1994). Altered cardiovascular function. In C. Betz, M. Hunsberger, & S. Wright (Eds.). *Family-centered nursing care of children* (2nd ed.). Philadelphia: WB Saunders; Disabato, J., & Wulf, J. (1994). Altered neurologic function. In C. Betz, M. Hunsberger, & S. Wright (Eds.). *Family-centered nursing care of children* (2nd ed.). Philadelphia: WB Saunders; Gans, B. (1993). Rehabilitation of the pediatric patient. In J.A. DeLisa & B.M. Gans (Eds.). *Rehabilitation medicine: principles and practice* (2nd ed.). Philadelphia: JB Lippincott; Hunsberger, M., & Feenan, L. (1994). Altered respiratory function. In C. Betz, M. Hunsberger, & S. Wright (Eds.). *Family-centered nursing care of children* (2nd ed.). Philadelphia: WB Saunders; Leonard, M. (1994). Altered hematologic function. In C. Betz, M. Hunsberger, & S. Wright, (Eds.). *Family-centered nursing care of children* (2nd ed.). Philadelphia: WB Saunders; Mason, K., & Wright, S. (1994). Altered musculoskeletal function. In C. Betz, M. Hunsberger, & S. Wright (Eds.). *Family-centered nursing care of children* (2nd ed.). Philadelphia: WB Saunders; Nicol, N., & Hill, M. (1994). Altered skin integrity. In C. Betz, M. Hunsberger, & S. Wright (Eds.). *Family-centered nursing care of children* (2nd ed.). Philadelphia: WB Saunders; Snyder, P. (1994). Fractures. In A. Maher, S. Salmond, & T. Pellino (Eds.). *Orthopedic nursing.* Philadelphia: WB Saunders; Vigneux, A., & Hunsberger, M. (1994). Altered gastrointestinal and renal function. In C. Betz, M. Hunsberger, & S. Wright (Eds.). *Family-centered nursing care of children* (2nd ed.). Philadelphia: WB Saunders.

ally leave little or no long-term sequelae. Static conditions are those that, once they occur, do not change with regard to the initial causative event, even though growth and development may cause changes in function. Progressive conditions result in deterioration of the affected system with progressive loss of function, and may end in death. Each type of condition requires a different focus of rehabilitation interventions. Examples of transient conditions are brachial plexus injury (congenital) and Guillain-Barré syndrome (acquired); examples of static conditions include cerebral palsy (congenital) and traumatic brain injury (acquired); and examples of progressive conditions include muscular dystrophy (congenital) and juvenile rheumatoid arthritis (acquired).

Children and adults differ with regard to the parameters to be measured at regular visits. In addition to height and weight, measurement of head circumference and, in very young children, chest circumference is necessary. Children's height, weight, and head circumference at different points in time are measured against standard growth charts to determine if physical growth is occurring at the rate and in the amount necessary for development of vital organs. Head growth is especially important because it implies adequate progression of brain development. Growth may vary from anticipated patterns, with a series of growth spurts and plateaus. The greatest changes in growth occur prenatally and during adolescence. Children grow more quickly during the summer months, which suggests that adjustments in orthotic and prosthetic equipment should be scheduled in the fall (Gans, 1993). Normal measurements for vital signs and other physiologic functions, including those measured by laboratory tests, change with age. In addition to measuring the child's progression of functional skills over time at each visit, comparison of the appropriateness of those skills with age-related norms is necessary to obtain a true picture of the child's developmental status.

Functional Areas of Difference Between Children and Adults

Mobility

With children, it is important to follow the developmental sequence with regard to mobility. For example, it is necessary to focus on development of head control before trunk control, trunk control before limb control, and gross motor control before fine motor control. Generally, children who are unable to walk independently will get braces around 1 to 2 years of age and will receive a mobility device, such as a wheelchair, at about 2 years of age. Most often, families and children put forth most effort developing mobility skills in the first 8 to 10 years of the child's life. Walking, in particular, is less energy intensive when the child's weight is lower than when it is higher. Therefore, it is typical for children with early onset disabilities, such as cerebral palsy and spina bifida, who were able to walk with braces during childhood, to move to wheelchair use in their early teens. A wheelchair is easier for adolescents to use than heavy leg braces.

It is generally accepted among rehabilitation specialists that facilitating a child's mobility by using assistive devices such as a manual or electric wheelchair does not frustrate the desire to walk; conversely, it allows the child to develop what mobility is possible and thus to develop more rapidly in other domains.

The ability to move and to explore the environment is crucial to learning and to development in all domains. Use of switch-controlled toys offers the mobility-limited child the opportunity for control and facilitates feelings of mastery and competence that are crucial to the development of self-esteem and social and academic skills. Therefore, mobility takes on the added importance of providing the crucial basis from which the child begins to learn about the world and his or her role in it.

At any age, especially the earlier years when growth changes occur rapidly, equipment must be changed frequently. This involves considerable expense to the family, both for frequent clinic visits and for new equipment. Assessment of the adequacy of size and strength of braces or other assistive devices must occur frequently and in a timely manner to prevent complications such as injuries, pressure ulcers, or joint deformity. In young children, assessment should occur at least every 6 months until school age, when regular assessments are performed on a yearly basis. Families are instructed to contact the provider whenever the earliest signs of problems are detected.

Self-Care

The earliest skills for young children involve meeting basic needs, such as eating, comfort, and protection. Getting needs met depends on the infant's ability to signal the caregiver and the caregiver's accurate interpretation of what each signal represents. Anyone who has experienced an infant's cry and a parent's response understands the complicated process of determining what that cry means—whether the child is hungry, lonely, wet, or scared—and how to adequately satisfy the need being expressed.

Because self-care in children is primarily provided by parents and other caregivers, much of the task of the pediatric rehabilitation nurse involves teaching parents to more accurately read the child's cues and provide just enough assistance to stimulate the child's development of self-care skills. Allowing the child to perform those skills that are developmentally appropriate for both the child's age as well as for his or her ability is crucial for progression of self-care skills. Teaching parents how to best support their child, without "overdoing" and while encouraging the development of independence, is often challenging. However, competency in self-care is developed through accurate assessments of a child's ability, coupled with the opportunity to fail sometimes and to learn from mistakes. Appropriate praise and encouragement facilitate the process. This is the way all children learn and develop mastery over self-care skills, whether or not they have disabilities.

Skin Care

Young children usually experience fewer problems with skin breakdown than do older children and adults. As infants, the greatest risk for skin breakdown is with diaper rash in infants with musculoskeletal problems requiring casts. Casts, especially body casts used for children with dislocated hips, which are common with early spinal cord dysfunction, may easily become soiled with stool or urine and are difficult to clean, resulting in skin breakdown underneath the cast. Infants with spinal cord dysfunction often leak stool constantly, resulting in severe diaper-area dermatitis and infection of surgical repair sites or the open lesions that may occur with myelomeningocele. As continence is established with appropriate bladder and bowel management, these skin problems decrease.

At any age, bony prominences present a risk for skin breakdown if exposed to undue pressure. Younger children, who are smaller and lighter, have less problems with skin breakdown. Children who wear leg braces or

limb prostheses may exhibit pressure areas or sores on bony prominences of the feet and legs or on the stump. Just as with adults, extremes of body weight, either overweight or underweight, contribute to an increased risk of skin breakdown. Another common site for skin breakdown in children who are kept supine after traumatic injury (e.g., the acute phase following cervical spinal cord injury) is the occiput of the head (Gans, 1993).

Children with sensory deficits of the skin are more prone to injury from burns. Hot liquids, such as coffee; sun exposure; objects that absorb heat, such as metal car seat belt buckles and metal playground equipment; heating sources, such as space heaters or radiators; and bath water that has not been checked for temperature, can all cause burns requiring medical care and even surgery. Additionally, winter brings the risk of frostbite if hands and feet are not adequately protected.

Increases in size and weight and hormonally mediated changes in skin and apocrine glands contribute to increased risk of pressure sores during puberty, particularly in wheelchair users. When children with spinal cord dysfunction switch from using leg braces to using a wheelchair for mobility, they are often unaware of the increased risks of unrelieved sitting and may develop large, deep pressure ulcers on the ischial tuberosities, sacrum, or trochanters.

Bowel and Bladder Care

Although there is a tendency to assume that infants with spinal cord dysfunction do not require bowel or bladder intervention because they will not develop control until around age 2 years, waiting until the typical maturational processes have occurred may result in life-long renal and intestinal complications. It is extremely important to evaluate the bladder and kidney function of young children to detect early signs of reflux, hydronephrosis, and sphincter-detrusor dys-synergia and for the pediatric rehabilitation nurse to be aware of the findings and integrate them into the care plan. Kidney damage from impaired bladder function can progress very quickly even in very young children and can jeopardize later kidney function as well as significantly shorten the life span (Badell, 1992). Infants with myelomeningocele have been diagnosed with urinary retention and reflux as young as 1 to 2 months of age.

Constipation is best addressed early in life. Young children with spinal cord dysfunction may experience chronic, lifelong problems with bowel management if early constipation is not corrected. Cerebral palsy and other neurologic conditions may affect smooth muscle as well as skeletal muscle, resulting in muscle weakness, flaccid colon, and chronic constipation. Nutritional deficits in young children with disabilities frequently complicate bowel dysfunction. Both bowel and bladder function suffer when children do not have adequate fluid intake.

Children with cognitive deficits benefit from timed bowel and bladder programs to aid in their awareness of bodily sensations and appropriately timed elimination. Even children with significant cognitive delays can learn from a consistent behavioral program.

Children should be on a consistent bowel and bladder program and out of diapers by school age at the latest. Strategies to achieve this may include medications, behavioral programs, surgical interventions, and devices such as external catheters or collectors and clean intermittent catheterization (Boyd & Perrin, 1992). As with other types of rehabilitative and assistive equipment, size is extremely important when considering the use of bowel and bladder aids. A wide range of supplies are available for urinary and bowel care, and careful selection of products and size of the products is recommended. Many assistive products come in pediatric sizes.

Spasticity

Children with neurologic deficits such as spinal cord injury, cerebral palsy, and neuromuscular disease are also at risk for spasticity and its complications. Children are more sensitive to side effects of medications such as Valium and baclofen, because the sedation effect may interfere with school achievement and learning. Other CNS side effects of medications for spasticity, such as hallucinations, are seen more frequently in children (Gans, 1993).

Physical modalities such as positioning, inhibitive casting, and bracing are more effective in children for reduction of spasticity. Other more invasive methods for managing spasticity in children include phenol or botulin toxin motor point blocks, selective dorsal rhizotomy for spasticity associated with cerebral palsy, and other surgical methods (Gans, 1993; Morrison, Hertzberg, Gourley, & Matthews, 1989).

Social Interaction and Behavior

Children often experience changes in coping, behavior, and developmental competence with hospitalization. These reactions to hospitalization may occur in children who enter the hospital due to traumatic injury resulting in disability or in children with a pre-existing disability who enter the hospital for corrective surgery or procedures. All children who are hospitalized for any reason experience many of the same stressors, such as separation from parents, other caregivers, and friends; pain and discomfort from the injury or illness and required treatments; loss of control, mobility, and competence; unknown and unfamiliar people and events and changes in usual daily routine; and unclear expectations (Wilson, 1994). When hospitalization occurs after trauma, these effects can be worsened as a result of the emotional stress of the initial injury, the changes in awareness of self and others that may result from the trauma, and the usually lengthy hospitalization. For children with disability, the loss of developing independence is often the most traumatic result of hospitalization. Reactions to hospitalization may take the form of developmental regression (more common in infants and young children); changes in temperament, such as an active aggressive child becoming passive and withdrawn; and changes in behavior and coping. Developmental regression is most often seen in young children or children with cognitive delay who enter the hospital for corrective surgery. Older children may use different behaviors to cope, ranging from aggression to withdrawal.

Development of social skills is jeopardized when children are absent from school and playmates for long periods during hospitalization and when opportunities for interaction with typically developing peers are lessened or lost by segregated school and community settings. Adolescents with disabilities are at greater risk for drug and alcohol abuse, dangerous sexual behavior, and gang involvement due to lack of appropriate social skills and low self-esteem. Body image is often significantly affected in adolescents with both visible and non-visible disabilities and chronic conditions, as are feelings of self-consciousness and inadequacy regarding sexuality (Davis, Anderson, Linkowski, Berger, & Feinstein, 1991). As peer relationships become increasingly important and looking and acting different become less acceptable, adolescent at-risk behavior increases (Hoeman, 1996).

Adolescents with disabilities or chronic conditions may choose "non-traditional" methods of asserting their independence, such as failing to perform self-care skills. Although in some cases failure to perform self-care becomes more of a nuisance for parents and health providers, it can also cause significant illness or complications in the adolescent, or may even lead to death. Social and psychological interventions may be required in these situations.

Cognitive Function and Learning

One of the most significant effects on the life prospects of the child with a disability is the impairment of learning in both academic and social arenas. Children with disabilities affecting cognition should receive special education consultation and should be included in typical classrooms with the supports they need to participate in the environment. With CNS injury or disability, difficulties with attention, visual and sensory perception, memory, and reasoning frequently occur. Speech problems significantly interfere with school performance and peer interaction. Every child who is unable to communicate through either verbal speech or some type of sign language should receive an evaluation for augmentative communication (Soifer, 1992).

Physiology

Children are more vulnerable to changes in physiologic stability during illness, injury, or hospitalization. Children in community settings who are dependent on mechanical ventilation or have suppressed immune systems due to their disability may be more vulnerable to illness or injury due to the combined effects of disability and physiologic immaturity. Especially in very young children, the effects of infection, fluid imbalance, and metabolic changes develop and progress much more rapidly than in adults. Hospital units, clinics, emergency departments, and other sites where children with disabilities receive health and rehabilitation services must be aware of these critical differences and have the proper equipment, staff training, and policies and procedures in place to care for this population.

Developmental differences in respiration include variations in both size and function. Diaphragmatic abdominal breathing predominates from the neonatal period through about 5 years of age. In very young infants, normal breathing is irregular and much more rapid than that in adults, even at rest. In infants, an early sign of increased respiratory effort can be identified by observing retractions, or pulling in of the skin around the ribs and sub-sternal and sub-clavicular area. Airways in children are much smaller than those in adults, creating four times the air resistance and increasing the risk of obstruction or collapse with respiratory insult. Children also exhibit higher oxygen consumption and increased heat loss, resulting in an increased metabolic rate. These differences result in an elevated risk of respiratory infection, anoxia, metabolic changes, and other airway problems in children with disabilities (Hunsberger & Feenan, 1994).

Cardiac function in children is affected both by the potential presence of congenital heart defects (which may be accompanied by congestive heart failure) and structural differences. Infants respond rapidly to changes in cardiac output with tachycardia, and they have much higher heart rates than older children and adults. Blood pressure varies with age, and cuffs should be sized appropriately for the size and the age of the child (Daberkow-Carson & Smith, 1994).

Fluid loss progresses more quickly than in adults because of the high ratio of body surface area to body volume in infants and young children. Even minor acute conditions that involve diarrhea and vomiting can cause rapid and severe dehydration. If the condition is accompanied by a fever, dehydration occurs even more rapidly, often within hours. Infants are unable to concentrate urine until 3 months of age, resulting in low specific gravities and an increased risk of dehydration. Additionally, young children cannot process large quantities of fluid and thus are at a greater risk for fluid volume excess when receiving intravenous fluids. Fluid and electrolyte losses must be made up carefully by following standard guidelines for pediatric fluid maintenance and rehydration (Vigneax & Hunsberger, 1994).

Infants have a diminished mucosal resistance to organisms, resulting in easy transmission of disease through mucous membranes by mouthing toys and other objects that other young children have come into contact with. Near-adult levels of disease resistance are reached by 2 to 5 years of age. Neonates are more susceptible to rapidly developing severe infections due to their immature immune response. A child younger than 4 months of age with a high fever and lethargy is generally evaluated for sepsis. Young children tend to respond to infection with an increased neutrophil count, greater than that seen in older children and adults. Laboratory values vary with age as well as with gender, and differ among neonates and infants, older children and adolescents, and adults (Nicol & Hill, 1994; Leonard, 1994).

Children of African-American, Mediterranean, Asian, Indian, and Middle Eastern descent are at risk for sickle cell disease. Cardio-vascular accident is a particularly severe complication of this genetic disease. If the child's sickle cell status is unknown and the child is in one of these high-risk groups, the issue of screening should be broached with the parents. In children who have sickle cell disease, a sickle cell crisis may be brought about by infection, dehydration, fever, or other physical and emotional stressors that may occur during hospitalization or rehabilitation (Leonard, 1994).

Altered gastric activity in infants predisposes them to increased motility, decreased gastric emptying, and gastroesophageal reflux. Infants' metabolic rate, which is already much higher than that in older children or adults, increases significantly with illness or injury and may result in the need for tube feedings or parenteral nutrition. The immature liver, most especially in infants, detoxifies substances inadequately. Medication administration requires careful monitoring and calculation of proper dosage by weight or body surface area (Cusson, 1994).

Neurologic status in infants and young children may change quickly, and such changes are difficult to detect. Often only behavioral changes such as lethargy, irritability, or anorexia are observed before serious illness sets in. A bulging fontanel in infants, nystagmus, and lethargy may be the only signs of increased intracranial pressure in a child with hydrocephalus. The terminus of the spinal cord changes in vertebral level from infancy to adulthood. In newborns, the cord terminates at L3, and in adults at L1-2; this may cause tethering and neurologic degeneration in children with dysfunction of the spinal cord. Brain wave patterns become more organized and rhythmic, increasing in frequency and decreasing in amplitude, as the child ages. Electroencephalogram readings that are normal for young children may suggest abnormalities in adolescents. In assessing coma in children up to 12 years of age, modified scales based on the Glasgow Coma Scale are used, such as the Glasgow Coma Scale for Verbal Response in Infants and the Rancho Los Amigos Pediatric Coma Scale (Gans, 1993; Disabato & Wulf, 1994).

Children's bones contain more cartilage and are more porous than the bones of adults, and they contain an active growth area known as the epiphyseal growth plate. Bones heal more quickly in children due to a thicker periosteum, which provides a rich blood supply. Due to the rich blood supply, callus forms more quickly. Bones remodel quickly after fracture, correcting some angulation deformities but not rotational deformities. Long bones are more likely to bow than fracture because they are able to absorb more energy before breaking, and greenstick fractures, with some intact periosteum, are more common in children than in adults. Sprains and dislocations are unusual with normal activity because soft tissues are more resilient in children. Radiologic evaluation of children's fractures is more difficult because of the large amount of cartilage present, and fractures may be missed (Mason & Wright, 1994; Snyder, 1994).

SUMMARY

This chapter reviews the basic concepts necessary to understand and implement quality, comprehensive pediatric rehabilitation nursing care. Current conceptual models used in interdisciplinary rehabilitation and habilitation services and research are presented. Outcomes and those factors contributing to outcomes in pediatric rehabilitation are discussed. Differences in considerations and interventions for children and adults with respect to rehabilitation care are reviewed. The unique effects of growth and development on the disabling process and habilitation and rehabilitation interventions for children are explored.

REFERENCES

Albrecht, G. (1992). *The disability business: rehabilitation in America.* Newberry Park, CA: Sage Publications.

Allen, B., & Ferguson, R. (1985). Cervical spine trauma in children. In D. Bradford & R. Hensinger (Eds.). *The pediatric spine.* New York: Thieme.

Allen, M. (1991). Prematurity. In A. Capute & P. Accardo (Eds.). *Developmental disabilities in infancy and childhood.* Baltimore: Paul H. Brookes.

Badell, A. (1992). Myelodysplasia. In G. Molnar (Ed.). *Pediatric rehabilitation.* Baltimore: Williams & Wilkins.

Badley, E. (1995). The genesis of handicap: definition, models of disablement, and role of external factors. *Disability and Rehabilitation, 17*(2), 53–62.

Bennett, F. (1984). Early intervention: rationales and practical guidelines to prevent or ameliorate developmental disabilities. *Children are Different: Behavioral Development Monograph Series Number 10.* Columbus, OH: Ross Laboratories.

Betz, C.L., Hunsberger, M., & Wright, S. (1994). Development of children. In C.L. Betz, M. Hunsberger, & S. Wright (Eds.). *Family-centered nursing care of children* (2nd ed.). Philadelphia: WB Saunders.

Boyd, J., & Perrin, J. (1992). Spinal cord injury. In G. Molnar (Ed.). *Pediatric rehabilitation.* Baltimore: Williams & Wilkins.

Campbell, A. (1977). Subjective measures of well-being. In G. Albee & J. Joffe (Eds.). *Primary prevention of psychopathology (vol. 1), the issues.* Hanover, NH: University Press of New England.

Cech, D., & Martin, S. (1995). *Functional movement development across the life span.* Philadelphia: WB Saunders.

Children's Defense Fund. (1995). *The state of America's children yearbook.* Washington, DC: Children's Defense Fund.

Coster, W., & Haley, S. (1992). Conceptualization and measurement of disablement in infants and young children. *Infants and Young Children,* 4(4): 11–22.

Cusson, R. (1994). Altered digestive function. In C.L. Betz, M. Hunsberger, & S. Wright (Eds.). *Family-centered nursing care of children* (2nd ed.). Philadelphia: WB Saunders.

Daberkow-Carson, E., & Smith, P. (1994). Altered cardiovascular function. In C.L. Betz, M. Hunsberger, & S. Wright (Eds.). *Family-centered nursing care of children* (2nd ed.). Philadelphia: WB Saunders.

Davis, S., Anderson, C., Linkowski, D., Berger, K., & Feinstein, C. (1991). Developmental tasks and transitions of adolescents with chronic illnesses and disabilities. In R. Marinelli & A. Dell Orto (Eds.). *The psychological and social impact of disability* (3rd ed.). New York: Springer.

Disabato, J., & Wulf, J. (1994). Altered neurologic function. In C.L. Betz, M. Hunsberger, & S. Wright (Eds.). *Family-centered nursing care of children* (2nd ed.). Philadelphia: WB Saunders

Farel, P., & Hooper, C. (1995). Biologic limits to behavioral recovery following injury to the central nervous system: implications for early intervention. *Infants and Young Children,* 8(1), 1–7.

Fletcher, J., Ewing-Cobbs, L., Francis, D., & Levin, H. (1995). In S. Broman & M. Michel (Eds.). *Traumatic head injury in children.* New York: Oxford University Press.

Gans, B. (1993). Rehabilitation of the pediatric patient. In J.A. DeLisa & B.M. Gans (Eds.). *Rehabilitation medicine: principles and practice* (2nd ed.). Philadelphia: JB Lippincott.

Gilfoyle, E., Grady, A., & Moore, J. (1990). *Children adapt.* Thorofare, NJ: Slack.

Goode, D. (1990). Thinking about and discussing quality of life. In R. Schalock & M. Bogale (Eds.). *Quality of life: perspectives and issues* (pp. 41–58). Washington, DC: American Association of Mental Retardation.

Guralnick, M. (1993). Second generation research on the effectiveness of early intervention. *Early Education and Development,* 4(4), 365–378.

Hens, M. (1989). Functional evaluation. In S. Dittmar (Ed.). *Rehabilitation nursing: process and application.* St. Louis: CV Mosby.

Hertzberg, D. (1993). The interdisciplinary team: the experience in the Armenia pediatric rehabilitation program. *Holistic Nursing Practice,* 7(4), 42–48.

Hoeman, S. (1996). Coping with chronic, disabling, or developmental disorders. In S. Hoeman (Ed.). *Rehabilitation nursing, process and application* (2nd ed.). St. Louis: Mosby–Year Book.

Hunsberger, M., & Feenan, L. (1994). Altered respiratory function. In C.L. Betz, M. Hunsberger, & S. Wright (Eds.). *Family-centered nursing care of children* (2nd ed.). Philadelphia: WB Saunders.

Johnston, M., Wilkerson, D., & Maney, M. (1993). Evaluation of the quality and outcomes of medical rehabilitation programs. In J.A. DeLisa & B.M. Gans (Eds.). *Rehabilitation medicine: principles and practice* (2nd. ed.) Philadelphia: JB Lippincott.

Leonard, M. (1994). Altered hematologic function. In C.L. Betz, M. Hunsberger, & S. Wright (Eds.). *Family-centered nursing care of children* (2nd ed.). Philadelphia: WB Saunders.

Marge, M. (1994). Toward a state of well-being: promoting health behaviors. In D. Lollar (Ed.). *Preventing secondary conditions associated with spina bifida or cerebral palsy: proceedings and recommendations of a symposium.* Washington, DC: Spina Bifida Association of America.

Maslow, A. (1970). *Motivation and personality* (2nd ed.). New York: Harper & Row.

Mason, K., & Wright, S. (1994). Altered musculoskeletal function. In C.L. Betz, M. Hunsberger, & S. Wright (Eds.) *Family-centered nursing care of children* (2nd ed.). Philadelphia: WB Saunders.

Michaud, L. (1995). Evaluating efficacy of rehabilitation. In S. Broman & M. Michel (Eds.). *Traumatic brain injury in children.* Baltimore: Oxford University Press.

Michaud, L., Rivara, F., Grady, M., & Reay, D. (1992). Predictors of survival and severity of disability after severe brain injury in children. *Neurosurgery,* 31, 254–264.

Miller, J., Steele, K., & Morse, J. (1994). Quality-of-life issues: the nurse's role. In P. Roth & J. Morse (Eds.). *A life-span approach to nursing care for individuals with developmental disabilities.* Baltimore: Paul H Brookes.

Molnar, G., & Kellerman, W. (1992). In G. Molnar (Ed.). *Pediatric rehabilitation.* Baltimore: Williams & Wilkins.

Morrison, J., Hertzberg, D., Gourley, S., & Matthews, D. (1989). Motor point blocks in children: a technique to relieve spasticity using phenol injections. *Journal of the Association of Operating Room Nurses,* 49(5), 1346–1354.

Morse, J. (1994). An overview of developmental disabilities nursing. In S. Roth & J. Morse (Eds.). *A life-span approach to nursing care for individuals with developmental disabilities.* Baltimore: Paul H. Brookes.

Nicol, N., & Hill, M. (1994). Altered skin integrity. In C.L. Betz, M. Hunsberger, & S. Wright (Eds.). *Family-centered nursing care of children* (2nd ed.). Philadelphia: WB Saunders.

Patrick, D., Richardson, M., Starks, H., & Rose, M. (1994). A framework for promoting the health of people with disabilities. In D. Lollar (Ed.). *Preventing secondary conditions associated with spina bifida or cerebral palsy: proceedings and recommendations of a symposium.* Washington, DC: Spina Bifida Association of America.

Pope, A.M., & Tarlov, A.R. (1991). *Disability in America: toward a national agenda for prevention.* Washington, DC: National Academy Press.

Rehabilitation Nursing Foundation. (1993). *The specialty practice of rehabilitation nursing, a core curriculum* (3rd ed.). Skokie, IL: Rehabilitation Nursing Foundation.

Russell, F., & Free, T. (1994). The nurse's role in habilitation. In P. Roth & J. Morse (Eds.). *A life-span approach to nursing care for individuals with developmental disabilities.* Baltimore: Paul H. Brookes.

Shapiro, J. (1993) *No pity.* New York: New York Times Books, Random House.

Snyder, P. (1994). Fractures. In A. Maher, S. Salmond, & T. Pellino (Eds.). *Orthopedic nursing.* Philadelphia: WB Saunders.

Soifer, L. (1992). Development and disorders of communication. In G. Molnar (Ed.). *Pediatric rehabilitation.* Baltimore: Williams & Wilkins.

Verbrugge, L, & Jette, A. (1993). The disablement process. *Social Science in Medicine,* 38(1), 1–14.

Vigneux, A., & Hunsberger, M. (1994). Altered gastrointestinal and renal function. In C.L. Betz, M. Hunsberger, & S. Wright (Eds.). *Family-centered nursing care of children* (2nd ed.). Philadelphia: WB Saunders.

White, M., Nichols, C., Cook, R., Spengler, P., Walker, B., & Look, K. (1995). Diagnostic overshadowing and mental retardation: a meta-analysis. *American Journal of Mental Retardation,* 100(3), 293–298.

Wilson, A.H. (1994). Nursing care during hospitalization. In C.L. Betz, M. Hunsberger, & S. Wright (Eds.). *Family-centered nursing care of children* (2nd ed.). Philadelphia: WB Saunders.

World Health Organization. (1980). *International classification of impairments, disabilities, and handicaps: a manual of classification relating to the consequences of disease.* Geneva, Switzerland: World Health Organization.

WHOQOL Group. (1995). The World Health Organization quality of life assessment (WHOQOL): position paper from the World Health Organization. *Social Science in Medicine,* 41(10), 1403–1409.

Wright, L. (1995). Genetic principles and disorders. In C.L. Betz, M. Hunsberger, & S. Wright (Eds.). *Family-centered nursing care of children* (2nd ed.). Philadelphia: WB Saunders.

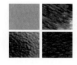

Chapter 8

Models for Practice and Service

Nancy M. Youngblood

The use of theories in practice furnishes the foundation for the planning and implementation of care to the child, family, and community. Within the framework of a theory, the nurse is able to provide holistic nursing interventions. Nursing theory provides a structure for the nurse to collect, organize, question, and clarify information regarding a situation. Through the use of a framework, the nurse is able to gather and interpret data in a systematic manner, thereby providing a perspective that gives meaning to the information and supplies direction for nursing interaction. Theories can be broadly applied to the clinical setting so that they can be used at many different levels. The theory can be used to structure administrative decisions as well as nursing interventions for a specific patient. Using a theory facilitates problem identification and informed decision making, which produce optimal outcomes. Nursing theory provides direction to nursing practice, ensuring that nursing actions are cohesive, systematic, consistent, and patient-focused across the spectrum of professional nursing experiences. This chapter presents the theories and models that are pertinent to the pediatric rehabilitation nurse.

INTERDISCIPLINARY TEAM AS A MODEL OF CARE

Definition of Interdisciplinary Team

The interdisciplinary team as a model of care is the hallmark of practice in rehabilitation. This model facilitates the delivery of services to patients and families in an orderly and cost-effective way. The value of the interdisciplinary team is particularly evident with children and families in pediatric rehabilitation settings, because these children have multiple physical, emotional, social, and developmental needs. These children and their families interact with numerous professional and paraprofessional people during the different phases of the rehabilitation process. Without a structured model of care, it would be very difficult, if not impossible, to achieve timely outcomes. The interdisciplinary team approach to care eliminates the problems encountered when care is fragmented and when professionals plan care in isolation. It ensures that the appropriate care is provided in the most effective manner without either unnecessary duplication of or gaps in the services required by the child and family.

An interdisciplinary team uses a collaborative team effort to achieve optimal outcomes. The team works together to establish goals that will meet the unique needs of each child with a disability or chronic illness and his or her family so that the child can reach his or her highest level of physical, social, and developmental functioning. The interdisciplinary team is a comprised of professionals that work together within a model that ensures the extensive sharing of individual expertise. The basis of the model is the ability of the group to collaborate on setting goals and implementing interventions that result in the best possible outcome for the child and family. The interaction of team members ensures that the needs of the child and family are addressed and that the treatment plan is developed with input from each member. Each team member shares the responsibility to implement a discipline-specific care plan that flows from the team plan. In focusing on the team plan, each discipline ensures that each intervention is implemented and team goals are attained. The strength of the interdisciplinary team is that each member understands and respects the strengths of the other team members and interacts in a manner that facilitates the group process.

The interdisciplinary team must be differentiated from multidisciplinary and transdisciplinary teams. The multidisciplinary team is composed of multiple professionals who assess and treat a child and family within the framework of their own disciplinary training. The multidisciplinary team differs from the interdisciplinary team in a number of ways. The multidisciplinary team is the model that has been used in the traditional delivery of health care. In this traditional model, each discipline functions in an independent manner and sets goals for the patient, and there is no attempt to coordinate these goals with those developed by another discipline. Any interaction that occurs between members of the different disciplines is coincidental and haphazard in design. Little thought is devoted to a specific plan for collaboration. Each discipline identifies discipline-specific goals, and not much effort is given to the coordination of these goals with those of other disciplines. Frequently, the goals of one discipline are met before another discipline begins to work with the child and family. The result is a situation in which services overlap, are duplicated, or are lacking in the provision of necessary services. These situations often develop because of the assumption that another discipline was responsible for and had taken care of the particular need.

The transdisciplinary team is similar to the interdisciplinary team in that the team is comprised of members of different disciplines. The team members develop goals for the child and family, and then one member is selected to carry out the interventions of all the team members. There are many advantages to this model. It is less stressful for the child and family to interact with only one person as opposed to a number of people. The team member is usually selected on the basis of child and family's identified needs. Once the goals are set by the team, the team identifies the member that will have the majority of treatment responsibilities toward meeting the team goals. The identified team member will then provide the treatment for all of the disciplines. The weakness in this model is the fact that a team member is not able to deliver the treatments of another discipline as well as a professional from that discipline. With this in mind, the team members monitor the child's progress toward goals and make any necessary changes in treatment when the child does not meet the interim goals by the dates set by the team. The transdisciplinary model is most effective when it is used in a setting in which the interventions of the team members do not vary greatly, so that one team member can provide all of the interventions without undue difficulty. This model has been used successfully in early intervention programs.

Goals of the Interdisciplinary Team

The interdisciplinary team has two primary goals. The first is the provision of care to the child and family. For the team to carry out this function, it is necessary for the team to maintain itself as a collaborative group of professionals. Therefore, the second goal of the team is self-maintenance. The interdisciplinary team is primarily a group of health care professionals that has been formed and continues to exist to provide care for a child and family. The team must be able to maintain itself before care can be provided. Team maintenance requires a strong commitment from all team members because of the tremendous amount of energy that it takes to interact on a professional level and at the same time develop a treatment plan for the child and family. The amount of effort that must be expended depends on the characteristics of collaborative practice. Collaborative practice is the essence of the interdisciplinary team. It is the endeavor whereby the diverse skills and expertise of team members are combined to develop and implement a treatment plan that ensures positive patient outcomes. Collaboration is the mutual communicating and decision-making process with the express goal of satisfying the wellness and illness needs of the child and family while respecting the unique qualities and abilities of each professional (Calluccio and Maguire, 1983). This definition implies that effective communication is the basis of the collaborative relationship. For communication to be effective, it must be based on mutual respect that allows each person to share openly their unique perceptions and expertise with the expectation that their contribution has equal merit and will be given serious consideration by the other team members. The notion of hierarchy does not have a place in a collaborative relationship. The traditional model that has dominated health care placed the physician at the top of the hierarchy, followed by other health care professionals at various levels. Position in the hierarchy determines the amount of power and influence of each team member. In this model, the physician makes all of the decisions and possibly even chooses the interventions of other disciplines involved in patient care. The situation is different when a collaborative relationship exists. Each member of the relationship has input into the decision-making process. When each member of the relationship has responsibility for decision making, the communication process must be clearly defined. The communication process must have two dimensions to ensure an effective exchange. First, the process should be one that allows each member an opportunity to participate. Second, each participant should be receptive to the contributions of other members. The success of the communication process in a collaborative relationship is determined by the willingness of team members to work on the communication process, which in turn results in the development of a strong collaborative relationship. Once the collaborative relationship is established, other components of the relationship must be in place for the relationship to be maintained. Arcangelo and colleagues identified the components that are necessary for success of the collaborative relationship; these include trust, knowledge, shared responsibility, mutual respect, good communication, cooperation, coordination, and optimism (Arcangelo et al., 1996, p. 107).

Trust   among all parties establishes a quality working relationship; it develops over time as the parties become more acquainted.

Knowledge   is a necessary component for the development of trust. Knowledge and trust remove the need for "supervision."

Shared responsibility   suggests joint decision making for patient care and outcomes and practice issues within the organizations.

Mutual respect   for the expertise of all members of the team is the norm. This respect is communicated to the patients.

Communication   that is not hierarchic but rather two-way ensures the sharing of patient information and knowledge. Questioning of the approach of care of either

partner cannot be delivered in a manner that is construed as criticism but as a method to enhance knowledge and improve patient care.

Cooperation and *coordination*   promote the use of the skills of all team members, prevent duplication of services, enhance knowledge, and improve patient care.

Optimism   that the collaborative relationship is the most effective method of delivery of quality care promotes success.

The process of maintaining the team takes place in tandem with the other goal of the interdisciplinary team: development of the treatment plan. This can be conceptualized as the task of the interdisciplinary team. To be successful in this task, the team must be patient-centered (Ducanis and Golin, 1979). Rehabilitation care is the reason for the team's existence; therefore, the child and family are the focus of the team efforts. The team has the task of assessing the child and family to identify the problems that have brought the patient to the attention of the team. The goals of the child and family are identified, and interventions are developed to help the patient meet the goals. Once each team member has contributed to the goals, they must then determine what responsibility each team member will have in enabling the child and family to meet the goals. The child and family members are considered the most important members of the team. Without their input into the development of the goals, the work of the team is without merit. The treatment plan will not be successful if the child and family members do not believe that the goals will help the patient reach a higher level of functioning. When the child and family members do not value the team goals, it is not likely that the goals will be achieved. Team goals are patient-specific and identify the level of function that the patient will achieve at the end of the interdisciplinary treatment. The time frame within which the goals are to be accomplished are set when the goals are established. The goals may be long term or short term, however, if long-term goals are established, short-term goals are necessary so that progress toward long-term goals can be monitored.

Description of Team Members

The interdisciplinary health care team is composed of a number of professionals from various disciplines. These professionals differ in educational preparation, professional expectations, and responsibilities. Pediatric rehabilitation team members usually consist of physicians, nurses, social workers, psychologists, physical and occupational therapists, therapeutic recreation specialists, and teachers. In the pediatric rehabilitation setting, team members need to have a strong grounding in developmental theory. In addition to health care professionals, the child and parents are the most important team members. If the child is cognitively and developmentally able to manage the team decision-making process, he or she is included. The following disciplines are those most commonly represented on the interdisciplinary team.

Family: The interdisciplinary team must be family-centered. The team must build a positive relationship with the family. The family's concerns and priorities must be reflected in the goals and treatment plan, and they should be encouraged to participate in team meetings. The family is the constant in the child's life whereas service systems and health care providers can fluctuate, and ultimately it is the family that will assume responsibility for the care of the child.

Physician: The physician on the interdisciplinary team is typically a physiatrist (a physician who specializes in physical medicine and rehabilitation). In the pediatric setting, the physician may also be a pediatrician specializing in the care of children with chronic illness or disability or a developmental specialist. The physician establishes the medical diagnosis and prescribes treatment in collaboration with the other team members. The physician also monitors the rehabilitation process with other team members to ensure the child's progress toward the goals.

Pediatric Rehabilitation Nurse: Pediatric rehabilitation nursing is a nursing specialty dedicated to the provision of care to the pediatric patient who has a disability or other chronic condition. The focus of nursing care is directed at improving quality of life for such children and their families. Nursing interventions are directed at improving or maintaining the child's level of function. Nursing care also focuses on preventing further debilitating conditions such as skin breakdown or contractures. The nurse provides care from a developmental perspective in conjunction with other members of the interdisciplinary

team. One of the major roles of the pediatric rehabilitation nurse is the education of the child and family and reinforcement of the teaching done by other team members. The nurse has the most frequent contact with the family and can report family progress and concerns to the rest of the team.

Physical Therapist: The physical therapist assists the child and family with functional restoration. The treatment plan of the physical therapist is aimed at maintaining joint range of motion, mobility, muscle strength, posture, gait, orthotic or prosthetic fit and function, and sensory/motor performance. The physical therapist uses treatment modalities such as heat, cold, hydrotherapy, ultrasound, electrical stimulation, joint mobilization, and therapeutic exercises.

Occupational Therapist: The occupational therapist focuses more specifically on activities of daily living and self-care activities such as eating, dressing, personal hygiene, grooming, perceptual-motor performance, and upper extremity orthotic or prosthetic fit and function. The occupational therapist evaluates the home and recommends modifications to provide a barrier-free environment, and provides training for community re-entry. The occupation therapist is concerned with the impact of a disability or chronic illness on the child's lifestyle.

Therapeutic Recreation Specialist: The recreation therapist uses recreational activities to increase self-confidence and develop socialization skills. These activities are also used to support muscle-strengthening therapies and improve endurance. The main goal of the recreation therapist is to provide activities that keep the patient occupied in a constructive manner. The pediatric recreation therapist provides experiences that are developmentally appropriate for the patient. The emphasis is on activities that will help the child master necessary developmental tasks.

Social Worker: The social worker helps the child and family to deal with problems that may arise when they are faced with a disability or chronic illness. The social worker assesses the quality of relationships among the child, family, and community and assists in resolving identified problems. The social worker acts as a liaison between the child-family unit and the community by contacting community agencies to ensure that services and equipment are in place so that the child will not have insufficient care.

Psychologist: The psychologist helps the child and family adapt to a disability or chronic illness by counseling the patient and family to strengthen coping skills. The child may also need treatment for behavioral problems. Many psychologists are trained to provide retraining for cognitive impairments.

Teacher: The teacher helps the child maintain the appropriate academic level and aids in cognitive development. The teacher interacts with the child's school to ensure that the instruction provided is compatible with the school curriculum. In addition, the teacher acts as a liaison between the interdisciplinary team and the child's school to facilitate a smooth transition back to school.

Phases of Team Development

Team building is a process that continues for the life of the team. Teams go through predictable stages and processes to reach the highest level of functioning. As the team develops, it passes thorough a number of distinct, natural phases. This is true for a newly developing team, and mature teams often revert to earlier levels of functioning when there is a change in team membership or structure. Regardless of the age of the team, smooth development and functioning depend on the degree to which team members understand the tasks that are completed at each stage. Lack of awareness of these tasks may result in a team becoming locked into a particular stage, unable to move forward. When the stages are understood, they become controllable. Some of the phases may be uncomfortable for team members, and the team may start to fragment and want to give up the idea of working as an effective team. It is of particular importance that the team leader recognize the particular stages of the group's development so that the team can be stabilized (Moxon, 1993). Team members can be reassured that the process is a natural part of development.

One of the classic models for team development that characterizes team stages was conceptualized by Tuckman (1965). This model can be used to characterize the types of behavior and issues faced by the team at each stage of development. The stages in this model are:

Stage I: Forming
Stage II: Storming
Stage III: Norming
Stage IV: Performing

Forming: This is the stage of identity development for the team. Individuals are getting to know each other. Group members are polite and avoid serious topics. Members tend to avoid exposure. Tasks are identified, and team members begin to determine how these tasks will be accomplished. The team returns to this stage whenever a new member joins the group.

Storming: This stage is characterized by competition and conflict (Moxon, 1993). Team members disagree over many aspects of team function. This is the most difficult stage in team development. Open conflict may cause many members to withdraw. Other members will use this time to dominate the group with their views. The group may be able to complete tasks during this phase, but there is a high expenditure of energy to reach a compromise. The group needs to move out of this destructive stage and establish an effective decision-making process. This stage cannot be skipped, however, because it is necessary to successfully move on to the third stage. Failure to complete this stage will result in failure of the team and a return to the first two stages until the power issue is resolved (Moxon, 1993).

Norming: At this stage, there is a distinct shift to a cohesive team. The team begins to define roles. The behaviors of group members start to change to those of active participation, active listening, and open exchange of ideas. During this phase, the group begins to identify its strengths and the unique talents of its members that can be used to achieve tasks. Collaborative relationships are formed, and high levels of trust are established.

Performing: Group members are committed to working together. A sense of loyalty has developed. Individual members are no longer a threat, and team resources are pooled. The group is creative, and a feeling of warmth exists. At this stage, the group is highly productive. From the outside, this group can appear closed. A new member may have difficulty gaining access to the group during this phase.

Team Leadership and Function

An interdisciplinary team's success depends on effective team meetings, when team members share assessments, set goals, and report progress toward goals. A formal leader is necessary to facilitate team effectiveness. The leadership role has traditionally been held by the physician; however, the team leader can be the case manager, social worker, or any team member appointed to the role. The physician is traditionally placed in this role because of his or her responsibility for medical treatment; however, anyone can assume the position of team leader if they have the ability to motivate and direct the team and integrate the input of all team members into the treatment plan. The team leader must have the skills to supervise the treatment team so that goals can be achieved. Effective leaders must have a clear understanding of the direction in which the team needs to move and have the ability to communicate that understanding to the team members. Parker (1994) describes an effective leader as an individual who can develop a sense of urgency about the team's work and can involve team members in goal setting and decision making.

Equally important to leadership is the ability of each team member to exhibit the willingness to coordinate, cooperate, and communicate with other team members.

The team meetings can be designed in such a way as to facilitate the team process. The structure tends to be the same for most interdisciplinary teams. In the most frequently used design, the focus is on the contribution of each discipline. A member from each discipline gives a progress report on each patient. The report may take the form of a narrative presentation on the patient's progress toward goals based on the discipline-specific interventions. This design works well because each member can concentrate on their efforts to help the child and family obtain the goals. Another approach is the problem-oriented plan. In this design, as each problem from the child's established list is presented, any discipline can comment and address their role in the management of the problem. This approach allows for a synergistic, interdisciplinary interaction, with one discipline's report building on the report of another.

The goal-oriented meeting is easier to manage because the reports are given in a specific order. In this approach, the team leader must be aware of the interventions of every team member so that the discussion can be facilitated in such a way that every discipline has a chance to report any relevant information. However, regardless of the design used, it is the team leader's responsibility to keep the team focused on the task. Personal discussions may dominate the conversation, and it is up to the team leader to keep the team focused, thereby preventing sidebar talk. The leader is also responsible to see that every idea is understood and that compromises are achieved when disagreement occurs between team members.

The team generally meets at a specific time every week according to a predetermined schedule. For example, the standard for a team may be to review every child's treatment plan at least every 2 weeks. Additionally, the team would have criteria to identify those patients needing to be reviewed on a weekly basis. Documentation of each meeting is necessary to record the child's progress toward goals. The record may take the form of a meeting summary in narrative form, or it may be a recording of a number code that indicates the child's progress toward goals. Team documentation becomes part of the permanent record. The documentation should contain team decisions and identify the person responsible for carrying out treatments. The target date for goal achievement is recorded when the goal is developed and updated if the child meets the goal early or fails to meet the goal by the date the team has set.

CASE MANAGEMENT

Definition of Case Management

The definition of case management that is approved by the Case Management Society of America (CMSA) is as follows:

> Case management is a collaborative process which assesses, plans, implements, coordinates, monitors, and evaluates options and services to meet an individual's health needs through communication and available resources to promote quality cost-effective outcomes.

The primary role of the case manager is to collaborate with the child, family and all members of the health care team so that needs are met in a timely. cost-effective manner. In the case management model, the expected course of the child's response to the interdisciplinary treatment plan and treatment goals are outlined. Once the outline is completed, the interventions are plotted for specific intervals (Zander, 1992). It is the responsibility of the case manager to coordinate the care provided by the health care team members to ensure that interventions are implemented as prescribed to prevent gaps in care. The case manager identifies additional patient problems and brings these issues to the interdisciplinary team for inclusion in the treatment plan. The most important attribute of the case manager is the ability to communicate effectively. The communication process ensures that individuals from various professional disciplines, the child, the family, community resource people, and the payor of the health care understand the treatment plan. The case manager facilitates the decision-making process by encouraging the appropriate use of resources by the child, family, and interdisciplinary team.

Two models of case management currently exist: the internal case manager and the external case manager. The internal case manager works within the treatment facility or program to oversee the delivery of care within the facility and ensure that the care is adequate as well as cost-effective. The internal case manager is generally the liaison for the payor and external resources to ensure a smooth transition into community living. The external case manager is most often found in insurance companies. The external case manager may also be an independent contractor who provides case management services without loyalty to the payor. Regardless of the external case manager's type of employment, the role is essentially the same—to oversee the delivery of services over the entire span of the illness or injury episode.

Evolution of Case Management

Case management has been around since the early 1900s. Case management was a model of care used in the early twentieth century by public health nurses and social workers who worked in the public health departments. Insurance companies began to use the case management model after World War II to manage the care of seriously injured soldiers returning from the war. The current model of case management evolved with Medicaid and Medicare changes in the 1980s and varied among organizations, depending on the needs of the clients and the services being rendered. As cost-containment became a critical concern in the health care industry, case management began to emerge as the model of care that would prevent the waste of health care dollars and yet provide adequate care for the patient. The modern concept of case management began to appear in the literature in the mid-1980s. Zander (1988) presented some of the original work in case manage-

ment that was carried out at New England Medical Center Hospital in Boston.

Interface of Case Manager With the Interdisciplinary Team

The case manager may or may not be a member of the interdisciplinary team or the person who spends the most time with the child and family, but may be the one that has the time available to communicate with other team members and coordinate care for the patient. The management of care ensures the cooperation of interdisciplinary team members with the initiation of the interdisciplinary treatment plan. Another dimension of the case manager role is that of liaison between team members and family members. The interaction of the case manager with team members facilitates creative problem solving so that maximum patient outcomes are ensured. To interact effectively with all members of the interdisciplinary team, the case manager must be knowledgeable and educated about the professional roles and responsibilities of the various team members and the types of services that each team member is capable of providing.

Case Manager as Child/Family Advocate

The case manager is an advocate for the child and family. As an advocate, the case manager must ensure that the child is receiving the necessary care. This is accomplished by negotiating with the payor and clearly presenting the reasons that outcomes cannot be achieved if specific treatments are not provided. The well-being of the child and family is the highest priority for the case manager. Family goals, needs, and resources are always considered when recommending care, and the treatment plan is developed within these parameters. The case manager frequently has a broader picture of health care resources than the family. Therefore, the case manager has the responsibility to educate the family about the necessary actions that will result in obtaining adequate services for the child. The case manager can ensure that the family understands the rationale for the treatment plan. Through the relationship with the family, the case manager can help the family set realistic goals for the child as well as themselves. The case manager can help family members care for themselves by obtaining family support services such as respite care or in-home health care services. The case manager is the person who can provide assistance in developing an educational plan for the child that will meet cognitive, physical, and psychosocial needs and ensure that this plan changes as the child changes so that developmental needs are met over the developmental continuum.

NURSING THEORIES AND MODELS OF PRACTICE

Characteristics of Theories

Nursing theory has progressed considerably since its beginning in 1860, when Florence Nightingale articulated the need for nurses to be educationally prepared to practice their profession and for the profession to be founded on research. Nursing theory has gradually come to be accepted as a beneficial mechanism through which nursing care can be carried out in an effective and consistent manner. The majority of nursing theories were developed from 1950 through 1975. Few theories have been developed since that time; emphasis has been on the use of the these theories in the educational, administrative, and clinical practice.

Fawcett (1989) noted four central concepts that provide the foundation for nursing theories:

- person
- environment
- health
- nursing

Each nursing theory uniquely defines these concepts and combines them to design a specific model. How the concepts are defined and the relationships between the concepts provide the structures that support nursing practice. The various theories that have been developed clarify information concerning the characteristics of the recipients of nursing care and the manner in which the care is provided. Different theories have different structures, objectives, and outcomes. Nursing theories vary in degree of complexity and level of usefulness. Because of variations in design, each theory has limitations in application. The strengths and weaknesses of a particular theory may make it useful in a particular setting but not in others. When selecting a nursing theory, it must be remembered that no one theory is universally applicable to all situations. The nurse must be knowledgeable enough to select from among the various theories. The decision regarding theory-based practice must include selection of a theory

that will support individual practice as well as a theory that can be used as the foundation for professional nursing practice in a health care setting.

When selecting a theory for practice, an assessment should reveal the characteristics of an organization or individual that are compatible with the nursing theory. The theory is then used to support practice. If characteristics, such as beliefs about the nature of humans, nursing, and health care, are in conflict with the nursing theory, application of the theory will be difficult. Any incongruence between the nursing practice and the theory creates a situation that will limit the effectiveness of nursing interventions. It may be necessary to use more than one theory. Theories can be combined so that the use of one or more theories can explain or direct the nursing plan of action and best explain the rationale for the nursing interventions. The theories can be complementary rather than competing. It is important for the nurse to be skilled in using different theories and adapting them to health-related encounters. The nurse must use different theories as tools to solve different health-related problems. Nursing is person-centered, not a series of tasks to be completed in a given time frame; therefore, combining nursing theories and other theories can support the nursing management of diverse health care situations.

Guidelines for Theory-Based Practice

Although a great deal of nursing research has been carried out in an attempt to strengthen the application of theory to the clinical setting, the actual use of theory in the clinical setting is limited. Nevertheless, it is the clinical setting that provides the true test of the effectiveness of a nursing theory. Repeated implementation of a theory enables the nurse to discern whether an unsatisfactory outcome is related to the theory itself, to the nature of the setting, or to the manner in which the theory was implemented. Theory-based practice supports the individual decision-making process and, additionally, strengthens the entire nursing profession.

Theories in Nursing

The nursing theories presented in this section are those that are more adaptable to the pediatric rehabilitation setting. Although many other nursing theories can be used, the following theories reflect the incorporation of developmentally appropriate nursing care for the child and family in pediatric rehabilitation settings.

Orem's Model of Self-Care

Orem's (1985) model focuses on the person's ability to perform self-care and is defined as "the practice of activities that individuals initiate and perform on their own behalf in maintaining life and well-being" (p. 35). Self-care involves the activities performed on one's own behalf to maintain life, health, and well-being. The ability to care for others is referred to as dependent-care. In Orem's model, the goal of nursing is to help people meet their own therapeutic self-care demands. Orem identified three types of nursing systems: wholly compensatory, where the nurse provides total care because the patient is totally unable to provide self-care; partially compensatory, where the nurse provides partial care because the patient has partial inability to care for self; and supportive–educative, where the nurse assists the patient in making decisions and acquiring skills and knowledge.

Orem (1995) identified *basic conditioning factors*, which are characteristic attributes, properties, or events, internal or external, that make each person unique in their self-care requisites. The following Case Study provides an application of this model. Basic conditioning factors can provide the essential structure for a pediatric rehabilitation nursing assessment. Once an assessment is completed, nursing diagnoses and interventions can be developed to meet the needs of a specific child and family.

CASE STUDY—Jasminia

AGE: 14-year-old child with the diagnosis of spina bifida

GENDER: Female

DEVELOPMENTAL STATE: developmental delay. Assessed at the cognitive level of a 9-year-old

HEALTH STATE:

PAST: Jasminia was born full-term following an uneventful pregnancy. She weighed 7 lbs., 3 oz. at birth. She was hospitalized until 1 month of age, at which time she underwent surgical repair of a myelomeningocele. She had an uneventful course after discharge. However, she has never been able to walk and is in a wheelchair ambulator. She was bottle-fed and progressed to table food at 3 years of age. Her immunizations are up to date. Jasminia started to menstruate 1 year ago and needs a great deal of support from her mother to manage her menses. She has no known allergies.

PRESENT: Jasminia is currently receiving services in an outpatient pediatric rehabilitation clinic for bowel and bladder training, self-catheterization teaching, and an evaluation for ambulation. She will attend the clinic for 4 hours every day during the summer. The goal is to prepare her to be more independent when she returns to school in the fall.

CHILD'S/FAMILY'S PERCEPTION OF HEALTH STATE:

CHILD: Is anxious but pleasant. States that she is afraid of the outpatient therapy because she does not think she can care for herself.

FAMILY: Parents are anxious and having difficulty giving up responsibility for the care of their daughter. The mother tells every member of the health care team that she does not believe that it is good for her daughter to have all of the pressure that will result from the teaching sessions.

SOCIOCULTURAL-SPIRITUAL ORIENTATION:

Jasminia and her family live in a neighborhood that is best described as predominantly black. Jasminia attends a public school for children with special educational needs. The bus picks her up at 7 AM and brings her home at 3 PM. It is difficult for her mother to get to the school for meetings because the family has one car and the father must use it to get to work. The family does not attend church and does not claim to have any religious beliefs. There are no relatives nearby, and the family tries to visit relatives in Tennessee whenever possible. The family has many friends in the neighborhood who frequently offer them help.

PATTERNS OF LIVING:

Jasminia is cared for by both parents, although the mother is the primary caregiver. Both parents worked until Jasminia was born, and then the mother had to quit her job to care for Jasminia. There are three children older than Jasminia, and they have assumed more of her care over the last 3 years because the mother has had two more children since Jasminia was born. She is also under treatment for depression and sometimes has difficulty managing the family.

ENVIRONMENT (CONDITIONS OF LIVING):
The family lives in a four-bedroom row house. The parents had to turn the living room into a bedroom for Jasminia because they can no longer carry her upstairs. The family does not have a yard, so the children play on the sidewalks. There is a public playground five blocks from the house and the mother tries to get Jasminia there on afternoons when the weather is pleasant.

AVAILABLE RESOURCES:
Financial resources are limited for the family. The father's income barely covers the bills, and any extra money usually is spent on equipment and supplies for Jasminia. The family is close and members communicate openly with each other. Their friends are available to help when the stress level becomes difficult for the family to manage. They all seem to love Jasminia and are happy when they can spend time with her (adapted from Dennis, 1997).

Rogers' Model of the Unitary Person

Rogers' (1986) model focuses on the individual as a unified whole in constant interaction with the environment. Rogers conceptualizes human beings as multidimensional energy fields that are in continuous mutual process with multidimensional environmental energy fields. The unitary person is viewed as an energy field that is more than and different from the sum of its biologic, physical, social, and psychologic parts. In the Rogerian system, human beings are continuously developing toward higher levels of diversity. Events in the life process provide opportunities for further development toward higher levels. Within this framework, there is an inherent assumption that human beings are desirous of continued self-growth. Nursing practice is directed at helping individuals achieve maximum well-being within their potential.

Neuman's Health Care Systems Model

Neuman's (1989) model focuses on the person as a complete system, the subparts of which are interrelated and include physiologic, psychologic, sociocultural, spiritual, and developmental factors. The person is viewed as an open system in interaction with the environment, maintaining balance and harmony between internal and external environments by adjusting to stress and by defending against tension-producing stimuli. Each person has a normal line of defense, which is a state of wellness, and flexible lines of defense, which protect the person from stressors. Lines of resistance are internal factors that help each person mount a stress response. Nurses act at levels of primary, secondary, and tertiary prevention. Primary prevention reduces the possibility of the individual's encounter with a stressor or strengthens the flexible lines of defense. Secondary prevention occurs when the stressor has penetrated the flexible line of defense and a reaction has occurred. At this level of care, the nurse focuses on symptom management and treatment. The goal of tertiary prevention is to maintain a degree of adaptation after reconstitution and stability have occurred.

Roy's Adaptation Model

In Roy's adaptation model (Roy & Andrews, 1991), humans are biopsychosocial adaptive systems who cope with environmental change through the process of adaptation. Roy has identified four subsystems of adaptation: physiologic needs, self-concept, role mastery, and interdependence. These subsystems make up adaptive modes that provide mechanisms for coping with environments, stimuli, and change. According to this model, the goal of nursing care is to facilitate the person's adaptation to the stressors that impact on the subsystems. Nursing interventions are directed at the regulation of the internal and external stimuli that affect adaptation.

Other Models Used in Nursing Practice

Health Belief Model

The Health Belief Model (HBM) is based on the premise that health-seeking behavior is determined by the person's perception of the threat that a pathologic condition presents to the existing state of health. The pathologic condition is managed by the actions that are valued in the resolution of the perceived health threat (Becker, 1974). The major components of the HBM include perceived susceptibility, perceived severity, perceived benefits and costs, motivation, and enabling or modifying factors.

Perceived susceptibility is the person's perception that the health threat is a reality and
may cause actual harm.

Perceived severity is the recognition that the
threat is potentially harmful enough to alter physical or physiologic well being.

Perceived benefits and costs refer to the person's perception of the health changes that
will result from treatment as weighed
against the potential problems that will result from the health problem.

Motivation is the desire that the person has
to comply with a treatment and the value
that health care has for the person.

The components of the HBM are modified
by factors such as personality variables, past
experiences with the health care system, cultural beliefs about health care, and sociodem-
ographic characteristics.

Functional Health Patterns

Gordon (1987) developed a data collection
system that provides the guidelines for a
comprehensive assessment. The system is
composed of 10 functional health patterns
that identify the areas of data collection necessary for the assessment of the patient's
health status. As a standardized model of
data collection, the nurse is assured that all
relevant data are collected and analyzed. The
10 patterns represent a composite of the individual's life experiences, including internal
and external forces. The following is a list of
these functional health patterns and a brief
description of the expected assessment information that is obtained through the use of
this model.

*Health perception–health management pat-
tern:* This pattern is the information gathered from the patient's and family's perception of health status and how health is
managed.

Nutritional–metabolic pattern: Information for
this pattern describes food and fluid consumption. Daily eating patterns as well as
likes and dislikes are assessed. Data about
height, weight, skin integrity, and condition of hair, nails, and teeth are obtained.

Elimination pattern: Excretory functions are
assessed. Laboratory analysis of specimens, output records, gross inspection of
urine and stool, and self-care abilities are
observed.

Activity–exercise pattern: This pattern describes the amount of time spent in exercise and sedentary activities. Gross and

fine motor skills are assessed and developmental level identified. Leisure activities
are described.

Sleep–rest pattern: Describes the patterns of
sleep, rest, and activity.

Cognitive–perceptual pattern: Cognitive functions such as language, memory, problem
solving, and decision making are assessed
in this pattern, as well as perceptual activities such as vision, hearing, touch, taste,
and smell.

Role-relationship pattern: This pattern describes the roles, formal and informal, that
a person has, as well as the relationships
that exist around these roles.

Sexuality-reproductive pattern: This pattern is
concerned with gender identity. Cultural
norms are an important part of this pattern. Secondary sex changes, sexual activity, and reproductive health are assessed.

Coping-stress-tolerance pattern: This pattern
describes general coping skills and the effectiveness of these skills.

Value-belief pattern: This pattern describes
patterns of values, including spiritual beliefs. Life goals are assessed, as well as the
guidelines and values that help a person
decide on specific life goals.

Systems Theory

The underlying assumption that supports
General Systems Theory (GST) is that a system must be understood as a whole rather
than in component parts. The system cannot
be understood by examining parts in isolation
(Bertalanffy, 1975). According to GST, the
whole is greater that the sum of its parts. This
statement implies an interdependence among
the components of a system. The parts of a
system are held together by a mutual relationship; thus, the behaviors of one component
influence the behaviors of the other components, and a change in one part of a system
causes a change in the other parts of the
system. Systems are separated from the environment by a boundary. This is an important
concept in GST, because to study a system it
is necessary to identify what is in the system
and what is not. Everything that is outside of
a boundary is the environment. Boundaries
are characterized by their relative amount of
permeability. The more permeable a system,
the greater the exchange with the environment. A system that freely interacts with the
environment is an open system. If no exchange occurs with the environment, the system is closed. Related concepts are input and

output. Matter, energy, and information may be taken in from the environment or transferred out of the system depending on the degree in which a system is open to the environment. Systems theory can be applied to any human group. It is commonly used to understand family relationships and the impact of the environment on the family system.

Maslow's Hierarchy of Needs

Maslow (1970) identified human needs according to a hierarchy. These needs are basic to all humans regardless of cultural influences on lifestyle. An inherent human trait is the need to move through the levels and become self-actualized. The five levels are physiologic needs, safety and security, love and belonging, self-esteem, and self-actualization. According to Maslow, the needs can be arranged according to hierarchic levels, and a person must meet their needs in an ascending order. Circumstances in a person's life may make it impossible to move to a higher level in the hierarchy. For example, living in extreme poverty would require so much energy to meet physiologic needs that the next level would be unobtainable. Physiologic needs are the highest priority and must be met first. Once a need is met, the person can seek fulfillment of higher-level needs. The person may move between the levels in response to life events. Also, a person may not stay at a level once achieved. A pathologic condition may return and cause the person to return to a lower level.

Stress Theory

Stress has traditionally been viewed as the body's response to an event. The idea of stress as a response gained attention through the work of Selye (1946), who defined stress as "the nonspecific response of the body to any demand made upon it to adapt whether that demand produces pain or pleasure" (p. 230). Stress theory is helpful in the understanding of the human response to any life event. The body's response is nonspecific because the body reacts as a whole organism regardless of the stress. Seyle called the body's generalized response to a stressor the general adaptation syndrome (GAS). The GAS has three distinct stages.

The alarm stage: In this stage the body prepares itself for flight or fight. The sympathetic nervous system stimulates the adrenal medulla, which secretes catecholamines, which are responsible for physiologic responses. These are increased heart rate, release of glucose, increased respiratory rate, and dilation of pupils.

The stage of resistance: During this phase, physiologic forces are mobilized to maintain an increased resistance to stressors. The body concentrates its activities on those organs that are most involved in the specific stress response. Successful adaptation implies a return to the normal state. If efforts are ineffectual, a state of maladaptation results. Chronic resistance eventually causes damage to the involved systems.

The stage of exhaustion: When the organs show evidence of deterioration, the body enters the third stage. Selye determined that the body exhibits a triad of symptoms: hypertrophy of the adrenal glands, ulceration in the gastrointestinal mucosa, and atrophy of the thymus gland. In this stage, energy for adaptation has been completely used, and the person is unable to further adapt. This stage is of concern to the pediatric rehabilitation nurse when caring for a child who has had a serious injury. It is often necessary to treat the problems that arise from stress as well as the direct injury. Parents also may exhibit signs of the stress reaction when faced with the task of caring for the child with disability or chronic illness.

THE NURSING PROCESS

The term *nursing process* emerged in the mid-1960s during a time when nursing was attempting to define itself as a profession. As the professional status of nursing became more recognized and respected, the need became acute for a system of ensuring accountability in nursing practice and evaluating the outcomes of nursing care. The nursing process emerged as a problem-solving approach that ensured that nursing care was based on a systematic series of steps. The nursing process provides the framework for nursing practice. It is a systematic approach used by nurses to collect information about the patient, identify patient problems, design and implement solutions to the problems, and evaluate patient responses to the nursing care. The patient can be defined as an individual, family, community, or society. The process can take place in a variety of settings, such as a hospital, clinic, school, home, or community. The phases of the nursing process include assessment, nursing diagnosis, planning, intervention, and evaluation.

Assessment: During the assessment phase of the nursing process, information is collected through a variety of methods. The collection of data may be objective and subjective. Subjective data should be gathered from the child as well as the parents. Data are gathered through the process of history taking, physical examination, and record review. Objective data also include any information that the nurse gathers through observation.

Nursing diagnosis: When assessment data have been collected and organized, they are analyzed to identify health problems that can be treated by nursing actions. The nursing diagnosis is the statement of the health alteration that has been identified through the nursing assessment. The nursing diagnosis describes the patient's response to a disease process, condition, or situation as opposed to a medical problem, which is written as a medical diagnosis. If the data indicate that a problem exists, the nurse uses that information to construct a nursing diagnosis. The nursing diagnosis is the actual or potential problem that affects the health status of the patient. The nursing diagnosis is a statement written in two parts. The first part is derived from the assessment data and is a statement of the patient health alteration, and the second part is the contributing factor to the health alteration. A nursing diagnosis may be written for an actual health alteration or for a potential problem. In the case of a potential problem, the patient is identified as having a high risk for the occurrence of a health alteration. Nursing diagnoses that lead to independent action should be distinguished from collaborative problems that necessitate the input of other disciplines. Examples of nursing diagnoses are:

- Impaired physical mobility related to muscle weakness
- Altered nutrition, less than the body requires, related to difficulty swallowing
- High risk for fluid volume deficit related to difficulty swallowing

Planning and intervention: During the planning phase, the nurse details the care that will help the child and family maintain or regain their optimal level of health. Each nursing diagnosis must have a number of interventions or specific actions to be taken to resolve the health alteration. The plan is goal oriented, with the expected outcomes clearly stated. Goals or expected outcomes are clear statements of the behaviors that will indicate that the health alteration has been resolved. For example, the outcome for the nursing diagnosis of impaired physical mobility might be "the child will bear his own weight for 10 minutes three times a day by [date]." The interventions for this outcome might be focused on leg-strengthening exercises or gradually increasing the time of weight bearing. The plan contains the specific nursing actions or interventions that will assist the child and family to achieve the identified goals. Several interventions are usually required for each diagnosis. Each intervention describes a specific action and the frequency that the action will be performed. The nursing intervention is written as a nursing order and it is the directions for care.

Evaluation: This phase involves the ongoing appraisal of the progress being made toward the goals. It is the assessment of the effectiveness of the nursing intervention plan. The evaluation phase of the nursing process provides the nurse with the opportunity to assess patient outcomes and decide if the nursing interventions have been effective. If the outcomes have not been obtained, then the nurse will have to revise the plan of care. The last phase of the nursing process requires a careful study of the outcomes for two reasons. First, it is important to document progress toward goals and the interventions that were successful. Second, it is important to document changes in the nursing interventions if the original ones have not been successful.

SUMMARY

As an emerging profession, nursing continues to develop a unique foundation of knowledge on which to base practice. Theories are tools or structures to be used by the pediatric rehabilitation nurse to give direction to nursing actions. Theory-based practice provides the underpinning from which clinical decisions are made and outcomes are evaluated. The nurse may choose to use one theory or develop an eclectic model on which to base practice. The nursing process is a problem-solving tool that supports theory-based nursing practice. The pediatric rehabilitation nurse must continually work on the development of critical-thinking skills, and it is through the use of the nursing process that critical thinking can be organized.

REFERENCES

Arcangelo, V., Fitzgerald, M., Carroll, D., & Plumb, J. (1996). Collaborative care between nurse practitioners and primary care physicians. *Primary Care, 23*(1), 103–113.

Becker, M. (1974). The health belief model and sick role behavior. *Nursing Digest, 6*, 35–40.

Bertalanffy, L. von. (1975). General systems theory. In D. Rubin & J. Yin (Eds.). *General systems theory and human communication.* Rochelle Park, NJ: Hayden Press.

Calluccio, M., & Maguire, P. (1983). Collaborative practice: becoming a reality through primary nursing. *Nursing Administration Quarterly, 7*, 59–63.

Dennis, C. (1997). *Self-care deficit theory of nursing: concepts and applications.* Baltimore: CV Mosby.

Ducanis, A., & Golin, A. (1979). *The interdisciplinary health care team: a handbook.* Germantown, MD: Aspen Publishers.

Fawcett, J. (1989). *Analysis and evaluation of conceptual models of nursing* (2nd ed.). Philadelphia: FA Davis.

Gordon, M. (1987). *Nursing diagnosis: process and application* (2nd ed.). New York: McGraw-Hill.

Maslow, A. (1970). *Motivation and personality.* New York: Harper & Row.

Moxon, P. (1993). *Building a better team: a handbook for managers and facilitators.* Hampshire, England: Gower.

Neuman, B. (1989). *The Neuman systems model* (2nd ed.). Norwalk, CT: Appleton & Lange.

Orem, D. (1985). *Concepts of practice* (3rd ed.). New York: McGraw-Hill.

Parker, G. (1994). *Cross-functional teams.* San Francisco: Jossey-Bass.

Rogers, M. (1986). Science of unitary human beings. In V. Malinski (Ed.). *Explorations on Martha Rogers' science of unitary human beings.* Norwalk, CT: Appleton-Century-Crofts.

Roy, C., Sr., & Andrews, H. (1991). *The Roy adaptation model: the definitive statement.* Norwalk, CT: Appleton & Lange.

Selye, H. (1946). General adaptation syndrome and diseases of adaptation. *Journal of Clinical Endocrinology, 6*, 117–230.

Tuckman, E. (1965). Development sequence in small groups. *Psychological Bulletin, 63*, 284–499.

Zander, K. (1988). Nursing case management: strategic management of cost and patient outcomes. *Journal of Nursing Administration, 18*(5), 23–30.

Zander, K. (1992). Focusing on patient care outcome: case management in the 90's. *Dimensions in Critical Care Nursing, 11*, 127–129.

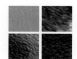

Part II

Perspectives on Children and Families and Their Environment

■

■

■

■

■

■

■

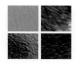

Chapter 9

Family-Centered Care

Nancy M. Youngblood

The family must be considered the primary unit for health care. The provision of care to the family unit is defined as family-centered care. Family-centered care is a philosophy of care "based on the belief that all families are deeply caring and want to nurture their children" (Edelman, 1991, p. 1). The nursing profession has acknowledged the family as the unit through which nursing care is administered to individuals or children. For the pediatric rehabilitation nurse to provide care for the family unit, it is necessary first to be able to define the family unit. With the large variation in cultures and lifestyles that exist in contemporary society, it is difficult to use one definition to conceptually describe the family unit. "Family" has different meanings to different people, depending on their culture, values, sexual orientation, developmental level, support systems, and financial resources. Jackson and Saunders (1993) provide a universal definition of family as "a group of human beings united by certain affiliations, including biologic, emotional, and legal" (p. 34). A family can be thought of as any human group that is held together by ties that arise from an emotional, biologic, or belief system basis. From the pediatric perspective, the family is the group of people who transmit biologic and cultural information that is intended to shape a child psychologically, emotionally, and socially and provide the basis for moral values.

FAMILY THEORY

A great deal of effort has been expended over the past three decades in an attempt to understand how families function and the forces that lead to family dysfunction. A number of relevant family theories have been developed and subjected to testing in clinical settings. Each theory presents a different aspect of family organization and relationships. Because of the diversity of families, no single theory applies to all families. The major themes are structural–functional, developmental, stress, and systems theory.

Structural–Functional

The structural–functional family nursing model emphasizes the organization or structure of the family and how the structure meets family needs (Friedman, 1992). This theory is concerned with the interdependence and integration between the family and society. *Structure* refers to the arrangement of roles and how members relate to each other. Other structural dimensions may include communication patterns, power structure, and support networks (Friedman, 1992). *Function* is the contribution made by an activity or task to the family as a whole and the consequences of the activity for the family as a whole. The family process is directed at maintaining a state of equilibrium among family roles. Internal relationships involve the identification of the tasks necessary to maintain the family unit and the distribution of responsibilities among family members to ensure survival of the family unit. Friedman (1992) defines five basic family functions.

Affective function: The maintenance of personalities of family members

Socialization and social placement function: Socializing the child to be a productive member of society

Reproductive function: Ensuring the continuity of the family and societal survival

Economic function: Providing and allocating adequate resources for the family

Health care function: Providing for physical needs, such as food, clothing, shelter, and high-level wellness

Structural–functional theory focuses on the integration of the family within the occupational system. The family roles are gender-specific. The expressive roles are seen as integrative, or the roles that bring family members together, such as hugging and meeting emotional needs. This role is usually assigned to the wife–mother. The instrumental roles are those that occur external to the family, such as earning an income. This is the role traditionally assigned to the husband–father. The instrumental roles are separate from family roles, and these roles become isolated from family function.

Developmental Theory: Family Life Cycle

Developmental theory views each family as evolving over time. This theory divides the life history of a family into expected stages of development. Each stage is characterized by developmental tasks relevant to that stage, and predictable crises associated with the achievement or non-achievement of specific developmental tasks.

Duvall (1977) developed one of the most systematic uses of the family life cycle approach to the study of families. Families are viewed as having universal tasks as well as specific developmental tasks that must be accomplished by the family at different stages. Duvall's (1977) theory assumes an intact family system as defined by marriage and children. Intact families pass through the same sequence of phases, most of which are marked by critical transition points such as marriage, birth of the first child, departure from home of the youngest child, empty-nest syndrome, retirement, and death. Duvall (1977) shows the typical life cycle of an intact family in terms of eight stages.

Stage 1. Marriage—the joining of families: The tasks that a couple must work through at this stage are the establishment of their identity as a couple and establishment of relationships with their extended families as a couple. At this stage the couple must also make decisions about parenthood.

Stage 2. Families with infants: During this stage, the couple must integrate an infant and assure the parenting role while still maintaining their relationship.

Stage 3. Families with preschool children: At this stage, the task is to socialize the children. The parents and children must begin to adjust to the children being with baby-sitters or other adults.

Stage 4. Families with school children: At this stage, children are developing peer relationships. Parents and children must adjust to longer periods of separation.

Stage 5. Families with adolescents: At this stage, teenagers are developing increasing autonomy. Parents are focusing on mid-life issues.

Stage 6. Families as launching centers: During this stage, the children leave home and become independent adults. The couple has to adjust their relationship as they are required to do less and less parenting.

Stage 7. Middle-aged parents: At this stage, the parents must adjust to living alone as the last child leaves home. They begin to prepare for retirement. The couple must develop new relationships with adult children and grandchildren.

Stage 8. The aging family: This stage begins as the couple enters retirement and ends at the death of one of the spouses. The couple begins to prepare for death and adjusts to the loss of friends and family members.

The life cycles defined by Duvall (1977) focus on the traditional nuclear family form. These life cycles cannot be used to describe many of the family units in contemporary society. Carter and McGoldrick (1989) recommend that additions be made to developmental theory frameworks so that they accurately reflect new lifestyle changes and can be used to study families of varying forms found in contemporary society. There are many dislocations of the family life cycle, such as divorce. These dislocations require changes to occur in a systematic manner if the family is to proceed developmentally. Carter and McGoldrick (1989) also stress that the family is a system passing through time in a social context that is also changing. Societal changes are reflected in the falling birth rate, increasing life expectancy, and rising divorce and re-marriage rates. Developmental frameworks need to reflect the impact of societal changes on family development. For example, a child in pediatric rehabilitation today is more likely to be from a single-parent family than in previous decades. The stresses and responsibilities of single parenting must be considered when making discharge plans and child care arrangements. A framework that delineates the family life stages can be useful for studying families because the needs of the family can be anticipated depending on the stage of the family.

Family Stress Theory

Family stress theory explains how families react to stressful situations. The theory focuses on the stressors that a family encounters, including normal life events, and the resources that are available to promote adaptation to the stressful event. Stressors are categorized as predictable (e.g., childbearing) and unpredictable (e.g., injury or death of a family member) (Wong, 1995). Stressors can be cumulative, and if too many stressful events happen in a short period of time, the family system may not be able to cope effectively. The amount of stress that a stressor creates for a family unit depends on the family's perceptions of the event. The ABCX model described by Boss (1988) identifies how factors A, B, and C can result in X. "A" is the stressful event with associated hardships. "B" refers to the family strengths or resources available to cope with the stressful event. Family resources may include finances, religious beliefs, social support, physical health, and family flexibility. Variable "C" refers to the family's view of the seriousness of the stressor event. "X" is the crisis or amount of disruption that an event causes in a family. Factors A, B, and C all influence the family's ability to prevent the changes associated with the stressor event. In the family stress model, nursing interventions target variables A, B, and C. Interventions are directed at enhancing family rescues or helping the family members adjust their perception of a stressful event.

Another family stress model is the double ABCX model, which is a derivation of the ABCX model (McCubbin & Patterson, 1982). The double ABCX model adds post-crisis variables to the original model to describe life stressors that accumulate over time as the family adapts to chronic illness. This model also adds social and psychologic factors that families use to successfully adapt to the illness event.

A more recent family stress model is the resiliency model (McCubbin & McCubbin, 1993), which builds on the ABCX model and double ABCX model. This model includes family types, capabilities, and strengths—all variables that are used to manage a stressful illness event—with emphasis on family adaptation (McCubbin & McCubbin, 1993). This model can be used in pediatric rehabilitation nursing practice because it focuses on the family's strengths and capabilities. Through the use of this model, the pediatric rehabilitation nurse can assess family adaptation and develop interventions that could further strengthen the family unit as they cope with the problems that arise from having a child with a chronic illness or disability.

Family Systems Theory

Family systems theory is derived from general systems theory (see Chap. 8). Family systems theory views an individual person as a complex being operating within a system. The focus is on the interactions of the members of the family system and the interaction of the family system with the environment (Friedman, 1992). The major assumptions of family systems theory are the following (Mercer, 1989):

The family system is greater than and different from the sum of its parts.

The family system is differentiated from the environment by boundaries.

The subsystems that exist in a family unit relate to each other in a logical hierarchy, and the family system interacts with systems in the environment.

Family systems change in response to stresses and strains from within as well as from the environment outside the family system boundaries.

A change in one family member creates a change in other members, which in turn results in a new change in the original member.

A problem or dysfunction does not lie in any one member but rather in the type of interactions used by the family.

Family systems have homeostatic features to maintain stable patterns.

Since it is the interactions, rather than the individual members, that are viewed as the source of the problem, the family becomes the patient, and the focus of care is the family unit. Therefore, the focus must be on the relationships between family members rather than on individual members. To effect positive change in a family, it is necessary to work with and through the subsystems of the family. When problems exist within the family, change can be effected by altering the interaction or feedback messages that perpetuate disruptive behavior. Feedback refers to processes within the family that help identify strengths and needs and determine how well goals are being accomplished. Positive feedback initiates change, whereas negative feedback resists change. When the family system is disrupted, change can occur at any point in the system. Consequently, it is not necessary to go back into the family history or an individual's life to find the cause of the problem (Wong, 1995). In family systems theory, the emphasis is on what is occurring now in the family and on intervening to change that pattern.

CASE STUDY 9–1
Assessment of a Family Based on Family Stress Theory

Michael, age 4 years, is being admitted to an acute pediatric rehabilitation hospital with the diagnosis of paraplegia from a motor vehicle accident. His family consists of his mother, who is a single parent, and a 6-year-old sister. His father has not been involved with Michael since birth. Michael's mother is an undocumented immigrant from Central America. However, because her children were born in America, she cannot be deported. Using the ABCX model (Boss, 1988), a family assessment will determine the level of crisis that Michael's disability means to the family. The assessment of this family is based on the premise that the family's ability to manage a stressful event depends on the family's perception of the event. Nursing interventions can be developed from the perceptions and needs that are identified from the assessment.

A (Stressful Event)

- Michael's disability
- Financial crisis
- Mother not working; lives on money she receives for the children
- Language barrier
- Mother unable to find child care for 6-year-old daughter
- Mother has no support systems
- Mother is frightened of Michael's care and will not attempt to touch or care for him
- Mother lives in an apartment that is not wheelchair accessible

B (Family Strengths)

- Mother has strong religious faith and attends Mass every Sunday
- Mother is very frugal
- Mother verbalizes a desire to keep her children with her

C (Family's View of Event)

- Mother was overwhelmed by health care system and expressed the belief that she could not manage her son's care
- Mother perceived the event as one that is out of her control

X (Crisis)

- The event is a major crisis for the family

The interdisciplinary team recommended that Michael go into foster care until his mother can develop the resources to care for him at home. The social worker set up a contract whereby Michael's mother would visit periodically and begin to work with the foster mother in learning his care. The social worker also began to look for different living arrangements for the family to accomodate Michael's disability.

FAMILY STRUCTURE

The families living in the United States today can no longer be defined as the traditional family consisting of a father, mother, and children in a situation where the father is the primary breadwinner. Although this structure does continue to exist as the dominant family structure within American culture, it cannot be considered the only structure. There currently are a number of family structures that represent the lifestyle changes that have occurred over the past four decades, as well as a new societal acceptance and openness that has developed in conjunction with these changes. Until recently, the model of the nuclear family was held as the most accepted structure, and failure to conform to this structure often placed a family on the fringes of the societal group. Because the threat of being ostracized could result in the destruction of the family unit, families may have been afraid to make their differences in family structure known to the public in general. The most common family structures currently encountered in the pediatric rehabilitation population are nuclear and extended families, single-parent families, blended families, gay/lesbian families, communal families, and empty-nest families.

Nuclear and Extended Families

The nuclear family, composed of husband, wife, and children who live in a common household, is the traditional representation of the family. In the past this structure was an economic necessity. For families to sustain themselves in an agrarian society, it was an economic necessity to have a family structure that could produce helpers or family members that could contribute to the family productivity by engaging in work on the farm. The more people available to work, the more the family would survive and prosper.

Currently, the nuclear family is relatively mobile and highly adaptable. Families are no longer bound to geographic areas for economic reasons and are no longer dependent on coordination with other family members for economic survival. Families frequently relocate for higher incomes or better employment opportunities. The mobility experienced by nuclear families makes it necessary for the family to purchase services once provided by extended family members. The extended family of the past was defined as consanguineous—family members of different generations living in the same household or in close proximity. The extended family could be counted on for such services as child care, care of an ill family member, or advice on family management issues. Although extended family members living in the same household have essentially disappeared, a majority of nuclear families maintain close contact with relatives through the use of modern technologic advances (Wong, 1995).

Single-Parent Families

The single-parent family is for the most part, a recent social phenomenon. A number of societal changes have been responsible for the change of family structure from nuclear to single parent. This type of family includes separated, divorced, and widowed parents; never-married individuals; single-parent adoptions; and foster parents. Wong (1995) identifies the women's rights movement as partially responsible for the emergence of the single-parent family. It is through this movement that women gained the autonomy to establish separate households. Divorce has become a commonplace event as a result of changes in laws and the change in social climate that makes divorce more acceptable today. Divorce has increased the number of children living in single-parent homes. It is becoming increasingly common for men as well as women to have primary guardianship of their children. It also is becoming more common for women to decide to have children and not marry. Both men and women are choosing to remain single and adopt children; however, the majority of single-parent families are headed by women. These families tend to be economically disadvantaged, because in many instances women earn considerably less income than men in our society, even though they may perform the same tasks. This lack of adequate earning power, plus a lack of financial support from the fathers of children of divorce, continues to plague single-parent families headed by women. Often these families are on welfare because of lack of skills or job training and because of expensive or non-existent child-care facilities.

A significant number of single-parent families result when a woman wishes to have a child but does not choose to marry. In the past, single mothers were expected to give their babies up for adoption. This is no longer a societal expectation, and many unmarried mothers often choose to keep and raise their children rather than place them for adoption. With the increasing independence of women as a whole and the increasing acceptability of illegitimacy in society, more women are deliberately choosing single parenthood (Wong, 1995). In the past 20 years, the number of unwed women bearing children has tripled, and a large percentage (32.7%) of these infants are born to women under age 19 years (U.S. Bureau of Census, 1987). Often, the young mother remains at home with her parents and raises the child in an extended family situation. Teens who become pregnant often lack knowledge about the importance of proper health care supervision during pregnancy. Fear of social stigma or lack of resources may cause the teenager to delay in obtaining prenatal care. Prenatal care may be more difficult for the pregnant teenager to obtain because of poverty, lack of availability, or lack of knowledge about where to go. This lack of care can lead to complications that go undetected. Complications during pregnancy may result in higher rates of premature births, congenital malformations, neonatal deaths, and higher infant and maternal morbidity and mortality rates among teens (Jackson & Saunders, 1993).

Blended Family

Blended families, also referred to as step-families (Ross & Cobb, 1990), are those that result from the marriage of individuals who remarry after divorce or death of a spouse. Frequently, the spouses bring children from previous unions together in one group. The families resulting from the joining of two families involve complex family structure. Every member of the new family has a past history, with experiences and expectations that affect family function. The major challenge to the blended family is to integrate past experiences and form a new family system that can satisfy all family members. In addition to the members of the family unit, there are extended family members, such as grandparents, aunts, and uncles, who must be considered when defining new rules and routines. Unlike nuclear families, in which members are added on a gradual basis, it is necessary for members of the blended family to begin functioning as a family without the advantage of time to work out relationships. Both formal and informal role patterns need to be examined and redefined. Childbearing decisions, financial concerns, and housekeeping tasks must be reconsidered, and conflicts can occur. It is very likely that some members of the blended family may continue to grieve over the loss of a parent or spouse and find it difficult to resolve the loss in a way that is healthy for the new family, thereby increasing the strain within the family. If the loss has been through separation or divorce, the grieving person may be constantly reminded of the loss every time there is interaction with the separated person. If the loss was through the death of a parent or spouse, there may be varied reactions. For example, the person who is deceased may be idealized. Once this person is viewed as being perfect, the replacement person may not be seen as an adequate substitute. Conversely, the person replacing the deceased family member may be viewed as a welcome member and integrated into the family unit with little difficulty.

Gay/Lesbian Family

The children that are part of a homosexual family are most commonly acquired through a previous heterosexual marriage of one of the partners (Wong, 1995). Gay men and lesbians marry partners of the opposite sex for a variety of reasons. Frequently, homosexual tendencies are not recognized at the time of their marriage or are not acknowledged until after the marriage has taken place. Others may marry hoping that a heterosexual relationship will abolish their homosexual desires. A gay man or lesbian may also enter into a heterosexual relationship for reasons that include love for the spouse, desire for children, family and peer pressure, desire for companionship, and fear of loneliness (Bozett, 1988).

Although most children in gay or lesbian households are the biologic child of a former legal marriage, homosexual couples who do not have children can use other means to bring children into the family. For example, the couple may become foster parents or choose to adopt children (Ricketts & Achtenberg, 1987). Lesbian mothers may conceive through artificial insemination or a sexual encounter with a man. As with heterosexual couples who are faced with infertility issues, the gay male couple may become parents through the use of a surrogate mother.

Increasingly, same-sex couples are demanding their rights in the legal system. They are attempting to legitimatize their union through the bonds of marriage, and in addition, they are exercising their right to become parents. These families face enormous challenges as they struggle with day-to-day problems that all families face. In addition, discrimination remains an issue that has a major impact on the lives of homosexual couples. The gay or lesbian family must also struggle with the challenges imposed on homosexual relationships by society.

Communal Family

When groups of individuals join together in one large household, farm, or community as a family unit, this is considered to be a communal family. These families most commonly emerge from a shared disenchantment with most contemporary life choices. Although the members of a commune share a mutual disregard for conventional family structures, they share common concerns and a willingness to work together to attain common goals. Communal living may take on a number of patterns. In one type of communal situation, couples may maintain a monogamous relationship, with childrearing a task jointly shared with all of the other adult members of the commune. In other communes, all of the adult members of the group are "married" to each other, with offspring belonging to the entire group. In communal families there is a strong reliance on other group members for emotional support. The group shares financial responsibilities, with every able-bodied member making a contribution to the well-being of the whole group. Material interdependence is expected, and the group mutually owns any material possessions. Family members provide collective security for nonproductive members, share homemaking and childrearing functions, and help each other with problems.

Empty-Nest and Return-to-the-Nest Syndromes

"Empty nest" is a term that is used to define a family structure that has changed because the children have grown up and left home. They may enter college, get married, or take an apartment with or without friends. "Return-to-nest" syndrome, or reverse empty nest, refers to the people who return to the home of origin after they have left to be independent of their parents. This syndrome has become increasingly common as adult children find financial independence very difficult to maintain. These children return at an older age to once again take up residence in the parental home. The reason for the return make be social, economic, or cultural. In the past, adult children rarely moved back in with their parents once they established their independence as self-supporting adults. Rates of unemployment or underemployment in some areas in the United States have resulted in the emergence of this type of family structure. Adults who have left home and established independent lifestyles may experience a loss of a job, divorce, or separation, or in some instances may find the cost of independent living greater than their salaries can support. Having few other choices, these adult children may return to their family of origin for a period of time. For the middle-aged or older parent, the return of the adult child can be both rewarding and frustrating. Lifestyles that were established after the adult left home may not be acceptable to the parents. Conflicts may occur because the parents no longer have control over the activities of the adult child. The conflict may be compounded when the returning children also have children of their own. Conflict may arise over discipline issues and child care responsibilities.

It is important for the pediatric rehabilitation nurse to understand that family structure may be very different from one family to the next. It is human nature to compare every family in the health care setting to one's own family of origin. In this situation, the pediatric rehabilitation nurse may judge the family as being unable to meet the challenges encountered when caring for a child with a disability or chronic illness. The nurse would not be able to support the family in a therapeutic manner. Once the nurse understands that each family unit is unique and has specific needs, nursing interventions can be developed to meet those needs.

FAMILY ROLES AND RELATIONSHIPS

Every individual occupies a variety of social positions within a given culture. The social positions held carry expectations of how a person is to behave toward others. The social positions are governed by rules, and these rules determine how a person will interact with the society in which they function. Rules govern the different roles that a person plays in a society and are learned as the individual is socialized by the family within a society. The socialization process begins at birth and is carried through all stages of development. Children learn that they have many roles. Each relationship carries with it a set of expectations that determine the interactions that will occur. For example, a person might have the roles of daughter, sister, granddaughter, aunt, and cousin at the same time. Each position held within the family and in society contains numerous roles to fulfill. The expectations of various roles are fulfilled according to the person's own understanding of what is expected. This understanding is determined by the culture of the society and is passed on to the child by the family, through the family's interpretation of cultural norms. What an individual actually does within a given role once it is learned from the family is called role enactment (Ross & Cobb, 1990).

Individuals may have difficulty in accomplishing the expectations of various roles. There are various reasons for this difficulty, such as incomplete socialization or interpersonal differences. This confusion about role expectations results in role stress or role strain. When an individual has many roles to fulfill, role overload may occur. An example of role overload can be found in two-career families in which the woman has the role of wife, mother, and employee and in addition has the responsibility for maintaining the home. In some cultures, children are socialized to behaviors that are not acceptable as an adult. Without an opportunity to learn adult roles, the child has difficulty assuming the new role. This is known as role discontinuity (Wong, 1995). When the child is socialized for behaviors that will continue throughout a lifetime, this is known as role continuity (Wong, 1995). An example of this would be a child that is socialized to be aggressive as a child and as an adult, as opposed to the child who is taught to be submissive as a child but aggressive as an adult.

Role conflict can emerge when the different roles that a person holds are in conflict or when the person's expectations of the role are different than those prescribed by the social group. Role conflict can create role strain. Because of the discomfort that role conflict and role strain create, the individual will make attempts to relieve the discomfort. The attempts to relieve the discomfort usually involve a manipulation or negotiations with another person, because roles never exist in isolation. A basic concept of role theory is that a particular role is joined with a reciprocal role held by another individual. Through interactions with one another, each individual influences the roles of others.

In analyzing role behaviors and expectations, one must be aware that roles may be either formal or informal. Society defines the roles; formal roles have explicit expectation, and informal roles are more subtle. Formal roles may be defined by society's expectations of the roles, such as father or mother, or the formal roles may be legally defined, such as the roles of physician, nurse, or teacher. Informal roles are learned as the child develops within the family system. The child may learn a dysfunctional role that is necessary to maintain the family unit. One family member may adopt the dysfunctional role of "bad child," which serves to divert the attention away from the discord that exists between the parents. If the role of bad child did not exist to consume the parents' attention, they would be faced with the problems that exist in their relationship.

During crisis situations, such as illness, hospitalizations, or death of a family member, role changes are usually required. This can be extremely stressful for family members, particularly if the role changes require behaviors that the individuals are not suited to or do not wish to assume. A period of instability may occur within the family until the necessary role changes have occurred. The period of instability can be extended indefinitely when the family has a child with a chronic illness or disability. In this situation, roles may need to be adjusted constantly as the needs of the child change. The mother may have to devote her time exclusively to the care of the child, thereby making it necessary for the husband to pick up the responsibility of home management, and another child may have to step into roles that they are not mature enough to assume. The process by which roles change over time is called role modification (Payne, 1988). Role modification may occur rapidly or slowly. The family members may have to adapt quickly to the role changes, or the changes may occur so slowly that the family members do not realize that roles have changed significantly. A family that is caring for a child with a disability or chronic illness usually experiences numerous role changes. The degree of change necessary will depend on the characteristics of the family members and the severity of the disability or chronic illness that the child has experienced.

CASE STUDY 9–2
Application of Role Theory

Ann is a 12-year-old girl with cerebral palsy. She attends a special needs program at the local public school. She has severe motor involvement and cannot care for herself without assistance. Her mother provides all of her care. Ann's father works in an accounting firm and believes that his responsibility is to provide financial support for the family. He wants his wife to care for the house and children. Ann has one older sibling and one younger sibling. Ann's father has never been involved in her care and does not attend school meetings or talk to therapists about equipment or treatment changes.

Ann's mother frequently expresses feelings of being overwhelmed with the responsibility of caring for Ann and her siblings. She does not have any activities outside of the home. Her husband feels she is a good wife because she manages family matters very efficiently. He is especially proud of the manner in which she manages holidays, which are celebrated in their home because he does not like to take Ann out because of the work involved. Generally, Ann's mother cooks for both extended families.

In this family the roles are traditional and inflexible. The family appears to be happy, but Ann's mother is stressed and does not have any relief from the constant stress. Her husband enforces the traditional roles, as do both of their families. The pediatric rehabilitation nurse is in a position to work with the family to find support that would not be offensive to family members.

—————

SOCIOCULTURAL INFLUENCES

In addition to an understanding of family structure and function, the pediatric rehabilitation nurse needs to be knowledgeable about the sociocultural influences that determine the structure and role relationships that a family exhibits. Each family unit functions within a culture that has expectations for how the members of a family should interact. The interactions may vary significantly among cultures. Some cultures may be difficult for the pediatric rehabilitation nurse to understand. It is important for the nurse to realize that nursing interventions can not be effective if the family's cultural beliefs are not taken into consideration when developing the plan of care. The nurse must endeavor to learn about cultural diversity and attempt to become culturally competent.

The Concept of Cultural Diversity

In recent years, there has been a dramatic increase of ethnic minority populations in the health care system. Providing health care for such a culturally diverse population can be a challenge to health care providers. To meet the needs of a culturally diverse population, it is important to understand how culture is defined. Culture can be defined as "the sum of socially learned and transmitted beliefs, concepts, and habits that shape human thought processes and characterize the work and the lifestyle of a community" (Niederhouser, 1989, p. 569). This definition can be simplified to the idea that culture is the way we live our lives. It is the mechanism by which we share our ideas, beliefs, and traditions. It is common for people to keep their cultural beliefs from generation to generation. In the United States, the notion of a mainstream culture has given way to a multicultural society. Brookins (1993) described the

United States as composed of "strata of ethnic groups that share common threads within the fabric of society while also holding . . . beliefs and practices peculiar to their ethnic group" (p. 1066). Nurses are more likely than ever before to have contact with culturally diverse families. To meet the total needs of children and families, nurses must become sensitive to their different cultural values, beliefs, and practices. It important for the nurse to understand the culture of each child, because it is their culture that strongly influences their behaviors and responses to health care. The provision of culturally sensitive care means that the nurse is able to understand a patient's behaviors and provide nursing care that reflects the patient's needs, thus resulting in positive patient outcomes.

Cultural Competence

The health care system traditionally has not responded to the needs of a culturally diverse population. However, health care providers should be sensitive to people who have cultural backgrounds that are different from those of the health care provider. Health care has traditionally been provided from an ethnocentric perspective. In the past, the patient was expected to conform to the rules and beliefs of the health care providers without regard for his or her own wishes. Health care providers should take the time to understand people from different cultures and not pass judgment on people viewed as different.

Changes are slowly being made that indicate that health care providers are becoming culturally competent by accepting the differences in beliefs and practices of children and families. There are several factors that can help in the development of cultural competence.

Practice self-awareness: by exploring one's own heritage. The more that one is able to understand his or her own beliefs and behaviors, the easier it is to understand people from other cultures.

Develop culture-specific awareness and understanding: by reading about different cultures. Articles about cultural diversity and cultural beliefs are starting to proliferate in the professional literature. Cultural awareness can be enhanced through interactions with people from different cultural backgrounds. Involvement with various cultures will allow one to develop sensitivity to people who are culturally different.

Consider the implications of cross-cultural communication: by learning the meanings that certain signs and symbols have for specific cultural groups. Nonverbal gestures, for example, have different meanings in different cultures, and what might be acceptable in one culture may be very offensive in another. Some cultures are very demonstrative and touch one another frequently, whereas in another culture, touching may offend the person being touched.

Consider the use of interpreters or translators. The inability to speak the same language is a major barrier to understanding a person from another culture. Every effort should be made to locate a translator. Family members can serve as translators, but care must be taken to ensure that cultural codes have not been broken by allowing a family member access to information that would not be shared under normal circumstances.

Collaborate with appropriate community agencies. Often, community agencies exist that can provide services for specific cultural populations. Connecting the patient and family with the appropriate agencies may result in easier access to and more appropriate health care for the family.

Above all, health care providers should ac-knowledge and respect cultural differences. Each person should be approached as an individual with unique characteristics and needs. Generalizations can result in insensitive interactions. Although a culture may have certain general characteristics, one cannot assume that every member of the culture shares the same beliefs. An overview of general cultural beliefs of the major ethnic groups are outlined in Table 9–1.

FAMILY RESPONSES TO A CHILD WITH A CHRONIC ILLNESS OR DISABILITY

All parents hope that their children will grow and develop free of physical and emotional problems. When a child is born with a physical disability or acquires a chronic illness, this expectation and all its attendant hopes are directly challenged. Responses to the diagnosis and the course of the illness vary among families; it may be an intense emotional upset for one family, but another family may be able to positively integrate the experience. Most families progress through a fairly predictable sequence of stages, regardless of the actual nature of the condition. Not all families experience the stages in a predictable order, and some families may go through more than one stage at a time. It is not unusual for a

Table 9–1 CULTURAL HEALTH PRACTICES RELATED TO HEALTH CARE OF CHILDREN AND FAMILIES

White American	Mexican American	Native American
Physician knows best	Cuaderos treat illness	Medicine men
Medicine makes it better	Herbs	Diviner
Influenced by the media	Rituals	Herbs
Costly	Religious artifacts	Rituals
	Make promises	Singers
African American	"Hot/cold" foods	
Self-care		**Southeast Asian American**
Folk medicine	**Puerto Rican American**	Herbalist
Root doctor	Espiritistas or panterios–folk healers	Family/friends
Prayer	Herbs	Diviners
Elders	Rituals	Priest
	"Hot/cold" treatments	Amulets
Haitian American	**Cuban American**	
Foods are "hot/cold"		
Home remedies	Eclectic health-seeking practices	
Voodoo priest	Folk medicine	
Amulets and prayer	Home remedies	
	Nutrition	

Adapted from Anderson, P., & Fenichel D. (1989). *Serving culturally diverse families of infants and toddlers with disabilities.* Washington, DC: National Center for Clinical Infant Programs; Geissler, E. M. (1994). *Pocket guide to cultural assessment.* St. Louis: CV Mosby; and Wong, D. (1995). *Whaley & Wong's nursing care of infants and children* (5th ed.). Philadelphia: CV Mosby.

family to return to earlier stages when faced with a change in the child's condition. These stages are:

Shock and denial: The initial response is one of disbelief and denial. The parents have difficulty accepting their child's diagnosis. Denial is a protective mechanism that helps the parents gradually accept the diagnosis. Denial becomes maladaptive when it prevents the recognition of the child's need for specific treatments. If the parents cannot accept the child's condition, they may not consent to treatment for the child. Shock and denial can last from days to many months (Wong, 1995). Denial may be manifested by behaviors such as minimizing the problems or trying to attribute the problems to a minor condition.

Grief: Grief is the response of an individual to a loss. In the case of chronic illness or disability, parents grieve the loss of their child's good health, loss of their own lifestyle, and perhaps ultimately the loss of the child. Grief begins as denial subsides. Grieving can be an intense and lengthy experience, marked by periods of denial, anger, bargaining, depression, and acceptance (Kübler-Ross, 1971). In this stage, parents are beginning to realize the reality of the situation. When the parents start to accept the child's disability or chronic condition, they may become angry. Anger is a normal reaction to the situation. The anger may be directed inward, and the parents may blame themselves for the child's condition. If the anger is directed inward, the parents may begin neglecting their own personal care, begin destructive behavior such as drinking alcohol, or become suicidal. Conversely, the anger may be directed outward. In this case the parents may lash out at their family members or health care personnel. The evolution of grief is not a linear, staged process but rather an emotional fluctuation among these states. Expressions of grief vary. Parents may cry, become angry, or block their feelings. Frequently parents withdraw from all other activities except those that center around the child. Regardless of their observable responses, the parents, siblings, and extended family members are in crisis, and their usual individual and emotional patterns are upset. The response of each parent and family member is unique. For example, the father of the child may be uncomfortable with or unable to handle his feelings and begin to withdraw from the child. The nurses may find his behavior upsetting because they believe that it is important for the child to have the parents present.

Adaptation: Over time, parents must gradually begin to accept the disability or chronic illness. They begin to have a renewed interest in life. The child is now viewed as an individual with a unique personality rather than a child with a problem. Routines are set up that include the child's special needs. For most parents, the child's diagnosis is the worst problem they will ever face. However, at the end of the grieving process, families can accept that life is forever different but realize that they have many strengths and the ability to go on with life (Lubkin, 1995).

CASE STUDY 9–3
Parental Response to Disability—Adaptation

Paul is a 10-year-old boy with a degenerative brain disease. At birth he was diagnosed with a hypoxic brain injury; however, he reached early milestones and then lost the ability to perform them. His motor ability began to reverse, and by 5 years of age he was in a vegetative state, unable to speak or move. When Paul was 2 years of age, his parents had another boy. Shortly after birth, the sibling was diagnosed with brain injury. At that time both children had extensive evaluations. They were diagnosed with congenital brain atrophy. Serial computed tomography scans revealed progressive brain atrophy. Both of the children were in a vegetative state.

The parents were both very concerned about the well-being of their children. Their goal was to make sure that the boys were comfortable and received the best care possible. They made it clear that if cardiac arrest occurred everything possible should be done for the boys. They insisted that the children be cared for at home; therefore, the boys were cared for at home by nurses and parents.

The parents were devout Catholics and said that the boys were angels that God gave them to care for on this earth and they were committed to fulfilling this role. Some of the nurses who cared for the boys had trouble agreeing with the family's philosophy. The pediatric rehabilitation nurse is in a position to help the other nurses understand the parent's belief system.

___

FAMILY ASSESSMENT

Family assessment is based on the principle that the family is the constant in the child's life and care must be family-centered to ensure successful outcomes. Although health care services and health care personnel fluctuate and change, the family, however it is composed, is the most consistent support for the child. To provide care or interventions that are family-centered and beneficial to the family unit, the family's strengths, individuality, different methods of coping, and needs should be identified. The identification process takes the form of family assessment. Bailey (1991) defines family assessment as the "ongoing and interactive process by which professionals gather information in order to determine priorities for goals and services" (p. 27). The purpose of a family assessment is to establish the family's needs and perceptions, which helps the professional determine the boundaries for intervention within the family unit (Youngblood & Hines, 1992). It is important to establish what families want for themselves and their children and to determine the professional support that they believe will help them achieve their goals. According to the definition, the assessment process is ongoing; the family is constantly evaluated for progress toward their goals, and adjustments are made as necessary to provide the interventions that will lead to a successful outcome. Information gathering in an assessment may be achieved in a number of ways. It is useful to have a clear framework or model that results in information about the family that is complete, systematic, and concise. Most models have a single focus for data gathering. The most common tools assess for the following: needs, strengths and capabilities, and social support and resources. The following lists the most commonly used tools.

FAMILY NEEDS

Family Needs Survey—Revised (Bailey & Simeonsson, 1990).
Family Needs Scale (Dunst, Trivette, & Deal, 1988).

Parent Needs Survey (Seligman & Benjamin-Darling, 1989).

FAMILY STRENGTHS AND CAPABILITIES

Family Strengths Inventory (Stinnett & DeFrain, 1985).

SOURCES OF SUPPORT AND RESOURCES

Family Support Scale (Dunst, Jenkins, & Trivette, 1984).
Personal Network Matrix (Trivette & Dunst, 1987).
Perceived Support Network Inventory (Oritt, Paul & Behman, 1985).

These family assessment frameworks and supporting data can be found by reviewing the references at the end of this chapter. Although these are just a few of the family assessment tools that are currently available, they represent the focus of most of the available tools. There is a proliferation of assessment frameworks available; however, most of the assessment tools are narrow in their approach to holistic family-centered care. For the pediatric rehabilitation nurse to function as a family advocate, there must be an eclectic approach to family assessment. A complete family assessment may be achieved by the adoption of parts of different frameworks when a single framework may be unnecessarily restrictive. The family assessment should be comprehensive and include the multiple aspects of family life rather than confining itself to a single point of view. Every conceptual framework is advantageous in some respects; however, basing family interventions on a narrow assessment of the family unit is not.

For the pediatric rehabilitation nurse to understand the family, an assessment should be completed. A family assessment can be part of the admission assessment, or it can be a separate form that is completed by the primary nurse or case manager after the initial meeting with the family. Having a written family assessment tool provides a basis for the development of family-centered interventions that are specific to the family and sensitive to the cultural background of the family. If a formal assessment tool is not available, the nurse should be concerned about the family's beliefs about health care and illness. The nurse who is sensitive to these issues will be able to ask a few appropriate questions so that a general understanding of the family unit can be obtained.

NURSING DIAGNOSIS FOR THE FAMILY WITH A CHILD WITH A DISABILITY OR CHRONIC ILLNESS

The nursing process (see Chap. 8) is the model that supports the practice of pediatric rehabilitation nursing. The nursing process begins with an assessment of family structure, relationships, and cultural background. From the assessment, the pediatric rehabilitation nurse can develop nursing diagnoses and interventions that meet the specific needs of the child and family. The nursing diagnoses for the family of the child with a disability or chronic illness will vary from situation to situation depending on the needs of the child and family. Some nursing diagnoses are more common in this situation and should be considered.

- Caregiver Role Strain
- Family Coping, Ineffective
- Parental Role Conflict
- Altered Parenting, High Risk for
- Altered Family Processes
- Grieving of Family Caregiver
- Social isolation, High risk for
- Family Caregivers' Health-Seeking Behaviors

ISSUES FOR A FAMILY MANAGING A CHILD WITH A CHRONIC DISABILITY OR ILLNESS

After the nursing diagnoses have been selected, interventions are developed. Regardless of the nature of the nursing interventions, there are certain issues that must be taken into consideration for every family that has a child with a disability or chronic illness. These issues include family education, support systems, support groups, and respite care. Every nursing diagnosis should address one or more of these issues.

These issues are important because of the underlying powerlessness that families feel when faced with the care of a child who has a disability or chronic illness. For many families, the feeling of powerlessness that occurs over the course of adjustment to the disability or chronic illness is never resolved. The inability to change the fact that the child has a disability (Smith, 1993) is very difficult for parents to accept. The sense of powerlessness is compounded by the fact that there is a loss of control over many parts of life. Health care providers tend to foster dependency in the families of children with a dis-

ability or chronic illness. There is currently a movement in health care for greater autonomy for the health care consumer; however, families are not always encouraged to take control of their children's health care, and it is easier for the family and health care provider when the health care providers are in control of the decision-making process. Unfortunately, dependency leads to feelings of helplessness, hopelessness, and isolation of the family unit, and these feelings lead to increased stress within the family unit.

The following list of requirements are common to families with a child who has a disability or chronic illness. If these requirements are addressed, the family may gain control and develop a power base from which to make decisions about matters critical to the family unit.

Parent education: Parents who understand the child's condition are better equipped to make informed decisions about the child's care. Parents should learn the health care terminology and its meanings so that they have a clear understanding of the child's needs and the goals of the treatment plan. Parents frequently learn much about the care of the child and become very proficient in providing this care. Parents should be taught to be proactive in seeking information and how to formulate questions and write down information so that they have a written record. Parents need to have written copies of all documentation from teachers, physicians, and therapists. The parents need a record-keeping system so that they have easy access to this information.

Support systems: Support systems can be identified within the family, in the extended family, and in the community. Families need to maintain the strengths that exist within the family unit. For example, one strength of a family may be open lines of communication between family members. This strength should be identified and supported, along with any other strengths that exist. Extended family members can provide support to the family by caring for siblings, grocery shopping, or providing transportation. In addition to the extended family, community members may volunteer to help the family with maintenance tasks. Community resources may be available for the child with a disability or chronic illness. Parents should be encouraged to find these resources and take advantage of them.

Support groups: Parents should be encouraged to develop relationships with other parents who have the same concerns. Talking to other parents can be a great source of support, and families may learn about treatment options and locations of resources. They also realize that they are not alone in their situation, which relieves feelings of isolation. The family can join a support group, which is a more formalized meeting with other families that have similar concerns. The support group provides the family members with a mechanism to resolve issues that increase family stress.

Respite: Families should learn to take care of their own needs, and having time away from the disabled individual is necessary to preserve physiologic well-being. Respite care provides the family with time away from the stress of caring for the child. Respite care may be in-home or out-of-home. In-home services provide care in the recipient's home and may involve skilled nursing care (Folden & Coffman, 1993). Out-of-home services vary from residential respite facilities to private family homes (Folden & Coffman, 1993).

Although respite care is clearly important for the families of disabled or chronically ill children, it may be a frightening experience for the family. Parents may be anxious about having others care for the child. They may not trust the skill level of the person providing the care and fear that the child may be injured while they are away. It is very difficult to find capable caretakers. Agencies are not always able to provide the number of skilled caretakers required for care of the child. Nurses in contact with the family must take an active role in finding respite services and carry out the role as family advocate.

SUMMARY

The pediatric rehabilitation nurse is a critical resource for the family of a child with a disability or chronic illness. The nurse needs a strong knowledge base in family theory and cultural diversity to provide maximum support to all family members. Nursing interventions should be developed to meet the unique needs of the child and family. To do this, it is imperative that the nursing plan of care be based on the nursing process, which should include an assessment of family relationships and cultural beliefs. When nursing interventions are family-centered, it is more likely that treatment goals will be valued by the family, and the family will be compliant with the management of the child with the disability or chronic illness.

REFERENCES

Bailey, D., Jr. (1991). Issues and perspectives on family assessment. *Infants and Young Children,* 4(1), 26–34.

Bailey, D., & Simeonsson, R. (1990). *The family needs survey—revised.* Chapel Hill, NC: Frank Porter Graham Child Development Center.

Boss, P. (1988). *Family stress management model.* Beverly Hills, CA: Sage Publications.

Bozett, F. (1988). Gay fatherhood. In P. Bronstein & C. Cowan (Eds.). *Fatherhood today: men's changing roles in the family.* New York: John Wiley & Sons.

Brookins, G. (1993). Culture, ethnicity, and bicultural competence: implications for children with chronic illness and disability. *Pediatrics,* 9(15), 1065–1072.

Carter, B., & McGoldrick, M. (1989). *The changing family life cycle: a framework for family therapy.* Needham Heights, MA: Allyn & Bacon.

Dunst, C., Trivette, C., Davis, M., & Cornwell, J. (1988). Enabling and empowering families of children with health impairments. *Children's Health Care,* 17(2), 71–81.

Dunst, C., Trivette, C., & Deal, A. (1988). *Enabling and empowering families: principles for practice.* Cambridge, MA: Brookline Books.

Duvall, H. (1977). *Marriage and family development.* Philadelphia: JB Lippincott.

Edelman, L. (Ed.). (1991). *Getting on board: training activities to promote the practice of family-centered care.* Bethesda, MD: Association for the Care of Children's Health.

Folden, S., & Coffman, S. (1993). Respite care for families of children with disabilities. *Journal of Pediatric Health Care,* 7, 103–110.

Friedman, M. (1992). *Family nursing: theory and practice* (3rd. ed.). Norwalk CT: Appleton-Century-Crofts.

Jackson, D., & Saunders, R. (1993). *Child health nursing: a comprehensive approach to the care of children and their families.* Philadelphia: JB Lippincott.

Kübler-Ross, E. (1971). *On death and dying.* New York: Macmillan.

Lubkin, I. (1995). *Chronic illness: impact and interventions.* Boston: Jones & Bartlett.

McCubbin, H., & Patterson, J. (1982). Family adaptation to crisis. In H. McCubbin, A. Cauble, & J. Patterson (Eds.). *Family stress, coping and social support.* Springfield, IL: Charles C Thomas.

McCubbin, M., & McCubbin, H. (1993). Families coping with illness: the resiliency model of family stress adjustment and adaptation. In C.B. Danielson, B. Hamel-Bissell, & P. Winstead-Fry (Eds.). *Families, health, and illness.* St. Louis: CV Mosby.

Mercer, R. (1989). Theoretical perspectives on the family. In C. Gilliss, B. Higley, B. Roberts, & I. Martinson (Eds.). *Toward a science of family nursing*. Menlo Park, CA: Addison-Wesley.

Niederhouser, V. (1989). Health care of immigrant children: incorporating culture into practice. *Pediatric Nursing*, 15(6), 569–574.

Oritt, E., Paul, S., & Behman, J. (1985). The perceived support network inventory. *American Journal of Community Psychology*, 13, 565–582.

Payne, M. (1988). Utilizing role theory to assist the family with sudden disability. *Rehabilitation Nursing*, 13(4), 191–194.

Ricketts, W., & Achtenberg, R. (1987). The adoptive and foster gay and lesbian parent. In F. Bozett (Ed.). *Gay and lesbian parents*. New York: Praeger.

Ross, B., & Cobb, K. (1990). *Family nursing: a nursing process approach*. Menlo Park, CA: Addison-Wesley.

Seligman, M., & Benjamin-Darling, R. (1989). *Ordinary families, special children: a systems approach to childhood disability*. New York: Gulford Press.

Smith, P. (1993). You are not alone: for parents when they learn that their child has a disability. *National Information Center for Children and Youth with Disabilities*, 111(1), 2–4.

Stinnett, N., & DeFrain, J. (1985). Family strengths inventory. In N. Stinnett & J. DeFrain (Eds.). *Secrets of strong families*. New York: Berkley Books.

U.S. Bureau of Census. (1987). *Vital statistics of the United States*. Washington, DC: U.S. Government Printing Office.

Wong, D. (1995). *Whaley & Wong's nursing care of infants and children* (5th. ed.). Philadelphia: CV Mosby.

Youngblood, N., & Hines, J. (1992). The influence of the family's perception of disability on rehabilitation outcomes, *Rehabilitation Nursing*, 17, 323–326.

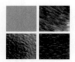

Chapter 10

Child Growth, Development, and Maturation

Dalice Hertzberg

■

FUNDAMENTALS OF DEVELOPMENT

The chief goal of pediatric rehabilitation nursing is to improve the functional capacity of the child so that the highest level of independence is reached and the child is included in the community as a productive member. For the child with an acquired disability from trauma or illness as well as the child who was born with a disabling condition, achievement of this goal requires that the nurse understand the developmental stages throughout childhood and into adulthood and the underlying physiologic processes that are responsible for growth and development. Likewise, a comprehensive understanding of the interactions among factors such as genetics, pre-natal environment and effects, and post-natal environment is necessary. This knowledge aids the nurse in supporting the child with a disability or chronic condition to accomplish new and ever more complex skills as growth and development progress.

Growth, development, and maturation are lifelong, dynamic processes that do not end when an individual reaches 21 years of age. Rather, these processes represent a continuum that begins with fertilization, progresses most rapidly during childhood, slows gradually through subsequent decades, and ends only with death. The younger the child, the more rapidly the processes of growth, development, and maturation occur. Although there is considerable variation in what is developmentally "normal" for each unique child, milestones in these processes are linked with the age at which they typically occur, making

the child's chronological age a critical component for understanding developmental events (Allen, 1991).

Central Developmental Concepts

Growth

Growth refers to an increase in size and weight. It is a quantitative change and is easily measurable. Growth is the net result of increases in cell numbers in the body as a whole and in various organs and structures.

Different organ systems have specific trajectories of growth marked by rapid cell differentiation and changes in form and influenced by environmental factors. Although individuals are unique regarding the exact timing of growth of organ systems, the sequential nature of the patterns are believed to be fairly consistent, barring interference by external factors or disease (Seidel, Ball, Daines, & Benedict, 1991). More recently, research and theory development has cast doubts on the contention that children reach motor milestones in the same sequence and by using the same strategies (Case-Smith, 1996). Changes in body composition at different ages results from differing rates of growth of organs and tissues. Body proportions change in relation to growth of organs and tissues as well as to the pattern of skeletal growth.

The relatively large size of the head compared with the body in infancy is an example of change in body proportion. Head growth is greatest during the fetal period and in the first 2 years of life, with half of the lifetime growth occurring by 1 year of age. Most neurons are formed pre-natally. About 100 billion neurons are contained in the fully developed brain (Hagerman, 1995). Most of the formation of neurons occurs in the first 3 months of fetal life, and about two thirds of brain cells are present at birth. Glial cells and myelin continue to develop after birth. By 10 months of age, new cell development in the brain is complete. After 2 years of age, head circumference increases only slightly, on an average of 2 cm/year during childhood. Cell size continues to increase, and at 2 years of age, 80% of brain growth is completed. Nine tenths of brain growth is complete by 7 years of age, and adult brain weight is reached by 10 years of age in the majority of children (Trauner, 1979; Seidel, Ball, Daines, & Benedict, 1991).

Brain size is estimated by head circumference, which generally provides a good measure of cell development. On average, neonatal head circumference is 34 cm, reaching 43 cm by the end of the first year and increasing about 0.5 cm/year until reaching an average adult circumference of 52 cm. Cells continue to increase in size for several years after birth. This growth occurs due to increasing white matter and synaptic connections. The cerebellum is very vulnerable to trauma during this early period of life.

All neurons and neural regions experience the same developmental events, but not all develop at the same rate. The neonatal spinal cord, located at the third lumbar vertebra, doubles its weight in the first year of life and increases to eight times its weight by adulthood. As the child grows, the spinal cord continues to move downward until it reaches the L1-L2 vertebral level by adulthood (Disabato & Wulf, 1994). Myelination of the central nervous system begins around the fourth pre-natal month and starts in the brain during the last trimester. The autonomic nervous system is myelinated and mature at birth, as are the cranial nerves. The cortex, the connection to the thalamus and basal ganglia, and the rest of the spinal cord do not become completely myelinated until about 2 years of age (Hagerman, 1995).

The most rapid overall growth occurs pre-natally and in the first 3 years of life, and the rate of growth remains relatively steady from about age 3 to 4 years until puberty. The rate of growth increases again during adolescence until adult height is reached. With the advent of walking, the infant's typical pot-bellied, bow-legged appearance begins to change to a more slender and taller physique, making locomotion easier and coordination better, partially due to changes in the center of gravity (Whaley & Wong, 1987). As the child grows, the limbs increase in length more rapidly than the trunk, and the trunk lengthens more rapidly than the head, giving the school-aged child a relatively adult head-to-body proportion. Both trunk and legs grow significantly during adolescence, when about 50% of the child's ideal weight is gained, skeletal mass and organ systems double in size, and secondary sex characteristics show their greatest predominance. The adolescent growth spurt results from the interaction of sex steroids and growth hormone (Seidel, Ball, Daines, & Benedict, 1991).

An infant's birth weight is largely determined by the mother's pre-pregnancy weight, the weight the mother gained during pregnancy, placental sufficiency, gestational influences, and genetics. Weight is related to height as well as development of organs and is largely determined by nutritional factors. The number and size of adipose cells are influenced by nutrition, and patterns of fat deposition are affected by age and gender. The amount of lymphatic tissue, which peaks at about 10 to 12 years of age at about double adult size, decreases during adolescence to the adult proportions (Seidel, Ball, Daines, & Benedict, 1991).

Gender also influences size and rate of growth. Newborn girls are shorter, lighter, and have less muscle and more fat than newborn boys. However, throughout pre-school and school years, girls grow and develop more rapidly. Growth rates and the timing of growth spurts differ somewhat between boys and girls, with girls growing faster than boys until adolescence, when boys catch up. During adolescence, the male growth spurt is more pronounced and lasts longer than that of the female (Seidel, Ball, Daines, & Benedict, 1991).

Bone growth is an important determinant of height. Different types of bones grow at different rates; for example, long bones grow more rapidly than flat bones or vertebrae. Ossification is the process of bone formation, which takes place in the diaphysis, the central area of long bones, and the epiphysis, or the end portion of the bone. Between these areas is located the epiphyseal plate, or growth plate, of the bone; this is where new growth occurs. Epiphyses that close prematurely due to trauma or disease stop the growth of the bone at that point and can contribute to limb-length discrepancy or other deformations of the skeleton. Skeletal age is determined by radiologic comparison of mineralization and ossification of bones to specific age-related standards and by timing of the closure of epiphyseal plates. Onset of menarche occurs at nearly the same time as closure of the epiphyses in the vertebrae and can be used as a marker for the cessation of spinal growth in girls. Skeletal growth is complete when the epiphyses of long bones are fused completely. In boys, this generally occurs at around 17.5 years of age and in females at about 15.5 years of age, or 2 years after menarche (Seidel, Ball, Daines, & Benedict, 1991).

Growth is dependent on a coordinated sequence of endocrine, genetic, constitutional, environmental, and nutritional influences. The pituitary gland secretes growth hormone, which stimulates DNA synthesis (primarily during late infancy and adolescence), which increases cell numbers. Insulin assists this process by promoting protein synthesis, which becomes the cytoplasm of the cells. Thyroxin, secreted by the thyroid gland, influences fetal and neonatal growth, affects skeletal growth and development, promotes sexual maturation, and influences mental development.

The developmental changes of puberty result from the interaction of the hypothalamus, the pituitary gland, and the gonads. During puberty, increased secretion of testosterone and estrogen lead to the development of secondary sex characteristics in boys and girls, respectively. Testosterone enhances muscular development and promotes bone maturation and epiphyseal closure. Estrogen stimulates linear growth by the acceleration of skeletal maturation and epiphyseal fusion. The growth and differentiation of the genitalia during the fetal period is also influenced by estrogen. Androgens secreted by the adrenal glands promote masculinization of secondary sex characteristics as well as skeletal maturation (Seidel, Ball, Daines, & Benedict, 1991). Both physical maturation and the changing levels of hormones help account for changes during adolescence that may lessen the effects of a disability (e.g., reduction in the number of fractures in children with osteogenesis imperfecta) or result in new concerns (e.g., skin care and changes in mobility in adolescents with spina bifida).

The rate and amount of growth is determined in part by environmental influences, which include nutrition; presence or absence of disease; exposure to toxic substances, either pre-natally or post-natally; and psycho-

social factors. A child's growth potential is inherited; body composition and height is individually programmed from the genes of both of the parents. The child who receives adequate nutrition while growing, especially in the first few years of life, is most likely to reach or slightly exceed that potential. Improved nutrition in the United States in the past 40 years has led to an increase in the average height and weight of children and adults.

Exposure to toxic substances in utero or after birth can affect growth through a variety of mechanisms. Mothers who smoke cigarettes during pregnancy place their infants at increased risk for low birth weight, prematurity, and greater rates of neonatal death (Rosenblith, 1992). Other substances used during pregnancy, such as cocaine and alcohol, also affect the size and growth potential as well as overall development of the child.

Deprivation has been shown to affect growth as well as development. The syndrome of psycho-social dwarfism is seen in emotionally deprived children who are neglected and do not receive the necessary care or nurturing. Children who grow up in orphanages without regular, loving caregivers or in extremely bleak surroundings do not reach their full growth potential.

The presence or absence of a variety of disease conditions can also affect growth, either directly or indirectly. Many conditions, such as cerebral palsy, contribute to malnutrition because spasticity and persistent primitive reflexes interfere with proper eating and swallowing. Children with sickle cell disease are often smaller than their age-matched peers, possibly because of anorexia during sickle cell crises. Metabolic bone diseases such as osteogenesis imperfecta influence size and body habitus due to continual fracture and re-fracture of brittle bones, making children and adults with this condition very small in stature. Conditions with a gastrointestinal component, such as cystic fibrosis, reduce the absorption of nutrients through the intestinal wall as a result of inadequate digestive enzymes, resulting in smaller stature and overall size. Prader-Willi syndrome, a genetic disorder affecting the endocrine system, predisposes affected children to eating disorders and obesity.

Unusual size and rate of growth, either more rapid or slower than usual, is often associated with the presence of disease. The relative proportions of the body may also vary with variations in growth. Individuals with Marfan syndrome, a genetic neuromuscular condition, are often very tall, with unusually long arms and large hands and feet. Children with achondroplastic dwarfism are not only small in overall stature but also have shorter relative limb length compared with trunk and head size.

Growth is evaluated by comparing the child's size and trajectory of growth to established norms. The modified growth charts standardized by the National Center for Health Statistics and available from Ross Laboratories (Seidel, Bell, Daines, & Benedict, 1991) are the most commonly used and the most widely validated for a variety of populations. However, even these growth standards do not clearly reflect the typical growth trends of children of various cultural groups or those who are affected by disabilities or chronic conditions. Additional information on growth assessment is included in Chapter 11.

Healthy, full-term newborns usually weigh between 2500 and 4000 g, double their birth weight by 5 months of age, and triple their birth weight by 12 months of age. Head circumference should be measured regularly until 2 years of age and then at least yearly until 6 years of age. Chest circumference can be used as a useful comparison when a problem with head size is suspected. Size for gestational age is categorized as appropriate for gestational age (AGA; within the 10th–90th percentile); small for gestational age (SGA; less than the 10th percentile); or large for gestational age (LGA; greater than the 90th percentile). Infants that are either SGA or LGA have an increased risk of morbidity and mortality, and these risks are increased if the infant is pre-term or post-term (Seidel, Ball, Daines, & Benedict, 1991). In addition, there are two types of SGA: symmetric and asymmetric. In the asymmetric type of SGA, the infant has had inadequate nutrition during the pre-natal period. The cause of the symmetric form of SGA is unknown, but this group of children does more poorly developmentally compared with the asymmetric SGA group.

Measurements taken at any point in time may reveal size for age that falls within the upper or lower 10th percentile, but these measurements are most meaningful when compared with the rate of growth over time. Measurements that have always been around the 50th percentile and then drop below the 10th percentile may indicate a serious deficiency in growth due to inadequate nutrition or disease. With children who exhibit failure to thrive, weight falls off first, then height, then head circumference. Small head circumference when compared with height and weight for age suggests inadequate brain growth. Discrepancies between height and weight percentiles may also indicate growth disorders. Obesity is determined by the progressive increase of weight compared with height or length and is generally considered to be weight 20% over the established norms for age.

The measurement techniques used to determine height, weight, and head circumference are crucial as they affect the accuracy of the result and the validity of the data. Children who are difficult to measure due to disabilities or chronic conditions often have inaccurate measurements. Children who use wheelchairs and cannot stand on a regular scale may be weighed on a wheelchair scale which weighs the wheelchair and the child or on a seated scale on which the child may sit. It may be difficult to measure the length of children with cerebral palsy because of spasticity and contractures of limbs and scoliosis. The method of measurement of growth can influence the information used to make recommendations for care by the rehabilitation team.

Maturation

Maturation is the internal regulatory mechanism that influences the emergence of skills and abilities in the developing child and is an important part of the processes of growth and development (Kuh, 1984). It is the process through which individual organ systems acquire function by producing physical changes (Seidel, Ball, Daines, & Benedict, 1991; Cech & Martin, 1995). Maturation is driven by genetics and influenced by environmental opportunity, resulting in movement from an immature state or function to a more fully developed state or function. Maturation moves in the direction of increased functionality and complexity. It cannot occur until the underlying biologic structures are present. The process of maturation is dependent on growth and differentiation of cells and underlies development. An example of the maturational process in development is the myelination and specialization of nerve cells combined with the muscular development and coordination necessary for urinary continence. Until the underlying maturational processes are in place, efforts to potty train a child are not successful (Betz, Hunsberger, & Wright, 1994).

Different organs and systems exhibit different markers of maturation. Closure of epiphyseal plates in the long bones represents a marker of skeletal maturation; puberty represents the beginning of endocrine system maturation. Reflexes and reactions disappear, as in the case of primitive reflexes, or appear as a result of central nervous system maturation. Myelination is an example of a maturational process that must occur before full neuromotor abilities are realized. Although myelination begins in utero, its progress is an indicator of functional efficiency and specificity of nerve transmission and is exemplified by increasing neuromotor capacity. Although the timing of myelination is largely under genetic control, recent research suggests that appropriate environmental stimuli can influence specific changes in the brain such as dendritic branching, creation of new synapses, and creation of new capillaries (Greenough, Black, & Wallace, 1993; Hallett & Proctor, 1996).

Development

Development represents the qualitative changes in function that result from mastering tasks and responding to challenges from the environment. These qualitative changes are more difficult to measure and are much more complex than the quantitative changes that occur with growth.

Each child has a unique trajectory of development based on the interaction of genetics and environment. Although children tend to develop according to a similar pattern, they do not necessarily develop at the same rate. An example of developmental variation is the child who learns to walk without ever crawling. Children may use different movement strategies to reach the same end—that of rolling over, reaching, or walking. Additionally, different domains of development, such as fine motor, gross motor, social, communication, and cognitive domains, do not all develop at the same rate. There is no strong relationship between the rate of development of one domain over another. For example, a child who is ahead of peers in motor development will not necessarily achieve the same level of development in speech or cognitive skills at the same time.

Although the rate of development varies in different domains, the progress of development among domains is closely interrelated. A strength, deficit, or challenge in one domain inevitably affects another domain. For example, the child who is limited in movement by paralysis and is unable to explore the environment independently will be limited in experience of the world and therefore is at much greater risk of limitations in cognitive, communicative, and social abilities. Any observation of one aspect of a child's development must be viewed in the perspective of all other aspects of that child's development, environment, and experience (Dixon, 1992).

Development is a series of stages, a process of gradual building of skills, one upon the other. Later stages build on the achievements of earlier stages. This process requires an enormous amount of energy on the part of the child and is a complex interaction between the child and the environment. Development does not occur in a smooth progression from one phase to another but rather in a series of "spurts and lulls" (Dixon, 1992). Periods of apparent disorganization in functioning may precede a developmental spurt. These periods of disorganization may be general or limited to the domain of development undergoing the most rapid change. The "lull" periods are believed to be times of refinement of skills (Dixon, 1992).

Development occurs in an orderly, predictable manner, following specific patterns: from simple to complex; from general or undifferentiated to specific; from head to toe, or cephalo-caudally; and from the midline out to the extremities, or proximo-distally. The norms that constitute developmental milestones are based on these predictable growth patterns and the average age at which they are reached. Within these predictable patterns, each child develops uniquely based on personal characteristics. Any deviations from the norm must be considered with regard to the general developmental patterns as well as the child's specific pattern or rate of development.

The ability of the young child to respond to stimuli is a good example of general to specific developmental progression. The young infant responds to a painful stimulus with undifferentiated gross movement, often pulling the entire body away from the stimulus, and crying and is unable to inhibit the reaction of crying after the stimulus is removed. The older toddler, however, is able to discriminate which part of the body the stimulus was applied to, pull that part out of the way, and continue with the previous activity. If the child cries out at the stimulus, the crying stops when the stimulus is removed, evidence of the ability to inhibit reaction to a painful stimulus. The ability to change and the rate of change from one activity to another and from one state to another is evidence of central nervous system development.

Progression from simple to complex is illustrated by the development of the pincer grasp. The 6-month-old infant reaches for a small object, such as a raisin, and scoops it up into the whole palm of the hand. A 9-month-old child delicately opposes thumb and forefinger to lift the raisin in a pincer grasp, using very specific, finely tuned movements unlike the generalized movement used by the infant. Similarly, the child's use of verbal language occurs first with single words, then progresses to formulation of two- to three-word phrases, and then to more complex sentences.

The principles of cephalo-caudal and proximo-distal development come into play with the direction of the development of muscle control. Head control comes before trunk control, and both are necessary for sitting, which involves a greater number of muscle groups and more coordinated movement. Gross motor development, such as rolling, sitting, or standing, occurs before fine motor development. Most children can roll at about 4 months of age and sit by around 6 months of age. Gross motor movements arise from muscular development of the head and trunk at the midline of the body. Fine motor movements, such as coordination of the small muscles of the hands, occur later, beginning around 8 months of age and continuing to progress through 6 years of age and later.

Sensitive periods are those developmental stages during which the child is most vulnerable to positive or negative environmental influences. Sensitive periods can be influenced either positively or negatively by external influences, such as lack of appropriate stimulation from the environment. Sensitive periods are the optimal times for positive environmental influences. Some developmental tasks will be mastered in the absence of the correct stimuli, but many will not.

Critical periods is the term used to describe the requirement for specific environmental stimulation, or an environmental trigger, to promote expected development. Critical periods require specific stimulation for the organism or child to achieve a distinct developmental task or skill. The development of a given system is modified by experiences that

result in physical alteration of the human cortex. Development, especially sensory development, can be interfered with by introducing a stimulus out of phase, or at the wrong time (Graven, 1996). Critical periods are generally those during which development occurs at a rapid rate (Craft & Denehy, 1990). An example of a critical period is the development of attachment. If the young child does not form an attachment within the first year of life with a reliable, nurturing caregiver, later social and emotional development will suffer. Another example of a critical period is the development of auditory function. Frequency discrimination and pattern recognition must be stimulated by sound from 28 weeks pre-natally to 3 or 4 weeks post-natally, or the infant will lack the ability to discriminate certain sounds (Graven, 1996). Although critical periods are most often used to refer to pre-natal development, they are believed to extend into early infancy. Developmental interactions that fail to occur during critical periods can prevent acquisition of a skill at a later time (Betz, Hunsberger, & Wright, 1994; Graven, 1996). During another period, the right combination of development, heredity, and environment may not have the same effect (Rosenblith, 1992). A depiction of developmental stages and critical periods during pre-natal development is provided in Figure 10–1.

Whaley and Wong (1987) describe the tendency for organisms to seek to achieve optimum developmental potential despite negative environmental influences. Periods of nutritional deficit, extreme stress, or deprivation that result in delays of growth and development may be overcome when the environment is more supportive. This period of "catch up" usually occurs until the child's individual growth and developmental pattern is reached. An example of this tendency is seen with premature infants, who often lag behind their same-age peers until approximately 1 to 2 years of age. Correspondingly, when young children who were premature are assessed developmentally, their age is adjusted by the number of weeks they were premature to more accurately represent their developmental achievements. Most children who were premature have "caught up" to their peers developmentally by pre-school. If they have not, the existing developmental lags are probably indicative of more general developmental problems. An overview of major landmarks in developmental phases is provided in Table 10–1.

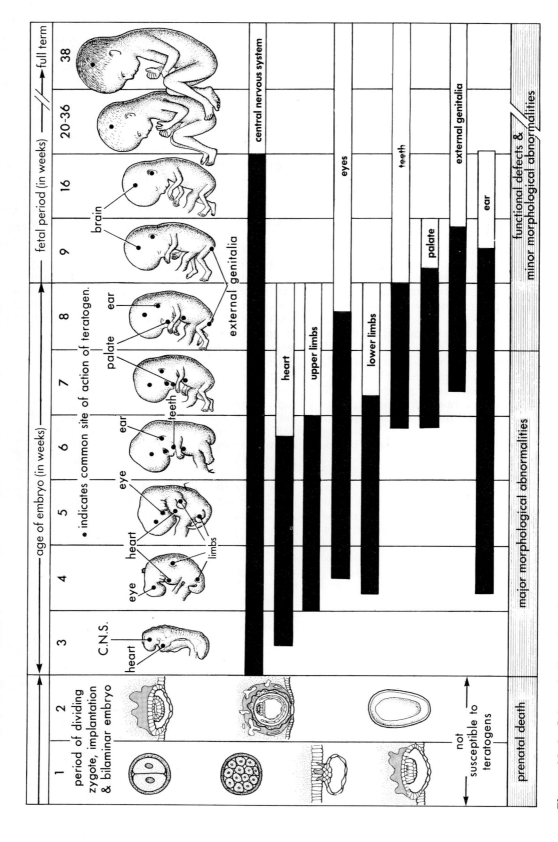

Figure 10–1 Schematic illustration of the critical periods in prenatal human development. (From Moore, K. [1989]. *Before We Are Born: Basic Embryology and Birth Defects*, 3rd edition. Philadelphia, PA: W.B. Saunders.)

Table 10-1 MAJOR LANDMARKS IN DEVELOPMENT

Age	Physical/Motor	Social/Affective	Cognitive
Conception to birth	Development of the body		
Birth	Digestion, respiration, circulation, basic functions, eye movements		
1–2 Months	Rhythms, cortical control, visual exploration	Smiling, eye contact	Learning: repetition produces memory
4–8 Months	Grasp, sitting, reaching	Smiling, response to strangers, development of fear and anxiety	Face recognition, capacity to discriminate caregivers from strangers
8–18 Months	Locomotion, feeding self	Attachment	Development of words, capacity to group
18 Months– 2 Years	Walking	Early socialization, toileting and other self-care, obedience	Move to pre-concrete operations, language begins
2½–5 Years	Better gross and fine motor control (running, climbing, games, drawing)	Issues include autonomy, peers, fears, frustration/ aggression management, imitation/modeling, dependency, identification, sex role typing, learning how to interact socially and to have friendships	Pre-conceptual thought gives way to development of intuition, a grasp of grammar and syntax, concept of negotiation/mediation
5–7 Years	Better motor control, increased size and coordination	Development of conscience, awareness of impact on others, learning how to get along outside of the home, in school, and with friends	Academic skills, reading, learning strategies, reasoning capacity
7–12 Years	At end of this period, beginnings of development of sexual characteristics and capacities	Development of reciprocal friendships, development of more differentiated conscience, self-image, view of others	Development of true concrete operational thinking capacity: class inclusion, serialization, conservation

Used with permission from Linda Iklé, Ph.D., University of Colorado Health Sciences Center, 1997.

Factors Affecting Development

According to Cech and Martin (1995) development is primarily influenced by four factors: genetics, maturation, environment, and culture. Genetics and the process of maturation govern the body's internal environment, all the components of which must be balanced to support growth and development. Environment and culture determine the experiences that the child is exposed to and help to define the specific repertoire of skills and competencies required to survive in that child's world. Values and beliefs about the world, child-rearing practices, family and community structure, and even availability and type of shelter and food are determined by culture and environment.

Genetics

The child's genetic make-up contributes the substrate for physical development; individual patterns of development; gender; and specific characteristics of appearance, personality, and vulnerabilities. Genetic inheritance is not the sole determinant of the child's characteristics; these are also modified by environmental influences. Genetic disorders caused by abnormalities of genes, chromosomes, and their component proteins and DNA occur in 15% to 16% of live births. Genetic disorders causing birth defects are the primary cause of infant mortality and a significant cause of reduced life span (Wright, 1994). Although most genetic disorders are identified immediately after birth or by the first year of life, new pre-natal diagnostic techniques such as chorionic villous sampling enable diagnosis of many genetic conditions by the 8th to 10th week of gestation (Batshaw & Perrett, 1986). A few genetic disorders, such as the muscular dystrophies, cystic fibrosis, and fragile X syndrome, are not diagnosed until later in childhood or adulthood.

The genotype is the term used to describe the genetic make-up of an individual. The phenotype is the unique expression of the genotype in a specific individual. Each human cell contains 46 chromosomes, or 23 pairs of chromosomes, which contain over 6 billion distinctive combinations of DNA called base pairs. The base pairs are arranged in a specific combination, making genes that code for particular proteins. It is usually the proteins coded for by the genes that produce a clinical effect. Proteins affect the organism in four broad categories: structural, which forms connective tissue such as bone and muscle; circulatory, which affects blood components; enzymatic, which affects enzymes needed to break down complex substances for metabolism; and transport, which affects moving substances across cell membranes. When the cell divides, the chromosomes divide also to replicate the exact pattern of DNA. During the division of reproductive cells, chromosomal abnormalities may occur spontaneously as part of the natural process of mutation, such as when maternal age is 35 years or older, or as a result of an external agent, such as radiation or chemical mutagens. Even a very tiny error in chromosomal material can cause serious and widespread biologic changes (Wright, 1995). The error may take the form of an extra or a missing chromosome (nondisjunction), a chromosome with a lost fragment that may or may not be attached to another chromosome (translocation), or a pre-existing error that may be repeated as is and passed down in successive generations.

Genetic disorders are classed into four major groups: chromosomal disorders, which include variations in chromosomal number, deletions of chromosomal material, and rearrangements of chromosomal material; sin-

gle-gene disorders, such as autosomal dominant, autosomal recessive and X-linked disorders; multifactorial disorders, including malformations and diseases; and nontraditional inheritance, such as mitochondrial inheritance, mosaicism, genetic imprinting, and uniparental disomy, which are relatively recent discoveries (Wright, 1995). It is important to try to determine the mode of transmission of the disorder to offer accurate genetic counseling to the family and to try and identify other family members who may be at risk for the disorder.

Single-gene disorders are variations at a particular location along a chromosome and usually have a relatively simple, definite inheritance pattern. These disorders are passed down through families according to a mendelian inheritance pattern. Each child inherits one gene per trait from each parent. The genes are either dominant or recessive and are responsible for a variety of genetic disorders, some of which are relatively minor and others of which cause significant disability (Whaley & Wong, 1987).

Autosomal dominant traits need only one gene from one parent to cause the disorder, and there is a 50% chance that the child will be affected. Examples of autosomal dominant disorders include osteogenesis imperfecta and Huntington disease. Autosomal recessive traits require that both parents contribute the same gene for the disorder to be expressed in the child, with possibility that the child may be a carrier of the disorder if only one affected gene is present. If the child is a carrier, the disorder will not be present, but the child will be capable of passing on the disorder or carrier status to a succeeding generation. With each pregnancy, if both parents are carriers, the child has a 25% chance of expressing the disorder, a 50% chance of being a carrier without showing symptoms of the disorder, or the child may not receive the gene at all. An example of an autosomal recessive disorder is cystic fibrosis.

In sex-linked disorders, the trait is carried on the sex chromosome, which is the X or Y chromosome that determines gender. Although the Y chromosome primarily contributes genes that cause male characteristics, the X chromosome carries many more genes, most of them related to traits other than gender. There are no Y-linked diseases, only X-linked diseases. X-linked conditions are either recessive or dominant, and X-linked dominant conditions occur much less frequently and are generally very severe. Recessive X-linked disorders are expressed in males but are almost never passed on by the father to a son, because the son receives the father's Y chromosome. Rather, the affected gene is transmitted through a carrier female to a son, who has a 50% chance of exhibiting the disease, or to a daughter, who has a 50% chance of being a carrier. Females who carry the gene are not usually affected by the condition, or if they are affected, the condition is expressed in a milder form. An example of a sex-linked recessive condition is Duchenne muscular dystrophy.

Dominant X-linked inheritance is similar to autosomal dominant disorders in that only one affected gene is needed for the child to exhibit the condition. A child of either gender has a 50% chance of inheriting the condition from the female parent. An affected male will give the gene to all daughters, but not to a son. Female children who receive the affected gene usually have a milder form of the condition, but some of these conditions are lethal to males. Familial hypophosphatemic rickets is an example of a dominant X-linked disorder.

Multifactorial inheritance combines a variety of genetic traits with environmental factors. Clinical expression of these disorders ranges along a continuum from mild to severe. There is a "threshold effect" when genetic and environmental influences overcome the ability of the organism to adapt and malformations occur. Because more than one gene is responsible for the disorder and environment plays a crucial role, multifactorial disorders are difficult to predict, and thus it is similarly difficult to counsel families regarding risk. Five principles are used by genetic counselors when establishing a pattern of risk for families affected by multifactorial disorders: incidence of specific genetic conditions may vary by race; the more severe the condition, the greater the risk of occurrence; the condition occurs more frequently in one gender than the other; the risk increases as the number of affected family members increase; and after one affected child is born, the recurrence risk is usually in the range of 3% to 5%. An example of a multifactorial disorder is spina bifida, or myelomeningocele, which is more common in individuals of Irish or English heritage than in individuals of Native American or Asian heritage (Wright, 1994).

Nontraditional inheritance accounts for other genetic mechanisms resulting in inherited disorders that, prior to advances in molecular genetics, were thought to have "familial" characteristics but no clear genetic cause. Mitochondrial inheritance accounts for disorders arising from genes found in the mitochondria of ovum and resulting in disorders causing blindness and neuromuscular disorders. Imprinting represents the differential expression of a specific gene, depending on whether inheritance came from the male or female parent. A good example of this type of inheritance is the differential expression of two disorders causing mental retardation: Prader-Willi syndrome and Angelman syndrome. Uniparental disomy occurs when two chromosomes of the same pair are inherited from the same parent, with no contribution of that chromosome from the other parent. This phenomenon does not appear to cause a unique disorder but rather is a variable mechanism of inheritance for other genetic disorders such as cystic fibrosis or hemophilia. Mosaicism occurs when cell lines that differ in genotype or karyotype arise from a single zygote. With mosaicism, a child may have chromosomes for a disorder in only some but not all of the body cells, as is typical with other forms of inheritance. Parents who have mosaicism may pass the genes to their child as well. Mosaicism results from an error of mitosis in the early stages of embryonic development and may result in differing numbers of chromosomes among different cells in the body. Some cells may have an extra chromosome, some may have a missing chromosome, and some cells may have the correct amount (Wright, 1994). Mosaicism is increasingly found to be relevant in a greater number of genetic conditions rather than primarily being seen in Down syndrome and Turner's syndrome. Research continues to reveal other mechanisms causing mutations.

The timing and patterns of maturational processes are primarily genetic in origin. The genetic make-up of the child in large part determines the child's underlying abilities to respond to the environment. The child's potential size, body shape, and temperament are genetically determined. The Human Genome Project, an international long-term research project to map the entire complement of human genes, has already suggested that some constituents of behavior and mood have genetic origins. Environmental opportunities and stimuli interact with the genetic attributes of the child to fulfill or stunt potential. As stated in earlier sections of this chapter, the child's interaction with the environment represents a continual feedback loop that increases and enhances learning and development in all domains.

Culture

The culture of the family that the child is born into affects more than child-rearing practices, family size and make-up, family lifestyle, social groups, and physical environment. Culture affects pre-natal development through the health beliefs of the mother and her ability to maintain health and adequate nutrition as well as to avoid disease, harmful substances, and trauma. Cultural practices direct the timing of emergence of skills and abilities through such practices as the amount of time an infant is held or allowed to move about independently, the use of swaddling or other close restraint that limits mobility, or the type and frequency of interaction between mother or other caregivers and the child. However, although child-rearing practices such as these may have some short-term influence on the development of motor skills or communication, they do not have long-term effects on development, and children raised in different cultural milieu show no differences from a developmental standpoint by late childhood. The influences of culture on the child with a disability or chronic conditions are explored in more detail in Chapters 7 and 9.

Nutrition

Children who receive less than adequate nutrition in utero experience intrauterine growth retardation and are often small for gestational age at birth and have low birth weight, which predisposes them to developmental delay and disability. Inadequate nutrition in the first few years of life, whether due to external factors, such as poverty or starvation, or internal factors, such as disease or a disabling condition, affects brain development. The earlier a nutritional deficit occurs, the more severe the brain damage and the less likely it is to be reversed. Nutritional deficits can be devastating if they occur during critical periods pre-natally or in the first 2 years of life. Nutritional deficits occurring early in development are time-specific in their effects and depend on the child's level of maturity at the time of the deficit. Thus, nutritional deprivation in the second trimester of pregnancy is likely to result in deficient neuronal numbers in the central nervous system. Deprivation in the last trimester of pregnancy and early neonatal life affects the number of glial cells and the maturation of neurons. Deprivation during 1 through 4 years of post-natal life primarily affects myelination and growth and extension of neurons. Conversely, the very lengthy periods of myelination and neuronal growth imply that nutritional rehabilitation for post-natal brain damage should be possible until at least 3 to 5 years of age and possibly later if the rehabilitation is continued over a long period. The most common nutritional problems facing the human fetus are inadequate supplies of energy and protein. In babies whose birth weight is low as a result of maternal nutritional deprivation, head size is smaller than expected for gestational age but normal for their body weight. The smaller the baby, the less the DNA content. Low-birth-weight infants may have brains that are less well myelinated than the brains of larger infants (Morgan & Gibson, 1991).

Children who are diagnosed with failure to thrive are often developmentally delayed and go on to develop more permanent disability. Nutritional factors do not only influence development and growth but may also contribute to disease, as in the case of kwashiorkor or rickets. Protective factors are provided by good nutrition as well, aiding in preventing disease such as atherosclerosis, minor acute and severe infections, and gastrointestinal problems. Adequate nutritional factors are critical to survival for children who experience trauma or burns.

Environment

Environmental stimulation and deprivation have profound effects on the developing child. The nature and severity of the defect produced as a result of environmental deprivation depends on the developmental events occurring at the time of the insult. Early studies of deprivation in children in orphanages and institutions have shown that neglected children have delayed and even impaired brain development. Environmental stimulation can lessen the detrimental impact of some insults and enhance recovery, especially if such therapy is instituted early. A variety of events can produce permanent and severe brain damage during the pre-natal period, including infection, the mother's neglect of her health, drugs, and metabolic disease. Post-natal infantile infections can also take a serious toll on the immature brain. Neuromalformations that occur during gestation are considered to be time-specific but stimulus–

non-specific. Thus, an insult of any kind during the first pre-natal month may result in neural tube defects, whereas insults at about 4 to 6 pre-natal months may result in deficient numbers of neurons and a pathologically small brain. The time-specific but stimulus–non-specific nature of pre-natal neuronal insults reflects neural maturational events. Those aspects of the brain actively maturing at the time of the insult suffer most.

Factors Affected by Development

Acquisition of Skills

Skill acquisition is dependent on growth, development, maturation, and the child's interaction with the environment. Maturation of the child is closely tied to learning and adaptation to the demands of the environment. Adaptation can occur on individual organ levels, internally (e.g., modeling of shape of the acetabulum and the femoral head with movement), or with the production of antibodies by the immune system following infection (Cech & Martin, 1995). The child adapts to the environment constantly by learning how to meet needs, whether by using muscles in a specific way to roll over and reach a toy or by smiling in response to a mother's voice and eye contact.

Betz, Hunsberger, and Wright (1994) describe development as involving competencies in three main areas: physical, intellectual, and emotional-social. Competency is generally thought of as the end result of skill development; therefore, competencies in different areas of development represent the level of skill necessary to survive and adapt successfully to the environment. Betz, Hunsberger, and Wright's (1994) description of competencies resembles the concept of domains of functioning in that development is broken down into interactive components.

Physical competency encompasses motor, neurologic, and biologic capacities needed to master self-care abilities. Factors such as physical health, size, strength, body build, rate of maturation, and motor skill performance combine in the child to produce functional mobility and manipulative skills.

Intellectual competency describes the development and use of communication and language skills, perceptual skills, and cognitive ability. Communication and language skills are inextricably bound to cognitive ability with regard to both comprehension and expression of ideas. Intellectual competency includes aspects such as problem solving, reasoning, abstract thought, memory, receptive and expressive language use, academic and work achievement, and intellectual quotient (IQ), or intelligence.

Development, as a process of change, balances the drive for the child to survive, organize, and adapt to the environment through the interaction of internal and external factors. None of the factors discussed in this chapter occur in isolation; they are wholly interdependent on each other and on environmental influences and opportunities for the child to achieve optimum potential.

Adaptation

Adaptation is an important concept in growth and development, encompassing both physiologic and psychologic domains. Adaptation occurs in areas of learning, such as language and cognitive development, as well as in behavior, motor areas, socialization, and all facets of development. Adaptation is the ability to adjust to internal and external environmental tensions and maintain homeostasis, or a steady state. According to Piagetian cognitive theory, adaptation is the tendency to cope with the environment, and it involves both accommodation and assimilation. Accommodation occurs when the child changes mental representations to include new information, and assimilation is when new information is incorporated into activities or ways of thinking (Betz, Hunsberger, & Wright, 1994). Coping is a form of cognitive and emotional adaptation used in the psychologic domain.

Adaptation to the environment is a dynamic process that forms the basis for learning and developing. As discussed previously, phases of maturation of organs and systems do not occur without specific environmental triggers such as light or sound. As the child develops, new skills are learned that enable the child to encounter more experiences and more stimuli for development. The sensorimotor system is a crucial factor in the child's ability to detect changes in the environment and to respond to them. Concepts of adaptation are based on the assumption that the child makes purposeful movements in an attempt to satisfy needs. These movements put the child in increasing contact with stimuli, which shape responses. Children who are limited in the sensorimotor domain have a reduced capacity to detect environmental changes and to respond to them. For example, the child who is deaf does not respond to sounds or speech, and development of communication is hampered.

Children with disabilities and chronic conditions must integrate the usual demands of age-related development as well as many non-normative demands related to the disability or chronic condition. These non-normative demands include recurrent severe illness; multiple hospitalizations; invasive interventions; prolonged therapies; physician appointments that interfere with social development and typical age-related activities, including school; use of assistive devices not used by peers; and physical differences. Children with disabilities or chronic conditions also may lack exposure to certain kinds of normative experiences. Each one of these demands creates a situation in which there is disequilibrium between the individual and the environment. Adaptation and coping are methods used by the child and the family to maintain or restore equilibrium. The level of adaptation and the coping styles used depend on several factors, both physiologic and psychologic, such as cognitive ability, developmental level, temperament, degree of resilience, past experiences, and the resources available.

Cognitive ability and developmental level affect coping and adaptation with regard to the number of prior experiences from which to learn and the ability to generalize from these experiences. Young children have fewer experiences and are less likely to be able to use complex thought process in problem solving. Their perceptions of situations differ markedly from those of an older child or an adult. Young children tend to use emotional strategies such as crying or tantrums to cope with a stressful situation, as do children who are cognitively delayed. The more developed the child's cognitive ability, the more likely they are to adapt successfully.

Developmental Domains and Theories

Development is divided conceptually into specific skill areas, or domains of development. The areas of motor development, development of communication and language skills, psychologic and cognitive development, and social development are interrelated, yet they may progress at different rates depending on the individual child and the environmental influences. For the purpose of this section, these four skill areas are used to describe the domains of development.

Although a myriad of theories addressing child development exist, many of these theories address only segments of development or do not fully address alterations in development. It is beyond the scope of this book to cover all of the existing developmental theories. Rather, this chapter focuses on selected theoretic approaches to development and presents them within the context of their application to the developmental domains, relevant to pediatric rehabilitation nursing.

Motor Development

Motor development includes the processes of gross motor development, fine motor development, and perceptual motor development, as well as the coordination and refinement of skills that accompany these processes. Two important motor skills that develop early in life are prehension, or the ability to grasp and hold an object; and locomotion, or the ability to move about. Motor development is closely tied to growth as well as to maturation of motor, sensory, and neurologic systems. Development of motor skills is dependent on the degree of maturation of the nervous and musculoskeletal systems as well as on the child's interaction with the environment. Gesell's theories remain some of the backbones of motor development approaches and are based on the idea that development follows maturation of systems (Gesell & Ilg, 1949). Neuromaturational theory, as described by Gesell, reflects the hierarchy of the central nervous system; that is, the development of the cortex, a higher level of the brain, replaces the immature and primitive influence of the lower levels of the brain, such as the brain stem. As the child matures, the increasing specialization and influence of the cortex affects the increasing specialization and complexity of the child's motor system (Case-Smith, 1996).

Development as a function of physical and neurologic maturation has long been a mainstay of developmental therapies. Pure maturationists believe that development is the result of genetic unfolding and that little that composes the child's characteristics is left to chance or influenced to any great degree by environment.

Gesell

Gesell (Gesell & Ilg, 1949) attributed development to genetically coded patterns that emerged as the child's central nervous systems matured. Gesell divided the child's development into distinct stages that govern behavior during those periods—what are now known as developmental stages. Gesell catalogued the physical and mental characteristics at each age level for the first two decades of life to determine what was "normal." Although Gesell took a multifaceted view of child development and acknowledged that environmental influences existed, the primary focus of the theory was genetic pre-destination of characteristics that emerged with age. Gesell also assigned physical body types to characteristics of children, called somatotypes, which are also genetically pre-determined. In Gesell's theories, function inevitably follows structure. The concept of critical and sensitive periods is based primarily on this approach. Many of the more recent theories and approaches to medical, physical therapy, and occupational therapy interventions are based on Gesell's theory, such as the neurodevelopmental treatment (NDT) approach used by physical therapists to treat children with cerebral palsy (Cech & Martin, 1995; Gesell & Ilg, 1949; Thomas, 1985; Wright, 1994).

Havighurst

Havighurst applied biologic principles to social and psychologic development and popularized the concept of developmental tasks (Thomas, 1985). According to Havighurst, the nature of developmental tasks varies somewhat among different cultures. Tasks can be seen either as single complex tasks or as a combination of small tasks. Havighurst divided the life span into six developmental stages, three of which occur during childhood or adolescence: birth through 5 years of age; 6 through 12 years of age; adolescence, 13 through 17 years of age; early adulthood, 18 through 30 years of age; middle age, 31 through 54 years of age; and later maturity, 55 years of age and older. The tasks of each stage are derived from biologic, cultural, and psychologic factors. Within each age group, a variety of sub-tasks exist in each of these three areas. Havighurst extended the generalization of critical periods to all realms of bio-psycho-social development in his developmental structure (Thomas, 1985).

Dynamic Systems Theory

Other more recently developed theories of motor development posit less dependence on the hierarchic nature of the central nervous system and more dependence on the responses of the child to environmental stimuli. Dynamic systems theory views motor behavior

> as the end product of a process of self organization, among the many elements comprising a system, including but not limited to the CNS. Movement is considered the "final common pathway" of the interaction among these subsystems, which are assembled purposefully to accomplish a specific task or goal. A basic assumption in this approach is that movement can never be isolated from the context of the functional task the child is performing. (Darrah & Bartlett, 1995, p. 53)

According to this theory, there are a variety of movement patterns that can be used to perform a functional task. The movement pattern that requires the least amount of energy and is the most efficient use of the involved systems is what is used by the child. It is the functional task that organizes the motor behavior, not just the organization of the central nervous system.

Application to Pediatric Rehabilitation Nursing

The maturational approach is widely supported by experts in child development and is the basis for a tremendous amount of research into both typical development and altered development. The use of developmental stages makes it easier to determine when a child's development is altered and in which areas it is altered. Interventions based on the desired behaviors and abilities at each age can be formulated. The neurodevelopmental perspective is the philosophic basis for developmental pediatrics (Caputo & Accardo, 1991). The concept of sensitive periods has been extensively researched and forms the basis for early intervention, pre-natal therapy, and the understanding of congenital disorders and neuropathology. Other developmental theorists, such as Piaget, use some aspects of the maturational perspective but not others.

The underlying principles of motor development can aid nurses in understanding of how children develop movement and differentiating movement patterns that are dysfunctional from those that are individual variations in normal movement. Assisting parents with anticipatory guidance, as well as in making sense of their child's behavior and characteristics, is an intervention performed by the pediatric rehabilitation nurse.

Development of Communication

Communication plays a central role in human society and is dependent on cognitive development. Language is the shared system of symbolic communication used to convey ideas. Language may be spoken, written, conveyed by gestures, or conveyed through the use of alternative or augmentative communication devices. Language is both receptive (i.e., perceived and understood) and expressive (i.e., conveyed to others). The purposes of language are to communicate with others, to exchange information, to maintain contact with other people, and to assist the individual in meeting needs and reaching goals. Speech is the vocal utterances used to convey language. Factors that are essential to communication include the setting in which the communication takes place, the speaker's and listener's expectations, shared knowledge, and extra-linguistic clues. These extra-linguistic contributions consist of gestures, facial expressions, and intonations (Nelms & Mullins, 1982; Soifer, 1992).

Children may communicate in a variety of ways but may not produce or understand actual speech. A communicative disorder occurs when the child is not able to convey language that can be understood by others or when the child is not able to understand and process information given to them by others. Communication disorders primarily affect psychologic and social areas of development and significantly affect learning and school achievement (Levine, Carey, & Crocker, 1992).

The components of language are content, form, and use. Language is mastered through integration and organization of these components. Content, or semantics, consists of the ideas the person wants to express. There are non-literal aspects of content, such as the use of idioms, metaphors, proverbs, or jokes. Advanced knowledge and use of semantics is necessary to understand the meaning of non-literal phrases. An example is the idiom "my hands are tied," which is not meant to be taken literally, but instead means one is unable to do anything about a situation. Development of semantic ability is closely intertwined with cognition. Developmental similarities exist in the language content of children of similar age groups, and individuality is derived from different experiences and culture.

The form of language is its apparent, observable feature of production. It is made up of sound systems (i.e., words and inflections) and grammar (i.e., syntax). These characteristics are acquired as a result of cognitive development and through experience. Use of language, or pragmatics, are the rules of language. These are based on norms of social interaction and relationships. The communicator must be aware of which words are correct to use in different social situations, taking into account the setting and the age, relationship, and cultural background of the listener (Soifer, 1992).

As the young child develops, language is acquired through spontaneous production of syllables, imitation, and comprehension, by relating a word or sound to an object. Development of speech and language skills are based on cognitive development, adequate development of the respiratory system, an intact oral cavity and larynx, intact hearing, absence of psychologic and emotional disturbance, and the appropriate stimulation, especially during sensitive periods. During most periods of speech and language development, the child's comprehension outstrips expression. The first types of words that are used are verbs, such as "go," as well as combination words, such as "bye-bye." As cognitive development progresses, the child begins to relate words to form first simple and then more complex sentences. Use of adjectives and adverbs begin, followed by use of pronouns and gender words such as "he" and "she." The child then begins to construct structurally complete yet simple sentences using five to seven words (Whaley & Wong, 1987).

The cry is the earliest form of vocal communication. As the muscles of the tongue develop, cooing emerges at about 2 months of age in both hearing and deaf children. Babbling begins around 6 months of age and is made up of consonants and vowels in single syllables. During this period, infants usually put together syllables that sound like "mama" and "dada." The first real word emerges at around 10 to 15 months of age in response to people or objects in the environment. This is referred to as "holophrasic speech" because the one word usually refers to a variety of objects or individuals.

Jargon is the term for linked syllables that do not have any apparent communicative meaning. This is the final stage of pre-linguistic speech. Two-word phrases that lack grammar but convey meaning are referred to as telegraphic sentences. Development of speech and language continues with improvements in vocabulary, articulation (i.e., the clarity with which the words are vocalized), and sentence structure. Sentence length and structure, quality of articulation, and vocabulary are often used to evaluate speech and language development. By the time the child is 6 to 7 years of age, his or her native language should be mastered with regard to both expression and comprehension.

Semantic development is the ability to communicate meaning. School-aged children are generally able to understand sentences that have the actor in the first part of the sentence. For example, the sentence "the cat chases the mouse" has the actor (the cat) in the beginning of the sentence. When the position of the actor is changed in the sentence, such as "it is the mouse that the cat chases," semantic ordering is reversed. Children continue to improve grammar and semantics into the pre-pubertal stages and often even into adulthood.

The environment and environmental stimulation are crucial to the child's speech and language development. Observation and imitation, coupled with underlying cognitive development, are the primary ways that children learn speech and language. Children who live in poverty, who have adolescent mothers or mothers with cognitive deficits, or whose parents do not understand the importance of verbal stimulation and interaction with their children are at greater risk for communication disorders. Children with disabilities and chronic conditions that affect their ability to hear or speak, their cognitive ability, or their ability to interact with the environment are also at significant risk for communication disorders.

Psychologic Development

Psychologic development includes intellectual or cognitive abilities, emotional development, personality development, and communication skills. Cognitive development is dependent on the maturation of the central nervous system; the development of the sensory system, which includes hearing, vision, proprioception, smell, and taste; the child's ability to move and interact with the environment; and the child's ability to learn, remember, and process information. Key to cognitive development and its measurement is the understanding and use of language in some form of communication. Communication may include oral language, sign language, gestures, or use of communication devices. Communication is also dependent on the child's neuromuscular development, whether it is the oral-motor skills needed to produce

speech or the fine motor coordination required to produce sign language or operate a communication device. In children, the ability to use language is a prerequisite for academic achievement. Piaget is the major theorist of cognitive development.

Development of personality depends on physical growth and maturation as well as genetics, and it interacts with the child's emotional and social development, including moral development. Freud and Erikson remain the most important theorists of personality development, whereas Piaget's theory of cognitive development is the most widely used. Piaget and Erikson postulated development of intelligence as based on a series of developmental tasks, with each succeeding level based on achievement of an earlier task. Failure to achieve one developmental task makes development of subsequent tasks more difficult or less likely. The developmental tasks are primarily based on resolution of conflict or overcoming a challenge. The challenge is derived from the child's need to master the environment combined with the child's lack of competence to achieve the mastery (Betz, Hunsberger, & Wright, 1994). With the guidance and support of adults, children mature and grow in experience and achieve the needed mastery. Erikson's infant state of "trust versus mistrust" requires that the infant resolve environmental challenges to develop a generally trusting nature. Piaget's school-aged child must learn to use symbols and the concepts they represent to achieve abstract thought processes (Betz, Hunsberger, & Wright, 1994).

The term "temperament" represents the behavioral style that an individual uses to relate to people and situations. Temperament is evident from birth and is an important component of personality (Betz, Hunsberger, & Wright, 1994). A child's temperament contributes to the way in which the child behaves and constitutes an individual quality separate from ability, motivation, or quality of behavior (Levine, Carey, Crocker, & Gross, 1983). Although a child's temperament is innate, it can be influenced by environmental experience. Temperament becomes less important as the child ages. As with other developmental characteristics, temperament is most amenable to influence during early childhood.

There are eight characteristics of temperament.

1. Activity level represents the motor component present in a child's functioning

throughout a 24-hour period. Factors such as movement during bathing, eating, playing, dressing, and handling are included in this characteristic, as are general mobility and movement while asleep.

2. Rhythmicity, or regularity, is used to describe the nature of repetitive biologic functions such as hunger, sleep-wake cycles, and elimination.

3. Approach or withdrawal refers to the nature of the child's initial response to a novel stimulus. Approach is a positive, accepting response, whereas withdrawal reactions are negative or rejecting.

4. Adaptability represents the nature of the child's modification of the response to new or altered stimuli, or how the child adjusts to the changed situation.

5. The threshold of responsiveness describes the level of intensity of stimulation that is needed to evoke a response from the child.

6. Intensity of reaction refers to the amount of energy involved in the child's response to stimulation.

7. The term "quality of mood" is used to describe the amount of pleasant or friendly behavior as opposed to unpleasant, crying, or negative behavior.

8. Attention span and persistence refer to the length of time an activity is pursued by the child and the continuation of activity in the face of obstacles, respectively (Levine, Carey, Crocker, & Gross, 1983).

Based on the above-mentioned characteristics, three temperamental constellations, or personality types, have been derived by researchers.

1. The easy child is characterized by regularity, positive approach responses, great adaptability to change, and a mild or moderately intense positive mood. Children who fall into this category are very easy to deal with; have regular patterns of sleeping, eating, and activity; are well adjusted psychologically and physically; are friendly; and usually exhibit positive mood. About 40% of children are included in this category, and about 18% develop some type of maladjustment.

2. The difficult child tends toward irregularity in biologic functions, is not very adaptable or is slow to adapt to change, shows negative withdrawal responses to new stimuli, and exhibits very intense and often negative mood. Children in this category are less dependent on other people and tend to be "loners." They are more likely to respond to frustration with a tantrum, and pleasure is expressed exuberantly, in an "all-or-nothing" reaction. The difficult child has a high level of activity in response to stress and is very competitive. Biologic functioning is characterized by irregular sleep and eating patterns. These children represent about 10% of all children, and 70% are thought to develop maladjustments.

3. The slow-to-warm-up child is one whose temperament is marked by negative responses to new stimuli that are of mild intensity. This child adapts slowly to change but does not have the extreme responses of the difficult child. The slow-to-warm-up child benefits from repeated opportunities to experience and master new situations. These children tend to be shy, to seek solitude, to mature late, and to be very sensitive. All reactions, whether positive or negative, tend to be mild and of low intensity. Mood tends to be fairly negative. This group represents 15% of children, and about 40% develop maladjustments (Levine, Carey, Crocker & Gross, 1983; Betz, Hunsberger, & Wright, 1994).

Although all children do not fall perfectly within these categories, and there is certainly wide variation of behavior among individuals, there is a tendency for these behavioral patterns to predominate in most children. Knowledge of these general personality traits can help the pediatric rehabilitation nurse make better judgments about nursing interventions, anticipatory guidance, behavioral interventions, and general parenting advice. The child's temperament will influence response to hospitalization, immobilization, treatment regimens, and illness or injury. Temperament is an important influencing factor in how a child adapts to a new disability or how a child with a developmental disability is able to adjust to and master the challenges of growth and development. Temperament prior to a disability that affects biologic regulation and activity level will influence the quality and quantity of behavioral change that occurs. For example, when a child who exhibits a "difficult" temperament receives a head injury, behaviors such as impulsivity, aggressiveness, hyperactivity, and erratic sleep and appetite patterns may be exacerbated.

Freud

According to Freud, human behavior is based on psychodynamic forces that are divided into the three components of personality—the id, the ego, and the superego. The id is driven by instincts and the goal of immediate gratification. The ego is the reality principle, which is the controlling self that helps to gratify the instinct and is able to intellectualize the drive of the id. The superego is the moral arbitrator and mediates the social order. Freud considered sexual instincts to be of great importance in the development of the personality, and formulated his five stages on the focus of pleasure-seeking that predominates during each age period. The presence of conflict at any stage may lead to arrest or impairment of development or regression to an earlier psycho-sexual stage. The oral stage occurs from birth to 1 year of age; the anal stage occurs from 2 to 3 years of age; the infantile-genital stage occurs from 3 to 4 years of age; the latency stage occurs from 4 or 5 years of age to puberty; and the mature-genital stage occurs from mid-adolescence to adulthood.

In the oral stage, the infant is focused on satisfying instinctual needs such as hunger. As such, the infant initially focuses on the mother's breast. Later, the infant uses his or her mouth to investigate the parts of the world that are accessible. The action of the infant frequently putting things into his or her mouth is an effort to incorporate and control the environment. Biting behaviors occur when the infant begins to sense ambivalent feelings, thus using the mouth to inflict pain. Personality traits that may occur in this stage include pessimism or optimism, determination or submission, gullibility or suspiciousness, admiration or envy, and over-confidence or self-belittlement.

The anal stage is concerned with issues of control. The child is attempting to control bodily functions, including bowel functions. Personality traits that are associated with this stage include stinginess or over-generosity, rigidity or flexibility, and orderliness or messiness.

During the infantile-genital stage, also known as the phallic stage, the child focuses on the genitals. Children become aware of sexual differences using the parents as examples, first identifying with the parent of the opposite gender and then the parent of the same gender. In this way the characteristics of masculine or feminine characteristics are developed, and the child begins to incorporate parental values and behaviors toward the opposite sex. In the Oedipus conflict, the male child fails to resolve sexual feelings for his mother; in the Electra complex, the female child fails to resolve sexual feelings for her father. Personality traits associated with this stage include brashness or bashfulness, courage or timidity, and gregariousness or isolationism.

During the latency stage, the child appears to forget earlier pleasures, repressing sexual feelings of earlier stages. Vigorous play and learning provide stimulation. Children relate to one another in same-sex groups. The superego functions as an internal representative of rules and values.

The final stage according to Freud is the mature-genital stage, which occurs during sexual maturation. The attention of both males and females turns back to the opposite gender, and they seek to satisfy sexual needs in a more adult manner. Although the ego, superego, and id are fairly mature, the rules of society may force the adolescent to sublimate sexual drive indirectly through artistic or philanthropic activities. The adolescent focuses energy on more mature friendships and opposite-gender relationships. (Whaley & Wong, 1987; DiCaprio, 1983).

Erikson

Erikson combined biologic needs and cultural expectations to form a psycho-social theory of human development (Cech & Martin, 1995). The entire life span is addressed in eight stages of psycho-social development based on a series of developmental and social challenges derived and refined from Freud's psycho-sexual theory. The individual must meet the challenge inherent in each stage to move on to the next. The mastery of the challenge is not an all-or-nothing proposition but rather a continuum of gradations that may be achieved. Each new challenge that is mastered contains within it the seeds of the next conflict or challenge. The first five of these stages address childhood through adolescence. Erikson's theory deals with three main goals of development: development of a healthy personality, socialization into a particular culture, and achievement of ego identity (Thomas, 1985).

The first psycho-social challenge for the infant is that of trust versus mistrust. The infant forms positive attachments to caregivers and positive contacts with the environment. For this to occur, the infant's needs must be predominantly met, including the need for affection. If these needs are not met in the first year of life, the child's ability to trust self and others is damaged. Erikson viewed trust as the ability to predict and to depend on the behavior of self and of others.

Autonomy versus shame and doubt is the second psycho-social crisis that occurs during the pre-school period. During this stage, punishment and discipline are more consistently applied, and this helps to form the stage. This stage is based on the child's ability or inability to control bodily functions such as bowel or bladder continence. Control of the body gives the child the ability to begin to do things independently, and the child exercises this new-found ability by testing the limits of autonomy and seeking balance between independence and parental control. The child's universe is based on the critical developmental tasks involved in learning to control. Over-control by others may result in an over-compulsive adult personality characterized by doubt and shame. Children of this age feel shame because they are developmentally unable to experience guilt. The goal in meeting this challenge is to achieve a sense of self-control without loss of self-esteem (Thomas, 1985).

During the period from 5 to 6 years of age, the conflict of initiative versus guilt leads ideally to development of self-regulation and a growing sense of identity. Mastery of important physical and social tasks helps the child to begin to rely on internalized value and reward systems (Cech & Martin, 1995). Lack of confidence is a negative outcome of this stage.

Children in the elementary school period face the psycho-social conflict of industry versus inferiority. Accomplishment of tasks that the child finds interesting and worthy lead to a sense of industry and confidence—of mastery. Feelings of inferiority result if the child's efforts are minimized or denigrated or if the task is beyond the child's abilities, resulting in failure (Thomas, 1985). Children with disabilities and chronic conditions have particular difficulty in keeping up with their peers academically during this stage and are at greater risk for failure to reach mastery of required tasks.

Identity versus identity diffusion is the psycho-social task of adolescence and one on which Erikson focused attention. Physical, cognitive, and hormonal changes result in changes in the individual's social roles and responsibilities. For the adolescent to successfully meet this challenge, a strong sense of self-identity, independent of family, must be formed. Erikson described ego identity as "the accrued confidence that one's ability to maintain inner sameness is matched by the sameness and continuity of one's meaning for others" (Erikson, 1959, p. 89). The opposite of a strong ego identity is identity diffusion, in which there is no strong sense of self and interactions are characterized by immaturity, intolerance, prejudice, and hero worship (Thomas, 1985).

Piaget

Piaget is perhaps the most widely accepted theorist of intellectual development in children. His theory poses four stages of cognitive development: sensorimotor, pre-operational, concrete operational, and formal operational. At each stage the child interacts with the environment differently based on increasing complexity of thought. Mastery of the environment is a primary goal of the child, according to Piaget (Flavell, 1977). Two basic functions operate within the child to achieve mastery. Assimilation is the ability to take in information, integrate it, and use or master it; accommodation is the ability to adapt to change. Piaget viewed knowledge not as an accumulation of information but as a process in which information is used in a physical or mental action. Thinking is an internalized action on a symbolic object (Thomas, 1985). Perception of events is modified by both the child's past experiences and stage of maturation. Individual differences in behavior are accounted for by the uniqueness of perception within each child. The objects, images, and symbols that the child uses to make sense of the world come from direct experience as well as from memory (Thomas, 1985).

In Piaget's first stage of development, the sensorimotor stage, the infant interacts with the environment to establish cause and effect and to eventually learn to anticipate the results of actions. People and objects come to be recognized and behavior becomes intentional. Active experimentation and manipulation of objects to attain a goal begins (Thomas, 1985; Cech & Martin, 1995).

The second stage, the pre-operational stage, is when the pre-schooler begins to expand the use of symbols, words, and objects to represent things that are not physically present. Language and vocabulary expand and assist the child in learning about the environment and interacting with it more satisfactorily. During this stage, children are egocentric and begin to show evidence of immature logic. As the child enters school, intuitive thought and the ability to see that more than one factor at a time influence an event begin to develop (Thomas, 1985). Egocentrism is decreased by about age 7 years as the child begins to realize that the world does not depend on the child's wishes or actions. However, at the end of this stage, the child is still largely dependent on perception as opposed to logic (Thomas, 1985; Cech & Martin, 1995).

Piaget's third stage, that of concrete operations, lasts from about age 7 to 11 years. During this stage, the child begins to solve concrete problems—that is, those problems that are directly related to objects. The child's thought processes are still perceptually based and not abstract. Although the child may be able to solve problems "in his or her head," those problems must involve real objects or pictures of objects. By the end of this stage, concepts of causation begin to be understood, and the processes that objects undergo during change are recognized (Thomas, 1985; Cech & Martin, 1995).

The fourth and final stage is that of formal operations. This stage begins at around age 11 years and is completed at about age 15 years. This stage is Piaget's highest level of cognitive development, in which the individual can solve problems in hypothetical as well as real situations. Logical decision making as well as the ability to think abstractly are characteristics of this stage (Cech & Martin, 1995). According to Piaget, this stage is not the end of the development of intellect, but it is the completion of the framework of cognitive functioning. Learning, as well as the ability to reason and solve problems, continues to develop as a result of experience. One significant difference between adolescents and adults identified by Piaget is the greater egocentrism that characterizes adolescents (Thomas, 1985). An overview of developmental states based on the theories of Erikson, Freud, and Piaget is contained in Table 10–2.

Fowler

Fowler's theory of faith development is based on the cognitive and psychologic theories of development of Piaget, Erikson, Kohlberg, and others. Beliefs are viewed as a system of order and activities rather than an inner spiritual process. The development of faith progresses through seven stages based on the child's cognitive development and, later, on the experiences and knowledge of the adult.

The primal stage begins in infancy, when attachment forms the basis for development of faith. The intuitive/projective stage is when the child of 2 to 6 years of age is dependent on the images, feelings, and symbols of the primary caregiver's beliefs. During the mythic/literal stage, at about 7 to 12 years of age, the child's beliefs begin to become more literal and are held more as a system of order and activity than an inner spiritual process. The synthetic convention stage occurs at adolescence and is when the individual synthesizes ideas about spirituality from significant others and life experiences. During this stage, self-reflection and insight occur. Through young adulthood to mid-life, the individual passes through three more stages in which beliefs are solidified, various dimensions of faith beliefs are integrated, and acceptance of other belief systems emerges. The final stage is characterized by unconditional regard and love for others (Betz, Hunsberger, & Wright, 1994).

Kohlberg

Kohlberg postulated three stages of moral development: a pre-moral or pre-conventional stage; a stage that involves conforming to society's conventions; and a post-conventional level based on personal, self-accepted moral principles. Each level contains two steps. In addition to these stages, there are 30 or more aspects of life about which moral judgments are made that fall under three general categories: modes of judgment of obligation and value, which include judgments of right, duty or obligation, or punishment and reward; elements of obligation and value, such as prudence, social welfare, love and respect, and justice as liberty or equality; and issues or institutions including social norms, personal conscience, and roles and issues of authority and democracy. The examples given are not all-encompassing, but they give a general idea of the types of decision making included in each of the three general areas (Thomas, 1985).

Kohlberg's stages exemplify a progression from lower levels of moral decision, such as those resulting from a fear of punishment, to higher levels of decision making that emphasize moral values and use universal principles that would apply to any individual in any situation (Thomas, 1985). In formulating this theory of moral development, Kohlberg believed that the child moves through the levels of moral judgment according to Piaget's prin-

Table 10-2 LEVELS OF COGNITIVE DEVELOPMENT IN PIAGETIAN TERMS

Level	Structure	Symbolization	Comments	Examples
I (birth)	Independent actions carried out by the infant	a, b	Each action is independent and unrelated to other actions; cannot construct connections. No control over responses. Operant conditioning would not work well, but classical conditioning would.	Child attempts to master simple physical movements by practice, learning to produce these actions at will.
II (6 months)	Uses one action to predict or produce another	$a \rightarrow b$	Learn connections between actions, able to predict the next event, able to anticipate, even somewhat able to emit an action to obtain a desired consequence.	Child would go to where he or she sees caregiver is, if he or she could move independently. Knows about sequences of activities, i.e., child cries, caregiver picks child up, then gives food. Child will stop crying when caregiver picks him up even though still hungry because child anticipates that food will be forthcoming.
III (1 year)	Understands reciprocity of action and consequence	$a \leftrightarrow b$	Learns of the two-way relationships between action and end. Behavior becomes more flexible.	Child begins to deliberately emit behaviors designed to produce desired reaction in caregiver to get needs met. Child does not realize that caregiver still exists when he or she cannot see him or her. To the child, he or she "produces" the caregiver by emitting certain behaviors such as crying. He can vary the crying behavior to bring the caregiver back more effectively. Separation anxiety begins here because of the child's ability to remember the caregiver's face long enough to compare it to a stranger's. Also can recognize, on seeing a stranger, that this is not a familiar face.

Table 10–2   LEVELS OF COGNITIVE DEVELOPMENT IN PIAGETIAN TERMS *Continued*

Level	Structure	Symbolization	Comments	Examples
IV (2–3 years)	Relates relationships	a ↔ b ↑ ↓ c ↔ d	Can understand that an action-end pair can be related to another action-end pair. Starts to mentally associate grouped behaviors together. Also starts to develop mental representations of actions or behaviors. These mental representations can then be manipulated cognitively in the absence of overt physical activity.	Object permanence emerges. Child now knows that caregiver still exists when he or she cannot see the caregiver. Child also begins to develop a self-concept. The concept of self and of caregiver are a product of a capacity or mentally represent something in the absence of concrete sensory input.
	Mental representations of single actions/ behaviors	A, B		
V (5 years)	Increasing complexity of mental representations	A → B	The child learns to mentally manipulate representations of actions/behaviors in the same sequence of increasing complexity as that followed with the learning of relationships and manipulations of actual actions/ behaviors.	One-directional mapping of systems.
VI (7–8 years)		A ↔ B		Reciprocal relationships of systems.
VII (12–15 years)	Development of abstract or formal operations.	A ↔ B ↑ ↓ C ↔ D		Abstractions. Use of abstract ideas to influence another person.

Used with permission from Linda Iklé, Ph.D., University of Colorado Health Sciences Center, 1995.

ciples of cognitive development. Therefore, the level of moral reasoning of which a child is capable is closely related to that child's level of cognitive development and ability to reason logically and abstractly. Culture and environment greatly influence the child's movement through the levels of moral development as well.

Application to Pediatric Rehabilitation Nursing

The psychologic approach to development has great application within pediatric rehabilitation nursing. According to Piaget and Erikson, the child must interact with the environment to learn and develop. Disability or chronic illness that interferes with that process affects the child's ability to learn and progress through the identified stages. Both of these theories provide a useful framework within which to understand the influence of disability, whether congenital or acquired, on child development. Piaget's stages of perception and learning can be used when teaching children self-care and during health education. Understanding the serial nature of learning can lead to developmentally appropriate nursing interventions. Erikson's theory of personality development can be applied to the development of nursing interventions to aid psychologic adaptation of the child to social and environmental challenges. Development of identity is key to the individual's understanding of and ability to perform a designated social role, most particularly in the presence of disability. Frequently, social role changes for the child and family occur with disability, and psychologic theories such as these help to put those changes into perspective for the nurse and family.

Pediatric rehabilitation nurses can help the family to better understand the behaviors and development of their children by using these theories. Each of these theories, particularly Piaget's, are the basis for other frameworks such as Fowler's approach to faith development and Kohlberg's moral development theory. Use of these psychologic theories can help families and caregivers better understand the scope and depth of the changes their child has experienced after a disabling injury or illness and provide a structure for therapeutic interaction with the child to facilitate development and to prevent the negative effects on the stage.

The theories of moral and spiritual development provide a framework for counseling children and adolescents and providing anticipatory guidance and counseling for families. These frameworks suggest guidelines for the type and amount of information the child requires and can help the nurse understand the child's perceptions and assess and intervene in relation to these perceptions (Betz, Hunsberger, & Wright, 1994).

Spiritual support of children and families is a neglected area of nursing care. Information about how children perceive and exhibit faith and spirituality can be very helpful to parents in supporting their child during long and difficult hospitalizations, traumatic injury, or terminal illness. Helping families to support siblings of the child with a disability or chronic condition is also an important area in which knowledge of faith development in children is useful.

Understanding moral development helps the pediatric rehabilitation nurse in setting realistic guidelines and having realistic expectations for the child based on his or her cognitive development rather than their chronological age. Older children with cognitive delays are often believed, based on their size and appearance, to have a more advanced intellect than they actually do. Counseling and supporting families in planning care and schooling for their child requires that the nurse integrate this knowledge with other developmental principles. Parents or other caregivers who do not have realistic expectations of their child's cognitive or behavioral abilities are at risk for child abuse or for placing their child in unsafe situations.

Knowledge of developmental differences in the way children apply standards of right and wrong is valuable when teaching the child ways to avoid misbehavior, emphasizing the rights and needs of others, and providing the child with opportunities to explore elements of moral problems and their potential solutions. Children with disabilities and chronic conditions are frequently faced with teasing or bullying in school or recreational situations and need to learn how to cope with these situations in an adaptive manner. Respect for other's ways of thinking and believing is a prerequisite for older children and adolescents to accept their peers who are different. The framework provided by these theories can be used to educate children with disabilities and chronic conditions with regard to problem solving and responding to the challenges of everyday life such as making decisions about peer groups, involvement with drugs, or other moral dilemmas (Betz, Hunsberger, & Wright, 1994; Thomas, 1985).

Social Development

Social development is dependent on both motor and cognitive development, as well as the interaction of the child with others, such as family, peers, and members of the community. One of the earliest aspects of social development is the ability to perform reciprocal interactions with primary caregivers such as the mother. Behaviors such as smiling, sucking, and the ability of the infant to be calmed by the mother's ministrations are all important factors leading to attachment. Attachment is the basis for the development of trust and the tendency to respond positively and in an accepting fashion to others, self, and cultural institutions. Infants who fail to attach to a significant caregiver often lose the ability to form lasting relationships later in life. Two of the key factors in the emergence of age-appropriate skills in this domain are experience and feedback from others. Children who are isolated from their peers do not learn appropriate social skills. Components of social-emotional development include attachment, social skills, the ability to make and maintain friendships, and moral and spiritual development.

This approach to development focuses primarily on the contribution of interaction with the environment to the development of cognitive ability and behavior. Interaction with the environment, objects as well as people, shapes the child as he or she reacts to events. A behavior is repeated as a result of prompts or reinforcements in the environment. This approach includes the behaviorists such as Skinner, as well as the social learning theorists such as Sears, Bandura, and Bronfenbenner.

Skinner—The Behavioral Approach

The strict behavioral approach applies the principles of operant conditioning to human behavior. Conditioning, by carefully applied positive or negative stimuli, results in behavior. All behavior is thought to occur by observation and imitation and can be shaped through reinforcement.

Sears and Bandura—The Social Learning Approach

Sears' theory of behavior is based on Skinner's model of stimulus and response and seeks to explain the early behavior of children by identifying the common reinforcers used to produce social behavior. This theory, called social learning theory, states that behavior is learned first from the parents, then the extended family, and then the peer group. Sears' theory emphasizes social variables as determinants of behavior and personality (Thomas, 1985).

Bandura took Sears' theory of social learning and improved upon it, adding the concept of modeling. Modeling is a type of cognitive patterning in which the child acquires simple skills and complex behaviors by observing patterns and copying them (Cech & Martin, 1995). Skills and behaviors may be learned purposefully or incidentally from adults in the environment or from other children or peers. Children not only imitate pure behaviors from others but are able to synthesize behaviors from a variety of observations, thus accounting for children exhibiting behaviors that they did not directly observe. Bandura believed that children are motivated to use modeled behaviors if the consequences of the behavior are desirable and that the desirability of consequences provides a regulatory effect on the performance of that behavior (Thomas, 1985).

Based on the theory of social learning, Bandura advocated use of behavior modification, believing that behavior can be changed by manipulating the consequences of the child's acts so the child finds it more rewarding to adopt acceptable behavior. This approach does not deal with the internal cause of behavior but seeks to change the behavior itself.

Bronfenbenner—The Ecological Approach

The ecologic systems approach offers a comprehensive framework for understanding the role of the environment in child development. Bronfenbenner focuses on the interacting systems of society—the family, community, and culture—and the relationship of these systems to the child. The model is an ever-widening series of spheres of influence with the child at the center and includes the microsystem surrounding the child, consisting of family, school, close friends, neighborhood, and direct health services; the mesosystem, or the area of interaction between spheres; the exosystem, or extended family, social, and health systems, the legal system, more peripheral friends and acquaintances, and mass media; and the larger macrosystem, which consists of the attitudes and ideologies of the culture (Cech & Martin, 1995).

Application to Pediatric Rehabilitation Nursing

A solid grounding in these theories of social development helps the nurse provide anticipatory guidance for parents, especially with regard to using modeling and observation to help the child learn desirable behaviors. This approach supports the philosophy of inclusion, in that children learn effectively from age-mates, especially behavior and social roles. Too often children with disabilities, chronic conditions, and cognitive delays are segregated into special classrooms, where they have little or no opportunity to learn from peers. As these children grow, their lack of appropriate social skills is often their greatest disability; it can prevent formation of friendships and cause difficulties in school and, later, in vocational situations.

Modeling of desirable behaviors by showing the child alternative actions may help him or her learn to cope better with difficult situations. In these theories, physical punishment is seen as modeling of aggressive behavior and is not a desirable method of discipline or behavior management. The focus on environmental influences has great implications for positive discipline and establishing a supportive structure for the child's behavior. Use of behavior modification, especially with children who are mentally retarded, can be a helpful approach to behavioral support of children with disabilities and chronic conditions. Many children with disabilities and chronic conditions and their families have great difficulty with the long and often arduous treatment regimens recommended by rehabilitation care providers. Understanding the influence of environment and social roles can aid the nurse in designing interventions

Table 10–3 COMPARISON OF DEVELOPMENTAL STAGES FROM VARIOUS THEORIES

Age	Erikson	Freud	Social Determinant	Piaget
Infancy	Trust/mistrust (predictability)	Oral	Dependence on mothering	Sensorimotor
Toddlerhood	Autonomy/shame and doubt	Anal	Becoming a separate individual (e.g., walking)	Early pre-operational
Pre-school	Initiative/guilt	Phallic	Becoming a social individual	Late pre-operational
Elementary school	Industry/inferiority	Latency	School or other skill acquisition	Concrete operational
Adolescence	Identity/role diffusion	Genital	Entering adulthood	Formal operational
Young adulthood	Intimacy/isolation		Entering sexual relationships and work relationships	
Adulthood	Generativity/stagnation		Fulfilling adult role in society: family and work	
Aging	Ego integrity/despair		Dealing with aging and death	

Used with permission from Linda Iklé, Ph.D., University of Colorado Health Sciences Center, 1995.

that support the family's and child's involvement with care. A comparison of developmental stages from selected theories is presented in Table 10–3.

OVERVIEW OF DEVELOPMENTAL MILESTONES BY AGE

The Neonate

Overview of Typical Development

The neonatal period is the first month of life. Physical development of the neonate is characterized by adjustments to the extrauterine environment and sets the stage for the child's future growth and development. Events that occur during the neonatal period, such as bonding with parents, and the ability of the neonate and the parents to successfully interact are crucial to the later emotional, psychologic, and social success of the child as well as the success of the family in providing for the child and meeting his or her needs. The two primary developmental tasks of the neonate are achievement of physiologic stability and development of attachment to parents and primary caregivers (Nelms & Mullins, 1982).

Innate characteristics present at birth allow the neonate to interact with the environment and prompt reciprocal interactions from the parents. Brazelton's Neonatal Behavioral Assessment scale measures many neonatal characteristics such as temperament, social behavior, orienting responses to stimuli, ability to cope with disturbing stimuli, state of arousal, and motor skills (Brazelton, 1984). The neonate is born with significant sensory abilities. Hearing is well-developed by birth, and the infant has a preference for speech. High-pitched tones which characterize the female voice, stimulate alertness, whereas more low-pitched tones such as in the male voice, are soothing to the infant. The neonate is able to recognize the mother's voice and discriminate it from other female voices. Behavioral manifestations of hearing that may be recognized easily are alerting (i.e., seeming to stop and listen), eye movements, startle reaction to sound from out of sight range, and crying. The ability to discriminate direction and origin of sound does not develop until a few weeks after birth (Delahoussaye, 1994; Hagerman, 1995).

The sense of smell is also well developed at birth and is used by the neonate to orient to the environment; the child shows a negative response to noxious smells and a positive response to pleasant smells. The smell of the mother and of the mother's breast is recognized by 1 week of age. Neonates have definite taste preferences at birth, have more taste buds than adults, and avoid bitter or aversive tastes (Hagerman, 1995).

Vision in neonates is somewhat less developed than other senses, with the retina more developed than the lens. By 2 months of age, fixation and tracking through the visual field are present. Although visual acuity is poor at birth, it improves in the first 6 months of life.

Very young infants prefer curved lines, bright colors, and high contrast, and they show a definite preference for the human face. Visual preference is described as the length of time the neonate fixates on a paired visual stimulus. Length of visual fixation in early infancy has been correlated with later cognitive development. Strabismus is often noted immediately after birth but should not be present after 3 months of age (Hagerman, 1995).

The sense of touch is present at birth, especially in the facial area, as it is necessary for rooting and sucking reflexes and behaviors. There is sensitivity to pain and extreme temperatures at birth, but discrimination does not occur until about the 10th day of life (Delahoussaye, 1994).

The neonate is born with a repertoire of reflexes that promote survival as well as complex sensory abilities. The preferred positioning of the neonate at birth is generally in flexion. Reflexes that are present at birth are the rooting reflex; the sucking reflex; the swallowing reflex; the palmar and plantar grasp reflexes; the traction response; the Moro reflex, or startle response; the yawn, stretch, and hiccup reflexes; the trunk incurvation reflex; the placing and stepping reflexes; the tonic neck reflex, or "fencing position"; and the Babinski reflex. These reflexes normally disappear from 8 weeks to 6 months of age. If they reappear or persist, they indicate neurologic compromise.

Neuromuscular maturity is rated by the amount of flexibility in posture using the Dubowitz Scale of Gestational Age. Based on the infant's response to the assessment items, a gestational age is determined (Delahoussaye, 1994; Dubowitz, Dubowitz, & Goldberg, 1970). Six states of arousal have been described for newborns: deep sleep; light sleep; drowsiness or semi-dozing; alertness; high activity level; and intense crying (Nelms & Mullins, 1982). States of arousal provide a good guide to the neonate's neurologic maturity. In addition, the stimuli used and the rapidity of state change in response to stimuli are also significant, especially in pre-term infants, who tend to react in immature or primitive ways to stimuli such as prolonged eye contact or touch. Responses that indicate neurologic immaturity include color change and cyanosis, yawning, and moving quickly into physiologic instability such as slowing of breathing and heart rate, even to the point of apnea and bradycardia and respiratory or cardiac arrest as responses to any kind of stress.

The cardiopulmonary system must change from fetal circulation to independent functioning. Skin mottling is often due to circulatory instability and is normal, as is acrocyanosis of the hands and feet in a cool environment. Excessive pallor, generalized cyanosis, and jaundice, especially during the first 24 hours, are abnormal findings and indicate illness or increased risk for illness (Nelms & Mullins, 1982).

The Apgar score provides an assessment tool that rates the infant's overall physical status and is a good predictor of later neurologic status. Five criteria are used in scoring: heart rate, respiratory effort and cry, muscle tone, reflex response, and color. These criteria are rated and scored at 1 minute after birth and at 5 minutes after birth, and the total score is the sum of the five criteria, rated on a scale of 0 to 10. The 1-minute score is usually lower than the 5-minute score because the physiologic depression of delivery peaks at 1 minute. By 5 minutes, most infants are fairly stable; a low score at this time is most predictive of later problems and usually reflects persistent hypoxia. The Apgar score is a useful tool for assessing contributing factors to childhood disability and chronic conditions. The neonate has very poor thermoregulation due to immaturity of the central nervous system and small amount of body fat (12%) (Delahoussaye, 1994). Vasomotor instability may result in variations in skin color from reddish to pale pink. The infant's racial background will gradually influence skin color (Nelms & Mullins, 1982).

The digestive system is functional but immature at birth. Very little saliva is produced, and spitting up is common due to a lax pyloric sphincter and relatively low muscle tone. The first stools of the neonate are meconium stools, which are dark green to black in color; these are present during the first 3 days of life and then change to transitional stool, which is greenish brown. Babies who are breast-fed tend to have two to four soft, yellow stools per day. Formula-fed neonates have paler, more formed stools with more odor (Delahoussaye, 1994).

Production of concentrated urine is limited in the newborn, leading to the need to excrete large volumes of water to eliminate solutes. Neonates first void during the first 12 hours of life. Urate crystals may be passed in the urine, and show as a pink staining in the diaper. It is important to discriminate urate from blood—urate crystals will wash out with water, but blood will not (Delahoussaye, 1994).

Developmental Concerns for Neonates With Disabilities and Chronic Conditions

Genetic conditions often cause disability or chronic illness that is recognized at birth, whereas some conditions may not be evident until later in life. An example of a genetic condition that is visible at birth is Down syndrome. Conditions that develop later include Duchenne muscular dystrophy. Congenital conditions caused by pre-natal events, maternal illness, or teratogens are also, for the most part, recognizable at birth. Maternal abuse of alcohol, cocaine, or other illegal drugs greatly influences neonatal behavior and physical make-up.

Prematurity is a significant concern whose consequences may last the child's lifetime. Premature infants are at risk for developmental delay, attention deficit disorder, and learning disabilities, at the least. More severe effects include neurologic disease, deafness, blindness, lifelong respiratory and cardiac conditions, and cognitive delay. Low birth weight, which usually occurs as a result of pre-term delivery and may occur in infants born at term, is defined as less than 2500 g, or 5 lb, 8 oz (Paneth, 1995). Very-low-birth-weight infants weigh 1000 g or less, and extremely-low-birth-weight infants weigh 800 g or less. Lowered birth weight increases the risk of developmental consequences (Fazzi et al., 1997; Bowen et al., 1996). For more information on prematurity, see the section Growth earlier in this chapter.

Another major concern for the neonate, especially the premature infant, is stress. Stress, such as that which occurs with hospitalization or illness, can affect the neonate's ability to achieve physiologic stability. Stress results from too much environmental stimulation, including interaction with caregivers, pain, neglect, noise, constant lighting with no periods of darkness or reduced light, and many other factors. Symptoms of stress in the neonate include stress ulcer, feeding difficulties, vomiting or diarrhea, irritability, sleep disruption, disturbance of the attachment process, and poor achievement and maintenance of states of arousal and rest (Nelms & Mullins, 1982). Due to the neonate's physiologic immaturity and poor thermoregulation, increased vulnerability to cold and heat loss is an important factor. The neonate's response to stress is related to his or her level of neurologic maturity; the more severe responses to stress are physiologic, such as slowed heart rate or breathing. For infants in neonatal intensive care units, a relatively new system of developmental care is increasingly being used that is designed to reduce the amount of stress premature infants and ill neonates experience, thereby reducing developmental risk (Als, 1992).

Disease represents a major risk to the neonate. Owing to the immaturity of the immune system and other systems such as the kidneys and the skin, neonates are at greater risk of infection than at any other time of life. Once an infection is acquired, it quickly overwhelms the newborn, resulting in sepsis, or central nervous system infection such as meningitis or encephalitis. Complicating the picture is the inability of the neonate's kidneys to concentrate urine, making the newborn more susceptible to dehydration. Any illness causing vomiting and diarrhea can result in life-threatening dehydration within hours. Respiratory disease puts the neonate, an obligatory nose-breather, at risk for anoxia.

The premature infant is also at great risk for disease and even is more vulnerable due to greater immaturity. In the neonatal intensive care unit, infections such as necrotizing enterocolitis, central nervous system infections, or infections related to invasive procedures may be deadly. Stress decreases the resistance of the premature infant. Systems of care delivery such as developmentally appropriate care decrease the stress of the neonatal intensive care unit and improve the infants chances of survival and intact neurologic function.

Development of attachment to the parents is a critical factor in the development of healthy social, emotional, and psychologic skills. Attachment also ensures that the neonate's needs are met during the least independent phase of life, childhood. Both the newborn and the parents are active participants in this process. Behaviors that elicit attention or contact with the parents include crying; eye-to-eye contact; sensory abilities such as feeling, smelling, and tasting; and hearing, which allows the newborn to respond to the environment and the parent's voice. Touch and proprioception also play important roles in calming the neonate, such as when the parent lifts the crying newborn and holds the child close. The vestibular stimulation of lifting and rocking the child provides a calming influence for the newborn (Nelms & Mullins, 1982). Neonates who are hospitalized for acute conditions or trauma or who are removed from the home due to maltreatment and placed in foster homes are at increased risk for attachment disorders. Additionally, neonates who are born with congenital conditions, were exposed in utero to alcohol or other drugs, or have neurologic impairments may be irritable, hard to feed and to handle, or have a high-pitched, constant cry that causes difficulty when parents attempt to bond to the child. Parents, especially teenage parents or mothers who are substance abusers, may not have the skills to manage the newborn with many special needs for attention and care.

Child maltreatment is a major cause of death and disability in young children. The younger the child, the more vulnerable he or she is. Neonates and very young infants are particularly susceptible to shaking injuries, which result in severe neurologic trauma. Young parents with new babies may not have the skills or supports to help them cope with the tiredness and stress of being a new parent. Neonates who were born with congenital conditions and whose care is more difficult and time consuming may be at greater risk for maltreatment.

Injury presents a significant risk to the neonate. The family and other caregivers must be aware of the proper use of car seats and placement of the seat in the car with regard to air bags and other adult-oriented safety devices. Suffocation presents a risk from plastic bags, leaving a newborn unattended while bathing, use of pillows or thick sheepskin pads in the crib, and using a crib and infant toys that do not meet safety specifications. Precautions such as avoiding propping the newborn's bottle, hanging a pacifier around the newborn's neck, and placing the newborn in supine or side-lying position after feeding can reduce the risk of suffocation (Delahoussaye, 1994). Neonates who are being treated for congenital disorders, especially orthopedic problems, may require casts, braces, or other devices that make transport more difficult. Approved adaptations of car seats or special-care seats can be helpful.

Nutritional inadequacies, whether stemming from feeding difficulties, neuromuscular conditions, cleft palate, illness or surgery, feeding the wrong kind or amount of formula, or starvation, present a significant risk to normal growth and development. Neonates require the proper amount of calories and combination of nutrients during this most rapid period of growth and development. Nutrition is very important to brain growth during this stage, and deficits may result in loss of cognitive potential as well as reduced weight and height. It is normal to lose some weight after birth, but that weight should be regained in the first few weeks of life. Lack of opportunity or ability to suck can lead to life-long feeding disorders. Neonates who are gavage-fed after surgical procedures or who have conditions that prevent them from taking a bottle or sucking require oral motor therapy to help them improve or to enhance the development of these skills.

The Infant

Overview of Typical Development

Infancy is a time of rapid developmental change for the child and requires adaptation by the parents to meet the changing needs of the infant. Infancy is the period from 1 month to 1 year of age. The infant starts this period very dependent and unable to walk, talk, or care for any needs independently. By one year of age, the infant is usually able to walk, to use beginning language and produce speech, and has a greatly expanded knowledge of the world. Physical changes occur quite rapidly, with corresponding changes in abilities. The infant's ability to interact with the environment is greatly enhanced (Nelms & Mullins, 1982). Play becomes an important method of learning about and interacting with the environment.

Physiologic changes include rapid physical growth. By 1 year of age, the infant's birth weight is expected to triple. Overriding sutures in the plates of the skull from the birth process resolve, and molding of the head from the birth process diminishes. The cardiopulmonary system stabilizes as fetal systems disappear. The infant's trunk grows in comparison to head and limbs, but the head still appears to be disproportionately large. The abdomen becomes protuberant, and the infant appears to have lordosis. The increase in subcutaneous tissue makes the infant appear fatter and rounder. Skin rashes, including diaper dermatitis, are frequent due to the infant's relatively thin skin and the loose attachment of the epidermis to the dermis. Infants who have spinal cord injury or spina bifida have a particularly difficult time with diaper dermatitis due to often continual leaking of stool and urine.

Vision improves with development of central vision and color preference. Depth perception is not present at birth and requires additional development of the cerebellum, which occurs at about 9 months of age. Hearing acuity and perception of multiple frequencies also improves in the first year of life. Exposure to various frequencies of sounds is necessary for hearing acuity to develop normally. Repeated otitis media, chronic serous effusion, or other types of hearing loss may delay language development and result in permanent speech and language difficulties.

Infants tend to have a more severe, generalized response to infection than older children; what would be a minor illness in an older child is much more serious in an infant. Nonspecific immunity continues to develop during early infancy, whereas specific immunity is dependent on exposure to antigens. Often, the first exposure to an antigen elicits a severe reaction, whereas the second exposure results in much less severe illness.

The respiratory system develops rapidly in the first 2 years of life, when size and number of alveoli increase. Any condition that decreases intrathoracic volume, such as congenital or infantile scoliosis or injury to the chest, decreases the number of alveoli and contributes to respiratory compromise (Nelms & Mullins, 1982).

Between 6 weeks and 6 months of age, the connections between the muscles of the pharynx and the brain mature so that voluntary swallowing is possible. This is when drooling decreases in normally developing children. Drooling beyond 6 to 8 months of age may indicate swallowing dysfunction. By the end of the first year, stools begin to firm up and become less frequent as the large intestine absorbs more water. Defecation is involuntary until about 2 years of age, when neuromuscular maturation makes sensing fullness and control of the sphincter possible. Maturation of the neurologic connections that make bowel control possible appears to be tied more to developmental level than chronological age (Nelms & Mullins, 1982).

As with bowel function, voiding is automatic in the infant. Sensation of fullness and muscular control increase through infancy, usually maturing earlier than bowel control. The infant is increasingly able to concentrate urine and regulate the acid-base balance. The infant's ureters are short, which complicates reflux into the kidneys for children with spinal cord dysfunction or ureteral or bladder anomalies.

The muscles grow rapidly during the infant period, faster than bone growth. As the neuromuscular system develops, the infant is able to exert increasingly more control over posture and movement. Bones are pliable and easily molded. Typically, the infant has bowed legs, and his or her feet turn inward. Infants usually have flat feet which pronate when they walk, but this changes with age. Any skeletal position that is unilateral or asymmetric may indicate orthopedic problems. Infants with low muscle tone or hypermobile joints may have more orthopedic structural dysfunction. During the first year of life, infantile, or primitive, reflexes disappear, and more mature postural, or defensive, reflexes begin to emerge. Although each primitive reflex typically disappears at different specific times, all of these reflexes are generally gone by 6 months of age and should be definitely gone by 1 year of age. A summary of infant growth and development is presented in Table 10–4.

Developmental Concerns for the Infant With a Disability or Chronic Condition

Infants with a severe acute illness, a chronic condition, or a disability have a significant risk for delays in growth and development. Infants who are hospitalized are stressed and often are separated from their parents for prolonged periods. They are exposed to frequent painful procedures and discomfort from their condition. Infants with chronic conditions often require lengthy treatments and procedures to maintain health and prevent further illness. Children with physical impairment and disability receive therapies at home, at the clinic, or in child care, which, although important, may diminish the time they spend with peers and engaged in family functions such as relaxation, recreation, or work. Parents or other caregivers may find it difficult to perform therapies at home if they are painful to the child or if the child has a negative response to the therapy. Invasive procedures such as gastrostomy tube feedings, tracheostomy care and suctioning, or clean intermittent catheterization of the bladder are time consuming and may be intimidating to perform. All of these procedures, although necessary to maintain physiologic stability, can interfere with growth and development.

For any infant identified with a congenital condition, early intervention remains the standard of care for treatment. For infants who experience delays during this stage of development, a variety of screening tools may be used to identify global or single-domain delays. If the screening indicates a score on a developmental task that is two deviations below the mean, referral for developmental testing and diagnosis is the next step. Testing identifies the scope and severity of the delays and allows the child to receive early intervention services through the state system under the Individuals With Disabilities Education Act (IDEA). More information on IDEA and early intervention are presented in Chapter 4.

The infant's condition, if it includes dysfunction of the motor system, can increase immobility and decrease the child's ability to explore the environment and to play. Infants with orthopedic conditions who need to wear a brace or cast that limits their mobility, especially for a long period of time, may experience motor and other delays as a result of their forced immobility. As stated earlier in this chapter, lack of the ability to explore the environment can affect sensory, cognitive, and neuromuscular development. Cause-and-effect play can help the older infant to manipulate the environment.

Caregiver support is crucial for the infant to develop trust. Parents or other caregivers who are unable to meet the infant's needs in a timely manner may interfere with this process, as well as with attachment. Maltreatment exacerbates the situation. Many children who experience maltreatment and who are removed from the home and put up for adoption have serious attachment problems and behavior and psychiatric difficulties.

Anxiety of the parent or caregiver can be translated to the child and enhance innate temperament characteristics. Anxiety or nervousness is easily transmitted to the infant or young child and results in anxiety and fear in the child. Additionally, anxiety in parents or caregivers may put them at increased risk for overprotecting the child, as well as for providing inadequate care. Overprotection can be an issue when the parents are so anxious about the child's well-being that the child is not allowed to interact with other children. Overprotection often may be an outgrowth of the very real risks to health and development that infants with disabilities or chronic conditions experience. In addition, parents and caregivers must be able to provide complex treatments and monitoring for children with multiple health and habilitative needs, as well as function as the child's service coordinator.

Safety is always a significant concern. As the infant's motor development improves and the child is able to explore the environment, safety risks such as poisoning, choking, and aspiration of small objects are a concern. Closely examining toys for removable parts that are smaller than the infant's trachea, avoiding toys that could be aspirated, and avoiding latex balloons can all help improve the environment of the infant with or without a disability or chronic condition.

The Toddler

Overview of Typical Development

The toddler period lasts from about 1 to 3 years of age. During this period, the child progresses from dependence in most areas to increasing independence but still requires a significant amount of support and assistance from caregivers. The toddler period is one of increasing exploration of the world and is characterized by curiosity, which produces serious safety risks for the child.

Size continues to increase, but not as much as during the infant period. The rate of development begins to slow during this period; significant changes in ability occur, but not as rapidly as during infancy. By the end of the toddler period, the child has slimmed down and his or her coordination has greatly improved. By 18 months of age, the anterior fontanel has completely closed.

Vision continues to develop concomitantly with neurologic development. Depth perception remains limited until around 3 years of age. The eustachian tubes are short and broad, as they are during infancy, and contribute to the frequency of ear infections in conjunction with respiratory infection or allergies. Changes in the sense of smell are related to the process of experience and learning, not physiologic changes. The toddler's neurologic system and muscles have matured to the point that swallowing is mature and drooling should not be present.

Maternal antibodies are generally no longer functioning in the child by 1 year of age; however, the combination of immune system maturity and immunization combine to offer the toddler significant protection. Young children who are cared for in group settings, such as child care and family child care homes, are at greater risk for minor acute infections than children who are cared for at home. However, as the toddler's exposure to pathogens increases, development of antibodies develops at a more rapid pace (Nelms & Mullins, 1982). Children who are cared for in child care centers experience an increase in ear infections. Group care such as child care

Table 10–4 SUMMARY OF INFANT GROWTH, DEVELOPMENT, AND HEALTH MAINTENANCE

Physical Competency	Intellectual Competency	Emotional-Social Competency
1–2 Months		
Holds head in alignment when prone; Moro reflex to loud sound; follows objects; smiles	Reflex activity; vowel sounds produced	Gratification through sucking and basic needs being promptly met; smiles at people
2–4 Months		
Turns back to side; raises head and chest 45–90 degrees off bed and supports weight on arms; reaches for objects; follows object through midline; drools; begins to localize sounds; prefers configuration of face	Reproduces behavior initially achieved by random activity; imitates behavior previously done. Visually studies objects; locates sounds; makes cooing sounds; does not look for objects removed from presence	Social responsiveness; awareness of those who are not primary caregiver; smiles in response to familiar face
4–6 Months		
Birth weight doubled; teeth eruption may begin; sits with stable head and back control; rolls from abdomen to back; picks up object with palmar grasp	Some intentional actions; some sense of object permanence, looks on same path for vanished object; recognizes partially hidden objects; more systematic in imitative behavior; babbles	Prefers primary caregiver; sucking needs decrease; laughs in pleasure
6–8 Months		
Turns back to stomach; sits alone; crawls; transfers objects from hand to hand; turns to sound behind	Continued development as in 4–6 months	Differentiated response to nonprimary caretakers; evidence of "stranger" or "separation" anxiety
8–10 Months		
Creeps; pulls to stand; pincer grasp	Actions more goal-directed; able to solve simple problems by using previously mastered responses. Actively searches for an object that disappears	Attachment process complete
10–12 Months		
Birth weight tripled; cruises; stands by self; may use spoon	Begins to imitate behavior done before but not seen self do. Understands words being said; may say 1–4 words. Intentionality is present.	Begins to explore and separate briefly from parent

Table 10–4   SUMMARY OF INFANT GROWTH, DEVELOPMENT, AND HEALTH MAINTENANCE *Continued*

Nutrition	Play	Safety
1–2 Months		
Breast-fed or fortified formula	Variety of positions; caretaker should hold and talk to infant; large, brightly colored objects	Car carrier; proper use of infant seat
2–4 Months		
As for 1–2 months	Talk to and hold; musical toys; rattle, mobile; variety of objects of different color, size, and texture; mirror, crib toys, variety of settings	Do not leave unattended on couch, bed, etc. Remove any small objects that infant could choke on
4–6 Months		
Introduction of solids; initial store of iron depleted	Talk to and hold; provide open space to move and objects to grasp	Keep environment free of safety hazards; check toys for sharp edges and small pieces that might break
6–8 Months		
Introduce finger foods; begin use of cup	Provide place to explore; stack toys, blocks; nursery rhymes	Check infant's expanding environment for hazards
8–10 Months		
As for 6–8 months	Games: hide-and-seek, peek-a-boo, pat-a-cake, looking at pictures in a book	Keep electrical outlets plugged, cords out of reach, stairs blocked, coffee and end tables cleared of hazards Do not leave alone in a bathtub Keep poisons out of reach and locked Continue use of safety seat in car
10–12 Months		
More solids than liquids; increasing use of cup; begin to wean	Increase space; read to infant; name and point to body parts; water; sand play; ball	As for 8–10 months

From Betz, C.L., Hunsberger, M., & Wright, S. (1994). Growth and development of the infant. In Betz, C.L., Hunsberger, M., & Wright, S. (Eds.). *Family-centered nursing care of children* (2nd ed.). Philadelphia: WB Saunders, p. 148–149.

may present significant risk for infection for children who have chronic conditions and are more vulnerable to infection.

Changes in the gastrointestinal system contribute to increasing hunger and the need for frequent, nutritional snacks. This is particularly important in young children who have chronic conditions or who are recovering from trauma, because they may require additional nutritional support to maintain growth and development and to recover from the injury. Although neuromuscular control improves throughout the toddler period, complete control of defecation may not occur until 3 years of age or later. In children with disabilities or chronic conditions, neurologic immaturity and resulting developmental delays in motor, cognitive, and communication areas frequently delay control of defecation until much later.

Urine output increases from 1 to 3 years of age, as does the ability to concentrate urine. Voiding continues to be involuntary, with control beginning in many children at around 2 years of age. However, when urinary distention reaches a certain point, the toddler will continue to void automatically (Nelms & Mullins, 1982).

Gross motor and fine motor muscular coordination improve as a result of increases in muscle size, maturation of the central nervous system, and the opportunity to explore and interact with the environment. Skeletal growth and maturation results in changes in physical characteristics. Genu varum ("bow legs"), metatarsus adductus ("toeing in"), and tibial torsion (internal rotation of the tibia) are all part of the normal growth pattern and are considered physiologic. Increases in myelination of nerves produces a more differentiated and refined motor response.

An area of social-emotional development of the toddler that is key to behavior is fear of separation. This characteristic demonstrates the toddler's emerging sense of object permanence as well as the strength of the relationship with the mother or primary caregiver. Separation anxiety begins with protest—crying, screaming, refusing to be comforted, and pushing the substitute caregiver away. Often the toddler will ignore the parent on return. Feelings of abandonment or waking at night may occur. Following this phase, if the separation continues, the child becomes withdrawn and may refuse food or sleep excessively. After longer separation, the toddler will appear to "recover" and be very affectionate, often inappropriately so, and

friendly with strangers. Separation anxiety can become a serious problem in the toddler hospitalized for a long period of time without one or both of the parents or the primary caregiver. Children who are hospitalized following a trauma in which one or both of the parents are also victims are at risk for this reaction. An overview of typical development in the toddler period is provided in Table 10–5.

Developmental Concerns for the Toddler With a Disability or Chronic Condition

Although toddlers are dependent for most of their self-care, they have improved enough in mobility and skills to explore their environment, producing multiple safety risks. Toddlers with disabilities or chronic conditions are not immune to these risks and may even be at greater risk because of delayed cognitive abilities or lack of intact hearing or vision. Young children who have delays in motor skills may continue to mouth objects much like an infant and may be at risk for choking and poisoning. Adapting safety procedures for the developmental level of the child, not necessarily their chronological age, is most appropriate.

Locating child care may be a real problem for parents of children with disabilities or chronic conditions. Often, children in this population will not achieve physiologic stability until the end of the first year of life or later. Some of these children, especially those with respiratory disorders or immune system deficits, may be too vulnerable to infection to risk group care. Children who require invasive procedures have a different problem—it may be very difficult to locate a child care or respite care provider that is willing or able to provide the technical care and monitoring the child requires. Many states prohibit delegation of nursing tasks by registered nurses, or in states which do permit delegation, locating a nurse who is both willing to delegate and knowledgeable about the process is very difficult. Additionally, families may have been dependent on skilled nursing settings earlier in the child's life which were covered by Medicaid or other public funding sources, and simply cannot afford regular child care. The great majority of child care is paid for out of the parent's pocket, and there is little access to public funding. Although the Americans With Disabilities Act makes it illegal for any public service agency or business to refuse service to children with disabilities or chronic conditions, many child care centers or family day care homes lack the financial resources and the skills to plan for a child requiring complex care.

Toddlers who are developing normally are at risk for accidents such as falls, motor vehicle–pedestrian accidents, and coming into contact with sharp objects. Burns are also a significant risk (see Chap. 21). Young children who are delayed in walking may have poorer balance and coordination, leading to a higher risk for falls. Child-proofing the environment and awareness of outdoor and playground safety can help prevent accidents.

The toddler period is when children with typical development gain control of bowel and bladder function. Children with disabilities or chronic conditions may be delayed in attaining this control due to cognitive deficits; lack of muscle control, balance, and coordination needed to sit on the toilet; or physiologic problems that interfere with normal functioning of the gastrointestinal and urologic systems. This delay in mastery of bowel and bladder control may lead to psycho-social conflict, according to Freud and Erikson. More information on management of delay in bowel and bladder control is presented in Chapter 12.

For the toddler to develop appropriately and acquire self-care skills, stimulation, interaction, play, and affection are necessary. A deficit in any of the areas may put the toddler's development in general and development of self-care skills at risk. Acquisition of literacy, or the ability to read, in children is related to the experience of parents or caregivers reading to the child. Children should be read developmentally appropriate materials in which the child has an opportunity to interact, such as saying words along with the reader, clapping hands, making faces, or other physical activities. The opportunity to observe and imitate adults performing self-care activities results in imprinting, so that the child can begin to imitate behaviors such as brushing teeth, washing hands, and other self-care activities.

Children with disabilities and chronic conditions are often not allowed to solve problems on their own, but are instead helped out of situations. The ability to practice simple problem solving and trial-and-error learning is crucial to cognitive development as well as emotional-social development. It is important at this point of development to begin to give the toddler simple choices whenever possible, for example, saying "Do you want the ball, or the doll?" Do not give a child an option that is not acceptable, such as asking whether or not the child wants medication.

Parents are often very sensitive about the onset of masturbation in the toddler. Sexual self-exploration is a part of the toddler's development of self as a sexual being and of gender roles. Negative reactions to masturbation such as threats or physical punishment can lead to negative feelings about sexuality and set up later conflicts. Parents who are tolerant of sex play among toddlers and are able to set appropriate limits will foster positive attitudes towards self, the body, and sexuality in the child. Sex play that is unsafe, such as placing objects in the urethra, vagina, or anus, or that is done in public places is unsafe and inappropriate. Sexual exploration and masturbation is best done in private, and it is necessary that the young child learn this societal limitation in a gentle, tolerant manner (Betz, Hunsberger, & Wright, 1994).

Children with disabilities or chronic conditions, especially those with cognitive delay, may display excessive interest in masturbation, particularly public masturbation. Any child who persists in this type of activity should be assessed to rule out vaginal infection, urinary tract infection, and possible sexual abuse. Although many children with cognitive delay may begin sexual self-exploration at a later age, it usually occurs according to their developmental level rather than their chronological age. A behavior reinforcement program can help limit these behaviors to appropriate times and places after infection or sexual abuse has been ruled out.

The Pre-schooler

Overview of Typical Development

The pre-school period extends from 3 to 5 years of age. During this period of slowing physical growth, refinement of skills continue until the 5-year-old child is able to perform more complex motor tasks such as skipping or skating. Fine motor coordination improves to the point that the letters of the alphabet can be copied, a two-part figure can be drawn, and a diamond can be copied. The pre-schooler's appearance changes, becoming more slender and proportioned more like that of an older child. The head is no longer as out of proportion to the body, and both trunk and limbs increase in length. A knock-kneed, flat-footed appearance is typical; however, extreme variations are best referred to a pediatric orthopedist. Speech and language con-

Table 10–5 SUMMARY OF TODDLER GROWTH, DEVELOPMENT, AND HEALTH MAINTENANCE

Physical Competency	Intellectual Competency	Emotional-Social Competency
General: 1–3 Years		

Gains 5 kg (11 lb)
Grows 20.3 cm (8 in)
12 Teeth erupt
Nutritional requirements
  Energy 100 Kcal/kg/day
  Fluid 115–125 mL/kg/day
  Protein 1.8 g/kg/day
	Learns by exploring and experimenting. Learns by imitating. Progresses from a vocabulary of 3–4 words at 12 months to about 900 words at 36 months.	Central crisis: to gain a sense of autonomy vs. doubt and shame. Demonstrates independent behaviors. Exhibits attachment behavior strongly and regularly until third birthday. Fears persist of strange people, objects, and places and of aloneness and being abandoned. Egocentric in play (parallel play). Imitation of parents in household tasks and activities of daily living.

15 Months		
Legs appear bowed. Walks alone, climbs, slides down stairs backward. Stacks two blocks. Scribbles spontaneously. Grasps spoon but rotates it, holds cup with both hands. Takes off socks and shoes.	Trial-and-error method of learning. Experiments to see what will happen. Says at least 3 words. Uses expressive jargon.	Shows independence by trying to feed self and helps in undressing.
18 Months		
Runs but still falls. Walks upstairs with help. Slides down stairs backward. Stacks three to four blocks. Clumsily throws a ball. Unzips a larger zipper. Takes off simple garments.	Begins to retain a mental image of an absent object. Concept of object permanence fully develops. Has vocabulary of 10 or more words. Holophrastic speech (1 word used to communicate whole ideas).	Fears the water. Temper tantrums may begin. Negativism and dawdling predominate. Bedtime rituals begin. Awareness of gender identity begins. Helps with undressing.
24 Months		
Runs quickly and with fewer falls. Pulls toys and walks sideways. Walks downstairs hanging on a rail (does not alternate feet). Stacks six blocks. Turns pages of a book. Imitates vertical and circular strokes. Uses spoon with little spilling. Can feed self. Puts on simple garments. Can turn door knobs.	Enters into pre-conceptual phase of pre-operational period: Symbolic thinking and symbolic play. Egocentric thinking, imagination, and pretending are common. Has vocabulary of about 300 words. Uses 2-word sentences (telegraphic speech). Engages in monologue.	Fears the dark and animals. Temper tantrums may continue. Negativism and dawdling continue. Bedtime rituals continue. Sleep resisted overtly. Usually shows readiness to begin bowel and bladder control. Explores genitalia. Brushes teeth with help. Helps with dressing and undressing.
36 Months		
Has set of deciduous teeth at about 30 months. Walks downstairs alternating feet. Rides tricycle. Walks with balance and runs well. Stacks eight to ten blocks. Can pour from a pitcher. Feeds self completely. Dresses self almost completely (does not know front from back). Cannot tie shoes.	Pre-conceptual phase of pre-operational period as for 24 months. Uses around 900 words. Constructs complete sentences and uses all parts of speech.	Temper tantrums subside. Negativism and dawdling subside. Bedtime rituals subside. Self-care in feeding, elimination, and dressing enhances self-esteem.

Table 10–5   SUMMARY OF TODDLER GROWTH, DEVELOPMENT, AND HEALTH MAINTENANCE *Continued*

Nutrition	Play	Safety
General: 1–3 Years		
Milk 16–24 oz. Appetite decreases. Wants to feed self. Has food jags. Never force food; give nutritious snacks. Give iron and vitamin supplementation only if intake is poor.	Books at all ages. Needs physical and quiet activities, does not need expensive toys.	Never leave alone in tub. Keep poisons, including detergents and cleaning products, out of reach. Use car seat. Have ipecac in house.
15 Months		
Vulnerable to iron deficiency anemia. Give table foods except for tough meat and hard vegetables. Wants to feed self.	Stuffed animals, dolls, music toys. Peek-a-boo, hide-and-seek. Water and sand play. Stacking toys. Roll ball on floor. Push toys on floor. Read to toddler.	Keep small items off floor (pins, buttons, clips). Child may choke on hard food. Cords and table cloths are a danger. Keep electrical outlets plugged and poisons locked away. Risk of kitchen accidents with toddler under foot.
18 Months		
Negativism may interfere with eating. Encourage self-feeding. Is easily distracted while eating. May play with food. High activity level interferes with eating.	Rocking horse. Nesting toys. Shape-sorting cube. Pencil or crayon. Pull toys. Four-wheeled toy to ride. Throw ball. Running and chasing games. Rough-housing. Puzzles. Blocks. Hammer and peg board.	Falls From riding toy In bathtub From running too fast Climbs up to get dangerous objects. Keep dangerous things out of wastebasket.
24 Months		
Requests certain foods, therefore snacks should be controlled. Imitates eating habits of others. May still play with food and especially with utensils and dish (pouring, stacking).	Clay and Play-Doh. Finger paint. Brush paint. Record player with record and story book and songs to sing along. Toys to take apart. Toy tea sets. Puppets. Puzzles.	May fall from outdoor large play equipment. Can reach farther than expected (knives, razors, and matches must be kept out of reach).
36 Months		
Sits in booster seat rather than highchair. Verbal about likes and dislikes.	Likes playing with other children, building toys, drawing and painting, doing puzzles. Imitation household objects for doll play. Nurse and doctor kits. Carpenter kits	Protect from Turning on hot water Falling from tricycle Striking matches

From Betz, C.L., Hunsberger, M., & Wright, S. (1994). Growth and development of the toddler. In Betz, C.L., Hunsberger, M., & Wright, S. (Eds.). *Family-centered nursing care of children* (2nd ed.). Philadelphia: WB Saunders, p. 190.

tinue to develop until a typically developing child can correctly name four colors, accurately describe a picture, and carry out three-part instructions by the end of the pre-school period. Vision improves so that visual acuity is nearly mature. Any strabismus is considered atypical at this point, and the child should be referred to an ophthalmologist for evaluation (Nelms & Mullins, 1982).

During the pre-school period, children develop a perception of the body and may view themselves as attractive or unattractive. Parental influence is very strong at this point, and the reactions and verbalizations of the parents will influence the child's self-perception for a lifetime. Children with disabilities are more vulnerable to negative messages at this time and can benefit from positive feedback about their bodies and themselves.

Pre-schoolers are cognitively able to focus on only one aspect of a situation. They have difficulty conceptualizing that objects do not have human qualities. During this period, the child begins to use symbolic play, or imaginative play, and often acts out experiences or situations with dolls or stuffed animals. Pre-schoolers also may have imaginary friends or fantasize in an attempt to gain mastery over a challenging situation. Using surrogates such as dolls can assist the nurse in teaching the child simple concepts about health education or hospitalization. Additionally, the pre-schooler is unable to conceptualize cause and effect; therefore, if the child has wished that a sibling would go away, and the sibling becomes ill, the toddler will attribute the illness to the wish and experience shame. These fears may have a significant impact on the child's behavior and need to be addressed by helping the child understand what actions are right or wrong while encouraging initiative. Emerging understanding of right and wrong and feeling rewarded for performing the right actions helps contribute to the pre-schooler's sense of self and mastery.

Development of gender identity continues through self-exploration and comparison with others, both physically and behaviorally. Pre-schooler's questions about their observations may be disconcerting for parents and are best answered in a clear, uncomplicated manner. More information on typical growth and development of the pre-schooler is provided in Table 10–6.

Developmental Concerns for the Pre-schooler With a Disability or Chronic Condition

Pre-schoolers have a lot of fears due to the fact that they do not completely understand the world and are unable to differentiate real and imagined dangers. Although fear can be protective, preventing children from taking risks, it can also be motivating and stimulating to curiosity. Pre-schoolers with disabilities may attribute their condition to bad behavior or thoughts or may think that other children who contract minor acute illness were somehow influenced by their condition. Pre-school children respond best when offered reassurance about and told that they are not responsible for their condition and the illnesses of others. Young children are not yet cognitively able to comprehend complex explanations and benefit from interventions that deal directly with immediate sensations, emotions, and experiences (Yoos, 1988).

Challenging behavior may begin to be noticed during the pre-school period. As pre-schoolers leave their home environment for group care settings or are involved in neighborhood play groups, issues with behavior may develop. Young children with challenging behavior due to an underlying disability or cognitive deficit often do better with one-to-one attention than when in a crowd. Hearing impairments, especially if they have not yet been identified, can prevent the child from communicating adequately with peers and adults and may lead to hitting or aggressive behavior in an attempt to have their needs met. Children with sensory-perceptual difficulties may be unable to tolerate the level of stimulation or noise in groups or public situations. The child may lash out, display withdrawn behavior, cry, scream, or run away. Coping behaviors during this period involve physical activities such as crying, hitting, and kicking, as well as more verbal behaviors such as name-calling or negative comments. Pre-schoolers may be taught to respond to situations in positive ways through input from parents and other caregivers. Children with disabilities may show coping behaviors that are less mature than their chronological age, but according to their cognitive or developmental level.

Safety issues for the pre-schooler are similar to those for the toddler. Motor vehicle–pedestrian accidents are more of a risk for pre-schoolers due to their improved motor ability combined with immature judgment. Pre-schoolers are more active explorers and are more likely to get themselves into risky situations, such as playing in old refrigerators or drainage pipes or accepting rides from unknown adults. Pre-schoolers continue to be at risk for poisoning and are more at risk for exposure to toxic substances that they may encounter in play in the yard or home. Drowning continues to be a risk. Pre-schoolers are old enough to learn how to swim, but they should never be left alone in any water situation. Children with tracheostomies should avoid water activities and water play, because they are particularly susceptible to drowning from getting water into the tracheostomy tube. Children with disabilities or chronic conditions who have been fitted with mobility devices, such as wheelchairs, should be taught safety precautions so that they do not back up off an elevated surface or injure other children with the wheelchair. Children should never be left alone in a house, whether they are in a wheelchair, use another type of assistive device, or are confined to a bed. These children are unable to respond to an emergency and may be trapped in the home should one arise.

The School-Aged Child

Overview of Typical Development

The family of the school-aged child must adapt to changes in roles, responsibilities, and peer groups. No longer is the family the primary controlling factor in the child's life, as the school takes responsibility for the child during the day. Social roles change for the child as well as for the family. Family members must relate with school personnel and adapt to the new influences in the child's life. Peers become more important, and other beliefs, values, and behaviors are available to the child. These new values and behaviors may be in conflict with those of the family, and the family must strive to reconcile the issues that arise as a result. Children are exposed to more competition, such as that of school mates for the teacher's attention. At this point in their lives, school-aged children tend to compare themselves with others and integrate that comparison as part of their self-concept and their perception of their own skill mastery. The roles of the child change, and although play remains important, it is now joined by school work as an important activity (Betz, Hunsberger, & Wright, 1994).

Physical development at this period varies greatly from child to child and between boys and girls. Children are slimmer and taller and look more like adults than like pre-schoolers. Skeletal deviations such as genu valgum, or knock-knees, and toeing-in tend to self-correct. School-aged children show considerable differences in height, weight, and body type, even when they are the same age. Boys develop physically somewhat more slowly than girls during this stage. Physical growth increases relatively slowly during the school-aged years. Body composition changes relatively little, and until puberty, boys' body composition is about the same as that of girls.

As the child grows older, the position of the eustachian tube changes and becomes more vertical, making ear infections less frequent. Changes in the lens of the eye may result in myopia and visual problems. Lymphoid tissue, such as the tonsils and adenoids, grows very rapidly during this developmental stage, finishing growth and then reducing in size by puberty. Illness is some what less frequent, with infection response similar to that of adults.

Continued refinement in the area of motor development occurs during this period. Basic skills have been acquired, and mastery of more complex gross and fine motor tasks takes place. Organized physical activity begins with games and sports. Activities become more physically complex the older the child becomes. During the later stages of the school-aged period, growth spurts may unbalance the child somewhat and cause more clumsiness than was previously noted (Betz, Hunsberger, & Wright, 1994).

Eye-hand and perceptual motor coordination in other areas improves with better performance of tasks such as writing, drawing, and other creative activities. Preference for the right or left hand emerges in the late pre-school period or early school-aged period. Most typically developing children are able to distinguish right from left on their bodies after handedness occurs. Accuracy and reaction time increases until about 9 to 10 years of age and then slows into adolescence and adulthood (Nelms & Mullins, 1982).

Academic achievement takes precedence over many other activities. The child starts school just prior to the beginning of Piaget's stage of concrete operations and begins to perceive and process more complex information. Cognitive development is constantly expanding, as are speech and language and other perceptual abilities. Understanding of the rules of games and expectations for behavior improve to the point that real information sharing can occur. The school-aged child begins to be able to analyze the problem-solving process, understand and order objects according to a variety of characteristics, and understand the concept of conservation of

Table 10–6 SUMMARY OF PRE-SCHOOLER GROWTH, DEVELOPMENT, AND HEALTH MAINTENANCE

Physical Competency	Intellectual Competency	Emotional-Social Competency
General Summary: 3–5 Years		

Gains 4.5 kg (10 lb)
Grows 15 cm (6 in)
20 Teeth present
Nutritional requirements
  Energy 1250–1600 cal/day
    (or 90–100 Kcal/kg/day)
  Fluid: 100–125 mL/kg/
    day
  Protein: 30 g/day (or 3 g/
    kg/day)
  Iron: 10 mg/day
	Becomes increasingly aware of self
	  and others
	Vocabulary increases from
	  900–2100 words
	Piaget's pre-operational/intuitive
	  period
		Freud's phallic stage
		  Oedipus complex—boy
		  Electra complex—girl
		Erikson's stage of initiative vs.
		  guilt
		Fowler's intuitive-projective
		  stage
		Kohlberg's pre-conventional
		  stage

3 Years		

Runs, stops suddenly
Walks backward
Climbs steps
Jumps
Pedals tricycle
Undresses self
Unbuttons front buttons
Feeds self well
	Knows own sex
	Desires to please
	Has sense of humor
	Language—900 words
	Follows simple direction
	Uses plurals
	Names figure in picture
	Uses adjectives/adverbs
		Shifts between reality and
		  imagination
		Engages in bedtime rituals
		Negativism decreases
		Animism and realism:
		  anything that moves is alive

4 Years		

Runs well, skips clumsily
Hops on one foot
Heel-toe walks
Goes up and down steps
  without holding rail
Jumps well
Dresses and undresses
Buttons well, needs help
  with zippers, bows
Brushes teeth
Bathes self
Draws with some form and
  meaning
	Is more aware of others
	Uses alibis to excuse behavior
	Is bossy
	Language—knows 1500 words
	Talks in sentences
	Knows nursery rhymes
	Counts to 5
	Is highly imaginative
	Uses name calling
		Focuses on present
		Egocentrism: unable to see the
		  viewpoint of others, unable
		  to understand another's
		  inability to see own
		  viewpoint
		Does not comprehend
		  anticipatory explanation
		Has sexual curiosity
		Shows evidence of Oedipus
		  complex
		Shows evidence of Electra
		  complex

5 Years		

Runs skillfully
Jumps three or four steps
Jumps rope, hops, skips
Begins to dance
Roller skates
Dresses without assistance
Ties shoelaces
Hits nail on head with
  hammer
Draws person—six parts
Prints first name
	Is aware of cultural differences
	Knows name and address
	Is more independent
	Is more sensible/less imaginative
	Copies triangle, draws rectangle
	Knows 4 or more colors
	Language—knows 2100 words,
	  meaningful sentences
	Understands kinship
	Counts to 10
		Continues in egocentrism
		Has fantasy and daydreams
		Resolves Oedipus/Electra
		  complex: girls identify with
		  mother, boys with father
		Body image and body
		  boundary are especially
		  important in illness
		Shows tension in nail biting,
		  nose picking, whining,
		  snuffling

Table 10–6 SUMMARY OF PRE-SCHOOLER GROWTH, DEVELOPMENT, AND HEALTH MAINTENANCE *Continued*

Nutrition	Play	Safety
General Summary: 3–5 Years		
Carbohydrate intake is approximately 40%–50% of calories Good food sources of essential vitamins and minerals are necessary Regular toothbrushing should be done Parents are seen as examples; if parent does not eat it, child will not	Reading books is important at all ages Balance highly physical activities with quiet times Quiet rest period takes the place of nap time Sturdy play materials should be provided	Never leave alone in bath or swimming pool Keep poisons in locked cupboard; learn what household items are poisonous Use car seats and seat belts Never leave child alone in car Remove doors from abandoned freezers and refrigerators
3 Years		
1250 cal/day Because of increased sex identity and imitation, child copies parents at table and will eat what they eat Different colors and shapes of foods can increase interest	Participates in simple games Cooperates, takes turns Plays with group Uses scissors, paper Likes crayons, coloring books Enjoys being read to and "reading" Plays "dress-up" and "house" Likes fire engines	Teach safety habits early Let water out of bathtub, do not stand in tub Caution against climbing in unsafe areas, onto or under cars, in unsafe buildings, in drainage pipes Insist on seat belts being worn at all times in cars
4 Years		
Good nutrition 1400 cal/day Nutritious between meal snacks are essential Emphasis is on quality not quantity of food eaten Mealtime should be enjoyable, not for criticism As dexterity improves, neatness increases	Has longer attention span with group activities Plays "dress-up" with more drama Draws, pounds, paints Likes to make paper chains, sewing cards, scrapbooks Likes being read to, records, and rhythmic play "Helps" adults	Teach to stay out of streets, alleys Continually teach safety; child understands Teach how to handle scissors Teach what items are poisons and why to avoid them Never allow to stand in moving car
5 Years		
Good nutrition 1600 cal/day Encourage regular toothbrushing Encourage quiet time before meals Child can learn to cut own meat Frequent illnesses from increased exposure increase nutritional needs	Plays with trucks, cars, soldiers, dolls Likes simple games with letters or numbers Engages in much gross motor activity: plays with water, mud, snow, leaves, rocks Plays matching picture games	Teach how to cross streets safely Teach not to speak to strangers or get into cars of strangers Insist on seat belts being worn Teach to swim

From Betz, C.L., Hunsberger, M., & Wright, S. (1994). Growth and development of the preschooler. In Betz, C.L., Hunsberger, M., & Wright, S. (Eds.). *Family-centered nursing care of children* (2nd ed.). Philadelphia: WB Saunders, pp. 235–236.

matter. This characteristic is exemplified by Piaget's classic experiment of moving the same quantity of water to a vessel of a different shape, then asking the child if there is more, less, or the same amount of water present. More advanced concepts of causality emerge around 8 to 9 years of age, and the child begins to pursue the physical and psychologic causes for events and experiences (Betz, Hunsberger, & Wright, 1994).

Concurrent with development of cognitive abilities is the progression of speech and language development. Speech is usually understandable by this period, with a few exceptions of specific sounds. By the time the child reaches adolescence, comprehension and expression of word meanings are similar to those of the adult. Vocabulary continues to increase, with improved understanding of multiple meanings and subtle connotations of words. The school-aged child enjoys humor and uses "knock-knock" jokes, word puzzles, and puns to manipulate language and demonstrate proficiency. Making jokes about others, such as adults, helps release tension and aggression toward adults, siblings, or other children and can delineate social groups.

Industry versus inferiority is Erikson's term for the developmental challenge of the school-aged years. Children like to become involved with others who *"know* things and *know how* to do things" (Betz, Hunsberger, & Wright, 1994, p. 294). Being useful and having information about people and objects is a primary goal and facilitates social relationships. The school-aged child's sense of self and of mastery rests to a large degree on these abilities and characteristics.

A part of social and role development is that of sexual behaviors. Young school-aged children often tease those of the opposite sex, and imaginative play moves frequently to male and female gender roles, as in playing "house" and "doctor." In middle school-aged children, both same-sex and opposite-sex relationships set the stage for more mature sex roles. Older school-aged children try out increasing physical contact, including hugging, kissing, or dancing with pre-adolescent children of the opposite gender. Sexually explicit language may be used by children at this stage, and interest in pictures, television shows, and movies with sexually explicit scenes increases.

Coping mechanisms most commonly used by school-aged children are information-seeking and controlling behaviors. According to Freud, the child's conscience, or superego,

emerges and provides more logical control for behaviors. The school-aged period is a balance between positive self-esteem and feelings of inferiority. Embarrassment becomes a fear. Alternate methods of dealing with fear and anger are helpful to children during this stage (Betz, Hunsberger, & Wright, 1994). More information on typical development of school-aged children is provided in Table 10–7.

Developmental Concerns for the School-Aged Child With a Disability or Chronic Condition

Children with disabilities and chronic conditions ideally have received early intervention and specialized pre-school services prior to entering the kindergarten-through-twelfth-grade school system. Transition planning is extremely important for children moving from pre-school to kindergarten, as the nature of the environment changes, the amount of time at school increases, and more academic and social demands are made on the child. Families often have a great deal of difficulty during this period as well, because they have gotten to know and become familiar with the pre-school staff and setting. At times, inclusive services are available in child care or pre-school, but segregated services such as "resource rooms" or special education classrooms may predominate during the school-aged period. Although federal legislation mandates a least restrictive environment for each child, that mandate is interpreted differently by different states, school systems, principals, and teachers. Individualized educational plans were formulated for children using public education services as opposed to private pre-schools, but during the post-kindergarten school years, the individualized educational plan is usually updated and reviewed yearly with complete academic and developmental testing occurring only once every 3 years. The school nurse is an integral part of the school team, providing assessment and services and operating as a valuable resource for pediatric rehabilitation nurses in both acute and other community settings.

Class sizes are larger in formal school, and teachers are often less willing to take on additional responsibilities for students with disabilities and chronic conditions because of lack of time and ability to deal with the needs of many diverse students. Children with physical needs often have an educational aide working with them to perform special care and help with academic work. Ideally, activities for the child with a disability or chronic condition are adapted to their abilities, and educational goals are realistic and tailored to the needs of the child. Learning disabilities may be subtle or obvious; many children with physical disabilities, such as those with spina bifida, exhibit subtle and difficult to identify learning problems that may be misconstrued as laziness or lack of motivation to succeed.

Children who are entering a school setting for the first time may have difficulty adjusting to peers, and peers may tease or bully them. It is important for children with disabilities and chronic conditions to be able to cope with these situations, and they will require advice and strategies in dealing with such occurrences. Peers may benefit from educational programs about people with disabilities or a class presentation from a health care provider and a parent about the child's specific disability. Children with challenging behaviors or significant cognitive delays are most likely to be segregated and thus to have the most difficulty in forming appropriate peer relations and being accepted by others. However, education and positive reinforcement and modeling of behaviors toward children with disabilities and chronic conditions can change the attitudes and behaviors of peers.

Depending on the child's disability or condition, physical involvement in games or motor activities may require considerable support. Adapting activities for the child with a disability, or adapting roles on the team such as assistant coach, can allow the child with a disability or chronic condition to participate in physical activities with peers. Adaptive sports programs out of school, such as disability field days, Special Olympics for children with primarily cognitive deficits (e.g., Down syndrome) and other adaptive sports programs can be very helpful in promoting mastery, acceptance by others, and individual self-esteem for the child with a disability or chronic condition. Physical education can also be adapted to the individual child's needs and abilities.

Social interaction is more difficult for children with communication delays and deficits and for children with cognitive deficits. Peers are very aware of differences in social behavior and language and are quick to label the child who behaves immaturely or inappropriately. Often the child with a disability or chronic condition may not be aware of the "different" behavior and does not understand why relationships are so hard to form and maintain. The child experiences loss and grief for failed relationships, which influences his or her sense of mastery and competence and may decrease self-esteem. Children with bowel and bladder incontinence may also have a more difficult time with social interaction if they use "baby-ish" methods such as diapers or if the odor of urine or stool is present.

Sexuality is also an interest for school-aged children with disabilities and chronic conditions, and masturbation may be the primary method of meeting their need for information and body exploration. Sex education is equally important for children with disabilities as for typically developing children and should include information on how the disability or condition affects or is affected by sexual feelings or behaviors. For children with cognitive delays who may not understand appropriate social behaviors, masturbation in public or inappropriate words, gestures, or actions such as touching other people's bodies must be curtailed by setting limits for behavior and providing alternative outlets for expression.

This stage of development is ideal for beginning to teach children with disabilities and chronic conditions about their bodies, health promotion behaviors, and their disability or condition. The developmental nature of information seeking during this stage facilitates learning. Teaching should always be tailored to the child's developmental or cognitive level rather than his or her chronological age, and information should be kept basic and concrete. Children need to hear more about how they are similar to other children than how they are different.

By this stage of development, children with disabilities or chronic conditions, with a few exceptions, should be participating in their self-care. Mastery over self-care skills is an important contributor to self-esteem and the development of competence. By this age, children with severe cerebral palsy should be managing a mobility device, such as an electric wheelchair, and should be working with some type of communication system that is appropriate to their cognitive and physical abilities. At around age 5 years, the child with spina bifida who does not have any upper extremity involvement should be taking part in self-catheterization by starting to help gather equipment, washing hands, and helping to clean up afterward. Depending on trunk control and fine motor coordination, the technique of self-catheterization may be taught. The child will still require assistance

Table 10–7 SUMMARY OF SCHOOL-AGED CHILD GROWTH, DEVELOPMENT, AND HEALTH MAINTENANCE

Physical Competency	Intellectual Competency	Emotional-Social Competency
General: 6–12 Years		
Gains an average of 2.5–3.2 kg/yr (5½–7 lbs/yr); overall height gains of 5.5 cm (2 in/yr); growth occurs in spurts and is mainly in trunk and extremities. Loses deciduous teeth, most of permanent teeth erupt. Is progressively more coordinated in both gross and fine motor skills; caloric needs increase with growth spurts.	Masters concrete operations. Moves from egocentrism; learns he or she is not always right. Learns grammar and expression of emotions and thoughts. Has vocabulary of 3000 words or more; handles complex sentences.	Central crisis; industry vs. inferiority; wants to do and make things. Progressive sex education needed. Wants to be like friends; competition important. Fears body mutilation, alterations in body image; earlier phobias may recur, also nightmares; fears death. Nervous habits common. Engages in constant activity. Enjoys group activities but no cooperative play. Temper tantrums used to express anger; is restless and indecisive.
6–7 Years		
Gross motor skill exceeds fine motor coordination. Balance and rhythm are good—child runs, skips, jumps, climbs, gallops; throws and catches ball; dresses self with little or no help.	Has vocabulary of 2500 words. Is learning to read and print; begins concrete concepts of numbers, general classification of items. Knows concepts of right and left; morning, afternoon, and evening; coinage. Has intuitive thought process. Is verbally aggressive, bossy, opinionated, argumentative. Likes simple games with basic rules. Has simple understanding of money.	Boisterous, outgoing, a know-it-all, whiney; parents should sidestep power struggles, offer choices. Becomes quiet and reflective during seventh year; very sensitive. Can use telephone. Likes to make things: starts many, finishes few. Give some responsibility for household duties. Uses words rather than physical means to express anger.
8–10 Years		
Myopia may appear. Secondary sex characteristics begin in girls. Hand-eye coordination and fine motor skills are well established. Movements are graceful, coordinated. Child cares for own physical needs completely; is constantly on move; plays and works hard. Enforce balance in rest and activity.	Is learning correct grammar and to express feelings in words. Likes books he or she can read alone; will read funny papers, scan newspaper. Enjoys making detailed drawings. Is mastering classification, seriation, spatial and temporal, numerical concepts. Uses language as a tool; likes riddles, jokes, chants, word games. Rules are guiding force in life now. Very interested in how things work, what and how weather, seasons, etc., are made.	Strong preference for same-sex peers; antagonizes opposite-sex peers. Self-assured and pragmatic at home; questions parental values and ideas. Has a strong sense of humor. Enjoys clubs, group projects, outings, large groups, camp. Modesty about own body increases over time; is sex-conscious. Works diligently to perfect skills he or she does best. Is happy, cooperative, relaxed, and casual in relationships, increasingly courteous and well-mannered with adults. Gang stage at a peak; secret codes and rituals prevail. Responds better to suggestion than dictatorial approach.
11–12 Years		
Vital signs approximate adult norms. Growth spurt occurs for girls. Inequalities between sexes are increasingly noticeable; boys have greater physical strength. Eruption of permanent teeth is complete except for third molars. Secondary sex characteristics begin in boys. Menstruation may begin.	Able to think about social problems and prejudices; see others' points of view. Enjoys reading mysteries, love stories. Begins playing with abstract ideas. Interested in "whys" of health measures and understands human reproduction. Very moralistic; religious commitment often made during this time.	Intense team loyalty; boys begin teasing girls and girls flirt with boys for attention; best friend period. Wants unreasonable independence. Rebellious about routines; wide mood swings; needs some time daily for privacy. Very critical of own work. Hero worship prevails. "Facts of life" chats with friends prevail; masturbation increases. Appears under constant tension.

Table 10-7 SUMMARY OF SCHOOL-AGED CHILD GROWTH, DEVELOPMENT, AND HEALTH MAINTENANCE *Continued*

Nutrition	Play	Safety
General: 6–12 Years		
Fluctuations in appetite due to uneven growth pattern and tendency to get involved in activities. Tendency to neglect breakfast owing to rush to get to school. Although school lunch is provided in most schools, child does not always eat it.	Plays in groups, mostly of same sex; "gang" activities predominate. Books read, all ages. Bicycles important, also sports equipment, cards, board and table games. Most of play is active games requiring little or no equipment.	Enforce continued use of seat belts during car travel. Bicycle safety must be taught and enforced. Enforce use of bicycle helmets. Teach safety related to hobbies, handicrafts, mechanical equipment.
6–7 Years		
Pre-school food dislikes persist. Tendency for deficiencies in iron, vitamin A, and riboflavin. Needs 100 mL/kg of water/day; 3 g/kg protein/day.	Still enjoys dolls, cars, and trucks. Plays well alone but enjoys small groups of both sexes; begins to prefer same-sex peers during 7th year. Is ready to learn how to ride a bicycle. Prefers imaginary, dramatic play with real costumes. Begins collecting for quantity, not quality. Enjoys active games such as hide-and-seek, tag, jump rope, roller skating, kickball. Ready for lessons in dancing, gymnastics, music. Restrict television time to 1–2 hr/day.	Teach and reinforce traffic safety. Still needs adult supervision of play. Teach to avoid strangers, never take anything from strangers. Teach illness prevention and reinforce continued practice of other health habits. Restrict bicycle use to home ground; no traffic areas; teach bicycle safety. Enforce use of bicycle helmets. Teach and set examples to prevent harmful use of drugs, alcohol, smoking.
8–10 Years		
Needs about 2100 calories/day; nutritious snacks. Tends to be too busy to bother to eat. Tendency for deficiencies in calcium, iron, and thiamine. Problem of obesity may begin now. Has good table manners. Is able to help with food preparation.	Likes hiking, sports. Enjoys cooking, woodworking, crafts. Enjoys cards and table games. Likes radio and records. Begins qualitative collecting now. Continue restriction on television time.	Stress safety with firearms. Keep them out of reach and allow use only with adult supervision. Know who the child's friends are; parents should still have some control over friend selection. Teach water safety; swimming should be supervised by an adult.
11–12 Years		
Male needs 2500 calories per day; female needs 2250 (70 cal/kg/day). Needs 75 mL/kg of water per day, 2 g/kg protein/day.	Enjoys projects and working with hands. Likes to do errands and jobs to earn money. Is very involved in sports, dancing, talking on phone. Enjoys all aspects of acting and drama.	Continue monitoring friends; stress bicycle safety on streets and in traffic.

From Betz, C.L., Hunsberger, M., & Wright, S. (1994). Growth and development of the school-age child. In Betz, C.L., Hunsberger, M., & Wright, S. (Eds.). *Family-centered nursing care of children* (2nd ed.). Philadelphia: WB Saunders, pp. 281–282.

and reminding about times for catheterization until cognitive development progresses to concrete operations.

The Adolescent

Overview of Typical Development

The adolescent is entering the last stage that leads to adulthood. Adult social and sex roles are increasingly tried out, sometimes with successful results, and sometimes with long-lasting consequences. During this stage, growth increases more than it has since birth. Both genders achieve their mature height and sexual development. The adolescent growth spurt lasts about 3 years and ends earlier for females than for males. Legs lengthen first, making for a disproportionate appearance. Uneven growth and development increases problems with motor coordination, but these problems disappear as final growth and development are reached. Lean body mass and fat double, with females developing more fat and males developing more muscle. As always, nutrition is important, but with the increased independence that accompanies this state, adolescents take more responsibility for their food intake and may not always make the healthiest choices. Weight consciousness appears, and adolescents tend to have misperceptions about the adequacy of their size, shape, and development compared with their peers.

Sexual maturation takes place at this stage, and primary sex characteristics that began to show in the late school-aged period become more prominent. Menarche begins at around 12 years of age in girls. Boys have had some sperm production since 3 years of age, but adult levels of sperm production do not begin until sexual maturity is almost complete. During adolescence, erections and nocturnal emissions begin, and although these are normal signs of sexual development, they are very embarrassing for boys (Betz, Hunsberger, & Wright, 1994).

Younger adolescents are still unable to separate other's interests from their own and tend to think that everyone is as interested in their lives as the adolescents themselves. This characteristic is termed adolescent egocentrism. This characteristic leads to feelings of uniqueness and "it can't happen to me" attitudes. The attitude of personal invulnerability leads to risk-taking behaviors and experimentation with illegal drugs and various types of lifestyles. By later adolescence, egocentrism fades.

During adolescence, abstract thinking begins to emerge. Adolescents are now able to "think about thinking" (Betz, Hunsberger, & Wright, 1994, p. 333) and are aware of other's thoughts and the fact that those thoughts are different from their own. They are able to question their own values and the values of others. Adolescents tend to be very preoccupied with themselves and may be very idealistic. Piaget's stage of formal operations encompasses the abstract thought typical of this period. One of the important cognitive functions during this stage is the ability to form a hypothesis, put together a plan to test the hypothesis, test the hypothesis, and draw conclusions. Understanding of symbolism in language is mature. A very descriptive statement from Betz, Hunsberger, and Wright (1994) describes this stage of thought as "a school age child can love a puppy and hate spiders, but a teen-ager can love peace and hate bigotry" (p. 334). Comprehension of the concept of future is possible, and adolescents can plan and reflect on hopes, fears, and goals. It is important to note that not all adolescents achieve the stage of formal operations and that some otherwise typical adults do not achieve this stage either.

Development of identity and body image are challenges for the adolescent. Hormonal changes make emotions more erratic, and physical changes complicate developing body image. The constant worry and comparison with others that adolescents typically go through is part of the process of adapting to changing bodies and feelings. The peer group is of primary importance to the younger adolescent, who is seeking to establish self-identity. Adopting different styles of dress, hairstyles and colors, and behavior or mannerisms is a method of "trying on" identity and may change rapidly. The experiences of adolescents from differing cultural groups vary somewhat from the experiences of adolescents from the dominant culture, and those differences may lead to misunderstandings and prejudices Adolescents from non-dominant cultures may internalize negative social attitudes, leading to poor self-esteem or emotional conflict. The process of separating one's self from the family involves considerable experimentation with roles, lifestyles, rebellion from families and from the "norms" of behavior, and identifying with the peer group or other social groups Some adolescents deal with the stresses of integrating and adapting to these changes by engaging in delinquent behavior (Betz, Hunsberger, & Wright, 1994).

Developing independence and emancipating from families usually peaks in later adolescence. Adolescents desire more responsibility and autonomy in decision making about friends, activities, driving the family car, and how late or how long they may stay at social events. Parents often feel that the adolescent has too much responsibility, and the balance between the adolescent's attitude and the parent's attitude is constantly shifting.

Sexuality is an important part of both identity development and seeking emancipation from family. As adolescents' bodies and feelings change with sexual maturation, they are bombarded with sexual messages from television, books, popular music, and movies. Sexual maturation comes with the risk of pregnancy, sexually transmitted diseases such as human immunodeficiency virus (HIV) and acquired immunodeficiency syndrome (AIDS), and emotional and psychologic conflicts. Early involvement in sexual activity exposes adolescents to these very real risks and affects formation of attitudes about sexuality and relationships. Homosexuality may become a preference at this time. Sexual activity for homosexual adolescents carries many of the same risks as those for heterosexual adolescents, but societal influences may make it more difficult for the adolescent to sort through sexual feelings and gain support for them. Early adolescents tend to relate to one another in groups, whereas older adolescents tend toward forming more mature relationships, and sexual behaviors become more explicit. More information on typical growth and development in adolescents is presented in Table 10–8.

Developmental Concerns for the Adolescent With a Disability or Chronic Condition

General health screening and well care is as important for the adolescent with a disability or chronic condition as it is for other adolescents. Weight and height for age are important to evaluate, as this population of adolescents may be overweight or underweight for many of the same reasons as others, in addition to the effects of limited mobility and decreased social opportunity. Just as with typically developing adolescents, this group has a need to understand how they compare with others physically and require reassurance that they are "normal" in these respects. Adolescents' self-identified health concerns center around social relationships and physical appearance, and they may be less concerned about health maintenance, dental care, nutrition, or prevention of sexually transmitted disease (Betz, Hunsberger, & Wright, 1994). Adolescents with disabilities and chronic conditions express similar concerns as typical adolescents.

Adolescence requires the greatest number of nutrients for growth and development than any other stage of development except for the first 3 years of life. Disabilities and chronic conditions may increase or decrease the number of nutrients needed as a result of altered levels of activity or metabolic needs of individuals with specific conditions. Adolescents with spinal cord injury require adequate nutrition to meet basic metabolic needs and to promote healing in the case of a new injury. However, with time, reduced activity levels may also cause calorie needs to decrease. Burn injuries increase the need for nutrients above the basic amount needed for growth and change requirements for specific nutrients and calories. Burns are discussed in more detail in Chapter 21. Adolescent boys with muscular dystrophy may have need for fewer calories as a result of their greatly decreased and decreasing activity level to prevent obesity, which will further reduce mobility and complicate attendant care.

Recreation and social opportunities are increasingly available for adolescents with disabilities or chronic conditions. Peer groups are very important during this developmental period, and activities that can be adapted for individuals with functional limitations are best performed in an inclusive environment that is integrated within the community. Camps for adolescents with specific chronic conditions or disabilities combine fun and exploration with education about self-care and the disability. These types of camps are, however, usually limited to adolescents with disabilities and are not attended by typical children. Adapted sports programs are increasing in number across the United States and include such activities as horseback riding, swimming, river rafting, boating, fishing, camping, skiing, and scuba diving. These programs are usually run by private centers, hospitals or rehabilitation centers, or sports centers that are open to the general public. Special Olympics programs are generally attended by children and adolescents with cognitive disabilities and less so by those with physical disabilities. Paralympics programs are structured sports competitions for older school-aged children, adolescents, and adults and generally attract those with physical disa-

Table 10–8 SUMMARY OF ADOLESCENT GROWTH, DEVELOPMENT, AND HEALTH MAINTENANCE

Physical Competency	Intellectual Competency	Emotional-Social Competency
General Summary: 12–21 Years		
Puberty begins 2 yrs earlier for girls than boys; girls stop growing sooner and have smaller increases in height and weight than boys During pubertal growth spurt, weight increases 50%; varies according to pubertal maturation, degree of adiposity, and size of muscle mass During puberty, growth spurt results in 15%–20% increase in height *Early Maturer:* About 80th percentile for weight for height at 12 yr *Late Maturer:* Below 20th percentile at 12 yr	Marked by Piaget's formal operations period, which includes hypotheticodeductive, combinational thinking, relativity, and objectivity.	Exhibits characteristics of Freud's genital stage, Erickson's stage of identity versus role confusion. Kohlberg's post-conventional level, and Fowler's state of individuation reflexive.
Early Adolescence: 12–14 Years		
Secondary sex characteristics develop. Testicular enlargement occurs first in 98% of boys (ejaculation occurs approximately 1 yr later with appearance of pubic hair). Breast budding occurs first in 84% of girls; menarche begins. There is an increase in body fat associated with each stage of pubertal development in females. Males become more muscular rather than fatter during puberty. Neurodevelopmental maturity is seen.	Has difficulty solving problems; thinks in present; cannot use past experience to control behavior. Exhibits a strong sense of invulnerability—society's rules don't apply to him or her. Becomes comfortable with own body: egocentric.	Struggle between dependent and independent behavior is obvious; begins forming peer alliances.
Middle Adolescence: 15–16 Years		
Growth spurt is evident (females: 8 cm/yr; males: 10 cm/yr). Sex patterns evident in growth, arms and legs of males are longer. Secondary sex characteristics are seen in females—menarche has begun; breast and areola enlarges; pubic hair coarsens, darkens, and covers the mons. The penis elongates and widens, testes enlarge, and scrotum pigment becomes evident in males. Both axillary and facial hair increase, along with body odor. No apparent neurodevelopmental growth.	Begins to solve problems through analysis and abstract thinking. Peak turmoil in child family relations; able to debate issues and use some logic, but not continuously.	"Tries out" adult-like behavior. Establishes peer group alliance with associated risk-taking behavior.
Late Adolescence: 17–21 Years		
Most of linear growth is achieved, secondary sex development completed, and adult genitalia attained. The male voice deepens. No neurodevelopmental changes are apparent.	Able to verbalize conceptually, deals with abstract moral concepts, makes decisions about future.	Aware of own strengths and limitations; establishes own values system. Peer group diminishes in importance; may develop first intimate relationship. Turbulence subsides. May move away from home. More adult-like friendship with parents.

Table 10-8   SUMMARY OF ADOLESCENT GROWTH, DEVELOPMENT, AND HEALTH MAINTENANCE *Continued*

Nutrition	Recreation	Safety
General Summary: 12–21 Years		
Caloric needs increase with size; growth can be influenced by dietary fads, diets, and drugs. Protein requirement is 12%–14% of daily total caloric intake. Zinc, calcium, and iron are three essential minerals needed during this period.	Romantic friendships emerge. Special talents and interests influence selection of activities. Social outings to the mall or beach are heavily influenced by desire to meet members of the opposite sex. Participation in group and individual competition can enhance social stature.	Educational programs for teens are vital. They should stress Prevention of substance abuse Sex education including prevention of sexually transmitted diseases (STDs) Sports injury prevention Driver safety Personal safety Anti-gang programs
Early Adolescence: 12–14 Years		
Male needs 2500 cal/day; female needs 2200 cal/day. Protein requirement for both is 0.29 g/cm of height/day.	Enjoys physical activity—bicycling, skateboarding, team/competitive sports, swimming. Quiet time focuses on books, computer games/videos.	Fact-based information should focus on prevention of Alcohol/drug abuse STDs/teen pregnancy Safe use should be stressed with Bicycles, skateboards, skates Automobile—seat belts, speed Athletic equipment Physical conditioning should be emphasized in relation to all intense physical activity (e.g., team sports).
Middle Adolescence: 15–16 Years		
Male needs 3000 cal/day; female needs 2200 cal/day. Protein requirement for males is 0.32 g/cm of height/day; 0.28 g/cm of height/day for females.	Enjoys dressing up, parties, and makeovers. Is preoccupied by computer games, videos, movies, and music. Likes outings to the mall, beach, or park. Driving and dancing are important pastimes.	Preventive education continues concerning Substance abuse Use of seat belts Use of safety equipment with bicycles, motorized scooter, motorcycles, and automobiles Physical conditioning related to sports injuries Athletic safety equipment Students Against Drunk Drivers (SADD) Date rape prevention
Late Adolescence: 17–21 Years		
Male needs 2900 cal/day; female needs 2200 cal/day. Protein requirement for males is 0.32 g/cm of height/day; 0.28 g/cm of height/day for females.	Continues to enjoy computer games and videos. Dating increases in importance. Other activities include athletic competition and sports, trips to the mall and beach, movies, dancing, teen nightclubs, and rock concerts.	Preventive education continues concerning Substance abuse Use of seat belts Driver safety Athletic safety equipment SADD Preseason physical conditioning Sex education Date rape prevention

From Betz, C.L., Hunsberger, M., & Wright, S. (1994). Growth and development of the adolescent. In Betz, C.L., Hunsberger, M., & Wright, S. (Eds.). *Family-centered nursing care of children* (2nd ed.). Philadelphia: WB Saunders, pp. 328–329.

bilities who are interested in athletic competition. Wheelchair tennis, basketball, and baseball are team sports that have been adapted for individuals who use wheelchairs.

Social activities vary in their accessibility to adolescents with disabilities or chronic conditions. The adolescent who is integrated in school and has friends in the neighborhood and home community is more likely to be included in typical adolescent social activities. It may be very difficult for an adolescent with a disability to "break in" to new social groups because of negative attitudes toward people with disabilities exacerbated by early adolescent tendencies toward sameness and conformity. Those individuals who have impaired speech, hearing, or other types of communication difficulties, who have delayed social skills and behave in an immature manner, or who have visible physical disabilities are less likely to be accepted into peer groups as new members at this stage of development. Promoting social skills in early childhood by including the child in typical community programs, schools, and neighborhood groups creates an atmosphere of acceptance on the part of other children and adolescents, facilitates the development of social skills, helps other children see beyond the disability, and gives children the opportunity to get to know each other and grow up together.

Safety issues for adolescents with disabilities or chronic conditions are similar to those of typically developing adolescents but may be complicated by differences in mobility, communication, or behavior. Adolescents who survived brain injury may have poor judgment and impulsive behavior that can contribute to safety risks such as running away, inappropriate sexual behavior, aggression, or operating dangerous machinery. For example, a 14-year-old child who had received a head injury in an automobile accident 2 years ago took his grandfather's snowmobile out for a ride without permission, flipped it, and broke his arm, receiving another mild head injury in the process. Adolescents who have an ataxic gait and slurred speech, such as some individuals with cerebral palsy or head injury, may be mistaken for being intoxicated and may be arrested by well-meaning but not very knowledgeable police officers. Both adolescents and their families should receive anticipatory guidance about these issues as well as teaching about risk management.

Substance abuse, including smoking, presents a serious health concern for adolescents with disabilities and chronic conditions as well as for general populations. For the adolescent seeking approval and acceptance into a peer group, smoking, drinking alcohol, or other substance abuse may represent a route to popularity. For adolescents with disabilities or chronic conditions who are experiencing role confusion, identity conflicts, or depression, substance abuse may also present a method of self-medication. These activities may increase health risks for adolescents if they have a condition that may be exacerbated by smoking, drinking, or illicit drugs or take medications that interact with drugs or alcohol. Adolescents who have difficulties with impulse control will find that impulsivity increases with the use of drugs or alcohol. Cigarette smoking increases the risk of cardiac disease in adolescents and adults with spinal cord injury over and above that of the general population and increases the risk of skin breakdown. Adolescents with disabilities or chronic conditions who are already substance abusers require counseling and treatment and may require psychiatric referral if symptoms of depression are present. Many adolescents acquire their disability as a result of drinking or drug use and motor vehicle accidents.

Along with the hormonal changes of adolescence, girls experience the onset of menarche and must cope with sanitary napkins, tampons, and added hygiene practices. Girls with a spinal cord injury or spina bifida are advised to use tampons only if they are changed frequently during the day and the girl is proficient at inserting and removing them. Adolescent girls with cognitive delays who have memory problems or who are unable to understand the importance of frequent changes to prevent infection and potential toxic shock syndrome should use sanitary napkins. Adolescent girls may need additional counseling and health teaching to manage cleanliness and prevent odor during menses.

Adolescent pregnancy occurs in girls with disabilities and chronic conditions as well as in typical adolescents. Girls with disabilities or chronic conditions may be more vulnerable to sexual invitation, believing that complying will increase their popularity and acceptance. The may wish to experience closeness and alleviate loneliness or even wish to become pregnant to create someone who will love them unconditionally. High-risk adolescents, whether typical or disabled, should receive counseling about birth control and the risks of unprotected sexual activity with regard to sexually transmitted diseases (STDs). Adolescents with disabilities or chronic conditions may have impaired judgment or cognitive abilities as well, exacerbating the problem and presenting additional risks for motherhood. Although women with disabilities are capable of being excellent mothers, young women with cognitive delays may lack the necessary abilities to properly care for the child without considerable support. Most adolescent girls have dreams of a loving relationship and having children; girls with disabilities are no different.

Boys with disabilities or chronic conditions are also at risk for joining gangs to increase acceptance and to gain a peer group. The presence of a disability does not prevent boys from taking part in petty crime and violent activities. Television, movies, books, and popular music encourage a "macho" attitude in males and condones and promotes violence. Adolescents with disabilities may have been involved in gangs before they acquired their disability; spinal cord and head injuries are increasing in frequency among members of gangs due to shootings, beatings, and other violent acts. The same conditions that lead to delinquency or gang membership in typically developing pre-adolescents and adolescents lead to similar behavior in those with disabilities. Those conditions include lack of family support, low socio-economic status, living in violent neighborhoods, and membership in a marginal societal group (Betz, Hunsberger, & Wright, 1994).

For adolescents with disabilities or chronic conditions, rebellion against parental authority may take the form of refusing or neglecting self-care regimes, therapies and treatments, or medications. Adolescents with spina bifida or spinal cord injury are at increased risk for pressure sores, urinary tract infections, and incontinence as a result of self-care refusal and maturation factors. For example, a 16-year-old boy with spina bifida acquired a large, deep pressure ulcer on his sacrum that required hospitalization for treatment. Whenever the rehabilitation team treatments reached the point of closing the wound and successfully promoting healing, the boy would pull out the stitches, tear the new tissue, or smear feces into the wound. This young man had very low self-esteem, exhibited self-destructive behavior, and was diagnosed with depression, and he required treatment at an inpatient psychiatric unit. Although most situations are not as extreme

as this example, adolescents may greatly compromise their health and functional ability by rebellion. Helping these individuals to find less destructive and more typical ways to rebel that will meet their developmental needs and promote independence and competence is a challenge and often requires team, client, and family problem solving.

Vocational education of adolescents with disabilities and chronic conditions begins in high school. Usually those individuals with cognitive deficits or whose physical disabilities are severe are most likely to receive vocational services. Adolescents with chronic health conditions that significantly limit their activity tolerance are also candidates for vocational education. Vocational education is frequently offered in combination with special education programs, and outcomes vary widely. Some programs give the adolescent and family few choices with regard to the type of work they find interesting or the adolescent's goals in life. Other programs prepare the adolescent with a disability with basic work skills that are adaptable to numerous situations. For students with disabilities or chronic conditions who may be behind in school or who need some extra educational time, their high school career can be extended to age 21 years. Many young adults with disabilities and chronic conditions are able to enter college or vocational school programs and do well. Some may need additional support to help with taking notes in class or doing homework or other tasks.

Transition out of school to adult services, especially health care services, can be a difficult process. All of their lives, children with disabilities and chronic conditions have received primary and specialty health care services from pediatric specialists and other health care providers, and the children and their families have gotten to know and feel comfortable with these providers. Although in many cases young adults with disabilities may continue with their pediatric specialists or pediatricians, these providers may not have the knowledge base necessary to meet the adult health care needs of their formerly pediatric clients. In many communities, especially rural communities, adult primary care providers may not have the experience to meet the special health needs of young adults with disabilities or may be unwilling to take on more Medicaid patients. Once they are emancipated from their parents, young adults with disabilities most often receive Medicaid for health services through some type of managed care plan. Young adults with developmental disabilities who qualify for services under state and federal legislation are entitled to receive support services and care coordination through the state. Other individuals with disabilities may not qualify for state funded services and remain "on their own" or continue to be dependent on family members.

DEVELOPMENTAL VARIATIONS

General Alterations in Growth and Development

Variations in growth and development represent a spectrum and a continuum of developmental disorders; there are a great variety of types of variations in development, and each type of variation falls somewhere along a continuum from mild to severe. According to the specialty of developmental pediatrics, there are three fundamental processes of developmental variation: delay, dissociation, and deviance (Capute & Accardo, 1991).

Delay represents a significant lag in one or more areas or domains of development, and a global delay is a delay across all domains of development. Delay is assessed using a standardized developmental assessment tool, such as the Bayley Scales of Infant Development (1993). Very significant delays are more likely to be caused by an organic problem, such as central nervous system damage, than by environmental factors.

Dissociation occurs when there is a difference between the developmental rates of different domains, with one domain being significantly more delayed than others. For example, a child with cerebral palsy may be considerably more delayed in the motor area than in other areas, even though other areas show delays also. A child who is deaf may display dissociation, because communication skills would initially fall significantly behind motor or even social skills.

Deviance represents a non-sequential nature to the achievement of developmental milestones; that is, milestones are not achieved or are achieved in a different order as a result of abnormal neuromaturation. For example, a 3-month-old infant who shows extreme arm strength in resistance to flexion, characteristic of a much older child, may actually be exhibiting the increased tone seen with severe cerebral palsy. Children who show deviance, by this definition, generally are characterized by neurologic dysfunction (Capute & Accardo, 1991).

Developmental regression occurs in the presence of degenerative neurologic disease such as a brain tumor or muscular dystrophy. True developmental regression almost always leads to a dire prognosis, because most of the causes are diseases that lead to early death. Some neurologic disorders characterized by developmental regression, such as infantile spasms, lead to severe developmental disability and mental retardation.

Molnar and Kellerman (1994) describe developmental diagnosis as the process of observation of behavioral and performance items in each domain of development as characterized by Gesell: gross motor, fine-motor adaptive, language, and personal-social areas. Developmental diagnosis is determined by standardized developmental diagnostic tests combined with expert observation. The basic premise of the rehabilitation approach is that disability is reflected as functional impairments. Although the underlying pathology is important, as is the medical diagnosis, functional assessment reveals the effects of the disability on the child's life.

Developmental diagnosis includes the process of careful history taking, comparison of the child's function with expected standards for age, and neurologic examination to detect any unusual variation in the functioning of the central nervous system. It also involves determination of the child's affect, quality of performance, and style of coping with a difficult or frustrating task. This information is combined with information from the child's parents and any other important caregivers. Finally, all of the information is summarized, and the pediatric rehabilitation team makes the diagnosis or diagnoses and formulates recommendations.

The patterns of functional variation that are identified in the child serve as a guide for further evaluation and determination of possible causes of the delays. Isolated delays of gross and fine motor function with minor or no other delays in the other domains suggests neuromuscular dysfunction. Cognitive deficit, or mental retardation, is usually characterized by delays in all areas, except perhaps motor and social abilities. Language delays or deficits suggest hearing loss or a specific language or affective disorder. Language function is probably the most helpful indicator of cognitive function in children with disabilities who may have delays in adaptive skills due to motor dysfunction. Any child with motor delays may also have difficulty with articulation of language as a result of the underlying motor dysfunction.

There are many similarities between the developmental pediatric approach to developmental diagnosis and the pediatric rehabilitation approach. Probably the most significant difference is the emphasis on age-appropriate functional evaluation that predominates in pediatric rehabilitation. There is also some difference in the population of children who are treated by each specialty area; developmental pediatricians focus more on children with primarily cognitive disabilities, and pediatric physiatrists focus more on the neuromotor aspects and functional aspects of the disability or chronic condition.

Prevention

Prevention is a global issue that affects all children. Simeonsson (1994) stated that the "prevention challenge faced by the major social institutions serving children in this country is to address the increasing number of children and youth at risk for significant physical, developmental, educational, and social problems" (p. 5). Many writers, researchers, and documents describe the great need for organized, coordinated programs that focus on prevention issues for children. Individual institutions or agencies operate various programs that seek to provide preventative services through health and safety education, screening, intervention programs, and tertiary care centers. Research continues to uncover more genetic, physiologic, and social causes of disability and chronic conditions as well as other influencing factors that lead to developmental disorders and maladjustment. Prevention goals that have been set by government and advocacy agencies that are important to children's health and well-being include *Healthy People 2000: National Health Promotion and Disease Prevention Objectives* (1991); *America 2000: An Education Strategy* (1991); the Institute of Medicine report (Pope & Tarlov, 1991); and the yearly reports and objectives of organizations such as the Children's Defense Fund (1996), the Child Welfare League (Merkel-Holguin & Sobel, 1993) and other private advocacy agencies.

Prevention of disability and chronic conditions in childhood takes into account the three levels of prevention. The goal of primary prevention is to reduce new occurrences of children with disabilities and chronic conditions, thereby changing the incidence of occurrence. This phase consists of population screening for genetic alterations that may cause disabilities or chronic conditions; pre-natal care emphasizing maternal nutrition, healthy lifestyle, and regular follow-up to prevent low-birth-weight and premature infants; and research to find the causes of congenital conditions in an effort to prevent them (Simeonsson, 1994). The research that determined the role of folic acid in neural tube defects that result in spina bifida or anencephaly and led to guidelines about folic acid supplementation prior to pregnancy is a good example. Safety guidelines and practices are powerful weapons against injury, yet compliance with safety measures is often poor on the part of business, agencies, and individuals.

Secondary prevention seeks to reduce the numbers of children with disabilities and chronic conditions by affecting prevalence (Simeonsson, 1994). This phase consists of activities such as immunization to prevent diseases such as polio, measles, mumps, chickenpox, and diphtheria. Treatment of strep infections prevents complications with the kidneys, heart, and central nervous system.

The goal of tertiary prevention is to reduce the sequelae and complications experienced by children who have been diagnosed with disabilities or chronic conditions (Simeonsson, 1994). This stage focuses on prevention of complications and secondary conditions such as respiratory infections that complicate pulmonary function; therapeutic techniques to prevent contractures of joints; early mobility to prevent the complications of bed rest, such as deep vein thrombosis; and surgical procedures to correct the biomechanics of bone and muscle and improve function

The pediatric rehabilitation nurse has a role in each of these levels of prevention. Teaching parents of children with disabilities and chronic conditions about routine child safety measures as well as assisting parents to adapt the environment to specific safety needs is a very effective primary prevention strategy. Engaging in prevention-focused research is also extremely important. Screening activities, whether they are performed on the acute care hospital unit or as part of a school program, are designed to identify children who have not yet been diagnosed with disabilities or chronic conditions. Tertiary level activities, such as maintaining range of motion to prevent contractures or taking steps to reduce the complications of immobility following corrective surgical procedures, can prevent development of secondary disability. These activities and many others suggest the extensive role the pediatric rehabilitation nurse plays in the prevention of disability and chronic conditions in children.

Risk and Vulnerability

Any factor—physical, environmental, or psychologic—that has the potential to negatively affect the child or family presents risk (Harkins, 1994). Risk factors may include prenatal effects of any category, such as genetic disorders, maternal malnutrition, and maternal substance use or disease; birth factors such as breech delivery, prolonged delivery, nuchal cord, fetal heart rate deceleration, and premature delivery; neonatal and early childhood factors such as size for gestational age, the amount of time the neonate spent in the intensive care unit, infection or other disease, and trauma; family factors, such as poverty, health beliefs, family cohesion, size and membership of the family, ability of the family to provide for the child's needs, and coping styles of the family; societal and social factors, such as the value the society gives to the family's cultural background and available social support; availability of systems that provide services, such as school, public protection, and health care; and the environment, including the presence of clean air and water, crowded living situation, noise, and sanitation or pollution.

The term "vulnerability" is often used to refer to risk and risk factors. Although there are many definitions, common components of these definitions all associate vulnerability with personal components, both constitutional and acquired. These personal components include inherited and intrinsic characteristics as well as acquired factors such as disease, injury, or those resulting from life events. The concepts of risk and vulnerability are closely related and are sometimes used interchangeably. Vulnerability focuses more on the personal attributes of the child or family, whereas risk includes personal as well as environmental attributes.

A basic understanding of the concepts of risk and vulnerability facilitates application of the levels of prevention for the individual child as well as for the population of children in general. Prevention strategies implemented for populations as well as individuals will benefit all children. Children with disabilities and chronic conditions are both more vulnerable and at greater risk than many other children; however, that does not suggest that their outcomes (i.e., the ultimate potential that is reached) or the quality of life that they obtain will be any worse than those of other children. The quality, timing, developmental appropriateness, and design of the prevention

(i.e., to the unique needs of the child) will influence the effectiveness of interventions. Although outcomes of services and other interventions are poorly supported by outcomes research, a coordinated national agenda with common definitions and conceptual models will greatly enhance the possibilities and the quality of life for children with disabilities and chronic conditions (Harkins, 1994; Simeonsson, 1994).

SUMMARY

This chapter reviews the definitions of growth, development, and maturation and describes their application to the care of children with disabilities and chronic conditions. Factors contributing to typical growth and development as well as those affecting atypical growth and development are discussed. Age and developmental stage–based concerns about children with disabilities and chronic conditions are explored and compared with typical developmental stages. Major developmental theories are reviewed with application to pediatric rehabilitation nursing. Knowledge regarding growth, development, and maturation in children with disabilities and chronic conditions is necessary for nursing assessment and planning and implementation of care and services, as well as for the role of the nurse on the pediatric rehabilitation team in acute or community settings.

REFERENCES

Allen, M. (199_). Preterm development. In A. Capute & P. Accardo (Eds.). *Developmental disabilities in infancy and childhood.* Baltimore: Paul H. Brookes.

Als, H. (1992). Individualized, family-focused developmental care for the very low-birthweight preterm infant in the NICU. In S. Friedman & M. Sigman (Eds.) *The psychological development of low birthweight children. Advances in applied developmental psychology,* Vol. 6. Norwood, CT: Ablex.

Batshaw, M., & Perrett, Y. (1986). *Children with handicaps: a medical primer.* Baltimore: Paul H. Brookes.

Bayley, N. (1993). *Bayley scales of infant development.* San Antonio, TX: Psychological Corp.

Betz, C.L., Hunsberger, M., & Wright, S. (eds.). (1994). *Family-centered nursing care of children,* (2nd ed.). Philadelphia: WB Saunders.

Bowen, J., Gibson, F., Leslie, G., Arnold, J., Ma, P., & Starte, F. (1996). Predictive value of the Griffith's assesment in extremely low birth weight infants. *Journal of Paediatrics and Child Health*, 32(1), 25–30.

Brazelton, T. (1984). *Neonatal behavioral assessment scale*, (2nd ed.). Philadelphia: JB Lippincott.

Capute, A., & Accardo, P. (1991). A neurodevelopmental perspective on the continuum of developmental disabilities. In A. Capute & P. Accardo (Eds.). *Developmental disabilities in infancy and childhood.* Baltimore: Paul H. Brookes.

Case-Smith, J. (1996). Analysis of current motor development theory and recently published infant motor assessment, *Infants and Young Children*, 9(1), 29–41.

Cech, D., & Martin, S. (1995). *Functional movement development across the life span.* Philadelphia: WB Saunders.

Children's Defense Fund. (1996). *The state of America's children yearbook.* Washington, DC: Children's Defense Fund.

Craft, M., & Denehy, J. (1990). *Nursing interventions for infants and children.* Philadelphia: WB Saunders.

Darrah, J., & Bartlett, D. (1995). Dynamic systems theory and management of children with cerebral palsy: unresolved issues. *Infants and Young Children*, 8(1), 52–59.

Delahoussaye, C. (1994). Families with neonates. In C. Betz, M. Hunsberger, & S. Wright (Eds.). *Family-centered nursing care of children* (2nd ed.). Philadelphia: WB Saunders.

DiCaprio, N. (1983). Personality theories: a guide to human nature (2nd ed.). New York: Holt, Rinehart & Winston.

Disabato, J., & Wulf, J. (1994). Altered neurologic function. In C. Betz, M. Hunsberger, & S. Wright (Eds.). *Family-centered nursing care of children* (2nd ed.). Philadelphia: WB Saunders.

Dixon, S. (1992). Basic perspectives: bias and format. In S. Dixon & M. Stein (Eds.). *Encounters with children—pediatric behavior and development* (2nd ed.). St. Louis: Mosby Year Book.

Dubowitz, L., Dubowitz, V., & Goldberg, C. (1970). Clinical assessment of gestational age in the newborn infant. *Journal of Pediatrics*, 77, 1–10.

Erikson, E. (1959). *Identity and the life cycle* in *psychological issues*, monograph 1(1). New York: International Universities Press.

Fazzi, R., Orcesi, S., Telesca, C., Ometto, A., Rondini, G., & Lanzi, G. (1997). Neurodevelopmental outcomes in very low birth weight infants at 24 months and 5 to 7 years of age: changing diagnosis. *Pediatric Neurology*, 17(3), 240–248.

Flavell, J. (1977). *Cognitive development.* Englewood Cliffs, NJ: Prentice-Hall, Inc.

Gesell, A., & Ilg, F. (1949). *Child development: an introduction to the study of human growth.* New York: Harper.

Graven, S. (1996). Current issues in the physical and developmental environment of the high risk newborn. *Pediatric Grand Rounds,* The Children's Hospital, Denver, CO, December 6, 1996.

Greenough, W., Black, J., & Wallace, C. (1993). Experience and brain development. In M. Johnson (Ed.). *Brain development and cognition: a reader.* Cambridge, MA: Blackwell Publishers.

Hagerman, H. (1995). Growth and development. In W. Hay Jr., J. Groothuis, A. Hayward, & M. Levin (Eds.). *Current pediatric diagnosis and treatment.* Norwalk, CT: Appleton & Lange.

Hallett, T., & Proctor, A. (1996). Maturation of the central nervous system related to communication and cognitive development. *Infants and Young Children*, 8(4), 1–15.

Harkins, A. (1994). Chronic illness. In C.L. Betz, M. Hunsberger, & S. Wright (Eds.). *Family-centered nursing care of children* (2nd ed.). Philadelphia: WB Saunders.

Healthy People 2000: national health promotion and disease prevention objectives. (1991). Washington, DC: National Academy Press.

Kuh, D. (1984). Cognitive development. In M. Bornstein & M. Lamb (Eds.). *Developmental psychology: an advanced textbook.* Hillsdale, NJ: Lawrence Erlbaum/Associates.

Levine, M., Carey, W., & Crocker, A. (1992). *Developmental–behavioral pediatrics.* Philadelphia: WB Saunders.

Merkel-Holguin, L., & Sobel, A. (1993). *The child welfare stat book.* Washington, DC: Child Welfare League of America.

Molnar, G., & Kellerman, W. (1994). History and examination. In G. Molnar (Ed.). *Pediatric rehabilitation.* Baltimore: Williams & Wilkins.

Moore, K. (1989). *Before we are born: basic embryology and birth defects* (3rd ed.). Philadelphia: WB Saunders.

Morgan, B., & Gibson, K. (1991). Nutritional and environmental interactions in brain development. In K. Gibson & A. Peterson (Eds.). *Brain maturation and cognitive development: comparative and cross-cultural perspectives.* New York: Aldine De Gruyter.

Nelms, B., & Mullins, R. (1982). *Growth and development: a primary health care approach.* Englewood Cliffs, NJ: Prentice-Hall, Inc.

Paneth, N. (1995). The problem of low birth weight. *The Future of Children*, 5(1), 19–34.

Pope, A., & Tarlov, A. (1991). *Disability in America: towards a neonatal agenda for prevention.* The National Institute of Medicine. Washington, DC: National Academy Press.

Rosenblith, J. (1992). *In the beginning: development from conception to age two* (2nd ed.). Newbury Park, CA: Sage.

Seidel, H., Ball, J., Daines, J., & Benedict, W. (1991). *Mosby's guide to physical examination.* St. Louis: Mosby Year Book.

Simeonsson, R. (1994). Promoting children's health, education and well-being. In R. Simeonsson (Ed.). *Risk, resilience and prevention: promoting the well-being of all children.* Baltimore: Paul H. Brookes.

Soifer, L. (1992). Development and disorders of communication. In G. Molnar (Ed.). *Pediatric rehabilitation* (2nd ed.). Baltimore: Williams & Wilkins.

Thomas, M. (1985). *Comparing theories of child development* (2nd ed.). Belmont, CA: Wadsworth.

Trauner, D.A. (1979). *Childhood neurological problems: a textbook for health professionals.* St. Louis: Year Book Medical.

U.S. Department of Education. (1991). *America 2000: an education strategy.* Washington DC: U.S. Department of Education.

Whaley, L., & Wong, D. (1987). *Nursing care of infants and children* (3rd ed.). St. Louis: CV Mosby.

Wright, L. (1994). Genetic principles and disorders. In C. Betz, M. Hunsberger, & S. Wright (Eds.). *Family-centered nursing care of children* (2nd ed.). Philadelphia: WB Saunders.

Yoos, L. (1988). Cognitive development and the chronically ill child. *Pediatric Nursing,* 14(5), 375–378.

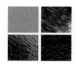

Chapter 11

Health Promotion and Health Management

Patricia A. Edwards

For the child with a disability or chronic condition and the family, effective health management is essential to fostering optimal growth and development and achieving the highest possible levels of independence. For children with diagnosed health problems, the pre-school years represent a time when special equipment, surgeries, and therapies are needed to eliminate a medical problem or reduce its later impact. Community-based, coordinated care is more responsive to the needs of families, as well as more cost-effective and efficient. This chapter focuses on the functional health pattern of "health perception—health management" and discusses how the pediatric rehabilitation nurse can help the child and family achieve the highest levels of wellness.

HEALTH AND WELLNESS

In 1946 the World Health Organization proposed the following definition of health: "Health is a state of complete physical, mental and social well-being, and not merely the absence of disease or infirmity." Since that time, others have proposed definitions that surpass the notion of health as merely a static condition. The term "health" has different and varied meanings for different people. Two well-known descriptions of health—the absence of disease and physical, mental, and social well-being—fall short of capturing the true meaning of the concept. Another concept of health is that health is a state in which an organism is functioning within normal limits, and this concept can be extended to describe a state in which an organism is enjoying a measure of well-being.

Dines and Cribb (1993) described health using the latter concept. It is a concept used to describe the functioning of a living organism and whether it is within normal limits. The organism may be described as unhealthy if its functioning is considered abnormal, or the organism may have some quality of life and sense of well-being. Dines and Cribb (1993) also stated that "health is created and lived by people within the settings of their everyday life; where they learn, work, play and love. Health is created by caring for oneself and others, by being able to make decisions and have control over one's life circumstances, and by ensuring that the society one lives in creates conditions that allow the attainment of health by all its members" (p. 209).

The First International Conference on Health Promotion in 1986 developed a charter for action aimed at health for all by the year 2000. In a subsequent document, *Healthy People 2000: National Health Promotion and Disease Prevention Objectives* (U.S. Public Health Service, 1990), health was described as a resource for everyday life, and some of its fundamental conditions included shelter, food, income, a stable ecosystem, sustainable resources, and education.

Another perspective is the definition of wellness by Hanak (1992) as "a dynamic, evolving process reflecting physical, psychological and social integration and growth within an individual, and an enhanced quality of life" (p. 4). In the pursuit of health, a person seeks growth-producing challenges, positive and flexible relationships with others, and health-enhancing activities. The concept of wellness involves an inter-relationship between the physical, psychological, and social dimensions of a person's life. Wellness promotion activities require a holistic perspective that addresses the inter-relationships between all other dimensions in a person's life.

A key assumption regarding health is that unless optimal levels of wellness are promoted, a child's potential to function in cognitive, psychosocial, and physical development may be adversely affected. Although children who are chronically ill or developmentally delayed may not be sick in the common sense of the term, the nature and extent of their disabilities may put them at higher risk for failure to thrive, recurrent illnesses, and secondary disabilities. The pediatric rehabilitation nurse must integrate the concept of wellness into the care and education of the child and family.

HEALTH PROMOTION

Health- and wellness-promotion activities must be a major focus of health care initiatives. Downie, Fyfe, and Tannahill (1990) described health promotion as "efforts to enhance positive health and prevent ill health, through the overlapping spheres of health education, prevention and health protection" (p. 2). These overlapping spheres included preventive services such as immunizations and screening; preventive health educational efforts to improve lifestyle; preventive health protection through legal and fiscal controls and regulations; health education for legislators and lobbying for legislation for preventive health protection; positive health education aimed at influencing behavior or developing positive health attributes; positive health protection through the implementation of workplace policies or commitment of public funds to accessible facilities; and health education aimed at positive health protection, raising awareness of the need and securing support for plans or policies. Health-promotion programs for people with disabilities can be viewed as an integral part of the rehabilitation process beginning early in the primary treatment phase and continuing throughout life. Nurses should find ways to empower the child and family to increase their control of essential activities and develop the skills needed to maintain and improve their health.

Achieving optimum wellness can be a major challenge for children and adolescents with disabilities or chronic conditions and their families. Rather than experiencing integration and growth in the various dimensions of their lives, they will likely face major disruptions. In addition, their abilities to use previous problem-solving, self-care, and coping skills may be severely compromised and their goals and personal relationships abruptly changed. Health services should be integrated into a network of supportive services, including occupational therapy, physical therapy, speech therapy, audiology, special education, psychology, nutrition, and social work. These interwoven services, in concert with active parental participation, augment carefully sequenced educational plans contributing to optimal growth and development to the extent of the individual child's abilities.

The pediatric rehabilitation nurse plays a central and coordinating role in helping children, adolescents, and their families identify how the child's disability or chronic condition has affected each dimension of their lives and learn the problem-solving and coping skills needed to successfully reintegrate these changed dimensions and achieve optimum wellness. As part of the advocacy role, there is also a need for health-promotion action. This means putting health on the agenda of policy-makers; working to create supporting environments; strengthening community action and development; enabling people to learn and develop personal skills; and reorienting health services.

"Across the nation, nurses are responding to children's health needs, providing skilled nursing care in homes, health education and primary care in schools, disease prevention in community clinics and health policy making in legislatures" (Igoe, 1993, p. 44). Nurses have developed models of care to meet the health needs of various populations of children, but the ultimate challenge is to reduce differences in health services and achieve access to primary care for all children.

HEALTH MODELS

A conceptual model described by Teague, Cipriano, and McGhee (1990) views health promotion programs as being integral to the rehabilitation process, beginning early in the primary care phase and continuing through all ages and stages. "The major objectives underlying health maintenance strategies are twofold: (1) teach the patient with a disability to become personally responsible for one's health and (2) to co-manage a large part of one's own rehabilitation program" (Teague, Cipriano, & McGhee, 1990, p. 55). The pediatric rehabilitation nurse assumes the roles of educator, collaborator, program provider, and researcher and focuses on initial health promotion strategies as well as the maintenance of change. As educator the nurse is responsible for teaching children and families about the health problem and the treatment plan, the importance of compliance, and the relationship between wellness and lifestyle. Health promotion programs should be provided that include information on the prevention of secondary disabilities with topics such as physical fitness, nutritional awareness, self-responsibility for health, and stress management. As collaborator the nurse is part of a network that requires coordination to be optimally effective, and as researcher the nurse is responsible for evaluating the effectiveness of the programs for health promotion and risk reduction.

Frye (1986) developed a model of wellness-seeking behavior that includes the theories of locus of control, self-efficacy, and hardiness as well as selected information on learned helplessness. This integration of source of control and levels of inner strength and self-confidence was applied to patients with spinal cord injury to determine a predictive profile of wellness-seeking behavior. This model can be applied to children with disabilities or chronic conditions to study the predictive value of the variables and develop teaching plans accordingly. The Health Belief Model and other nursing models are described and explained in relation to pediatric rehabilitation nursing in Chapter 8.

Values and culture influence the child and family's response to health-promotion activities. Some behaviors that might be observed relate to the degree that individuals feel they can effect change in their lives; whether the culture views human nature as good or bad; group norms about privacy preferences and the openness of the family unit; orientation to time, whether present or future; and beliefs about health, illness, rituals, and special traditions (Hanak, 1992).

The influence of attitudes and beliefs on pediatric rehabilitation nursing care is explored in depth in Chapter 1. Attitudes are central to health promotion because they tie together feelings and beliefs. They are acquired through personal experiences with family, friends, and school and peer groups.

Attitudes can be changed by a challenge to the knowledge base or by altering behavior, and these approaches can be part of health-promotion activities.

An interdisciplinary care continuum model (Broughton & Lutner, 1995) was developed as a cultural model for community practice, the main theme being "that the child and family should receive culturally sensitive care in the community" (p. 320). This model is designed to help achieve outcomes in the areas of prevention, education, and rehabilitation and to bring the interdisciplinary team and the community together to enhance education, rehabilitation interventions, and prevention strategies. The interdisciplinary team includes nurses, therapists, physicians, teachers, case managers, social workers, and clergy. Community outreach to areas such as shelters, churches, support groups, and counseling services was included, as well as mobile immunizations and cable TV programming. The goal was to have children and families enter the care continuum and have their needs assessed in a health care environment where cultural barriers have been overcome.

Health education is one route to the improvement of people's health. It "encompasses activities aimed at enhancing positive health and preventing or diminishing ill-health" by "influencing the beliefs, attitudes and behavior of individuals and of the community at large" (Downie, Fyfe, & Tannahill, 1990, p. 28). Many different groups of people have a role to play in health education.

> To be effective health education must be developmentally appropriate. . . . Decision making skills, the basic pre-requisite for the development of preventive health behaviors, must be learned and used as children encounter choices about lifestyle and health risk-taking behaviors during the formative years. . . . All effective pediatric health promotion programs are based on understanding children's developmental comprehension of time, the body, health, clinical procedures, illness and death. (Igoe, 1993, pp. 44–45)

Each child should have a primary care provider who performs appropriate health screening, treatment, and referral and who provides age-appropriate health counseling and health education. Nurses in public health, school health, community clinics, and primary care settings can develop programs to meet the identified health needs of the nation's children. Schools are the logical setting in which to educate youngsters about health risks and health-promoting behaviors. "Successful health promotion and disease prevention programs follow these steps: 1) conduct needs assessments, 2) develop performance objectives, 3) use a variety of learning activities, 4) break course content into manageable sections, and 5) evaluate the results (learning and behavior changes)" (Igoe, 1993, p. 50).

HEALTH AND DEVELOPMENTAL CONTINUUM

Prevention and screening are the core services envisioned as a major shift occurs from illness to wellness care. When balancing technologic imperatives and disease prevention, the intervention of choice whenever and wherever possible should be prevention. In this way, nurses sustain and extend lives and teach children and families how to protect themselves from disease and injury.

The four foci for prevention according to Downie, Fyfe, and Tannahill (1990, p. 50) are:

Prevention of the onset or first manifestation of a disease process, or some other first occurrence through risk reduction. Accident prevention through reducing hazards or risk taking behavior is an example.

Prevention of the progression of a disease process or other unwanted state through early detection when this favorably affects outcome

Prevention of avoidable complications of an irreversible, manifest disease or some other unwanted state. Attempts to prevent pressure sores or urinary tract infections are examples.

Prevention of recurrence of an illness or other unwanted phenomenon.

Pediatric rehabilitation nurses provide an individualized continuum of care along three levels of prevention: primary, secondary, and tertiary. Primary prevention, or health promoting, reduces the incidence of disease, prevents the occurrence of disease or illness, and encourages healthy patterns of living. Secondary prevention, or health supporting, concerns early detection and prompts intervention to curb or retard illness or disease progression, supports the development of new behaviors, or modifies existing stressors. Tertiary prevention, or health restoring, includes medical surveillance to prevent complications and maintenance and rehabilitation designed to minimize illness or disease impact, potentially return the individual to the community, and modify or reduce the nega-

tive impact of illness or disease (*Standards of Nursing Practice for the Care of Children and Adolescents With Special Health and Development Needs*, 1994). This health and developmental continuum is depicted in Table 11–1.

According to Hunsberger (1994), primary prevention is promotion of health and protection against problems; secondary prevention includes early identification of problems and prompt interventions resulting in decreased duration and severity; and tertiary prevention is the provision of rehabilitative services to restore an individual to optimal functioning within the constraints of the disability.

Primary care interventions focus on the prevention of illnesses by educating the parents and child about disease transmission and how to prevent problems by immunizing and avoiding infectious contacts. Secondary care interventions include early recognition of conditions that may lead to disability and their management if required, as well as referral for additional services. Tertiary care interventions include managing existing disabilities, including ongoing serial assessments, evaluation of progress in growth and development, teaching about and monitoring the administration of medications, and managing other procedures and treatments specific to the individual child (Russell & Free, 1994).

To improve the lives of children and their families, one pediatric rehabilitation facility developed a "Primary Care Model" for their growing population of physically challenged children (Children's Specialized Hospital Foundation [CSHF], 1996). Through this model, the routine health care and physical, mental, and developmental growth of the child are mapped and tracked through a scheduled regimen of care with constant observation. A team, headed by a primary care physician and including other medical specialists and professionals, works with children and families in this model. If intervention is needed, an acute care hospital with proven strengths in pediatric care participates as a resource (CSHF, 1996). The pediatric rehabilitation nurse is a valuable member of this team.

PRIMARY HEALTH CARE

"Pre-schoolers and school-age youth are the healthiest segment of the population. Most of their illnesses and injuries are preventable if complete immunization, acceptable living conditions and adequate parenting are provided" (Igoe, 1993, p. 41). "Primary health

Table 11–1   HEALTH AND DEVELOPMENTAL CONTINUUM

Levels of Prevention	Optimal Health and Development Primary Prevention (Health Promoting)	Risks to Optimal Health and Development Secondary Prevention (Health Supporting)	Diagnosis or Symptoms of Health or Developmental Problems Present Tertiary Prevention (Health Restoring)
	Core Public Health Functions		
Examples of nursing care at the individual or family level	Provision of anticipatory guidance designed to support the health and development of infants, children, adolescents, and their families	Health and developmental assessment	Nursing interventions (direct or delegated) on behalf of children, adolescents, or their families
		Risk reduction education and counseling	Care coordination (service or resource coordination)
		Referral to other disciplines as needed, with monitoring of referral outcomes	Consultation with multidisciplinary/ interdisciplinary team members and/or referral
Examples of nursing care at the community level (population-based)	Public awareness programs to promote child/adolescent health, development, nutrition, and safety	Population-based screening to identify infants with potential/ actual developmental delays	Development of standards, policies, procedures, and monitoring and evaluation systems for child care or school-based services for children who require invasive procedures
		Risk reduction education and counseling for a group of children with asthma	
		Development of primary health care services for children with special health care needs	

From *Standards of nursing practice for the care of children and adolescents with special health and developmental needs* p. 28 (1994). Lexington, KY: University of Kentucky Chandler Medical Center.

care encompasses routine health care (health histories, measurements, developmental and behavioral assessments, screening, examinations, routine laboratory tests and physical examinations), anticipatory guidance and health education. The aim of primary care is to promote optimal health habits so disease does not occur, as well as to identify possible problems early" (Urbano, 1992, pp. 160–161).

Primary care consists of three components: first-contact care, continuous care, and comprehensive care. The primary care prac-

titioner is a pivotal member of the team in managing care of a child with a disability or chronic illness and the family and may be the one person who remains in continuous contact with the child as he or she matures. Early identification of problems, developmental screening, well child and routine health maintenance care, and ongoing, continuous monitoring of the child's program and progress are all integral parts of the primary care role. During the school-aged years, when problems occur it is important to rule out medical conditions that may be affecting school performance and then schedule appropriate evaluations and collaborate with the school system to design appropriate educational plans (Marquis, 1991).

Routine health care should occur according to a pre-determined schedule beginning at 1 month of age. The visits should include general health information as well as address any illnesses or accidents. Objective measurements of growth (e.g., height, weight, head circumference) should be obtained, and screening (e.g., vision, hearing) should be done to identify problems early. Head-to-toe physical examinations assess physical appearance and also provide time to elicit concerns and questions and provide information about the expected sequences of growth and development and anticipatory guidance.

Immunizations should be given according to the recommended schedule, although this schedule may need to be altered if the child has frequent illness or other problems. It is necessary to weigh the potential risk from the immunization against the potential effect of the illness. Immunization should be part of the routine preventive care to promote wellness. Although the majority of children receive adequate protection through immunization, some children are still vulnerable to influenza, pneumonia, and meningitis.

Safety is important because accidents are a common cause of injury and death in children, and those with a disability or chronic condition may be even more vulnerable because of decreased strength and coordination. Pediatric rehabilitation nurses have the responsibility not only to provide a safe environment for the child but to teach parents and others about safety hazards and the appropriate preventive measures. Areas of special concern include car restraints; smoke detectors; home environment modification to prevent burns, falls, aspiration, or poisoning; and teaching first aid for injuries.

All children need adequate amounts of *rest, sleep, and exercise,* but those with disabilities or chronic conditions may require longer or more frequent periods of sleep and rest as well as modifications to facilitate adequate exercise. Assessment of the child's patterns is helpful in providing clues to areas needing intervention and insight into specific behaviors.

Dental health is important because many children have dental problems related to poor care, trauma, medications, or other conditions. Parents need to learn the techniques of good oral hygiene and be referred to a dentist while the child is young to avoid later problems.

Attempts should be made to identify signs of delay early, and developmental screening should be an important part of primary care. Promotion of *optimal growth and development* is the responsibility of the interdisciplinary team, and intervention strategies should be designed to decrease the effects of the condition. Developmental screening tests are useful when developing interventions and recommending stimulating activities. A holistic approach with normalization of experiences facilitates development (Urbano, 1992).

Play and recreation must be incorporated into the child's life. "Play is a spontaneous and active process in which thinking, feeling and doing can flourish since they are separated from the fear of failure or disastrous consequences. . . . Play is a way of assimilating new information and making it part of ourselves" (McMahon, 1992, p. 1). In play children can practice being in charge of their world and act out their feelings, images, and desires, thus coming to terms with them in their own way. A sense of mastery can be achieved, and the child can learn new skills. The child's ability to play follows a predictable pattern related to his or her physical and psychosocial development. To use play appropriately, the pediatric rehabilitation nurse must assess the developmental level of the child and provide experiences that are appropriate to the level and abilities of the child. For example, play for the toddler might involve climbing and exploring the physical world as well as imitative play. The preschooler enjoys tricycle riding and sand and water play as well as activities that involve cooperative play with domestic themes. If the child has a physical disability that limits or restricts purposeful movement, equipment and activities must be adapted to their needs if play is to be used appropriately (McMahon, 1992).

Young children may be integrated in nursery or pre-school play groups, in special play and opportunity groups, or receive services at home, in a hospital setting, or at a child development center. Older children may have adaptive activities in schools, including special activities at holidays and adventure playgrounds designed for children with physical limitations. "Play is far more than a technique to foster intellectual development. It is essential to the development of autonomy and mastery" (McMahon, 1992, p. 118). A child who is unable to participate in spontaneous play should receive help from an adult who fosters all of the attributes of spontaneous play at the child's developmental level rather than taking them away. The child and adult can take turns as active playmates, sharing the fun of the play activities and thus equalizing the relationship.

ROLE OF THE PRIMARY CARE PROVIDER

The position of nurses in health care allows them to have a major impact on wellness, health promotion, and disease prevention. The pediatric rehabilitation nurse plays an integral role in helping children and families identify how their disabilities and conditions have affected each dimension of their lives and in learning the problem-solving, self-care, and psychosocial skills needed to successfully reintegrate these changed dimensions and achieve optimum wellness.

"Clinical preventive services (CPS) are widely seen as an important part of the daily primary care practice. CPS include counseling interventions, screening tests to detect disease, immunizations and chemoprophylactic regimens" (Griffith & DiGuiseppi, 1994, p. 25). Guidelines for clinical preventive services, including counseling, screening, and immunizations, are important to nurse practitioner practice, education, and research. Delivery of clinical preventive services can be improved by the use of evidence-based guidelines, which provide recommendations on what services should be provided and who should receive them.

As medical management becomes increasingly complex with the advent of new knowledge and technology, and as the financial system continues to try to contain health care costs, efficiency and effectiveness will continue to be central concerns. Primary care providers, in the role of case managers, are needed to provide services to children and families and to assess and document the effectiveness of the treatment and programs. The case manager role was incorporated into Public Law 99-457 as described in Chapter 4, and reimbursement for these services is provided. "This formal federal recognition of the benefits and necessity of case management for children with chronic conditions and the need for reimbursement for these services hopefully portends more movement in this direction" (Jackson, 1992, p. 9). The pediatric rehabilitation nurse in advanced practice has the knowledge and skills to manage the care of the child with a disability or chronic condition. The advanced practice nurse must "promote independent problem solving by the family, be available to support the family, and foster self-care of the illness" (Chow, Durand, Feldman, & Mills, 1984, p. 574). Four essential considerations are continuity of care, collaboration, promotion of self-care skills, and community resources.

Continuity of Care

Regularly scheduled visits that enable the family to develop a trusting relationship with the nurse are essential. Time should be allotted for comprehensive assessment, any necessary treatment, the development of a plan of care, and evaluation and modification of the plan as necessary. During the nurse's visits, time should be allowed for the child and family to express feelings of frustration and sadness. The family should be given information on how to contact the primary provider and a list of telephone numbers.

Collaboration

The advanced practice nurse serves as primary coordinator of the treatment plan and makes referral to specialists depending on the needs and problems of the child and family. As the child and family adjust to the disability or chronic condition, sensitive, collaborative care by professionals is essential.

Promotion of Self-Care Skills

The advanced practice nurse facilitates the development of self-care skills to increase the confidence of the child and family and minimize the anxiety they may have in relation to the disability or chronic condition. Areas of self-care include breathing, feeding, nutrition, elimination, rest and exercise, social interaction, personal hygiene, safety, and the promotion of normalcy. The nurse assists the child and family in developing the skills to problem solve and make decisions that help meet the child's personal needs.

Community Resources

The advanced practice nurse collaborates with other health professionals and a network of persons and organizations to identify community resources for the family. These vary according to the perceived needs of the child and family, their immediate environment (e.g., home, school, and community), and their economic situation. Familiarity with current community resources is essential; assistance with financial aid, social services, and resources directed to parents, such as support groups, and to children, such as summer camps and clubs, can assist in providing needed information and personal and financial support (Chow, Durand, Feldman, & Mills, 1984).

BARRIERS TO OPTIMAL HEALTH CARE

Health practices and the use of health care services vary tremendously from family to family. Family differences in both conceptualization of what constitutes health and illness and the degree of motivation needed to seek health care services and improve health constitute the main reasons for the observed diversity of health care practices. (Friedman, 1992)

A useful tool for looking at the factors related to health care services is the Health Belief Model described in Chapter 8.

Children with disabilities or chronic conditions have unique needs, and their conditions are subject to exacerbations and remissions that occur according to their changing growth and development. For this reason it is recommended that comprehensive, coordinated care be provided to minimize the impact of the condition and allow the child to develop to his or her maximum potential. Many barriers exist to providing this necessary level of health care, and these can be divided into three categories: financial barriers, system barriers, and knowledge barriers. These barriers include lack of payment for services, lack of time to provide services, and lack of knowledge about resources and new techniques. (Jackson, 1992). For families to become an effective health resource, they must be involved in the total therapeutic process in an equal relationship with health care providers. This is true whether curative and rehabilitative needs are under consideration or preventive health services are needed (Friedman, 1992).

Financial

Children with disabilities who are covered by health insurance are more likely to receive physician care than those children not covered by insurance. In children with chronic conditions this lack of regular care frequently results in aggravation of the chronic condition. (Jackson, 1992, p. 5)

As mentioned in Chapter 5, although public programs such as Medicaid and Supplemental Security Income (SSI) allow access to health care for many families, restrictions on benefits and eligibility may vary significantly, and the families may have limited access to providers. If the family and child are covered by private insurance, access may be improved, but other medical expenses may need to be covered by family funds. The cost of caring for a child with a chronic condition is not limited to medical expenses. Expenses in addition to medical needs may include "transportation costs, special diets, clothing, day care or respite care, dental and visual services, or home remodeling. Frequently the care required by the child necessitates that one parent be home with the child, reducing time at work with subsequent loss of income and possibly insurance coverage" (Jackson, 1992, p. 5).

System

The current system of public and private agencies designed to provide services makes access even more difficult for families. Each agency has its own bureaucracy with specific regulations, and services may be dependent on geographic availability. Often it is the active involvement of medical personnel or disease-oriented voluntary organizations that help meet the families' needs.

Knowledge

Both the family and the practitioners may lack knowledge. Early intervention and initiation of care may be delayed by not recognizing their need or value. Practitioners must know how to access services and be sensitive to the cultural heritage of the family or they may inadvertently undermine the resources that are available. Practitioners may also find it difficult to keep abreast of current management techniques because of the rapid growth of medical knowledge and constant advances in technology (Jackson, 1992).

SCREENING AND ASSESSMENT

The pediatric rehabilitation nurse should include screening for developmental disabilities as an essential component of child care, and when problems are detected, the nurse should assist the child and family to obtain comprehensive assessment and treatment. With the prevalence of developmental disorders in the general pediatric population estimated at 5% to 10%, these are the most common conditions for which a child is screened (Marquis, 1991). The nurse can identify children at risk and monitor their early development closely.

> Developmental screening of infants aims primarily at detecting sensory deficits and major developmental handicaps associated with central nervous system dysfunction. . . . Other developmental disabilities screened for in the first year of life include cerebral palsy and moderate to severe mental retardation. The nurse can identify infants who are at high risk and monitor the early development of these infants closely. (Marquis, 1991, p. 134)

Obvious physical defects can be easy to detect, but those that are more subtle require close examination. The nurse should look for the presence of abnormal head circumference and asymmetry of motor function. An infant's cry, muscle tone, reflexes, and the achievement of developmental milestones should all be evaluated and any abnormalities further assessed (Cohen, 1991).

The pediatric rehabilitation nurse in advanced practice can be instrumental in providing screening services through the Early and Periodic Screening, Diagnosis and Treatment Program (EPSDT). It provides for wellness-oriented screenings as well as problem-oriented check-ups and for the necessary treatment services for identified health problems.

> The full checkup includes a health history; an unclothed physical exam; assessment of nutrition; and assessment of developmental, mental and behavioral status. Assessment of immunization status, with provision of any needed immunizations also is required (Tesh, Selby-Harrington, Corey, & Cross, 1995, p. 70).

Children with disabilities or chronic conditions should be assessed at regular intervals along the health care continuum. Assessments can be done in a variety of settings, including hospitals, clinics, rehabilitation facilities, the home, or the school. Assessment is a critical element in the nursing process; therefore, every pediatric rehabilitation nurse should use it as the basis for planning therapeutic interventions. Assessments are holistic, encompassing all aspects of a child's life, and they take place within the context of the family system (Ricci-Balich & Behm, 1996).

The process and procedures for screening and assessment of young children can take many forms. The process called "Child Find" is a public awareness activity designed to alert the community to available intervention programs and describe some signs that might encourage parents to seek further services. Table 11–2 describes the purpose and activities of Child Find as well as three other types of assessment activities, including developmental and health screening, diagnostic assessment, and individual program-planning activities. Developmental and health screening encompasses activities for early identification of children at high risk for delayed or abnormal development. Diagnostic assessments are used to ascertain the nature of the delay and its cause and to propose intervention strategies. Assessments for individual program planning "are criterion-referenced, focusing on a child's mastery of skills or tasks rather than the child's relative standing in comparison to some normative group" (Meisels & Provence, 1989, p. 14).

Characteristics of the screening and assessment process include parental participation, clinical interviewing, observation, and setting. The active participation of parents in the screening and assessment is essential. The nurse should enable parents to convey information productively by creating a climate in which emotions such as anxiety, guilt, or anger can be expressed. Clinical skills such as listening to parents and being sensitive to their spoken and unspoken needs and problems can be a source of data and a major guide for future interactions with the family. Observation, especially of child behavior at play and in interaction with others, provides information about the child's growth and development. The setting in which screening or assessment takes place is also very important. Informal, stress-free settings are ideal, especially if they can include observations of parent-child interactions (Meisels & Provence, 1989).

Benner (1992) identified four broad categories for assessment: identification and diagnosis, program planning, program evaluation, and multipurpose assessment.

> Identification and diagnosis includes case finding, screening and the diagnostic process that infants, toddlers and young children typically proceed through on their way to receiving early intervention. Program planning incorporates competence assessment, identification of family strengths and needs, environmental or ecological assessment and mastery motivation. The third purpose of assessment, program evalua-

Table 11–2 LEVELS OF ASSESSMENT ACTIVITIES

	Purpose	Personnel	Activities
Child Find	To create awareness of typical and atypical child development among the general public	State personnel, public health professionals, volunteers, community members, early childhood personnel, parents, caregivers	Census taking, posters, brochures, media publicity
Developmental and health screening	To identify children who may need further diagnostic assessment	Parents, professionals, lay professionals	Administration of screening instruments, medical examinations, hearing and vision testing, parent questionnaires, and review of records
Diagnostic assessment	To determine existence of delay or disability, to identify child and family strengths and needs, and to propose possible strategies for interventions	Multidisciplinary team of educators, psychologists, parents, clinicians, physicians, social workers, therapists, nurses	Formal testing, parent interview, home observation, team meetings
Individual program planning	To determine individual educational/family services plan, program placement, and remedial activities	Parents, teachers, assessment team personnel, other professionals	Home and/or program observation, informal assessment, development of remedial objectives

From Meisels, S., & Provence, S. (1989). *Screening and assessment: guidelines for identifying young disabled and developmentally vulnerable children and their families* p. 13. Washington, DC: National Center for Clinical Infant programs.

tion, is aimed at the determination of program efficacy. Finally, assessments can be designed to achieve multiple purposes. (Benner, 1992, p. 24)

Benner (1992) also outlined the sequence of activities in the assessment process to ensure that the required information is obtained. These are planning, assessing, interpreting, and evaluating. The planning stage, which includes both parents and professionals, is the time to identify the purpose or purposes of the assessment, the specific information needed, and where and when assessments will take place. Initial decisions about the assessment instruments to be used are also made during the planning stage. Assessment is the second stage and includes child assessments, environmental assessments, and a determination of family strengths and needs. When all the necessary data have been gathered, the results are interpreted and recom-

mendations formulated. The final stage is when professionals and parents review the process and determine the quality of the information obtained.

The History and Physical Examination

The Encounter

Most people can probably conjure up visual images and even smells from their first pediatric encounter with a primary care provider. It might be the kind smile of the family "Doc" or the more frightening image of running from the person who held the needle. Over the years these encounters have changed, and as needs have evolved, so has the approach to the health care of children and adolescents. The "check-up" is now referred to as "health care maintenance," and the concept itself has also become more complex. Algranati (1992) identified the components of child health maintenance:

> Establish a trusting and two-way working relationship with the patient and family.
> Obtain a history to assess physical and developmental progress of the patient. Assess family wellness and the impact of family problems on the patient.
> Perform a physical examination to assess wellness (including growth and development) and pick up hidden problems.
> Provide appropriate screening tests and immunizations.
> Provide anticipatory guidance.
> Provide diagnostic and therapeutic intervention when necessary. (Algranati, 1992, p. 7)

Pediatric Health History

Obtaining a pediatric health history begins with the assessment of the child's physical and developmental progress and the family wellness. Review of the history-taking format and the previous medical records enables the health care provider to make observations while conversing with the parents and child. General categories that should be included are daily care activities; affective, cognitive, and physical development and milestones; general health, with an update on past history and a systems review; and family and psycho-social wellness. It is important to establish a trusting working relationship with the child and the family. Ask the parents to tell you about the child's problem and symptoms and listen to the child's point of view. If the child is old enough to provide information, some of the interview may even be conducted separately from the rest of the family, depending on the abilities and age of the child. During the interview, remember to also share information with the child and parents (Algranati, 1992). "The interview of the child with a disability and his or her family requires particular attention to the functional abilities of that child. One open ended question that often elicits critical information is 'Describe a typical day'" (Burkett, 1989, p. 241).

Physical Assessment

During the physical examination, the trusting relationship with the child and family must continue to be developed. Securing the cooperation of the child helps to obtain accurate and complete assessments. Because each child progresses along the developmental continuum at his or her own unique rate, findings are measured using established norms, comparing the child with a one-point-in-time reference. Norms have been established for height, weight, head circumference, skin fold thickness, blood pressure, and developmental milestones, but any deviations from the norm should be evaluated in the context of the whole child. The sequence of the assessment depends on the child's age and usually proceeds from head to toe. Examinations that are uncomfortable may be left until later, and sometimes it is beneficial to begin with respiratory and cardiac assessments while the child is quiet and relaxed. "Start with a general assessment gathered by observation and take measurements, plotting these findings on charts to begin to interpret how the child is doing" (Algranati, 1992). Observation of the child during play gives the nurse an opportunity to assess any obvious abnormalities as well as social responsiveness and interactions. "Particular attention should be given to the motor abilities of the child including observation of any primitive reflexes, abnormal muscle tone, and altered sensation. These are common problem areas for a child with a disability" (Burkett, 1989, p. 241).

Psychological Assessment

"It is important to assess the child's mental abilities since they impact directly on expectations of the child's behavioral, social and functional capacity. One question often asked is 'What age does your child act?'" (Burkett, 1989, p. 241). If testing needs to be done, equipment that the child needs to communicate must be obtained and used. Some children with disabilities and chronic conditions may present a challenge to psychological assessment because their physical and intellectual abilities are continually changing.

Growth and Development

Assessment of growth and development is an integral part of the history and physical examination. As you gather information, use observation of the child to confirm or modify your evaluation. Because basic knowledge of growth and development is essential to the complete assessment of the child, review the age-related information in Chapter 10 before beginning the process. As mentioned previously, screening tools may aid in the early detection of delayed development, but if more specific assessments are required, there are several tools that can be used in both rehabilitation and home settings. These are described further later in this chapter. Screening tools "are best utilized as a basis for discussion and as a guideline for what changes a family can anticipate in the developmental progress and functional abilities of their child" (Burkett, 1989, p. 240).

Child and Family Adjustment

> It has been suggested that a mourning period for the "loss" of the perfect child is necessary for parents to mobilize resources for effectively living with and managing the child with a disability. This loss can change to a feeling of "chronic sorrow" that varies in intensity at selected developmental milestones or crisis points. (Burkett, 1989, p. 245)

The children will have to deal with different issues as they grow and develop, and their adjustment will be influenced by the way their parents handle the effects of the disability or condition. An environment that is consistent and stimulating seems to enable a child's growth and development, and he or she adjusts with minimal problems in such an environment. As mentioned previously, parents must be made equal partners in the child's care and management, and pediatric rehabilitation nurses should serve as resources, offering accurate information and providing anticipatory guidance regarding expected changes.

Transdisciplinary Play-Based Assessment

Linder (1993) described a natural, functional approach to assessment through play. The Transdisciplinary Play-Based Assessment (TPBA) "involves the child in structured and unstructured play situations with, at varying times, a facilitating adult, the parent(s), and another child or children" (Linder, 1993, p. 1). This instrument provides an opportunity for developmental observations of children from infancy to 6 years of age and includes cognitive, social-emotional, communication and language, and sensorimotor areas. The child's developmental skills and processes, learning style, and interaction patterns are examined. "The model is less stressful for the child, less intimidating to the family and results in meaningful information that translates into objectives and strategies for intervention"

(Linder, 1993, p. 1). The information obtained is useful for educational and therapeutic program development, and inclusion of the parent in the process leads to more reliable information and greater teaming with the family in the selected interventions. "The process is individualized for each child who is assessed using interests, motivation, learning style and optimal interaction patterns" (Miller, 1994, p. 89).

MEASURES OF DISABILITY

> Conceptualization of health and disability as a hierarchical structure: the first level is general health or the absence of illness, the second level is basic performance of self-care and mobility activities that are critical for independence and the third level is the ability to perform and maintain these complex activities and roles associated with a meaningful life. (Kelly-Hayes, 1995, p. 145)

Using this approach to rehabilitation, interventions and outcome measures are aimed at the level of limitation and disability and address a range of functional performance from basic self-care to community reintegration. The assessment process is the basis for planned interventions and should include all aspects that affect "normal functioning." Measures of disability might include:

Barthel Index: A widely established measure to monitor function, independence, and the amount of care needed. It scores items such as feeding, bathing, dressing, grooming, continence, toileting, transfer, and mobility based on the amount of assistance needed: supervision, direction, or personal assistance. It is used for screening as well as formal assessment and has excellent validity and reliability.

Functional Independence Measure (FIM): An assessment instrument of functional status with 18 items relative to self-care, sphincter management, mobility, locomotion, communication, and social cognition. The seven levels of scoring, from complete independence to complete dependence, can detect incremental change. It is widely used in rehabilitation because it is appropriate for screening and formal assessment as well as program evaluation. It is used clinically as an outcome measure and is part of the Uniform Data Set (UDS) for medical rehabilitation, which is discussed in Chapter 25.

Patient Evaluation and Conference System (PECS): These are discipline-specific evaluations with a broad range of categories, evaluating 79 items that are divided into sub-scales including medications, nutrition, assistive devices, pain, pulmonary rehabilitation, and vocational-educational, as well as medicine, nursing, and activities of daily living. The scale ranges from most dependent to independent and documents functional status and progress toward rehabilitation goals.

Level of Rehabilitation Scale (LORS II): An instrument for measuring broad functional outcomes in five areas: mobility, activities of daily living, communication, memory, and cognitive ability. A nurse or therapist rates the client on a scale of cannot/will not perform the activity to performs normally. It was designed to meet Commission on Accreditation of Rehabilitation Facilities (CARF) criteria.

Other measures that might be used are the Katz Index of Activities of Daily Living and the PULSES profile (Cole, Finch, Gowland, & Mayo, 1995).

FUNCTIONAL ASSESSMENT INSTRUMENTS FOR CHILDREN

Functional assessment is an effort to systematically describe and measure a child's abilities and limitations when performing the activities of daily living. With this information, professionals can plan and assess rehabilitative and habilitative care. Because the plan of care to promote functional independence evolves directly from the assessment, it is imperative that the tool effectively defines and measures the relevant construct, that is, function rather than development. (McCabe & Granger, 1990, p. 120)

The process of early intervention assessment includes

Case finding: locating those infants and toddlers who might be eligible for early intervention

Screening: identifying infants and toddlers needing in-depth assessment

In-depth assessment: assessments that verify a problem and determine its nature and the types of appropriate services needed

Assessment for planning intervention: gathering information to determine the current functional level and strengths and weaknesses, as well as to identify useful intervention objectives, strategies, and outcomes

Monitoring change: tracking the rate of progress and the effectiveness of intervention strategies

Program evaluation: gathering information to determine program effectiveness

Early intervention assessment can be accomplished through procedures that include direct testing by objective measures, naturalistic observation of various behaviors, review of various records (e.g., medical, previous assessments, and developmental), and interviews with parents and caregivers (Widerstrom, Mowder, & Sandall, 1991).

With increased emphasis on functionally focused interventions, a concept to describe the functional performance of infants and young children is needed. This model must address two issues: a developmental framework and contextual influences. Performance must be measured in relation to the order and timing of appearance of functional skills and the changes occurring with maturation and learning. The model must also reflect the inter-relation between function and the social and physical environment.

Almost all children's functional activities take place under the supervision or instruction of others and in environments set up and controlled by adults. The functional performance must therefore be characterized as a transactional process, not just as a set of fixed skills that the child either does or does not have. It is necessary to incorporate a distinction between disability and social role performance into a pediatric framework. (Coster & Haley, 1992, p. 15)

The measurement of change in a clinical setting should be guided by a system that organizes information about a child or group of children and includes the appropriate ways to measure the effectiveness of intervention. A model called the Pediatric Evaluation of Disability Inventory (PEDI) "incorporates four levels of impairment, functional limitations, disability and social role performance as well as developmental and contextual influences" (Coster & Haley, 1992, p. 21). This instrument, appropriate for ages 6 months to 7 years, includes social outcome measures as well as measures of activities of daily living in part I, and caregiver assistance and modifications in parts II and III. The functional skills content of the PEDI is divided into three domains: self-care, mobility, and social function, as shown in Table 11–3. These domains were chosen to have reasonably broad applicability across home and school contexts for infants and young children. A feature that makes the PEDI a very usable tool is its flexibility in administration. A sample form for

Table 11–3 FUNCTIONAL SKILLS CONTENT OF THE PEDIATRIC EVALUATION OF DISABILITY INVENTORY

Self-Care Domain	Mobility Domain	Social Function Domain
Types of food textures	Toilet transfers	Comprehension of word meanings
Use of utensils	Chair/wheelchair transfers	Comprehension of sentence complexity
Use of drinking containers	Car transfers	Functional use of expressive
Tooth brushing	Bed mobility/transfers	communication
Hair brushing	Tub transfers	Complexity of expressive
Nose care	Method of indoor locomotion	communication
Handwashing	Distance/speed indoors	Problem resolution
Washing body and face	Pulls/carries objects	Social interactive play
Pullover/front-opening	Method of outdoor locomotion	Peer interactions
garments	Distance/speed outdoors	Self-information
Fasteners	Outdoor surfaces	Time orientation
Pants	Upstairs	Household chores
Shoes/socks	Downstairs	Self-protection
Toileting tasks		Community function
Management of bladder		
Management of bowel		

From Haley, S., Coster, W., Ludlow, L., Holtiwanger, J., & Andrellos, P. (1992). *Pediatric evaluation of disability inventory (PEDI) version 1.0 development, standardization and administration manual* p. 13. Boston: New England Medical Center Hospitals.

scoring the PEDI is found in the Appendix. The PEDI can be administered by a team of professionals, by structured parent interview, or by a combination of both, and it is also useful as a supplement to other scales so that the child's abilities can be related to functional performance. The Case Study documents the PEDI results for one child and also compares these results with three other scales.

The PEDI can provide an evaluation tool for pediatric rehabilitation programs; an evaluation instrument for therapy services, school programs, and community agencies; and a uniform mechanism for documenting functional disability for data banks and outcome evaluation research. "It is designed to identify the child's functional ability along three scales: 1) typical functional skill level; 2) modifications or adaptive equipment used (i.e. braces, motorized wheelchair); and 3) physical assistance required of the caregiver" (Feldman, Haley, & Coryell, 1990, p. 603). The three scales are depicted in Table 11–4, with specific rating criteria given for each.

The Functional Independence Measure for Children, also called the WeeFIM, was developed by the Research Foundation—SUNY in 1991 for use with children ages 6 months to 7 years and older. It can be used for older children if their disability limits certain behaviors. It mimics the FIM used for adults but reflects the functional differences seen in children due to their age. The WeeFIM is a basic indicator of severity of disability, using

a seven-level scale to represent gradations in behavior. The scale ranges from 7, independent, to 1, maximal dependence. Eighteen sub-domains, representing the six domains of self-care, sphincter control, mobility, locomotion, communication, and social cognition, are incorporated in the tool (McCabe & Granger, 1990). The WeeFIM measures what the child actually does and includes the efforts of others as well as the use of tangible goods. The tool can be scored by direct observation or parent report and is usable by any trained clinician. Nurses have adapted it for use in documentation as well as in admission assessment and reassessment, daily patient classification, and outcome evaluation both at discharge and follow-up.

Pediatric rehabilitation nurses working with children and families in a variety of settings must also be cognizant of the other screening and assessment instruments available for use. The ones most frequently seen are listed and described in Table 11–5. In developing intervention strategies for the child with a disability or chronic condition, it is important that the team consider all available information. Results from these tests can provide valuable information to incorporate into the plan when setting goals and determining outcomes. Table 11–6 lists some other screening and assessment tools that might be part of the information provided and gives a brief description of the purpose and the appropriate age group for each test.

Table 11–4   RATING CRITERIA FOR THE THREE TYPES OF MEASUREMENT SCALES

Part I: Functional Skills	Part II: Caregiver Assistance	Part III: Modifications
197 Discrete items of functional skills Self-care, mobility, social function 0 = Unable or limited in capability to perform item in most situations 1 = Capable of performing item in most situations, or item has been previously mastered and functional skills have progresses beyond this level	20 Complex functional activities Self-care, mobility, social function 5 = Independent 4 = Supervise/prompt/monitor 3 = Minimal assistance 2 = Moderate assistance 1 = Maximal assistance 0 = Total assistance	20 Complex functional activities Self-care, mobility, social function N = no modifications C = child-oriented (non-specialized) R = rehabilitation equipment E = extensive modifications

From Haley, S., Coster, W., Ludlow, L., Holtiwanger, J., & Andrellos, P. (1992). *Pediatric evaluation of disability inventory (PEDI) version 1.0 development, standardization and administration manual* p. 16. Boston: New England Medical Center Hospitals.

SUMMARY

A major focus of health care initiatives in the years ahead must be on prevention and screening services. The shift in focus from illness to wellness will provide a framework for the design and delivery of health care services that assist children and families to develop health-enhancing behaviors. Pediatric rehabilitation nurses are in a position to have a major impact on health promotion and disease prevention. The nurse knows the child and family well and can tap into the resources of the community, so it is imperative that he or she assume leadership in the complex health care management of children with disabilities or chronic conditions.

CASE STUDY

Fernando is a 7-year-old Hispanic boy. In his household there is a 4-year-old half brother, his mother, and an uncle. The family had just moved to a new apartment the day before his accident. Prior to the accident he was attending school in a regular first-grade class and had no reported problems. He understands and speaks both English and Spanish but his mother's English is limited, so an interpreter is used for assessment and teaching. Birth and early development were normal according to the mother's report. He has been seen for routine care at the neighborhood health center. His prior medical history is unremarkable, all immunizations are up to date, and his growth and development was proceeding at the expected pace until his accident. He was hit by a car as a pedestrian, found in the road unresponsive and unconscious, and admitted to the pediatric intensive care unit with a severe closed head injury and right tibial open fracture. While in the acute hospital he had an open reduction of the fracture with pin placement and casting, a craniotomy with a ventriculo-peritoneal shunt placed, and a gastrostomy tube placed for ease of feeding. He began to show improvement with multidisciplinary intervention and was transferred to the acute rehabilitation hospital. At the time of admission for pediatric rehabilitation he was still very dependent in most activities of daily living. Initially, his mother performed all activities but allowed for more independence as she began to understand the nature of his head injury and the resulting deficits. She initially thought that when his leg healed from the fracture he would begin to walk again normally and did not understand the severe deficits to his right hand and leg resulting from the injury to his brain. Taking him home on a leave of absence a few times increased her awareness of his needs. Feeding and eating improved, and the gastrostomy tube was removed. The leg cast was replaced with a lighter splint and gait training begun. Occupational therapy prescribed a stabilizer splint for the right hand, but progress was slow. Verbal ability improved but was hindered by memory deficits and low tolerance for frustration. At discharge, he was referred for continued out-patient therapy and evaluation in school.

Table 11-5 FREQUENTLY USED SCREENING AND ASSESSMENT TOOLS

Tool	Description
Bayley Scales of Infant Development II (Psychomotor Scale)	Birth–36 months. Basis for early diagnosis of developmental delay. One of the most widely used tests of infant development. Motor and mental scales. Mental scale (Mental Development Index) includes object permanence, memory, manipulation, problem solving, verbal communication, and comprehension. Motor scale (Psychomotor Development Index) includes fine and gross motor function, hand function, posture, and locomotion. Behavior rating scale (Infant Behavior Record) includes observed behavior and social and objective orientation toward the environment. Can be used clinically and for research. Individually administered, takes approximately 30–60 minutes
Vineland Adaptive Behavior Scales	Birth to adult. Measures adaptive behavior needed for personal and social self-sufficiency. Evaluate typical level of independence in usual environment. Domains: communication, daily living skills, socialization, and motor skills. Semi-structured interview with parent or caregiver.
Peabody Picture Vocabulary Test—Revised	Under 2.6 years: "point to" response test. Measures hearing vocabulary for standard American English. From 2.6–4 years: verbal and non-verbal response, changes in receptive vocabulary. From 2.6–18 years: expressive language scale, general concept of abilities.
Peabody Developmental Motor Scales and Activity Cards	Birth–6.11 years (83 months). Assess motor skills. Gross motor: reflexes, balance, non-locomotor, locomotor, receipt and propulsion of objects. Fine motor: grasp, hand function, eye-hand coordination, manual dexterity. Direct testing and observation. Can be used to design therapeutic interventions by linking assessment items and activity cards. Useful in screening, evaluation, and program planning.
Test of Early Language Development	From 2–8 years. Assesses receptive and expressive syntax and morphology. Score based on form and content.
Uzgiris-Hunt Ordinal Scales of Development	Birth–24 months. Assessment provides information on psychological infant development, 7 sensorimotor branches based on Piaget. Visual pursuit, object permanence, means-end, vocal imitation, gesture imitation, operational causality, schemes for relating to objects. Strengths and weaknesses on each sensorimotor scale.
Denver Developmental Screening II	From 1 week–6 years. Identifies developmental lags. Developmental screening, minimal equipment, available in Spanish. Four domains: personal-social, fine motor–adaptive, language, and gross motor. Screens for developmental deviations. Individually administered and takes approximately 20–35 minutes.
Miller Assessment for Preschoolers (MAP)	From 2 years, 9 months–6 years 2 months. Identifies children at risk for developmental delays. Assesses cognitive, communication, physical, social-emotional, and adaptive function. Individually administered, takes approximately 30–40 minutes.
Hawaii Early Learning Profile (HELP)	Birth–36 months, and 3–6 years. Checklist for developmental screening. Cognitive, language, gross motor, fine motor, social, self-help skills.
Home Observation for Measurement of the Environment (HOME) (1984)	Birth to elementary age. Two forms: infant/toddler and pre-school. Observation and interview. Report and direct observation of interactions and environment and consistency of stimuli. Subscales measure quality and quantity of social, emotional, and cognitive support in the home. Emotional and verbal responsiveness of mother, avoidance of restriction and punishment, organization of the environment, provision of appropriate play material, maternal involvement with the child, opportunity for variety in daily stimulation.

Table 11–6   OTHER SCREENING AND ASSESSMENT TOOLS

Gesell Developmental Schedules	Birth–6 years. Assesses adaptive, gross and fine motor, language, and personal-social development.
Bruininks-Oseretsky Test of Motor Proficiency (BOTMP)	From 4.6–14.6 years. Assesses gross and fine motor functioning—running, speed and agility, balance, coordination, strength, visual-motor. Designed for screening and identifying physical problems.
McCarthy Scales of Children's Abilities	From 2.6–8.6 years. Measures six aspects of children's thinking, motor and mental ability.
AAMR Adaptive Behavior Scale	From 3–16 years. Screening tool and institutional planning. Behavior domains and maladaptive behavior. Informants.
Bender Gestalt Tests	Under 3 years, evaluation tool for developmental problems. From 5–10 years, assesses visual motor function.

Minnesota Developmental Inventories	Infant
	   Birth–15 months. Measures developmental areas: gross motor, fine motor, language, comprehension and personal social.
	Child
	   From 6 months–6 years. General development, gross and fine motor, expressive language, comprehension, conceptual, self-help, personal social.

Early Intervention Developmental Profile	Birth–36 months. Aid for individual program planning. Specific developmental strengths and weaknesses. Complete developmental assessment linked to team assessment.
Sequenced Inventory of Communication Development—Revised	From 4–48 months. Measures communication development in children.
Infant and Toddler Temperament Questionnaires	Infant, 4–8 months, toddler, 12–36 months. Assesses general patterns of behavior.
Gross Motor Function Measure	From 5 months–16 years. Change in gross motor function over time in children with cerebral palsy. Observation of five dimensions: lying and rolling; sitting; crawling and kneeling; standing; and walking, running, and jumping.
Leiter International Performance Scale	From 2 years–adult. Nonverbal test of intelligence. Areas include perceptual, symbolic transformation, quantitative discrimination, spatial imagery, genus matching, immediate recall.
Test of Visual Motor Skills	From 2–13 years. Measures eye/hand coordination, eye/hand motor accuracy, motor control, and motor coordination through copying figures.
Toddler and Infant Motor Evaluation	Birth–42 months. Comprehensive diagnostic assessment of mobility, stability, motor organization, functional performance, social/emotional abilities.
Brigance Inventory of Early Development—Revised	Birth–7 years. Developmental readiness and early academic skill inventory.
Milani-Comparetti Motor Development Screening Test	Birth–3 years. Neurodevelopmental examination to assess motor development. Evaluate changes in primitive reflexes and parachute, righting and equilibrium, reactions with emerging motor behavior.

PEDI Results—In the functional skills domain, the highest score was in social function, followed by self-care and mobility. Caregiver assistance was most needed in the area of social function, and modifications were most needed for mobility. When all areas—functional skills, caregiver assistance, and modifications—were totaled, they ranged within 5% of each other. This scale is most helpful in that it gives a picture of the actual functional skills and behaviors, as well as the modifications needed and the amount of caregiver assistance required. Three other scales (Vineland, American Association on Mental Deficiency [AAMD] Adaptive Behavior Scale, and WeeFIM) were used for comparison purposes, and it was very interesting to see the similarities in scores received on the different scales when the same areas were assessed and to note how differently each scale assessed similar areas of information. Probably the most comprehensive tool for assessing this child would be a combination of many scales, although the PEDI was most helpful because it included the ratings for caregiver assistance and modifications and provided good information for comparisons over time.

REFERENCES

Algranati, P. (1992). *The pediatric patient: an approach to history and physical examination*. Philadelphia: Williams & Wilkins.

Benner, S. (1992). *Assessing young children with special needs: an ecological perspective*. New York: Longman.

Betz, C.L., Hunsberger, M., & Wright, S. (1994). *Family-centered nursing care of children* (2nd ed.). Philadelphia: WB Saunders.

Broughton, B., & Lutner, N. (1995). Childhood chronic illness: a nursing health-promotion model for rehabilitation in the community. *Rehabilitation Nursing*, 20(6), 318–322.

Burkett, K. (1989). Trends in pediatric rehabilitation. *Nursing Clinics of North America*, 24(1), 239–255.

Children's Specialized Hospital Foundation. (1996). *Primary care for chronically ill children and children with disabilities: The Children's 21st Century Challenge*, Mountainside, NJ: Children's Specialized Hospital.

Chow, M., Durand, B., Feldman, M., & Mills, M. (1984). *Handbook of pediatric primary care* (2nd ed.). New York: John Wiley & Sons.

Cohen, H. (1991). Services for young children with disabilities: new directions and emerging issues. *Physical Medicine and Rehabilitation: State of the Art Reviews*, 5(2), 427–441.

Cole, B., Finch, E., Gowland, C., & Mayo, N. (1995). *Physical rehabilitation outcome measures*. Philadelphia: Williams & Wilkins.

Coster, W., & Haley, S. (1992). Conceptualization and measurement of disablement in infants and young children. *Infants and Young Children* 4(4), 11–22.

Dines, A., & Cribb, A. (Eds.). (1993). *Health promotion concepts and practice*. Boston: Blackwell Scientific Publications.

Downie, R., Fyfe, C., & Tannahill, A. (1990). Health promotion models and values. New York: Oxford University Press.

Feldman, A., Haley, S., & Coryell, J. (1990). Concurrent and construct validity of the pediatric evaluation of disability inventory. *Physical Therapy*, 70(10), 602–610.

Friedman, M. (1992). *Family nursing theory and practice* (3rd ed.). Norwalk, CT: Appleton & Lange.

Frye, B. (1986). A model of wellness seeking behavior in traumatic spinal cord injury victims. *Rehabilitation Nursing*, 11(5), 6–7, 14.

Griffith, H., & DiGuiseppi, C. (1994). Guidelines for clinical preventive services. *Nurse Practitioner*, 19(9), 25, 27–28, 31, 35.

Hanak, M. (1992). *Rehabilitation nursing for the neurological patient*. New York: Springer.

Hunsberger, M. (1994). Health concepts: children's perceptions and behaviors. In C.L. Betz, M. Hunsberger, & S. Wright (Eds.). *Family-centered nursing care of children* (2nd ed.), pp. 379–410. Philadelphia: WB Saunders.

Igoe, J. (1993). Prevention: child health. In American Nurses Association Council of Community Health Nursing (Ed.). *Prevention across the life span: healthy people for the twenty-first century*. Washington, DC: American Nurses Publishing.

Jackson, P. (1992). The primary care provider and children with chronic conditions. In P. Jackson & J. Vessey (Eds.). *Primary care of the child with a chronic condition*. Boston: Mosby–Yearbook.

Kelly-Hayes, M. (1995). Functional evaluation in rehabilitation nursing. In S. Hoeman (Ed.). *Rehabilitation nursing process and application* (2nd ed.). Boston: Mosby.

Linder, T. (1993). *Transdisciplinary play-based assessment: a functional approach to working with young children, revised*. Baltimore: Paul H. Brookes.

Marquis, P. (1991). Developmental disabilities in primary care. In A. Capute & P. Accardo (Eds.). *Developmental disabilities in infancy and childhood*, pp. 133–137. Baltimore: Paul H. Brookes.

McCabe, M., & Granger, C. (1990). *Content validity of a pediatric functional independence measure: research briefs*. Philadelphia: WB Saunders.

McMahon, L. (1992). *The handbook of play therapy*. New York: Tavisock/Routledge.

Meisels, S., & Provence, S. (1989). *Screening and assessment: guidelines for identifying young disabled and developmentally vulnerable children and their families*. Washington, DC: National Center for Clinical Infant Programs.

Miller, L. (1994). *Assessment instruments: review of instruments for evaluating children ages birth to three years*. Denver, CO: Colorado State Department of Education.

Ricci-Balich, J., & Behm, J. (1996). Pediatric rehabilitation nursing. In S. Hoeman (Ed.). *Rehabilitation nursing process and application* (2nd ed.). Boston: Mosby.

Russell, F., & Free, T. (1994). The nurse's role in habilitation. In S. Roth & J. Morse (Eds.). *A lifespan approach to nursing care for individuals with developmental disabilities*. Baltimore: Paul H. Brookes.

Standards of Nursing Practice for the Care of Children and Adolescents with Special Health and Developments Needs. (1994). Lexington, KY: University of Kentucky Chandler Medical Center.

Teague, M., Cipriano, R., & McGhee, V. (1990). Health promotion as a rehabilitation service for people with disabilities. *Journal of Rehabilitation*, Jan/Feb/Mar, 52–56.

Tesh, A., Selby-Harrington, M., Corey, V., & Cross, A. (1995). The early and periodic screening, diagnosis and treatment program: opportunities for nurse practitioners. *Nurse Practitioner*, 20(8), 68–73.

Urbano, M. (1992). *Pre school children with special*

health care needs. San Diego, CA: Singular Publishing Group Inc.

Widerstom, A., Mowder, B., & Sandall, S. (1991). *At-risk and handicapped newborns and infants: development assessment and intervention.* Englewood Cliffs, NJ: Prentice-Hall.

ADDITIONAL RESOURCES

Brown, C., & Seklemian, P. (1993). The individualized functional assessment process for young children with disabilities: lessons from the Zebley decision. *Journal of Early Intervention,* 17(3), 239–252.

Campbell, S. (Ed.). (1994). *Physical therapy for children,* Philadelphia: WB Saunders.

Haley, S., Coster, W., Ludlow, L., Haltiwanger, J., & Andrellos, P. (1992*). Pediatric evaluation of disability inventory.* Boston: New England Medical Center.

Igoe, J., & Giordano, B. (1992). *Expanding school health services to serve families in the 21st century.* Washington, DC: American Nurses Publishing.

Logogian, M., & Ward, J. (Eds.). (1989). *Pediatric rehabilitation: a team approach for therapists.* Boston: Little Brown & Co.

Lord, J., Taggart, P., & Molnar, G. (1991). Assessment instruments for evaluation of motor skills in children. *Physicial Medicine and Rehabilitation: State of the Art Reviews,* 5(2), 389–384.

Rubin, I., & Crocker, A. (1989). *Developmental disabilities: delivery of medical care for children and adults.* Philadelphia: Lea & Febiger.

VanDeusen, J., & Brunt, D. (1997). *Assessment in occupational therapy & physical therapy.* Philadelphia: WB Saunders.

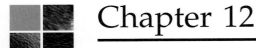

Chapter 12

Physical Health Care Patterns and Nursing Interventions

Susanne R. Hays

The functional health patterns developed by Gordon (1994) provide a data collection system for a comprehensive assessment of the child or adolescent with a disability or chronic condition and their family. This system is explained in Chapter 8 and a brief description provided about the assessment information obtained for each pattern. This chapter covers four physical patterns: nutritional-metabolic, elimination, activity-exercise, and sleep-rest. Issues relating to skin maintenance, which transcends the four areas, are provided to assist in assessment and management of alterations in skin integrity. Each functional pattern is discussed briefly in relation to the child's normal development, specific alterations in development related to that pattern, and the pediatric rehabilitation nursing management. It is paramount that the pediatric rehabilitation nurse have knowledge of the expected development and physiology of the child or adolescent prior to assessment and the establishment of interventions. Selected information regarding each functional health pattern is provided that is valuable for the nurse as clinical decision-making skills are used to provide care to the child or adolescent and family in the hospital, clinic, home, school, and community.

NUTRITIONAL-METABOLIC PATTERN

This pattern includes food and fluid intake and how this affects the child's metabolic condition. Specific areas of assessment to determine the child's nutritional health patterns include types and amounts of food and fluid intake, eating patterns, likes and dislikes, oral-motor skills, anthropometric data, and condition of the skin, mucous membranes, teeth, hair, and nails (Gordon, 1994).

Children with developmental delays, disabilities, or chronic conditions are at high risk for nutritional difficulties and alterations in feeding. Some reasons for feeding alterations include

- Anatomical conditions—cranial facial anomalies, cleft lip or palate, or trauma
- Developmental sensory neuromotor conditions that cause delay in development of oral skills, difficulty with coordination of oral-motor movements, or difficulty experiencing oral sensations
- Psychosocial environmental issues—failure to thrive (FTT) or maternal deprivation

Early recognition of problems is paramount. Failure to thrive, delayed oral-motor skill development, and family stress can be minimized through appropriate early identification and intervention. Nourishing the child is one of the family's main goals, and resources, interventions, and appropriate health care providers may not be readily identified. This can be a very frustrating and lonely experience. The causes of alterations in nutrition and growth can be any of the following: chronic illness, developmental delays and disabilities, metabolic and genetic disorders, feeding and swallowing disorders, medications, and psychosocial or environmental situations.

The expression of nutrition alterations generally is represented by either slow growth,

FTT, or obesity. For children with delays and disabilities, slow growth or FTT usually is related to poor organization of the ability to manage fluids and solids in the mouth and to successfully swallow them, or related to a specific condition that has growth failure as a component. For children with a chronic condition, often the ability to manage fluids and solids is well developed but the caloric needs are much greater than the child is willing or able to consume; therefore, they have growth delays. Children with nutritional alterations leading to obesity may be overfed via a tube, have a syndrome that has obesity as a component, be inactive and thus consume more calories than needed for growth and health, or have a combination of problems.

Development of Feeding Skills

The development of the ability to suck, swallow, and breathe, and thus successfully feed, begins in the intrauterine environment. At 34 to 35 weeks gestation, the infant can successfully organize all components and reflexively suck, swallow, and breathe. Organization of sucking is a very complicated and valuable early skill. Sucking not only allows the infant to receive nutrition, but also supports self-calming and sensory neurodevelopmental organization. Oral reflex skills also allow the infant to explore the environment, as in early play, and set the stage for early control over physiologic needs and psycho-social interactions. During infancy a tongue thrust is normal, and the tongue will push solids from the mouth.

As the sensory neuromuscular system matures, the reflexes that support early suck, swallow, and breathing patterns fade and development of a coordinated control of feeding begins to be identified. This transformation normally is noted between 4 and 6 months. At this point, one can see the child making up and down munching movements with the mouth, the tongue can transfer foods from the front of the mouth to the back for swallowing without gagging, and small amounts of liquid can be taken from a cup. The infant has oral skills that make it possible to manage pureed foods, progressing to blended table foods and mashed lumpy foods, and can start drinking from a cup with assistance.

By 9 months of age, the child is starting to lateralize tongue movements and can control the position of food in the mouth. Rotary chewing starts to develop and makes it possible for the child to manage ground, finely chopped, and small pieces of soft foods. Interest in the spoon as a tool for feeding begins, but finger and hand feeding is preferred.

At 1 year of age, the child is able to chew chopped foods and cooked table foods, and can drink from a cup with less assistance. Over the next year the child's oral skills continue to refine, allowing for chewing of tougher textures and successful cup drinking. At 2½ to 3 years of age, the child has matured oral skills that should make it possible to manage almost all textures successfully. It is still important, however, to monitor the child's eating and to avoid small pieces that could easily be aspirated, such as peanuts, grapes, and hot dogs. Table 12–1 outlines the development and physiology of nutrition and feeding for each age group from infant/toddler through adolescence.

Nutrition for Health and Growth

Brain growth is related to body growth; therefore, adequate nutrients during the most rapid growth of the brain in the intrauterine environment as well as in the first 2 to 3 years of life are very important (Vaughn & Litt, 1990). It is well known that disabilities can be prevented if the mother nourishes herself well prior to conception, during pregnancy, and during the breast-feeding period, as well as abstaining from addictive substances such as cigarettes, alcohol, and drugs. Adequate nutrients plus water are, however, only part of what is necessary for the health and wellness and growth and development for the child. The most important component necessary is loving nurturance, for without it, the child can become depressed and refuse to eat.

Infants are believed to be nourished best by mother's milk. If that is not possible, it is recommended that they receive iron-fortified formula during their first year of life. According to Satter (1987), normal eating is related to emotions, hunger, schedule, and proximity of food, and children learn what to eat and how to behave during meals by observing the adults in their environment. Specific dietary preferences in the United States continue to include the consumption of animal protein. Some families prefer vegetarianism; if this type of diet is used, it is important that the child and family are knowledgeable about how best to establish a nutrient-dense diet to support the high-energy demands of the growing child. Guidelines for a nutritionally sound vegetarian diet include

Table 12–1 AGES AND STAGES: DEVELOPMENT AND PHYSIOLOGY OF NUTRITION AND FEEDING

INFANT/TODDLER
Has organized reflex pattern of suck, swallow, breathe by 34 to 35 weeks gestation
Has normal tongue thrust reflex until about 4 to 6 months of age
Starts hand-to-mouth skills useful for finger feeding at about 4 to 6 months of age
Starts pureed solids by spoon at 5 to 6 months of age when able to open mouth for spoon, indicate
   fullness by turning away and have head and neck control
Introduces liquid by cup
Needs supported semireclining feeding position
Starts munching movements when food is presented
Requires 108 kcal/kg/24 hours from birth to 6 months of age
Sits in highchair with back at 90 degrees by 7 months of age but may still need external support
Starts rotary chewing at 8 to 9 months of age
Has 6 to 8 teeth by 1 year of age
Requires 100 kcal/kg/24 hours by 1 year of age
Requires 102 kcal/kg/24 hours between 1 and 3 years of age
Toddlers often have food jags or refuse to eat
Appetite changes with energy needs and developmental focus

PRESCHOOLER
Continues to have fluctuating appetite
May be labeled as "picky" eater

SCHOOL-AGED CHILD
Requires 90 calories/kg/day, age 6 to 7 years
Requires 70 calories/kg/day, age 7 to 10 years
Requires 30 to 74 calories/kg/day, over 10 years
Begins weight gain leading to obesity during this age
Begins eruption of permanent teeth

ADOLESCENT
Has erratic eating behaviors
Eruption of second molars
Requires 50 to 75 calories/kg/day for males and 40 to 55 calories/kg/day for females
Needs guidance regarding nutritional needs if pregnant

Sources: Ekvall, 1993; Vaughn & Litt, 1990; Morris & Klein, 1987.

Ensure a balance of dietary protein; legumes and grains
Supplement the diet with products containing vitamin B12
Provide dietary sources of vitamin C
Follow the principles of the food groups
Stress a wide variety of food intake (Ott, 1994)

Alterations

Malnutrition can limit brain and skeletal growth and the overall development of the child. Embryonic growth especially is susceptible to a decrease in nutrients, which may occur if the mother has poor dietary habits, is ill, or engages in poor self-care practices during pregnancy. Although much is known about severe malnutrition, the science of borderline nutrition and its effect on the development and physiology of the child is very complex and not well understood (Vaughn & Litt, 1990).

Obesity, a significant health concern for children in the United States, is an imbalance in the amount of energy expended and the amount of calories consumed. A child is considered obese when body weight is 20% above the standard desired 'ideal' body weight (Dietz, 1987). The child with obesity may also suffer from inadequate nutrition. Risk factors for obesity in a child with developmental delays, disabilities, or chronic conditions include

- Inability to clearly demonstrate satiation by turning away
- Being overfed when sustained by tube feedings
- Continuing to get standard calories for age when calories should be decreased because of a specific disability or decrease in activity level

Nutrition: Less Than Body Requirements

Nutritional concerns related to decreased caloric intake can be caused by oral-facial abnormalities, such as clefting; oral-motor functioning difficulties, such as those seen in children with hyper- or hypotonicity; and oral aversions found in children with delayed oral feeding experiences. Psycho-social/emotional concerns such as depression and environmental and socioeconomic issues, such as inadequate food available during high-growth times, can also cause decreased caloric intake. Children born with central nervous system (CNS) impairment often have slowed or delayed growth. This may be related to a specific condition, such as fetal alcohol syndrome, or to the fact that the child is unable to take in enough calories because of dysfunctional sensory neuromotor systems.

Children with cerebral palsy are often smaller than normal children their age; many are below the third percentile on the weight-for-height charts. This may be related to chronic malnutrition or a congenial conditions, but there is inadequate information regarding energy requirements for children with cerebral palsy, so it is important to individually determine their needs based on their growth parameters, activity, type of cerebral palsy, and other conditions, such as feeding difficulties and illness (Bandini, Patterson, & Ekvall, 1993).

When children have a CNS impairment from trauma after birth, they may become severely malnourished because of an inability to consume calories and a greater need for certain nutrients essential in the healing process. Abdominal injuries may delay the safe passage of foods; therefore the child is provided limited calories through peripheral intervenors, alimentation, or enteral feedings. Once there is the possibility of safe oral feedings, the presence of dysphagia, aspiration, and behavioral issues may present themselves, further complicating the nutritional status.

Nutrition: More Than Body Requirements

For children with disabilities, obesity may be a concern; defining when a disabled child is obese is somewhat more complex. Standardized growth charts are not available for each disability, and often there is difficulty obtaining accurate measurements of growth parameters. It usually is thought that a child is obese when actual weight exceeds the 'ideal' by 20% or is at or above the 75th percentile weight for height (Rallison, 1986). Obesity may cause the child with a disability to be at increased risk for skin breakdown, to have difficulty with mobility and transfers, or to have difficulty with fitting of wheelchairs and other adaptive equipment (for example, a child with muscular dystrophy whose activity level progresses from ambulation without equipment to wearing braces and eventually using an electric wheelchair for mobility). For the child who has a severe injury or for infants who are extremely premature, overfeeding may have metabolic consequences, affecting the respiratory system and hepatic functioning and increasing the risk of mortality (Chwals, 1994).

Nutrition Related to Disability or Chronic Illness

Increased need for calories is documented as important to support adequate growth and health for children with chronic lung disease, cardiac defects, infection, trauma, burns, or who must take medications that are known to depress the appetite, such as methylphenidate (Ritalin). Children born with conditions that include atrophy and paralysis of the lower extremities, such as spina bifida and sacral agenesis, are at high risk for becoming obese. This is thought to occur because the lower-limb atrophy does not allow them to be as active. Therefore, they do not need the same number of calories as normal children their age, and the calories they consume may be an overabundance. See Chapter 15 for more complete information on the management of the child with spina bifida. Children born with conditions such as Down syndrome and spinal muscle atrophy with hypotonicity as a component are thought to need less calories to grow because of delayed mobility, immobility, and decreased activity. Therefore, these children are also at high risk for obesity (Ekvall, Bandini, & Ekvall, 1993).

For children with infections and fever, caloric expenditure increases 7% for each degree Fahrenheit above normal. Fevers also place the child at higher risk for dehydration and can increase protein utilization; therefore, these children need to increase fluid and protein intake. Respiratory infections and pneumonia can dramatically increase energy expenditure as well as cause difficulties with intake of liquids and nutrients (Rallison, 1986).

The child who has experienced major burns presents a nutritional challenge. Providing adequate nutritional reserves for metabolic stress, fluid and electrolyte balances, healing, changing caloric needs, and normal developmental growth requires consistent monitoring. Having a pediatric registered dietitian on the team to provide this sophisticated nutritional management for the child minimizes complications and provides for optimal nutritional support for healing, as well as normal growth (Hutsler, 1991). See Chapter 21 for more complete information on the management of the child with burns.

Children with acquired immune deficiency syndrome (AIDS) are at high risk for nutritional deficits and malnutrition. Protein-calorie malnutrition, deficits in vitamins and minerals, and a decrease in lean body mass all have a detrimental effect on their immune systems (Thorn, 1995). See Chapter 19 for more complete information on the management of the child with human immunodeficiency virus (HIV).

Recently, more attention has been given to the use of specific dietary regimes as well as megavitamin and mineral supplements for treatment of children with developmental disabilities and chronic conditions. It is important that the pediatric rehabilitation nurse and the multidisciplinary team are aware of these alternative therapies and can discuss the use of them openly with the family (Nickel, 1996).

Food Allergies and Intolerance

Allergic reactions to food can occur at any age, but infants are at the greatest risk, because they have immature immune capability as well as immature digestive systems. It is the absorption of incompletely catabolized proteins that can allow for an antigenic reaction and thus a true food hypersensitivity that can lead to anaphylaxis. Food intolerance can be mistaken for a food allergy and may even resemble antigenic reactions. The most common adverse reactions to foods are gastrointestinal symptoms, such as vomiting, diarrhea, gas, and bloating, or skin irritations, rashes, and redness. Clinically, common foods that cause allergic or intolerance reactions are eggs, cow's milk, peanuts, wheat, and soy (Anderson, 1994).

Physiology of Feeding Difficulties

Anatomic

Changes in anatomic structures necessary for successful feeding include those seen in max-illa-oral-facial conditions such as clefting, conditions that effect the structure of the trachea and esophagus such as tracheoesophageal fistula (TEF), or those affecting the stomach. The major anomaly affecting early feeding abilities is oral-facial clefting. Infants with these conditions are at high risk for feeding difficulties related to the anatomic defect in oral structures; thus, they have difficulty creating the adequate suction needed for pulling milk from the breast or bottle.

Infants with cleft of the lip only may not have a problem, but those with clefting of the palate and/or alveolar ridge have difficulty establishing adequate suction to pull milk from the breast or nipple. The infant still has a mechanical feeding problem even with an intact suck-and-bite reflex necessary for feeding and no damage to the CNS. Feeding will be altered until surgical repair is completed and the child fully recovers from the surgery, at which time normal feeding is possible.

Often, the child is sent home from the hospital soon after birth without the establishment of a successful oral feeding plan and without a continuity-of-care plan that supports the family and monitors the infant's growth. Many mothers are encouraged to breast feed; however, those infants with clefting of the palate will not be able to develop adequate suction because of the opening between the mouth and nose. With an effective feeding plan, these infants can receive adequate calories for growth. If there is a palate defect, the child is also at higher risk for middle ear disease. Infections, such as middle ear disease, need to be treated for adequate growth to continue. See Chapter 16 for more information on management of children born with craniofacial anomalies.

For infants with syndromes that include clefting and CNS or cardiopulmonary alterations, successful oral feeding skills are even more difficult to establish. Depending on the severity of the condition, their diets may need to be supplemented with non-oral methods of nutrition, and they need to be managed by a multidisciplinary team of professionals who have the skills necessary to maximize the child's potential for oral feeding.

Trauma occurring later in a child's life can also affect the structure, and thus the function, of the oral cavity and the child's ability to eat. Recovery of feeding skills is directly related to healing of the structures, unless that trauma includes the CNS. If problems with the central or peripheral nervous system are evident, successful oral feeding will be directly related to recovery of that system.

Sensory Neurodevelopmental

Pathophysiology of the CNS affects function and development of the sensory neuromotor processes needed for successful feeding skills. See Table 12–2 for a summary of signs of sensory neurodevelopmental dysfunction related to feeding. Dysphagia or impaired swallowing decreases the child's ability to pass liquids or solids safely from the mouth to the stomach. This condition often is seen following CNS damage, as in severe traumatic brain injury, anoxia or infectious brain injury, prematurity, or other conditions that affect oral-motor functioning.

To determine the parameters of dysphagia, it is paramount that normal developmental oral-motor skills necessary for feeding be well understood. Some of the signs thought to be related to dysphagia are gagging, coughing, or vomiting related to feeding attempts; refusing certain foods such as those with pieces, or those that are very thin, like water; failure to thrive or weight loss; pneumonia related to aspiration; or absence of gag reflex activity. It is possible to miss symptoms of dysphagia until the child has been diagnosed with aspiration pneumonia.

Children with cerebral palsy are at very high risk for feeding difficulties, which can be the first sign that the infant has some type of problem or condition. These children may have poor oral skills with difficulty chewing and organizing an effective swallow, as well as retained early reflexes such as tongue thrust, bite reflex, asymmetric tonic neck reflex (ATNR), and suck-swallow. These poor oral skills, combined with poor head, neck, and trunk control, create increased difficulty with oral-motor skills necessary for feeding.

There are occasions when children born with spina bifida and hydrocephalus also have the Chiari II malformation. These children may have feeding difficulties related to bulbar palsy and thus, if the condition is not managed early, have failure to thrive. It is therefore very important to have the child's feeding skills assessed on a regular basis, especially during growth spurts.

Psycho-social—Environmental

Feeding difficulties related to psycho-social-environmental issues are always multifaceted and complex and the infant or child may be diagnosed as FTT. There are three categories of FTT: organic (related to physical factors), non-organic (related to environmental-interactional factors), and mixed or a combination of both (Ott, 1994). Most, if not all, children with FTT can be classified in the mixed category. As more is learned about the complex human system and the dynamics of interactions, it is discovered that caregiver-infant interactions are very complex and affected by many factors involving both persons (Lobo, Barnard, & Coombs, 1992).

There is often a component of psycho-social-environmental feeding difficulties with children who have chronic illness and or disability, as shown in the following case study.

Table 12–2   SIGNS OF SENSORY NEURODEVELOPMENTAL DYSFUNCTION RELATED TO FEEDING

Oral hyper- or hyposensitivity

Excessive gagging or no gag reflex

Motor incoordination with dysphagia, impaired swallowing

Excessive drooling

Poor organization of the child's general level of arousal state and behavior necessary for processing environmental stimuli during feeding

Aspiration pneumonia

Slow growth not related to illnesses or other known conditions

CASE STUDY

One little girl, 9-month-old Sara, was diagnosed with cerebral palsy including oral-motor feeding difficulties. She had done well with oral-motor therapy and was able to take in solids from a spoon, preferring high sweet flavors and smooth textures, but was inconsistent and sometimes fussy at the time of her feedings. She was also able to take milk from a bottle adequately even though she had a somewhat ineffective suck. She was not strong enough for sitting in a highchair, but sat well in her car seat for spoon feedings. Her weight gain was slow but had developed along the fifth percentile.

One week, her weight was 8 ounces less than the previous week, even though she had been well. Her mother said she had not been able to get her to eat solids. After much listening, the nurse realized that the mother was expressing signs of depression and had also not been able to eat much that week. She finally said she just didn't have enough energy to "fight with Sara and make her eat solids." Sara's mother, because of her depression, did not have enough energy to spoon-feed Sara, and therefore the little girl had lost weight.

The advanced practice nurse who was providing the home-based therapy identified the following interventions:

- Discuss with the mother her feelings about and problems with feeding Sara and attempt to establish a feeding program that could be easier for mother and Sara
- Set specific, realistic timeframes and amounts of solids and milk that Sara needs every 24 hours for adequate growth
- Encourage mother to use other adults in the home such as the father to assist with feeding Sara
- Encourage mother to utilize the grandmother, who is willing to care for Sara one day on the weekend, so the mother can have some time to herself
- Encourage mother to see her primary care physician for evaluation and referral for counseling
- Refer Sara to an early intervention program for assistance with respite care, parent group interaction, and developmental therapy
- Offer to see Sara twice a week for therapy during this difficult time (obtain an order from the physician) and train other adults who may be willing to care for Sara

Outcome:

1. Mother, with encouragement from family, started drinking enriched supplements every time she fed Sara solids.

2. Sara started to slowly gain weight over the next month. .

3. Involvement with the early intervention parent group provided emotional support for the mother and reasons for outings, which assisted in resolving mother's depression.

4. Other family members began to assist with feeding Sara on a regular basis.

Other Conditions that Affect Feeding

Gastroesophageal reflux (GER) is a normal phenomenon that in some instances can be-

come severe. This abnormal reflux condition causes esophagitis, dysmotility, respiratory disease, reflux associated apnea, bradycardia, and often is part of vomiting and rumination. Children who have GER associate feeding with pain and discomfort, and refuse feedings. Conditions often observed when GER is present are

- Low birth weight
- Neurologic disease, especially with associated hypotonia, hypertonia, and spasticity
- Chronic respiratory disease
- Congenital esophageal anomalies
- Chronically increased abdominal pressure, as in obesity or hiatal hernia
- Rapid bolus feeding through a tube
- Vagal injury or dysfunction (Orenstein, 1994)

Due to the complexity of gastroesophageal reflux and lack of clear management strategies, a multidisciplinary team approach, including a clinical psychologist, the child, and family, is imperative.

Rehabilitation Nursing Management

The role of the pediatric rehabilitation nurse in relation to nutrition and metabolic needs includes a thorough assessment of the child's nutritional status, the family's knowledge of foods and the changing nutritional needs of their growing child, and provision of interventions and referrals as needed. It must be understood that the recommended dietary allowances (RDAs) are to be used as a guideline for the child's needs and that there is a wide variety of food and feeding practices that are safe and effective for the child. Cultural values and traditions as well as religious practices must be respected and acknowledged. Some food traditions that the nurse should consider are

- Spanish and Native American—use of beans and rice
- Chinese—rice, soybean products, food in small pieces cooked quickly
- Japanese—raw fish, little meat
- Middle Eastern—yogurt, ground meat (lamb) mixed with rice and spices; religious dietary preferences

The child who experiences a developmental delay, disability, or chronic illness must be seen as a unique individual with potentially complex nutritional and feeding concerns.

Assessment

Assessment of feeding and nutrition status must include assessment, or at least a screening, of the child's overall development, information about the child's primary diagnosis and other health conditions, plus thorough information about the family's concerns and questions. This information is very important in order to assist the nurse in adequately assessing the child's feeding and nutrition status. For example, many times a parent has concerns about a child who, at the age of 8 months, gags with the beginning of third foods or foods that have a thinner base with chunks of solid foods included. For a typically developing child, this can be a short-term behavior until rotary chewing is learned. However, if the child also has delays in development, the gagging may also be a sign that an oral-motor feeding assessment is needed as well as a complete developmental evaluation.

Clinical

- General physical condition, appearance, state of hydration, sensory status
- Presence of defects, syndromes, degree of impairment
- Developmental screening and observation of feeding process, including strength of oral musculature and gag and swallow ability
- Three-day diet history of caloric intake—more accurate than recall
- Skin condition, irritations, excessive dryness, bruises, rashes
- Dermatitis, hair loss, condition of oral mucosa and teeth
- Observation of current feeding skills and behaviors
- Family concerns regarding feeding and nutrition
- Behavioral feeding issues determine whether the problem is organic (related to physical factors) or non-organic (related to environmental interactional factors), or a combination of both
- History of vomiting, regurgitation, rumination, reflux, refusal to eat, or cardiorespiratory symptoms related to vomiting

Anthropometric

- Height—supine if possible; if not able to extend out because of contracture, measure in steps; i.e., head to base of spine, hip to knee, knee to foot
- Weight—without any clothing if there is a concern about weight gain, with light clothing if there is no specific concern
- Head circumference for children 36 months of age or less or for those suspected of being microcephalic
- Triceps and subscapular skinfolds—assess changes in total body fat

All of these parameters should be compared against accepted reference data to provide information about how the child is growing (Ekvall, 1993). Weight for height is a very valuable indicator of malnutrition or obesity and can be used to assess changes over time. The National Center for Health Statistics (NCHS) has developed growth charts for American children. For infants who are at high risk for feeding difficulties and growth delays and children with chronic illness and developmental disabilities, assessment of their growth must be done on a routine basis as one part of the regular health assessment, or more frequently if there is heightened concern about adequate nutrition.

When doing the anthropometric assessment, the nurse must consider the child's ethnicity as a factor. The NCHS growth charts were based on growth of black and white children in America. Children of Mexican, Chinese, or Japanese parents or other ethnic groups may show some group differences when plotted on the NCHS charts (Chumlea, 1993). Growth charts have been validated for some groups of children with special conditions such as Down syndrome, spina bifida, Prader-Willi syndrome, sickle cell disease, and Turner syndrome. These charts are available in pediatric nutrition textbooks.

Diagnostic/Laboratory

Determining the need for laboratory tests should be the role of the primary care provider in conjunction with the specific interdisciplinary team. Laboratory tests that might be used are complete blood count and urinalysis to detect marginal deficiencies before physical signs and symptoms are present. A registered dietitian should be available for assessment and management of children with complex conditions. Other methods of assessment include

- Videofluoroscopic barium swallow study for assessment of the swallowing process
- Ultrasonography for imaging the oral cavity
- pH probe study, barium radiography, endoscopy to assess presence and severity of gastroesophageal reflux disease (GERD)

- Manometry to document peristalsis of swallow process
- Nuclear medicine studies to evaluate food transit time, GERD, and stomach emptying (Kramer & Eicher, 1993)

Nursing Diagnoses

Major nursing diagnoses that relate to this functional health pattern are

Altered nutrition: less than body requirements

Altered nutrition: more than body requirements or potential for more than body requirements

Impaired swallowing

Altered growth and development

Ineffective infant feeding pattern

If the diagnosis of "impaired swallowing" is identified, the nursing plan of care found in Table 12–3 can be used after the assessment is complete and it is individualized for the child and family.

Expected Outcomes

The desired outcomes for the child and family include

- Maximize the nutritional status of the child and prevent nutritional deficiencies and growth failure related to oral-motor feeding alterations
- Demonstrate safe, effective swallowing of developmental age-appropriate foods and liquids without aspiration
- Demonstrate oral-motor skills and feeding skills at optimal developmental skill level
- Achieve weight for height between the 25th and 75th percentile while maintaining optimal health and wellness
- Demonstrate knowledge of specific nutritional and caloric needs according to activ-

Table 12–3   NURSING PLAN OF CARE

Nursing diagnosis: Impaired swallowing
Related to: Neuromuscular impairment
      Obstruction such as edema, tracheal tube

Altered level of consciousness
Fatigue

Goals	Nursing Inverventions/Teaching
Maintain airway and prevent aspiration	Use correct positioning with head and trunk in midline and head slightly flexed forward Use appropriate texture of foods and liquids to avoid aspiration or compromised airway Place food in mouth correctly Refer for consultation with therapist experienced in feeding difficulties if necessary Refer for positioning consultation and equipment if necessary Suction as necessary Teach emergency measures for choking
Feeding techniques correctly utilized	Provide feeding program based on oral motor development Appropriate utensils are used for solids and liquids Foods should be appealing and of correct temperature and consistency Avoid fatigue or feeding when drowsy from medications Provide cognitive cues; minimize distractions Coordinate with speech language pathologist or occupational therapist to enhance oral motor skills necessary for swallowing Teach feeding techniques and swallowing exercises Monitor weight Administer good oral hygiene after each feeding Consult with dietitian for assistance with diet plan Assure optimal caloric and fluid intake

Expected Outcomes

Liquids and solids pass from mouth to stomach
Appropriate feeding methods are demonstrated
Adequate hydration and body weight are maintained

ity level, type of disability, type of chronic disease when ill and well

- Verbalize and demonstrate skills necessary for use of specific feeding equipment such as tubes, pumps, special spoons and cups
- Have adequate nutrition and fluids for successful growth
- Maintain a safe, pleasurable feeding environment
- Achievement of effective oral hygiene

Interventions and Teaching to Meet Caloric Needs

Each child has an individual system of metabolism based on physical condition, genetic makeup, activity level, and health wellness pattern. Because of the multiplicity of conditions, a variety of options for assuring that the child has adequate calories to meet nutritional needs may be necessary. A registered dietitian with experience and knowledge in management of children with chronic conditions or developmental delays must be consulted in order to maximize the pediatric rehabilitation nurse's intervention strategies.

After a complete assessment of the child's nutritional status has determined that an increase in calories is necessary, there are still many decisions that need to be made. For the child who has oral-motor feeding skills adequate for safe effective oral feeding, the simplest intervention for increasing calories without increasing the intake volume is to maximize calories in all food intake and to increase the number of snacks with calorie-dense foods. Caution must be taken when increases in caloric density are considered. High osmolality and renal solute loads may lead to dehydration and diarrhea, especially in young infants. Some children are being fed foods that are not calorie dense, such as yogurt, meals with decreased fat content, or low-fat milk. Foods sometimes used to increase a child's calories and protein include cheese, strained baby food meats, powdered skim or evaporated milk, instant breakfast, vegetable oils, and powdered polycose.

As part of the intervention, the family needs to be taught to read the labels on foods and make high-calorie selections for the child. The child's oral skills, developmental age, and additional caloric needs must be considered before making a selection of food types and amounts. Consultation with the child's rehabilitation team or dietitian is recommended. For children who have significant oral-motor feeding difficulties that affect the oral intake of nutrition, the team may need to use other methods of ensuring the child is getting calorie-dense foods. This may mean using nasogastric, gastrostomy, or jejunostomy tubes. If the situation seems to be a temporary one, nasogastric tubes usually are selected.

The family must be an active member of the team, consulted for thoughts and ideas regarding the use of tubes. It is the parents who usually will be following through with the intervention after discharge. They often have had contact with other families with similar experiences and may have made a decision as to the intervention for their child. Often the parents feel they have failed in their role of nourishing their child when the team presents the idea of inserting a tube for additional feeding. These feelings must be acknowledged and respected. However, in situations when the child's life is threatened because of lack of nutrition, there may not be time for a complete process that allows the family to feel comfortable with the decision, so continued discussion and support is essential.

Frequent adjustment of the amount and type of nutritional intake for the child who has experienced acute trauma, such as burns, is necessary to support healing of the wounds and the health of the immune system, the effective responses to stress, and the needed nutrients for continued growth of the developing child (Hutsler, 1991).

The use of parenteral nutrition to meet the caloric needs of children with chronic illness is very complex and necessitates an interdisciplinary team that includes a clinical pharmacist, registered dietitian, and other professionals. There are many complications associated with this process, including infection, mechanical problems with the system, and metabolic disorders (Cochran, Phelps, & Helms, 1988).

Management of Dysphagia

Dysphagia requires a specialized interdisciplinary approach. The pediatric rehabilitation nurse must be able to recognize the early warning signs of dysphagia and, along with the family, may be the first to suspect this condition. With appropriate assessment, a specific treatment plan will be initiated by the team; the nurse, with knowledge and skills in feeding, is often the professional who follows through on a daily basis with the feeding program and teaches the family.

Positioning, food texture, the child's state of arousal and hunger, and the nutritional needs are all very important components of a treatment plan. For infants who are developmentally delayed and may not be able to demonstrate good neck and head control or turning away, starting solids needs to occur at approximately the same time chronologically as it would for a child who has normal development. Positioning for safe, effective feeding and assessment of satiation by other cues, such as keeping the mouth closed or other behaviors, is important. With many children, a delay in starting solids further compromises their willingness and ability to manage foods and other new textures.

For children who demonstrate dysphagia related to increasing the texture of foods, the problem may be related to poorly developed oral skills and continued use of the suck-swallow pattern for managing foods. Adequate assessment of the child's feeding skills is necessary with active oral-motor feeding intervention to teach the child to chew. It is well known that the child needs to be able to make up and down chewing movements and move food to the side of the mouth before textures that require chewing can be managed. The focus of the intervention is to develop chewing skills. See Table 12–4 for suggestions for teaching a child to chew.

Transitions from tube feeding to oral intake can be slow and labor intensive but important for the child's overall motor development and speech production. Readiness is related to the child's health and nutritional status, oral-motor and swallowing skills, family desires, and resolution of the original problem that necessitated use of a feeding tube. The major interventions needed to make the transition are (1) normalization of the meal and hunger cycles, (2) nutritional support, (3) normalization of oral-motor and swallowing skills, (4) management of the feeding behavior problems, (5) education of the family and other care providers, and (6) continued assessment and program modifications as changes occur (Glass & Lucas, 1990).

Management of Reflux, Vomiting, and Rumination

There are three basic methods of managing GER, all of which are controversial and not always effective. The most conservative management is dietary modification and positioning. It is recommended that smaller, frequent feedings with thickened formula may decrease reflux. Avoiding positioning that allows the infant or child to slump or be supine is thought to be beneficial in decreasing the incidence of reflux. Medications that improve the peristaltic function and gastric emptying, such as cisapride (Propulsid), metoclopramide (Reglan) or omeprazole (Prilosec), and those that neutralize gastric acidity such as famotidine (Pepcid), ranitidine hydrochloride (Zantac), cimetidine (Tagamet), or magnesium and aluminum hydroxide (Maalox and Mylanta), have been beneficial for some children.

The third and most drastic intervention is fundoplication surgery. This procedure wraps the fundus of the stomach around the lower esophageal sphincter and may be done in conjunction with placement of a gastrostomy tube. Even with this form of treatment, the

---

Table 12–4 SUGGESTIONS FOR TEACHING A CHILD TO CHEW

1. Provide oral play with teething toys that have a variety of textures. Stimulate all areas of the mouth, especially the tongue, sides of the mouth, and gum surfaces. Avoid gagging the child.

2. Offer small pieces of graham cracker, soft cheese puffs, or other foods that will melt in the side of the mouth over the molars (if present), over the gums, and inside the cheek by the molar gum area. This will stimulate the child to move the tongue laterally and to munch the food. Peanut butter should be avoided due to the high risk of choking and allergic reactions.

3. Encourage the child to imitate munching movements by using a mirror and demonstration. This is a fun activity for siblings.

4. When the child can demonstrate munching movements with food placed in the sides of the mouth, try placing the food in the front or have the child bite off a piece for moving to the side and munching.

5. Once the child is able to manage foods that melt, try adding small pieces of solids for stimulation of chewing. Crispy rice cereals are a good product for this type of therapy, because it stimulates chewing and makes a sound that gives the child feedback.

6. Using foods that have high flavor and are cold may also be of value when teaching a child to learn to chew.

child already may have learned to associate feedings with pain and discomfort and have difficulty eating. This surgical procedure also decreases the size of the stomach, necessitating smaller feedings. Children who have this procedure usually are not able to vomit and may have vomiting behaviors without producing any emesis. They also may gag if too full from gastrostomy tube feedings or if an unpleasant tasting substance is put in their stomach through the tube. Understanding the pathophysiology and management of GER and the outcomes of various treatment modalities will further refine the procedures used for this disorder (Orenstein, 1994).

Vomiting and rumination may be part of GER or may be separate behaviors that are self-induced. Once medical conditions have been ruled out, the team usually turns to a behavioral psychologist to assist in the development of a treatment plan. Many children who ruminate are seeking sensory stimulation, and some type of substitute stimulation added to their activities may be beneficial.

Management of Behavioral Feeding Issues

The most significant difference in intervention for pediatric as opposed to adult feeding and nutrition issues is the need to acknowledge the dynamics of physical and behavioral development. Many children with developmental disabilities or chronic conditions have feeding disorders related to organic issues. There also may be conditions related to nonorganic issues, and most often there is a multiplicity of issues that necessitate a skilled interdisciplinary group of professionals to assess and provide successful intervention.

For many children, the use of a developmental behavioral management program is the most effective on a long-term basis for improving oral feeding skills. There are many issues to be considered when choosing the type of intervention. These include (1) the ability to provide intervention consistently; (2) the child's psychosocial, cognitive, and motor development level; (3) specific oral-motor skills; (4) specific conditions that have affected successful oral feeding in the past; (5) the family's concerns and wishes regarding the feeding issues; (6) the child's current nutritional status and type of feeding program; (7) availability of a specialized experienced team of professionals to develop, monitor, and teach the strategies; and (8) avoidance of placing blame.

Dorsey and Diehl (1992) described the establishment of a behavior modification program for a 5-year-old child who had experienced burns and had significant weight loss. A program was established that incorporated developmental issues and the child's need to regain control over life, and that effectively shaped his food consumption behaviors and established a positive weight gain pattern. The program was interdisciplinary in nature, and long-term follow-up demonstrated that this child's eating behaviors continued to remain positive even after the behavior modification program was no longer being implemented.

Management of Oral Care

Children with developmental disabilities or chronic conditions are at higher risk for poor oral hygiene. They often have increased medications for the medical management of their condition and may require sweeteners to be added to their diet for increased calorie intake. In addition to the problem of increased sugar in the mouth, many children with disabilities do not have effective suck-swallow skills and food pockets develop in the mouth around the teeth. Also, it may be difficult to care for the child's oral cavity and dentition because of oral hypersensitivity, time required for hygiene, and expense related to seeing a dentist. Difficulty locating a dentist who is comfortable and willing to treat children with disabilities can also be a problem (Kenny & Judd, 1988). Some suggestions for prevention of dental caries include

- Start an oral care routine that includes cleansing the gums with a soft wet cloth on the end of a finger before teeth erupt
- Ask for sugar-free medications and follow the medication with water
- Brush the child's teeth or clean the gums before and after medication
- Avoid giving medications just before a nap or bed time
- Avoid trauma to the teeth
- Consult a dentist as needed for care

SUMMARY

Nutrition and feeding patterns for the child with a disability or a chronic condition must be assessed and appropriate treatment plans implemented. Health and wellness and growth and development all benefit from adequate nutrition. The pediatric rehabilitation nurse working in any setting must be capable of early identification, assessment, and intervention, including referrals for therapy and dietary management. Treatment is best managed by a multidisciplinary team. If specialists are not available to provide more complete evaluations and treatment, the rehabilitation nurse may need to consult with specialists at pediatric rehabilitation centers or early intervention programs to develop a treatment plan for the child and family. The goal is for the child to have a positive nutritional pattern and competent oral-motor skills that contribute to health and development.

ELIMINATION

This pattern includes bowel and bladder elimination functions (Gordon, 1994). Information regarding the child's expected bowel and bladder functioning, difficulties in toilet learning due to developmental delays and neurogenic bowel and bladder conditions, and autonomic dysreflexia management is included.

According to Dunn (1996), bowel and bladder control for the typical child "presents some of the most problematic and yet easily resolved issues for parents and health care providers" (p. 277). Social and cultural beliefs about what are "normal" elimination patterns for children may create the belief that there is a problem when none exists (Dunn, 1996). This situation, combined with the information about what is expected to be normal for a child with a disability, may create a very difficult situation that requires collaboration from a team with knowledge about what is normal and what is anticipated because of the type of disability.

An example occurred with a child who was born with spina bifida. She was breast fed, and during her first few weeks she stooled with each feeding. When she was about 6 weeks of age, her stooling pattern changed to several days between stools. When she did have a stool, it was yellow and seedy, having a somewhat liquid consistency, the typical type for an infant fed solely with breast milk. She used at least 10 diapers per day and her urine was dilute. The rehabilitation team had taught the mother that infants with spina bifida are at high risk for impaction and constipation, so she was very concerned about this infrequent stooling. The nursing assessment determined that the infant was not having a problem with impaction and constipation, but her stooling pattern was typical for some infants who are breast fed.

Chronic and disabling health conditions af-fect elimination in different ways. Cognitive deficits slow the child's perception of body cues such as bladder or rectal fullness. Learning when and where to use the bathroom may be a slow process. Conditions such as spina bifida, spinal cord injury, or other neuromuscular diseases affect sensory and motor nerves and result in neurogenic bowel and bladder. Traumatic brain injury or cerebral palsy rarely directly affect bowel and bladder function, but the conscious control of elimination may be affected. Other conditions, such as diabetes, cardiac disease, or autoimmune conditions do not directly affect bowel and bladder function. Medications taken for these conditions, such as diuretics (which cause increased urine output) or pain medication (which causes constipation), may alter bowel and bladder function. Side effects of the condition, such as increased risk of urinary tract infection with glycosuria, often occur.

Expected Development and Physiology

The development of effective bowel and bladder control is a task that is of high priority for the child, family, and society. It indicates successful growth toward adulthood. When the child has difficulty with this major task, shame and embarrassment can be part of the psychologic impact. This not only affects the family but also the child, for society expects control over that area of the body by 3 to 4 years of age. See Table 12–5 for a summary of ages and stages for elimination development.

Toilet Training

Early in the infant's life, each elimination pattern is reflexly controlled. The bladder empties when the fullness stimuli creates the need to empty. The bowel empties in relation to the gastro-colic reflex, a peristalsis movement induced by stomach fullness. As the infant matures neurologically, these reflexes become organized as part of the coordinated control system. Thus holding on and letting go develops and matures to effectively establish an individual pattern of elimination. However, there is a very wide range of normal elimination patterns for children (Dunn, 1996).

After the first meconium stools of the neonate, the stool color and frequency depends on food types. For infants who are breast fed, the stools are unformed, soft, bright, golden-yellow to slightly light yellow in color. They have many small stools per day early in life, with stools changing to a range of one per

Table 12–5   AGES AND STAGES: ELIMINATION DEVELOPMENT

Infant/Toddler
   Early elimination pattern reflexly controlled
   Breast-fed infants have unformed, soft, bright, golden yellow to slightly light green stools, several
      small stools per day, changing to a normal range of 1 per day to 1 every 10–14 days
   Formula-fed infants have firmer stools that are dark yellow to brown, depending on the formula and
      iron supplement, with 2–4 per day, changing to 1–3 per day after 1 month
   Stool color and consistency change as solids are introduced
   Well-hydrated infants urinate from 6 to 12 small amounts in 24 hours
   Starting toilet training—may be completed both day and night

Preschooler
   Bowel evacuation on regular pattern, 1 to 3 per day to 1 every 3 to 4 days
   Urination 8 to 14 times per day
   May be toilet trained day and night

School-aged child
   Toilet trained completely

day to as infrequent as one every 10 to 14 days. Infants who are formula fed have firmer, more formed stools that are dark yellow to brown, depending on the type of formula and iron supplements. They initially have more stools per day the first few weeks of life, then usually have one to three per day by the first month of life (Deloian, 1996).

At approximately 1 year of age, many children are able to be trip scheduled—taken to the toilet on a regular basis—for bowel and bladder elimination and can stay dry. This depends on an adult consistently being attentive to the child's non-verbal signals that indicate that the need to evacuate the bowel or empty the bladder and taking the child to the toilet quickly so that he or she can let go in the toilet. Some children still remain unpredictable in the number and times of stooling, which makes trip scheduling much more difficult, unless there are very attentive adults.

Many cultures are able to facilitate the child's being continent at an early age because of their expectations for success. In countries where disposable diapers of all sizes are readily available and used because of convenience, children may develop continence much later. Control during the day may come sooner than at night, because of convenience and expectation. The desire for parents and children to get an uninterrupted night of sleep, thus choosing not to be disturbed, may delay the night-time drive to be trained.

The child's system generally is ready for training with the maturation of sphincter muscles and myelination of the pyramidal tracts at about the time he or she can sit and walk well, or between 12 to 18 months. The child must also cognitively be able to understand the desire to eliminate and be able to communicate that awareness to an adult. Psychologic readiness includes the desire to please the parent by holding on and letting go at the appropriate times, as well as a desire to be autonomous and in control of that process.

Alterations and Pathophysiology

Children with major bowel and bladder alterations fit into three broad categories: those children with normal sensation and bowel and bladder functioning who are developmentally delayed in cognition, language, and skills necessary for understanding the meaning of the messages coming from the body about bowel and bladder functioning and expectations regarding becoming continent; those with conditions that cause neurogenic bowel and bladder dysfunction, such as spina bifida and spinal cord injury; and those children with psychosocial environment concerns not specifically related to delays or chronic illness. Usually the difficulty in learning to be continent is multifaceted.

Alterations Related to Developmental Delays

Children with delays in the development of skills necessary for understanding toilet training at the chronological age that society expects children to be continent often eventually develop continence when their cognitive functioning reaches the age of 3 or 4 years. The major reason for their inability to respond to toilet training at the chronological age when children are expected to be continent is that they are not cognitively and motorially mature enough to accomplish that task. Other issues for children with delays that may create difficulty in toilet training are problems with constipation, diarrhea, night-time liquid nutrition feedings, motor delays affecting the child's ability to care for the diaper area of the body, and adults assuming responsibility for the child's diapering needs and not teaching the child step-by-step self-care for changing needs. Other issues include complex sensory integration and processing problems that affect the child's ability to perceive messages of fullness and need to empty; bladder infections; lack of proper equipment to support sitting; disposable diapers made for older children that are so absorbent the child has no sensation of wetness or being uncomfortable.

Alterations Related to Neurogenic Bowel and Bladder Dysfunction

The bladder, urinary outlet and sphincter, rectal musculature, and the rectal sphincter are controlled by somatic and autonomic nerves exiting the spinal cord at the sacral level. In addition, conscious control of micturition and defecation occur at the cerebral level. Neurologic conditions that affect the reflex and conscious functions of the brain and spinal cord frequently result in neurogenic bowel and bladder. Children and adolescents with bowel and bladder incontinence related to neurogenic conditions require a interdisciplinary team approach.

Neurogenic Bladder

Each child with neurogenic bladder dysfunction should have the benefit of regular evaluations by a pediatric urologist to determine the function and condition of the urologic system and to establish the most appropriate techniques for management of the child's incontinence. Urologic testing may include ultrasonography to determine the status of the bladder, ureters, and kidneys and to rule out complications such as bladder stones, bladder diverticulae, vesicoureteral reflux, renal damage, or lesions such as cysts or tumors. An intravenous pyelogram (IVP) may give more definition to structures if abnormalities are found, as well as defining functional capacities of the urinary tract. Bladder pressure is evaluated with a voiding cystourethrogram, and vesicoureteral reflux can be identified. A cystoscopy, or internal examination of the bladder, can identify irregularities of the bladder wall, as well as stones. Regular evaluation and monitoring for urinary tract infection (UTI) is also necessary, because UTIs are common in children with neurogenic bladder. Blood urea nitrogen (BUN) and serum creatinine also are performed on a regular basis to evaluate kidney function.

For normal micturition to occur, the brain and spinal cord must work in a coordinated manner. Parasympathetic, sympathetic and somatic pathways carry messages through the spinal cord at the S2-3-4 level to the sacral micturition center. If not interrupted by disease or injury, sensory messages continue up the spinal cord to the brainstem and the frontal cortex. If inhibition occurs due to voluntary control, micturition does not occur. If there is no inhibition from the cerebral cortex, micturition occurs. Without cerebral control, the reflex arc extending from the bladder to the sacral micturition center and back again causes a reflex response to bladder fullness of urination (Pires, 1995). Higher cerebral functions provide coordination of bladder contraction with sphincter relaxation, as well as taking into account the sociocultural aspects of the situation, such as the appropriate time and place to urinate. If there is interruption of this complex process by neurologic damage, then incontinence, increased bladder pressure, or inadequate emptying of the bladder may occur. Symptoms that eventually result include UTI, vesicoureteral reflux and renal damage, bladder stones and diverticulae, as well as social embarrassment and skin breakdown from chronic wetness. See Table 12–6 for summary of the types of neurogenic bowel and bladder dysfunction. Many chil-

---

Table 12–6 TYPES OF NEUROGENIC BOWEL AND BLADDER DYSFUNCTION

1. Uninhibited neurogenic—uninhibited contractions cause complete emptying of bowel and/or bladder

2. Reflex neurogenic (upper motor neuron or spastic)—uncoordinated contractions cause partial emptying of bowel and/or bladder

3. Autonomous neurogenic (lower motor neuron or flaccid)—hypotonic or absent reflexes cause partial emptying of bowel and/or bladder with overflow, may have continuous leakage of urine or feces

4. Sensory or motor paralytic—empties bowel and bladder with timed schedule

dren with neurogenic bladder dysfunction do not have a single type of dysfunction, but mixed types.

Neurogenic Bowel

Evaluation of bowel function is performed by history and physical examination, by digital examination of the rectum to rule out impaction, by abdominal radiographs to determine presence of stool in the colon, and occasionally by rectal sphincter electromyographic measurements to determine the degree of sphincter function. It is important to obtain a diet history and list of current medications. Often the physiatrist on the interdisciplinary team is involved in bowel evaluation and management, whereas children with more complex symptomatology may be referred to a gastroenterologist.

Bowel function, as with bladder function, depends on the coordinated actions of the nervous system and abdominal and rectal musculature, with sensory and motor messages conveyed by the spinal cord tracts. The gastrointestinal (GI) system is unique in that it has its own nervous system, the enteric nervous system, that allows the GI system to function separately from conscious control. Moderation of this functioning can be effected by autonomic nervous system stimulation from the brain (Gender, 1996). Digestion and movement of a bolus of food through the GI tract occurs without conscious control. The defecation reflex occurs when the fecal mass enters the rectum, and is strengthened by a reflex arc from the rectum through the sacral spinal cord. The sensation of rectal fullness stimulates the conscious response to hold or to defecate by inhibiting or not inhibiting the external rectal sphincter. Recruitment of abdominal muscles is used to aid in defecation and is under voluntary control. The internal sphincter of the rectum is not controlled voluntarily, whereas the external sphincter is controlled voluntarily. Most children with neurogenic bladder also have neurogenic bowel, because the enervation of both structures arises from the sacral spinal cord level. Cerebral coordination of defecation also is a factor that may be affected by cognitive deficits.

Upper motor neuron lesions are those above the T12-L1 level, and the reflex arc remains intact. Lower motor neuron lesions occur below this level, and reflexive activity is lacking. An intact reflex arc usually results in automatic emptying of the bowel every 2 to 3 days or according to a regular program.

An areflexive bowel is associated with flaccid internal and external sphincters and frequent emptying of stool. Children with this type of neurogenic bowel generally require a daily bowel program (Edwards-Beckett & King, 1996).

Alterations Related to Psychosocial Concerns

Bowel and bladder elimination problems related to psycho-social concerns are most common with the child who is developing typically but has either not established age-appropriate continence or for some reason has become incontinent. Stress within the family is often the cause; however, there are times when a child chooses not to become continent because of secondary gains.

The child with a disability may have a psychosocial problem that causes continence to be more difficult to achieve. For example, Tim, a 9-year-old with cerebral palsy, was able to be bowel and bladder continent until his family moved and he was placed in a new neighborhood school. The stress of moving and attending a new school was just enough of a psychosocial stressor for him to become incontinent. The fact that there were sources of new stimuli and thus distractions from the environment caused Tim to become less focused on his newly learned skill of continence. Once he had settled into the new school and routine, he was able to become continent again.

Possible Complications in Elimination Pattern

Constipation

Constipation occurs when the stool consists of small, dry, hard, formed balls that are hard to pass. Absence of stool for several days or straining to pass stool can be misinterpreted in an infant as constipation. Infants who receive breast milk may have long periods between stooling, especially after the first month, when the gastrocolic reflex has diminished. If the stools are infrequent but soft, it is not seen as constipation.

Usually in infants, actual constipation is seen when they are not taking in enough fluids. This could be caused by a variety of conditions: (1) poor oral motor skills, (2) lethargy related to illness, (3) low muscle toner, (4) medications, (5) inexperienced or uninformed mothers, (6) illnesses that change the characteristics of the stool, or (7) intestinal and rectal malformations. For infants who are using formula, mothers report constipation related to iron-fortified formula. There is no evidence from research that this causes constipation, however, many mothers continue to believe that it does and seek to remedy this situation by changing formula to low-iron or from milk-based to soy-based formula.

Constipation in older children easily can be related to poor intake of fluids, increased loss of body fluids as in increased drooling, or colds, poor diets, decreased activity, withholding because of painful experiences with passing stool, or illness. Children with conditions such as cerebral palsy, delayed motor development, Down syndrome, spina bifida, and dystrophies and atrophies that cause low muscle tone and thus decreased activity levels are at very high risk for constipation. Children who have experienced physical or sexual abuse are also at high risk for constipation.

Constipation over a long period of time can create sustained stretching of the intestinal wall, which makes intervention much more long-term and problematic. Often by the time a family seeks assistance and locates a professional with experience plus adequate knowledge for long-term intervention, the child has started producing hard stools that are the size of baseballs. This, of course, causes micro tearing of the rectal mucosa, increasing the likelihood of the development of hemorrhoids, pain and fear with passing if sensation is present, poor appetite, and possibly vomiting, bloating of the abdomen, low-grade fever, irritability, and sometimes passing of small amounts of liquid stool. Constipation also may cause difficulty with bladder functioning and bladder programs because of the increased pressure in the lower abdominal cavity.

Impaction is defined as lack of ability to pass stool, with the transverse colon distended with hard stool. Sometimes the first indication of an impaction is the passage of liquid stool with small pieces of hard stool. Essentially what has happened is the outer layer of the hard stool is sloughing off and pieces of the hard core are being passed with it. This process can be misinterpreted as diarrhea and treated thus, causing increased problems with the impaction.

Medications also can cause increased risk for constipation. The anticholenergics often given to children with neurogenic bladder conditions are noted to dry out the mucus membrane and increase the risk of constipation.

Infants who are breast fed and are already at high risk because of disability or chronic conditions may experience problems with constipation when they are first started on rice cereal and bananas. Green, watery stools are a sign of diarrhea, and the infant's primary health care provider must be contacted.

Anticipatory guidance and prevention are related to educating the mother/parents to avoid giving the infant foods such as bananas, which may cause constipation. When rice cereal is started, the mother can be alerted to also start small amounts of dilute juice in order to avoid constipation. Research shows that milk is the only food found to be constipating, so for children over the age of 1 year, milk intake can be limited to 16 to 24 ounces per day (Schmitt & Mauro, 1992).

Prevention of constipation is the most effective treatment. Infants and children who experience low muscle tone such as those with Down syndrome, spina bifida, muscle diseases, and cerebral palsy are at high risk. The nurse must diligently educate the family regarding adequate fluid and fiber intake, causes of constipation, preventive measures, and professionals to contact, if necessary, for further treatments. In addition to the diagnosis of low muscle tone, there are many possible situations that may place the child at risk for constipation. See Table 12–7 for a summary of causes of constipation for children who are at risk.

Programs used to manage constipation must be very finely tuned to each child's needs and condition. Inadequate intake of fluids is a major cause of constipation. If the child will not drink water, then use of frozen juice bars, Jello, and foods that contain high contents of water may be the best choice. The fiber and fluid intake may cause the child to feel full and thus disrupt the intake of adequate calories for growth. Adding unprocessed bran to cereals or other foods may be the best solution. If this method is used, the intake of fluids must also be monitored because adding bran to the child's diet may put him or her at higher risk for constipation if fluid intake is not adequate. Sometimes there is no simple technique for increasing the intake of fiber foods or fluid intake, and medications need to be used.

For example, J.J. was a 6-year-old with pervasive developmental delays who had severe constipation and stooled about every 2 weeks. His abdomen would become distended, he would significantly decrease his intake, and he would first pass liquid, then hard stool.

Table 12–7   POSSIBLE CAUSES OF CONSTIPATION FOR CHILDREN WHO ARE AT RISK

Change from breast milk to formula or other milk

Introduction of bananas and/or rice cereal

Excessive drooling related to teething and/or difficulty keeping mouth closed

Illness and fever without compensation of increased fluid intake

Change in diet, fluid intake, exercise, bowel habit patterns, or caretakers

Transition times such as starting school, vacations, hospitalizations, and surgeries that may interrupt the bowel and fluid intake routine

Change of caretakers and patterns for children who are dependent on an adult for feeding of foods and fluids

Use of medications, i.e., those for bladder management, pain, or decongestants

Increased loss of fluids related to respiratory illnesses and allergies

His intake consisted of ice-cream bars, cereal of certain types, milk, white bread, mashed potatoes, and pasta without vegetables. His only intake of fruit was small amounts of applesauce, which he took with medications used for management of seizures and activity. He refused to try any new foods or liquids. The only option that was effective was to add Senokot to applesauce each morning and evening. Gradually, over about a 6-month period of time, J.J. started stooling every other day. The pediatric rehabilitation nurse working with this family had to maintain weekly contact to adjust the amount of medication and monitor J.J.'s stooling pattern. If he became ill or had situations where he did not get the usual amounts of liquid, further difficulties with the bowel program would occur. See Table 12–8 for management of constipation.

Dysreflexia

Autonomic dysreflexia, a life-threatening condition, is seen most often in children with complete spinal cord lesions at or above the thoracic sympathetic outflow (T6 or T7). With a lesion at or above this level, the system that provides feedback between the sympathetic and parasympathetic branches of the autonomic nervous system is disrupted. Therefore, if overstimulation of the autonomic system occurs because of an irritant, such as a distended bowel or bladder or skin stimuli such as heat, cold, pressure, or pain below the spinal cord injury, a sympathetic response develops.

The symptoms of the response are acute and result in a significant increase in blood pressure; a pounding headache; feelings of anxiety with sensations of nausea; sweating profusely above the level of injury but "goose bumps" below; blotchy, flushed skin on the face and neck; blurred vision; stuffy nose plus cardiac and respiratory irregularities; increased spasticity; and possible seizures (Huston & Boelman, 1995; Pires, 1995). Children are not able to alert their care-givers when the symptoms of autonomic dysreflexia occur. The pediatric rehabilitation nurse must be vigilant to detect the signs and take the appropriate steps to reduce symptoms immediately as well as to teach interventions to all care providers.

Interdisciplinary Management of Bowel and Bladder Dysfunction

Bladder Dysfunction

Although management of bladder dysfunction is the responsibility of the interdisciplinary team, it is most often the pediatric rehabilitation nurse who works most closely with the family and the child in establishing the program. The bladder program most often is formulated and prescribed by a urologist, or sometimes the physiatrist or pediatrician.

Bladder management for the child with a disability or chronic condition is based on the type of dysfunction that is present. Types of bladder management methods include (1) timed programs; (2) intermittent catheterization of the bladder, either clean or sterile; (3) indwelling urinary catheters; and (4) surgical interventions.

Timed programs most commonly are used for children with developmental delays, with cognitive deficits, and who do not have spinal cord involvement. A timed program consists of placing the child on the toilet at intervals to encourage urination. Determination of the child's pattern and frequency of urination, as well as the child's readiness to learn and interest in the process, is important. Positive reinforcement for the desired response, combined with a matter-of-fact attitude rather

Table 12–8   CONSTIPATION MANAGEMENT

Dietary management with an increase in food with fiber, such as whole grains and whole-grain products, raw or cooked vegetables, preferably with skins, fruits, especially prunes, plums, and apricots, and nuts and seeds if chewing ability is well developed. Avoidance of foods that increase tendency toward constipation—those used sometimes to manage diarrhea as in the BRAT diet (bananas, rice, applesauce, and toast)—foods low in water and fiber such as cheese and white bread.

Increased intake of fluids: children need about 1.5 ounces of fluid per pound each day and should develop the habit of drinking water.

Increase in activity and exercise with attention to regular meals, activity, and sleep patterns.

Massage of the abdomen and the gluteal muscles, combined with supporting the infant's legs and hips in a flexed position on the abdomen during stooling, can provide additional pressure to assist with passage of stool.

Herbal remedies and cultural practices for management of or prevention of constipation should be explored and respected if safe.

Clearing the colon of impactions with enemas, laxatives, etc., prior to establishing a program of prevention.

Use of stool softeners to facilitate bowel evacuations.

Avoidance of long-term use of mineral oil, because it decreases the absorption of fat-soluble vitamins.

Use of supporitories to facilitate evacuation, such as glycerine, which provides lubrication, or bisacodyl (Dulcolax), which stimulates evacuation.

---

than punishment for accidents, is a hallmark of this method. To begin a timed program, the child must be able to sit on the toilet and show other signs of readiness, such as the ability to perceive wetness or a full bladder, and some interest in the process.

Because there are times in development when the child is interested in bowel and bladder training activities, it is important for the family, with guidance, to encourage the child to learn the program. One of the first places to start is when the child is developing hand functioning and can learn to remove the tabs from the disposable diaper. The child also can retrieve a clean diaper before changes. This should all take place in the bathroom, so the child gets the idea that this is the place for toileting. As the child's motor and cognitive skills progress, more responsibilities can be added to the program. An important part of involving the child in the program is assisting the child to become comfortable touching themselves in the diaper area, and to assume responsibility for that part of the body.

Intermittent catheterization (IC) is used for children with neurogenic bladder resulting from spinal cord dysfunction or neuromuscular disease. This procedure also may be used for children with traumatic brain injury in the acute phase of treatment. Insertion of a clean or sterile plastic or Teflon-coated catheter into the bladder at intervals empties the bladder and prevents retention of urine. In most cases, IC produces continence. Children with a spastic bladder may experience leakage of urine as well as vesicoureteral reflux. Use of medications to relax the bladder may be helpful, and may or may not be used along with medications to increase sphincter tone. Although IC generally is done as a clean procedure, children with frequent UTIs may be instructed by the urologist to use a sterile procedure. Also, children with immunodeficiencies or who are hospitalized may use sterile catheterizations. Although most children with a neurogenic bladder have a high bacterial count in the bladder, insertion of a nonsterile catheter is not believed to increase bacteruria or to cause infection. Frequent emptying of the bladder, in most cases, prevents high concentrations of bacteria that result in infection. Most children who use IC to manage their bladder dysfunction catheterize four to six times a day.

With IC, care must be taken to use the correct size and type of catheter. Many children with spina bifida are allergic to latex, so latex catheters are not recommended. Infants are usually catheterized with 4- to 5-French feeding tubes. Older toddlers and preschoolers may be catheterized with feeding tubes or

6- to 10-French catheters. School-age children tolerate 8- to 12-French straight catheters. In adolescent males, the prostate enlarges and a coudé catheter, which is slightly bent at the tip, may be preferred. The coudé catheter is also used for children with urethral angulation (Gray, 1996). The size and type of catheter usually is prescribed by the urologist.

Indwelling urinary catheters are used infrequently in children for long-term bladder management, because they provide a nidus for infection. The catheter may be placed in the urethra or suprapubic area of the lower abdomen. Most often, indwelling catheters are used temporarily following bladder surgery. Some spinal cord injury centers place suprapubic catheters in adolescents with cervical injuries resulting in poor hand function or loss of hand function.

Advances in surgical management of urinary dysfunction have greatly benefited children with neurogenic bladder. The use of the artificial urinary sphincter has resulted in achievement of continence for some children who would not otherwise be continent. The artificial urinary sphincter has been most useful in boys older than 8 years with spina bifida or spinal cord injury.

A more recent method, called an appendico-vesicostomy, or continent vesicostomy, uses the appendix to connect the bladder to the abdominal wall. This procedure is also known as the Mitrofanoff catheterizable channel (Kurtz, VanZandt, & Sapp, 1996). The child or parent can then catheterize the vesicostomy at regular intervals. Formation of a one-way valve prevents leakage from the vesicostomy (Kurtz, VanZandt, & Sapp, 1996). This method of catheterization is easier to manage for many children with spina bifida or spinal cord injury, and reduces the problems of reflux and bladder spasticity while maintaining continence. Frequently, the bladder is augmented with bowel or stomach tissue to increase the bladder capacity and reduce spasticity (Liptak, 1997). Procedures to tighten the internal bladder sphincter or to correct reflux may also be performed (Kurtz, VanZandt, & Sapp, 1996). The use of vesicostomy, minus the catheterizable channel, has been used for many years to reduce bladder pressures in infants and young children with spina bifida who are born with reflux or develop reflux very early.

Adolescents or adults with spina bifida or spinal cord injury who have renal damage from severe reflux may have an ileal conduit, where the bladder is connected to the abdominal wall, and urine drains into a collection bag. This procedure is rarely performed, but may be seen in older individuals. The ostomy bag is difficult to manage for many children with spina bifida, and may leak and cause odor and skin breakdown,

All children with neurogenic bladder, regardless of their management method, are at risk for UTIs. Signs of UTI in children may include

- Foul-smelling urine
- Concentrated urine
- Hematuria
- Fever
- Leaking between voids when the child usually is continent

The child with sensation will experience flank pain, abdominal pain, and a sensation of burning and pressure on urination. There are age-related differences in symptomatology of UTI in children, with younger children more likely to exhibit systemic symptoms such as sepsis, failure to thrive, irritability or lethargy, and vomiting. Older children, both school-aged and adolescents, are more likely to experience strong-smelling urine, hematuria, abdominal pain, frequency and urgency, and enuresis. All ages exhibit fever, diarrhea, vomiting, and personality or behavioral change (Miller, 1996). UTIs should be treated promptly and completely. Some children with frequent infections may take a prophylactic antibiotic or urine antiseptic medication.

Bowel Dysfunction

Establishing a regular time for bowel evacuation is important. Usually morning and evening times, after a meal, are chosen to avoid therapy and school programs, and also to capitalize on the effect of the gastro-colic reflex, which stimulates the colon to empty. Many factors affect the consistency of the stool and therefore cause constipation or diarrhea. Stool consistency affects the bowel program, and can make continence easier or more difficult to achieve. Stool consistency changes result from diet, medications, stress, and presence or absence of disease, such as colitis. Establishment of a bowel program takes into account the child's developmental level, physical abilities, and the child's and family's unique emotional and cultural needs (Edwards-Beckett & King, 1996).

For example, one child learned that eating fresh green grapes could cause him to have diarrhea, so he then balanced that out with eating bananas, which were constipating. Another young man managed his bowel program by maintaining constipation during the week, not have an evacuation at all. On Friday night he would eat spicy chili and drink at least two beers, and spend most of Saturday morning in the bathroom. He was not interested in another type of program because he had a job and this program worked for him.

A thorough assessment to determine the cause of the bowel incontinence is necessary, as well as to determine the child's usual pattern and consistency of stool. As infants, defecation occurs reflexively, and this may continue in the absence of cerebral control, such as after traumatic brain injury, spinal cord injury, or with neurologic conditions. Frequently, children with developmental delays or cognitive deficits such as occur with traumatic brain injury may be placed on a timed program, set up on a regular schedule following a meal. Children with these types of conditions often are able to "tune in" on their body cues and establish bowel continence. Presence of constipation or diarrhea may complicate the picture, and use of a glycerin suppository, at first, may be necessary to aid bowel evacuation.

Children with neurogenic bowel may have a more difficult time establishing continence. Frequently, children with neuromuscular disease are constipated, and the constipation must be corrected before the bowel program is initiated. Generally, this is done by cleaning out the bowel with an enema or an oral laxative. Depending on the amount of rectal tone and the child's diet, stool softeners may also be needed in the long term. Ideally, stool consistency is managed with adequate fluid and fiber intake, but many children with spina bifida, neuromuscular disease, or spinal cord injury are very picky eaters and tend not to choose high-fiber foods. It is best to start out children early with a high-fiber diet to develop as many desirable food habits as possible.

Once the bowel is cleaned out, a program is begun that consists of sitting on the toilet at the same time every day. Again, after a meal, in the morning or the evening, is generally best. Children with poor rectal tone may need to use a medicated suppository such as bisacodyl (Dulcolax) to stimulate rectal contractions. Some children with spina bifida and many children with spinal cord injury use a method called digital stimulation, where the defecation reflex is stimulated by a gentle, circular movement of a gloved finger inserted a short way into the rectum. Children with an intact reflex may benefit from this method. A complete record of the amount, characteristics, and frequency of the child's stool should be kept to monitor for problems, such as diarrhea or constipation, and to determine the child's pattern.

For children who are born with neurologic conditions that affect bowel function, interventions to maintain bowel tone and prevent constipation begin in infancy. Frequently, children with spina bifida already have a history of constipation with enlarged colon and rectum by the time they start school. Beginning prevention early by teaching the parents what types of stools constitute constipation, and intervening when necessary with dietary measures or medications when necessary, will help to maintain bowel tone and aid in establishing a bowel program that the child can perform independently.

Developing Independence in Bowel and Bladder Care

The child should be involved in the performance of the bowel and bladder program as young as possible. Participation, in the form of helping to gather supplies, assistance in the removal of clothing, and becoming familiar with the routine, is a good place to start, and depending on the child's physical and cognitive abilities, may begin as early as 2 to 3 years of age. By age 8 or 9 years, most children should be performing the majority of their bowel and bladder program, including timing, frequency, gathering the necessary materials, cleaning up, and keeping track of the size and consistency of the stool (Edwards-Beckett & King, 1996).

Establishment of a behavioral program supports the child's performance of independent bowel and bladder care and serves as a motivator for the child. Positive reinforcement of desired behaviors and rewards that are appropriate to the child's likes and dislikes are helpful. Modeling of positive toileting behaviors by parents is a good learning experience for young children. Punishment is counter-productive.

Often, children who have limited sensation may fail to take an interest in the bowel and bladder program, especially if they are not involved with the program early in life. Many times it is easier for the parents to just get the program completed and move on to one of many other tasks they need to perform. Although this may be easier at the time, it creates more difficulties in the long run. In children with congenital or early occurring disabilities that affect bowel and bladder function, the older the children when they start becoming involved in the program, the more difficult it is to establish independence. Participation in self-care camps and sports programs, where other children or young adults with disabilities can model independence in self-care, can be of great help in this situation.

Rehabilitation Nursing Management

Assessment

Assessment of the child or adolescent for excretory function and altered bowel and bladder elimination includes

- Child's developmental level and motor functioning skills
- Child's behavioral functioning patterns
- Past and present elimination patterns
- Past and current variations in elimination patterns and usual method of management, including successes and failures
- Present health status related to elimination, focusing on the cause for altered elimination
- Dietary habits including fiber and fluid intake
- Medications related to elimination and other problems/conditions
- Child's and family's commitment to an ongoing daily management plan
- Presence of complicating factors such as frequent UTIs, reflux, or kidney disease or anomalies
- Child's cognitive and physical capabilities and family's abilities to follow through with a daily management plan
- Other resources necessary to assist the child and family in effective management, i.e., equipment, consultation
- Referrals necessary for effective management of altered elimination

If dysreflexia is present, include

- Knowledge of dysreflexia symptoms and prevention
- Identify the symptoms and determine the cause of the autonomic nervous system overstimulation
- Monitor vital blood pressure

Nursing Diagnoses

In the area of elimination, several nursing diagnoses must be considered:

Altered bowel elimination
  Constipation
  Diarrhea
  Bowel incontinence
Altered urinary elimination
  Urinary retention
  Incontinence (total, functional, reflex, urge, stress)
  Dysreflexia

Expected Outcomes

The overall expected outcomes for the child and family include

- Elimination patterns normal for child with a disability and or chronic condition
- Use of technology as necessary for accomplishing normal elimination patterns
- Prevention of dysreflexia with health maintenance practices
- Prevention of bladder infections
- Prevention of constipation
- Socially acceptable elimination program

Intervention—Teaching

Specific areas of nursing intervention and teaching related to altered bowel and bladder elimination include

- Teach self-care skills as the child grows and develops
- Encourage child to become responsible for bowel and bladder management as soon as developmentally capable
- Teach bowel and bladder retraining when appropriate
- Establish intermittent catheterization program for urinary incontinence when appropriate
- Establish bowel program that includes a specific daily time for evacuation, adequate fluids and foods with fiber, and medications, suppositories, or use of digital stimulation when appropriate
- Resolve psychosocial concerns before implementing a continence program; may require referral to behavioral therapist

If dysreflexia is a problem:

- Elevate head of bed
- Remove the source of overstimulation immediately (empty the bladder, check the rectum and remove fecal material, check for other sources of skin overstimulation)
- Use local anesthetic for catheterization of bladder or catheterize bladder without local anesthetic

- Use topical anesthetic ointment to remove fecal material in bowel
- Teach prevention to children at high risk for dysreflexia as well as their families and all caregivers (Huston & Boelman, 1995; Pires, 1995)

SUMMARY

For many children, the problems of bowel and bladder incontinence are ignored until the child enters school and it becomes a social problem. An interdisciplinary team of professionals must establish an effective continence program and support the child and family while they are learning the protocol. The pediatric rehabilitation nurse may be the key professional to provide the ongoing support, to teach the child and family, and to be available for consultation and intervention when problems occur. Although early education of the components of continence and skin care is important, effective skin care may also be taught during the continence program.

SKIN INTEGRITY

The key functions of the skin are to protect the body from injury and microorganisms, assist with temperature regulation, provide for sensation of touch, protect from cold and trauma, provide calorie storage, excrete toxins from the body, and provide a place for expression of emotions through blushing and sweating. It is the largest organ of the body (Barber, 1996).

Expected Development and Physiology

Management of skin integrity problems for the child without delays, disabilities, or chronic conditions accounts for about 20% to 30% of all visits to a pediatrician's office (Hurwitz, 1993). Conditions such as rashes, bacterial infections, furuncles (boils), impetigo, yeast infections such as thrush, and herpes simplex infections are the most common conditions. The development of the skin continues throughout life (Rudy, 1991).

The three major layers of the skin are (1) the epidermis, which is the barrier layer; (2) the dermis, which is the supportive structure for body tissues; and (3) the subcutaneous fat layer, which assists in insulating the body as well as providing a cushion from trauma. The epidermis can regenerate new skin cells every 28 days (Nicol & Hill, 1994). The skin of infants has the adult melanin level by 1 year of age, and vascularization is well developed by age 3 years. Eccrine sweat glands are fully functional in the preschooler, the sebaceous glands become active during the school-age years, and the adolescent has active apocrine glands and continued development of cutaneous nerves. More information on the anatomy and physiology of the skin can be found in Chapter 21.

Alterations and Pathophysiology

Pressure Sores

Pressure sores are the most common skin integrity problem seen in pediatric rehabilitation and are the most serious healthcare problem in the United States. These sores are caused by unrelieved pressure, shearing, or friction. They are related to immobility, lack of skin sensation, poor nutrition, age, circulatory dysfunction, incontinence, medications, and psychosocial issues (Braden and Bergstrom, 1989).

Skin breakdown is most common with children who have insensate skin, such as those with myelodysplasia or spinal cord injury. However, skin breakdown is also seen in children who have skin sensation but are immobile and therefore cannot change their position to relieve the pressure, such as children with dystrophies and atrophies, as well as the child with severe developmental delay. Even children too ill to move or be moved may have pressure ulcers.

Although the location of the skin breakdown usually is over a bony prominence where there is insensate skin, it can also develop in other areas, especially where the skin barrier has been broken by trauma. Children with immune deficiency are also at high risk for skin breakdown difficulties. For the infant with myelodysplasia, the first problem with skin breakdown may occur after surgical repair of the back when the infant is immobilized and positioned to protect the surgical site. Once home, the older infant may experience skin breakdown when starting to pull along the floor on the tummy. Because the child does not have lower extremity strength to crawl, the unprotected insensate toes, malleolus, or knees are dragged along, creating a friction-type ulceration. Children with braces are also at high risk for skin breakdown over a bony prominence. Later, when the child spends more time in a wheelchair, skin breakdown may develop due to lack of pressure relief measures.

Heat and cold can cause skin breakdown, as well as injuries. Burns can result from hot metal playground equipment, indoor heaters, very hot drinks, and hot water. Heat lamps, hair dryers (to dry moist skin), and heating pads should not be used on children with insensate skin. Exposure to the cold may cause frostbite, which can result in loss of toes, particularly if children do not wear adequate shoes and stockings.

Infants with neurogenic bowel and bladder may leak urine or stool constantly and are at risk for development of severe diaper rash. Older children who wear diapers are also at risk for skin breakdown from wetness and should be changed frequently, no matter what the bladder and bowel management program. Other causes of wetness for children with insensate skin include wet swimming clothes and perspiration.

Other Skin Conditions

The pediatric rehabilitation nurse must not overlook the conditions caused by other factors. For children who develop a rash and are being treated with a new anticonvulsant, the nurse must be concerned about an allergic reaction to the medication and take appropriate steps to assess the situation.

Often, children with frequent antibiotic treatment or prolonged use of systemic steroids develop Candida infections. The skin located in warm and moist areas, such as diaper areas, oral mucosa, and areas around tubes such as gastrostomies or tracheostomies, is the most susceptible (Harvey, 1996).

Chronic Skin Conditions

A chronic skin condition, epidermolysis bullosa (EB), which is a group of genetic diseases, varies from mild to life-threatening. Blistering of the skin and mucous membrane occurs with even slight trauma, as well as spontaneously. Skin care regimes begin at birth, usually because the birthing process causes the first blisters. Although this is a very rare condition, the pediatric rehabilitation nurse, especially in the community, may have an opportunity to provide care, teaching, and case management for children with this condition. These children are at very high risk for infections, growth and developmental concerns, feeding problems related to friction caused by sucking, continuous specialized skin care management, and psychosocial isolation (Gibbons, 1990).

Preventative Skin Care

Prevention of skin breakdown begins with maintaining a clean, dry skin surface. Moist skin should be avoided, as it contributes to maceration of the skin and breakdown. The use of powders to dry moist skin is not recommended, particularly in infants, who can inhale the powder, resulting in respiratory distress. However, very dry skin may crack and lead to skin breakdown. Skin should be supple, well hydrated, and maintain a healthy color for the child's skin tone. Use of massage over and around bony prominences has not been found to be an effective method of pressure sore prevention (Buss, Halfens, & Abu-Saad, 1997).

Wrinkles in clothing or bedclothes or heavy seams in clothing should be avoided to prevent red, irritated areas. Socks should be pulled smooth, again avoiding wrinkles or lumps, before shoes or braces are applied. Tight clothing, such as tight jeans, are not recommended in order to prevent pinching of the skin and undue pressure. Shearing and friction, the sliding of skin against other surfaces, can result in burns and skin breakdown. When transferring children, or moving them in bed, do not drag them, but lift or roll them, supporting all joints and parts of the body. Use of a turning sheet or sliding board may be helpful.

Frequent changes of position to avoid prolonged pressure on bony prominences is recommended, particularly for children who lack skin sensation and for children who are unable to change position themselves. Children with spinal cord injury may need to build up skin tolerance after injury, and increase the amount of time they can sit or lie in one position. The use of bridging pillows or rectangular pillows to position around bony prominences in order to relieve the pressure can be very helpful and can prolong the time spent in one position. All children who are unable to move by themselves, regardless of their diagnosis, should be positioned with proper body alignment when lying or sitting, to prevent formation of contractures and skin breakdown.

Nutritional factors may increase risk for skin breakdown. The child who is very obese or the child who is very underweight are both at risk. Nutrients must be available in adequate amounts both to prevent skin breakdown and to promote healing. Adequate amounts of B-complex vitamins; vitamins D, E, A, and C; trace minerals such as iron, zinc,

Teaching Box: Prevention of Skin Breakdown

Avoidance of High-Risk Situations

- Heat—keep child away from heat sources such as heaters, hot water pipes, fireplaces, metal playground equipment that has been in the sun, very hot beverages; test bathing water carefully before putting the child into the water (see Chapter 21 for information on burns). Do not use heating pads, heat lamps, or hair dryers on insensate skin areas.
- Cold—be sure that children wear adequate socks and shoes in cold weather and that they are not exposed to the weather for long periods, such as when waiting for the bus. Children who take part in winter sports should take special care when dressing to protect vulnerable feet, especially toes, and take frequent breaks inside in a warm environment, checking for color change and signs of frostbite in extremities.

Consistent Skin Care and Monitoring

- Check areas of insensate skin at least daily, preferably morning and night, to detect changes. Skin should be inspected for presence of redness, change in temperature, blistering, or breaks in the skin. If an area is red, apply pressure to check for promptness of capillary refill. If the color does not return to the skin promptly, damage has extended into the deeper tissues and the child's health care provider should be notified. Areas on the buttocks or back of the legs should be inspected using a mirror.
- Skin should be kept clean and dry at all times. Light-weight clothing with good air circulation is best for hot climates.

- Avoid shearing and friction when moving on surfaces.
- Clothing should be applied without wrinkles. Very tight clothing should be avoided. Socks should be smoothed to prevent wrinkles, taking care not to compress the toes. Shoes should fit well and not pinch.
- Braces should be removed at regular intervals and skin underneath checked for pressure areas, especially when new or with young children. This procedure should also be followed if there is any damage to the braces.
- When sitting in a wheelchair, weight shifts are performed every 1 to 2 hours, more frequently if there is a history of skin breakdown. Weight shifts may consist of a 'push up,' pushing on the arms of the chair so as to lift the buttocks off the seat; side shifts, where the child leans to one side or another, enough to lift partially off the seat, or a forward lean, which takes the weight off the tailbone. Each weight shift should be held for at least 10 seconds.
- Wheelchair cushions come in various types and are made of a number of different substances. Whichever type is chosen, the cushion should be regularly checked to ensure that it remains in good repair.
- When lying down, turn to change position regularly. Some children may need to use bridging cushions to position bony prominences off of the bed surface. Maintain proper body alignment using pillows as necessary. Use of pressure-relieving mattresses or overlays such as sheepskin, eggcrate cushion, or other devices may be necessary.

Teaching Box: Prevention of Skin Breakdown *Continued*

Maintain Good Overall Health
- Maintain or improve range of motion in joints. Contractures may contribute to skin breakdown.

- Assist the child to maintain an average body weight and good nutrition. Extremes of weight, either very heavy or very thin, increase risk of skin breakdown.
- An active, involved life promotes overall health and can decrease the risk and severity of skin breakdown.

---

and copper; and magnesium and calcium are particularly important (Kunz, 1996). Adequate protein also is necessary.

Children who have joint contractures are also at risk for skin breakdown. The contracture may prevent proper positioning of the limb and contribute to pressure. Spasticity, resulting in intermittent, involuntary movement of a limb, such as rubbing on a sheet, can cause a friction burn and result in skin breakdown. Spasticity may also result in body movement that causes poor positioning or moves the child out of the proper position.

Pressure-relieving devices such as wheelchair cushions and mattresses can also relieve pressure and prevent skin breakdown from occurring. A variety of devices are on the market, some as simple and inexpensive as a foam eggcrate mattress, to an air-filled bed that continually alternates pressure. Wheelchair cushions also come in a range of designs and prices, ranging from a high-density foam cushion, a gel cushion that mimics natural tissue, and high-priced alternating pressure cushions. No matter what type of mattress or wheelchair cushion is used, maintenance and regular inspection of the equipment itself is necessary to identify failure or malfunction that can result in pressure sores.

Rehabilitation Nursing Management

Assessment

All skin surfaces, especially those over bony prominences, should be examined at least daily, more frequently if the child has multiple risk factors or has an existing pressure sore. Skin areas where there were prior pressure sores are at a higher risk for skin breakdown due to the presence of scar tissue. As the hormonal changes of adolescence begin, skin increases in oil production and the risk of skin breakdown increases. Children most

likely to have difficulty with skin breakdown are those with spina bifida, spinal cord injury, or other neuromuscular conditions that alter mobility and sensation. Vascular ulcers are unusual in children, with most skin breakdown resulting from friction, unrelieved pressure, or extreme heat or cold.

Redness of the skin, a differential in warmth between one skin area and another, or an open area necessitate further assessment and intervention. If the skin area is reddened, put slight pressure on the reddened area to check for capillary refill. A rapid return to color is indicative of early stages of skin breakdown and prolonged blanching suggests deeper injury and interruption of circulation. Palpation of the area may indicate boggy areas or hardened areas, also indicative of tissue breakdown or inflammation extending beneath the skin. The appearance of the area of skin breakdown should be fully documented including the size of the lesion, the shape, the approximate depth or extent of the lesion, and the appearance of the tissue. Exact measurement is preferred over estimation.

Pressure ulcers are classified to more accurately and consistently determine extent and severity. One of the most common systems is that of the National Pressure Ulcer Advisory Panel (NPUAP), which grades pressure sores according to four stages. The grades are

- Stage I: erythema of intact skin that does not blanch
- Stage II: partial-thickness skin loss; superficial ulceration; abrasion, blister, shallow crater may be present
- Stage III: full-thickness skin loss; damage involves underlying subcutaneous tissue, but remains superficial to deep fascia
- Stage IV: full-thickness skin loss with deep, extensive destruction of tissues to the muscle, bone, and support structures (NPUAP, 1989)

Expected Outcomes

The desired outcomes for the child and family include

- Prevention of skin breakdown
- Education about specific skin care technology and its use
- Appropriate utilization of skin care technology
- Elimination of skin integrity alterations at Stage I

Interventions

La Mantia (1996) lists four priorities of nursing interventions for skin breakdown, which are adapted here for the child and adolescent.

1. Eliminate or reduce the effects of primary and secondary factors for skin breakdown and development of the wound
2. Provide the optimal microenvironment for the skin
3. Provide support to the child and family during treatment
4. Ensure the education of the child according to developmental level and communication needs, and educate the family in prevention and care

The cause of the pressure ulcer or other skin breakdown must be identified and addressed before healing can commence. Incontinence, other sources of moisture or soiling, spasticity or contractures, nutritional status, and sources of pressure and irritation are all potential causes. Wound healing occurs from the bottom, or deepest area of the wound, to the skin surface. Cleansing the wound, debridement of necrotic tissue, and treatment of any infection present is necessary. Wounds or ulcers often produce a large quantity of exudate, which must be absorbed. Moistness of the skin is critical to healing, because the natural tissue environment is moist. Absorptive dressings that loosely pack the wound serve to fill in any open areas. Covering the wound helps to maintain the natural environment and keep out any foreign substances, as well as protect the area (La Mantia, 1996).

A large variety of different types of wound care products and dressings exist, designed to maintain the natural tissue environment and to promote healing. Most products provide protection for the wound, differing amounts of absorption of exudate, and different types of wound "filler." Although discussion of the many types of wound care products are beyond the scope of this section, it is advisable to investigate the properties of the various products before using one of them.

Other options for treatment of persistent or difficult to heal pressure ulcers include the use of hyperbaric oxygenation and electrical stimulation. Surgical management of pressure ulcers is usually considered for stage III or stage IV ulcers, those that are very large, or for children who require early mobilization or who have osteomyelitis. If osteomyelitis is present, intravenous antibiotics are necessary and, in severe cases, surgical debridement may be required before a skin flap can be used to surgically cover the ulcer. Postsurgical care of the child requires an interdisciplinary team approach. Although chronic or very severe osteomyelitis resulting from pressure ulcers is unusual in children, it may occur in the presence of complicating factors such as extreme neglect of care on the part of the child or caregiver.

When considering which type of product or dressing to use, take into account the following factors:

- The appearance and stage of the ulcer or wound
- The child's general health and other risk factors, such as presence of spasticity that may dislodge some types of dressings or the condition of the skin around the area of breakdown that may not support adhesive dressings
- The cost and availability of the product or treatment method
- If the child or family are to provide wound care at home, the ease or difficulty involved in applying and monitoring the product
- Frequency of clinic or home visits to monitor wound healing

Once the area of skin breakdown or pressure ulcer has healed, care must be taken to build up the skin tolerance by reintroducing pressure cautiously. Increased frequency of weight shifts or position change is often required, and the area must be inspected several times a day to detect unfavorable changes. It is imperative that the child and family put into practice preventative interventions.

SUMMARY

Although most children with disabilities and chronic conditions are less vulnerable to skin breakdown from pressure than adults with similar conditions, children experience alterations in skin integrity that interfere with the rehabilitation process and threaten their health. Effective prevention, treatment, and follow-up for skin breakdown in children includes knowledge of skin care and interventions, as well as developmental factors. Nurses contribute greatly to the care and treatment of children with skin breakdown through assessment, intervention, and education.

ACTIVITY—EXERCISE PATTERN

Movement, and activities that result from movement, are very important to the child's overall development. This functional pattern includes not only mobility but also activities of daily living and leisure and recreational activities. Play for the developing child is the major form of leisure and recreation (Gordon, 1994). Mastery of early motor skills, beginning with head control, is necessary for self-care skill development. Activity for the developing child is important for healthy functioning of the physical body and motor learning and for cognitive and psychologic development.

This functional health pattern includes activities that require expenditure of energy, such as mobility, exercise, and activities of daily living (Gordon, 1994). The patterns of activity that get established during childhood may have long-term effects upon the health and well being of the person as an adult (Burns, 1996). For children with disabilities and or chronic conditions, the development of healthy patterns of activities and exercise can be very important, because they may need these to compensate for other areas.

Healthy People 2000: National Health Promotion and Disease Prevention Objectives for the Year 2000 (U.S. Department of Health and Human Services, 1990) includes objectives for the child and adolescent with a disability. These objectives focus on reduction of the number of children who are overweight, who do not participate in leisure time physical activity, who experience adverse health effects from stress, and who sustain a secondary disability after a serious head or spinal cord injury. Objectives also focus on increasing of the proportion of newborn screenings by state-sponsored programs for genetic disorders and other disabling conditions and the number of service systems and preschools for children with, or at risk for, chronic conditions and disability.

It has been written that the youth of the United States are not as fit as those of other countries (Kuntzleman, 1993). This also includes those children with developmental delays, disabilities, and chronic conditions. There are often no opportunities for these children to be involved in sports or other activities. Special Olympics International, perhaps the best known group, has sports training and athletic competition programs for children with mental retardation, which may include other types of disabilities and chronic conditions. There are also other recreation and sports organizations that make it possible for the child to be active and competitive. Sometimes the best activities are created by willing parents and coaches in the community in which the child lives and goes to school. Many children also have the opportunity to participate in adaptive sports and physical education programs in the schools.

Expected Development and Physiology

Movement and development of motor skills may be an insurmountable task for the child who is physically limited or restricted by disability. Adaptive devices and therapy must be provided to assist with compensation so children can progress along a developmental path. Learning through movement is a major aspect of development; therefore, exploration of the environment by activity must be readily available to the child.

Toddlers, for example, often are seen as "little motor creatures," and when a gross motor task such as walking is being learned, other developmental tasks stop or slow in their progress. All of the child's energy is directed toward the gross motor learning. At an older age, the child still is controlled by motor movement and not cognitive assessment of the situation. For example, the child who is running into the street for a ball is not able to problem solve what to do about the possibility of cars and danger. Movement is in charge and going for the ball is the priority. Only words in the "danger voice" of an adult may call a halt to the running.

Have you seen a young child learning to drive an electric wheelchair? They go charging ahead no matter what the obstacles. They take such delight in being able to move that they just cannot attend to what may be in their way, so the path must be cleared so that their need to move is not restricted. With learning, they are able to incorporate the wheelchair into their sense of self and become mindful of not "hurting it," just as a child learns to walk around obstacles in his or her way. This happens at about 2½ to 3 years of age. See Table 12–9 for a summary of the expected development of motor skills.

Alterations

For the child with a disability or chronic condition, learning to be independent in self-care requires being developmentally ready at the optimal time to learn a skill, having the energy and motivation, having assistance available to teach the child and family, and having adaptive equipment to allow the child to be as independent as possible. If the developmental time for learning is not used, the child may not feel responsible for self-care activities.

Children born with disabilities may not have the needed sensory input and muscular control for bowel and bladder continence, and it is this deficit that complicates the toilet training process. However, these children do go through a normal developmental stage where they want to assist with taking their diapers off, sit on the potty chair, or stand to void just like other males in their home. Showing interest in the process of eliminating like other members of the family, or like peers in child care or pre-school, provides developmental cues that the child is ready to move on with independence skills.

Developmental cues must be taken as direction for further independence in self-care skills, with bowel and bladder programs created to reinforce the child's developmental drives. Often when bowel and bladder continence with adaptations is needed because of societal expectations such as starting kindergarten, and the child has not been encouraged up to that point to become as independent as possible, the child may not be interested in learning the skill because energy is focused on learning other tasks. Adolescence is a time for self-care independence with the ability to integrate complex cognitive functioning skills.

Table 12–9 AGES AND STAGES: DEVELOPMENT OF MOTOR SKILLS

Infant/toddler
   Fading of general reflexes such as moro, startle, asymmetric tonic neck, and those involving the extremities such as palmar and plantar grasp and Babinski, which controls movement early in life
   Movement from totally dependent on adult for all self-care needs to being able to cooperate with dressing by extending arms and legs, and removing socks and hat
   Movement from dependent in ability to change positions to walking without support
   Movement from hands fisted to open with the ability to open and close hand, use eye-hand coordination for play with objects
   Throws ball forward
   Rides tricycle using pedals alternately
   Runs, jumps, walks stairs (up and down) using feet alternately
   Dresses with supervision and assistance for fasteners
   Self-care skill development
   Uses spoon
   Washes and dries hands

Preschooler
   Refinement of gross and fine motor skills
   Runs through obstacles, still bumping into them
   Copies letters and numbers
   Takes responsibility for toileting needs, may still need help with wiping
   Uses fork and napkin
   Bathes when reminded
   Self-care skill learning completed with refinement continuing

School-aged child
   Fine motor skills necessary for school work
   Disappearance of gross and fine motor awkwardness
   Refinement of movement in space, such as jumping while clapping hands

Adolescence
   Use fine and gross motor skills in competitive sports
   Assumes responsibility for self-care skills and decisions, focusing on their management

Sources: Vaughn & Litt, 1990; Betz, Hunsberger, & Wright, 1994.

Chronic conditions, such as cardiac and pulmonary diseases, may limit the child's energy for certain diversional activities. This may create a social problem because the child feels unable to participate in the physical activities. It is the responsibility of the family and the rehabilitation team to assist the child in making adaptations to continue to be active and participate.

Risk of Injury

Injury continues to be the leading cause of death in children 19 years and younger (Betz, Hunsberger, & Wright, 1994). Children with developmental delays and or chronic conditions are also at general risk for injury, as well as injury related to their specific disability. For children who have delays in their ability to problem solve, who are impulsive and very active, injuries can occur because of the inability to be safe in their environment. Injury prevention is an essential component in the plan of care.

For example, one child who was severely cognitively delayed but ambulatory enjoyed playing outdoors. The school staff had been working on teaching him how to rotate his hand, a skill needed for opening doors. One day he came home from school and his mother thought he was safe from going outside because he couldn't open doors. Her usual routine was to allow him to play in his room before dinner. After several minutes of silence, she went to check on him and he was nowhere to be found. He had used his new skill and opened the door, going out to play without supervision. In situations where risk of injury is possible, communication and consistency between all providers of care is very important. What may seem a big accomplishment for a child and his or her therapist may make added stress for the family in their environment, so communication is extremely important.

Children who have sustained traumatic brain injuries and those with learning disabilities (LD) and attention deficit hyperactive disorder (ADHD) are at high risk for other injuries. They usually have impulsivity, poor motor planning, and memory problems that cause them to be at high risk for other injuries.

Children using mobility equipment are at risk of injury, and rolling their wheelchair off the curb or over a bump can increase risk for falls. Proper safety equipment must be made available and the child instructed in the correct, safe use of all equipment. A conflict may exist between the desire to allow the child more independence with the wheelchair and the desire to reduce the risk of accidents. Parents and professionals must use their best judgment to help promote independence while maintaining reasonable safety.

Children with chronic medical conditions or disabilities are sometimes overprotected and kept from beneficial activities because of fear of injury. Certainly children with cardiac conditions must be under the care of a cardiologist and have specific exercise prescriptions. Children with respiratory conditions may be restricted from exercise, but properly managed asthma, for example, should not preclude participation in exercise.

Safety and prevention of injury must be a part of the treatment plan and shared with all caregivers and school personnel. Children with seizures usually are encouraged to exercise, but choice of activities must be made with information regarding usual seizure activity and control. It is important to exclude children from activities that would put themselves or others at risk if they had a seizure, such as swimming, other water activities, or climbing activities (Burns, 1996).

Sometimes children unknowingly are prevented from an activity because of fear of injury. This occurs with a young child just learning how to climb or move against gravity. Because of the fear of falling, the child is restricted from attempting and learning how to motor plan a new task. Good motor planning skills are essential to moving safely.

Families are often fearful for a child who has recovered from surgery for hydrocephalus. Questions about the restriction must be well spelled out through consultation with the physician or surgeon. If the child's head needs to be protected, there are lightweight helmets that can be used, allowing the child to continue to explore the world without risk of injury and without restriction of motor learning.

Rehabilitation Nursing Management

Assessment

The pediatric rehabilitation nurse's role is to teach the child and family, foster interventions established by other team members, and assess areas of need from a developmental and health care perspective. Included in the assessment would be the following areas:

- Developmental level, cognitive ability, and motivation to perform own self-care activities and be mobile
- Caregiver's desire to have the child as independent as possible or to infantilize the child
- Need for adaptive/assistive equipment
- Need for physical therapy (PT) and occupational therapy (OT) assessment and treatment
- Energy available for mobility, transfers, self-care activities, sports, leisure activities
- Usual daily routine including self-care, exercise, and leisure time activities
- Child and family goals specific to functional activity
- Physical examination and observation of activities—screening for need to be referred to other rehabilitation professionals
- Comprehensive assessment of cardiopulmonary and neuromuscular ability as necessary
- Use of functional ability measurement scales

Nursing Diagnoses

Self-care deficit
  Feeding
  Toileting
  Bathing/hygiene
  Dressing/grooming
Activity intolerance
Diversional activity deficit
Impaired physical mobility
Disuse syndrome

Desired Outcomes

The desired outcomes for the child and family include

- Activities and self-care will be appropriate for developmental age
- Variety of activities will contribute to overall growth and development
- Technology and equipment will be used when necessary to provide the support for the child to accomplish developmental tasks and participate in a variety of physical activities

Each child is a unique individual who presents challenges for the multidisciplinary team, especially in the areas of mobility and self-care. In the functional areas of mobility and self-care, specialized equipment and technology can often effectively facilitate a ther level of independence, which then supports the child in achieving a higher level of developmental success (Trefler, Hobson, Taylor, Monahan, & Shaw, 1993).

Mobility is of most importance in relation to development. The infant learns about the world by movement and eventually becomes able to differentiate the self from the world. It is important that every person has the ability to be independent in mobility. For children with severe neuromotor impairment, without the ability to move, cognitive, perceptual, and functional development is limited. Therefore, effective means of self-propelled mobility must be a priority. Decisions must be made regarding the type of device based on the child's developmental skills, energy available for mobility, and their environment. When they are cognitively aware of their space and want to be in different positions and places for exploration, they need the ability to move at will. If movement of a system uses all the child's energy and leaves none for other functional activities or play, then it is important to consider a motorized system. Research and clinical experience indicate that children around 15 months cognitively can safely manage motorized mobility devices (Bailey & Gilbert, 1989).

Even an infant younger than 6 months realizes that sitting upright to view the world is more interesting than being flat and seeing only the ceiling or suspended toys. For the young child who is still in the home, self-propelled systems may be appropriate, but as the child's world expands into group settings, playgrounds, and the community, a powered system may be advantageous.

To be able to move as fast as everyone else in your peer group is important and supports self-esteem. Even the child with a high level spinal cord injury may want to play baseball with his wheelchair as an extension of himself. Thus it is important for the child to be able to power the chair over the field rapidly and successfully, just as if the child were running. Accessibility, transportation, and cost may be seen as impossible challenges, but the child's needs should be of utmost importance. With a focused, creative, and motivated rehabilitation team, the challenges can be overcome, freeing the child to achieve mastery over mobility difficulties. Chapter 14 provides additional information on assistive technology.

For children with neuromotor difficulties, appropriate positioning for effective mobility may also be a challenge. There is a large variety of seating systems and also teams of specialists who can be resources to the child and family. The nurse must be knowledgeable and able to make referrals to centers for specialized mobility and seating systems that are the most effective in meeting the child's individual needs.

Play has been described in Chapter 11 as a method of assessing and evaluating a child's level of functioning and determining how the environment fosters development. Observation of patterns of play provides information about stress and coping, present level of functioning, themes of separation, and boundary problems. Play can be used as a method of skill development or to strengthen existing motor and self-care abilities. It is important to have an understanding of the play activities appropriate at each level of development and to create an environment that optimizes the child's potential for growth. Some of the functions of play are

- Assessment of a child's perceptions and feelings
- Help the child make sense of experiences, especially painful ones
- Facilitate ability to cope and release tension
- Provide an escape into diversional activity

As part of the nursing process, the pediatric rehabilitation nurse can assess the child's need to play, develop a "play play," and integrate it with other aspects of rehabilitation care and treatment. This plan should include

- Provision of appropriate opportunities to play
- Encouraging expression of emotions and feelings
- Adapting the environment and equipment to the abilities of the child
- Preparation of parents to participate in play and continue it in the home environment

The nurse must assist all caregivers to include play that is developmentally appropriate as the child matures and to create an environment where play is encouraged.

SUMMARY

For the child with a disability or chronic condition, the task of learning to be independent in self-care may be seen as difficult and time consuming. However, through the use of developmentally staged play and other fun activities, care can be successfully learned. As the child becomes independent in care and mobility, the stage is set to participate in sports and leisure activities.

SLEEP–REST

Sleep, rest, and relaxation are included in this pattern (Gordon, 1994). Children must have a balance of sleep, rest, and relaxation to be able to grow and develop. The physical, psycho-social, and environmental factors of the child all combine to provide the opportunity for this balance. The stages in the development of sleep-rest patterns are found in Table 12–10.

Expected Development

Sleep Patterns

Sleeping through the night is viewed as a sign of maturation and growth. Parents say a baby who sleeps long is a good baby. In the current family lifestyle, with all of the adults working, stress increases if the baby awakens during the night after about 3 months. Children initiate many behaviors that support their ability to self-calm and get themselves to sleep. If children have the opportunity to get themselves to sleep, their ability to return to sleep when awakened during the night is greater. Children who are placed in their cribs asleep have not had that opportunity and often are less able to get themselves back to sleep. Some normal behaviors young children use to assist with getting themselves to sleep are repetitive, rhythmic activity such as head turning and body rocking; sucking a pacifier, thumb, or blanket; using transitional objects such as a favorite blanket, toy, or pillow; and music (Feber & Kryger, 1995).

When a child is old enough cognitively to understand separation from mother, sleep is viewed as separation. Because separation is perceived as stressful, transitional objects are of great assistance to help the child go to sleep. As the child matures, gaining control over the body is a major task and affects sleep patterns. The child, if permitted, will decide to set the sleep time. That may not coincide with the family's pattern. Depending on the family's discipline patterns, the child's temperament, and other stressors in the child's life, this control issue may become a major stressor for both parents and child.

Consistency of method and interventions is most important. As cited in many childcare books and articles in popular parent magazines, sleep problems are perceived as very disruptive and parents often seek assistance managing them. At times all families are in need of education, anticipatory guidance, and even intervention to alleviate the stress pro-

Table 12–10   AGES AND STAGES: DEVELOPMENT OF SLEEP-REST PATTERNS

Infant/toddler
   Newborn sleeps 10 to 23 hours/day with no diurnal pattern
   By 2 months may start to sleep through the night for 10 hours with 3 daytime naps
   Breast-fed infants may be slower to sleep through the night than bottle fed
   REM sleep ⅓, deep sleep ⅔ by 3 months
   By 6 months most infants sleep through the night
   Twenty-five percent who sleep through the night may start awakening between 6 to 12 months
      during REM sleep
   Organization of sleep with light/dark cycle by 1 month
   Use rhythmic stimulation to assist with soothing and falling asleep—either by caregiver or self-
      induced, such as sucking, head or body rocking
   Tend to sleep on back or stomach
   Use transitional objects 9 months to 3 years for self-calming and getting to sleep

Preschooler
   Give up daytime napping
   Gradual decrease in body shifting at night
   Tend to sleep on their sides

School-aged child
   Average 8 to 9.5 hours in bed, asleep 95% of the time
   Have average of one to three brief awakenings
   Fall asleep in 20 to 25 minutes

Adolescent
   Often sleep long hours and short hours
   Wide range of needed sleep over 24 hours
   May need to enforce regular sleep routine
   May need more sleep but get less
   Tend to stay up later at night and sleep later in the morning

Sources: Betz, Hunsberger & Wright, 1994; Feber & Kryger, 1995; Vaughn & Litt, 1990.

duced by a child who has taken charge and refuses to go to sleep at the expected time, stay asleep, return to sleep when awakened, or sleep in the expected place.

Positioning for Sleep During Infancy

The American Academy of Pediatrics (AAP) recommends that infants use the side-lying or supine position for all sleep during the first 6 months of life, unless that is contraindicated by a medical condition (AAP Task Force on Infant Positioning and SIDS, 1992). This position significantly decreases the incidence of sudden infant death syndrome (SIDS) (Spiers & Guntheroth, 1994).

Alterations

Infants and children with developmental disabilities or chronic conditions are at high risk for sleep pattern disturbances. They may have been unable to develop a successful pattern due to disruptions while in the hospital early in life or they may have their patterns disrupted by hospitalizations, medical or sur-

gical interventions, family stress, extra feedings, repositioning, or treatments.

Premature infants have a different sleep pattern. They awaken as often as every 2 hours until the corrected age of 4 months, and many are not able to sleep 8 hours without awakening until the corrected age of 8 months (Gorski, 1988). Other studies indicate that for premature infants without medical complications, disorganized sleep has not been noted (Feber & Kryger, 1995).

Infants born with oral-facial defects may experience sleep difficulties of varying degrees. Infants born with cleft lip and palate or cleft palate have noisy breathing, especially before the surgical repair of the cleft, when they are congested due to upper airway infections, or after surgery because of short-term localized edema. Usually this type of difficulty does not cause obstructive apnea. However, it is important for the infant to be clinically assessed and positioned to allow for successful air exchange. Those with Pierre Robin syndrome may have sleep pattern disturbances because of obstructive apnea.

Children with cerebral palsy or those who

have been exposed to cocaine prenatally may have a very disrupted sleep pattern related to neurologic immaturity or damage to the sensory-perceptual and regulatory systems. They awaken during the night, which may cause them to hyperextend their body and extremities, thus becoming overaroused. Their situation, combined with their difficulty in self-calming, causes them to have problems returning to sleep without adult intervention.

Usually, the adult has developed a routine to assist the child to get to sleep during the first part of the night, so the same routine needs to be carried out to assist them in getting back to sleep. The child also may be very sensitive to overstimulation from the environment, so little sound may cause awakening. One example of this occurred with a little girl, Nellie, who was 9 months old. She had been noted to be developmentally delayed but had not been diagnosed with a specific condition. When the pediatric rehabilitation nurse was completing an assessment in the home, she learned that Nellie had difficulty sleeping through the night. Her mother had already learned that Nellie needed to be wrapped tightly and placed on her back between three pillows, one touching the top of her head and one at each side for her to settle. She had also learned that any light, even a small night light, would awaken Nellie and that sometimes hunger awakened her, especially if she did not eat enough during the day. Another factor in Nellie's sleeping problem was very active play with her older sister shortly before bedtime. The nurse discussed with the mother how stimulating active play right before putting the child in bed to sleep could be and mentioned other activities that might be incorporated into the bedtime routine to help Nellie begin to sleep through the night.

Children with spina bifida and Chiari II malformation are at high risk for sleep apnea, snoring, and stridor. These children are also at risk for sudden respiratory arrest. Use of a cardiac/apnea monitor is recommended and the parents must be trained to perform cardiopulmonary resuscitation (CPR). Interruption of sleep patterns may also occur because of the child's need for repositioning to prevent pressure areas and skin breakdown. Cardiopulmonary conditions easily can produce restlessness and sleepless nights, especially in children with respiratory conditions who may awaken with coughing. Anoxia, chronic or acute, can also disturb sleep.

Seizures may be a cause for sleep disturbances. If the seizures occur at night, it is important to avoid the risk of apnea or respiratory difficulty. Children with seizures may need to be electronically monitored at night for safety. If the seizures are during the day and the child has a pattern of post-ictal sleep, their night-time patterns may be disrupted. Attempts to interrupt the post-ictal state usually are not successful (Feber & Kryger, 1995).

Children who experience trauma, such as brain injury, may have significantly altered sleep-wake patterns. These usually result from acute management of the trauma, which interrupts the sleep pattern. Medications often used for children with ADHD may cause difficulty with falling asleep. If that is a problem, the timing of the medication must be reassessed and adjusted.

If normal night wakening becomes a problem for the family, the situation needs to be assessed to determine if the child's response to wakening is the problem, as opposed to the wakening itself (Feber & Kryger, 1995). Caregiver fatigue may be a tremendous stressor for families who have a child who needs treatments, observations, and feedings during the night long after the child should have been expected to be able to sleep through the night. The caregiver's fatigue increases even more if the child has difficulty returning to sleep or establishing a successful sleep pattern after being awakened for nightly treatments. Sleep disturbance problems are highly related to maternal stress (Quine, 1991). Table 12–11 lists other causes of sleep alterations in children.

Rehabilitation Nursing Management

The pediatric rehabilitation nurse working in the hospital and community must be alert to the problems that sleep disturbances can create within the family and be able to assist with meaningful intervention.

Admission to the hospital places the child in a very strange environment. For the child who needs structure to feel secure and successful, sleep routines are very significant. Often the family has established a routine that is effective for them and their child and, if at all possible, the nurses within the hospital need to be sensitive to continuing those routines. Experiencing an extended hospitalization after birth, trauma, surgery, or active rehabilitation, the infant or child may sleep on the hospital schedule and need familiar hospital routines, sounds, lighting, positioning, and swaddling to effectively sleep. That may

Table 12–11 CAUSES OF ALTERATIONS IN SLEEP

Hunger, especially in children with feeding difficulties and congenital heart conditions

Coughing from respiratory conditions

Fatigue related to illnesses or anemia

Inconsistent patterns of family responses to awakening, sleeplessness, and late sleeping

Separation anxiety and abandonment issues

Anxiety, fears, stress, night terrors, and nightmares

Need for treatments or medications during the night

Overprotection by parents

Specific conditions that make self-calming difficult to learn, such as difficulty getting the hands to the
mouth for sucking, poorly modulated sensory systems that affect the child's ability to habituate to
auditory, visual, or tactile stimuli, or extensor tone that may cause overarousal

Pain or general discomfort

Medications with stimulation, agitation, or euphoric effects such as corticosteroids, caffeine, and those
used for attention deficit disorders

Sleep apnea related to obstruction, positioning, or central apnea

---

be difficult to recreate at home and may seriously disturb family life and integration of the child into the home. Monitors can also be an added stressor and affect sleep for the entire family. In some situations, the mother and father started sleeping in separate rooms because of the child's needs and later were able to return to sleeping together.

Assessment

Some sleep disturbances are part of normal development. The role of assessment for sleep pattern disturbances is to determine (1) if the problem is a part of normal development; (2) if it is occurring because of a temporary situation such as pain, hospitalization, or family stress; (3) if it is a problem because of some medical condition such as sleep apnea, seizures, or ear infections; or (4) if it is a problem because of lack of successful self-calming activities, sensory overload, or lack of training for successful sleep. There are several critical times when sleep must be part of the rehabilitation assessment. Table 12–12 outlines the specific areas to be included when assessing sleep patterns.

Discharge planning is a most important component of preventing sleep alterations. Evaluation of the night routines related to treatments, medications, and procedures routinely given at night must be reassessed and moved to a schedule that more closely ap-

proximates and supports family life. This may be the role of the case manager, the family, or the nursing staff; no matter who initiates the transition, it must not be overlooked or left until the day before the child is being discharged. Many infants and children are able to habituate to the sounds and lights of the hospital and establish regular sleep patterns; however, many do not and need intervention even in the hospital setting.

Nursing Diagnosis

Sleep pattern disturbance

Expected Outcomes

The desired outcomes for the child and family include

- Child receives enough sleep, rest, and relaxation to meet individual developmental needs
- Child's environment supports meeting these needs

Intervention—Teaching

Understanding the causes of sleep alterations and establishing a successful intervention can be very complex and requires a interdisciplinary team approach, including the family and child. There may be times when the nurse

Table 12–12   ASSESSMENT FOR SLEEP CONCERNS

General medical history and physical examination

Social and psychologic history

Developmental screening and complete assessment, if necessary

Sleep history including sleep log for 2 weeks if possible

Environment—where the child sleeps

Parent-child interactions

Cultural practices

Family's perception of the sleep alterations, current, past, and onset of problem (best to talk to all adults involved with sleep problem)

Child's description of sleep problem (if old enough to respond)

Treatment already attempted, what worked, what didn't

Problems at night or nap (if still napping)

Predictability of problem by preceding events during the day or child's condition at bedtime (occurs only when overtired, illness, transitions such as starting school, stress within family)

Related to bed wetting

If reliable history difficult to obtain, discussion should be continued until family and child can provide information (this may be very time consuming, but data are important to determine cause and appropriate interventions)

Sleep studies in a pediatric sleep laboratory

Table 12–13   SUGGESTED METHODS OF SUPPORTING SUCCESSFUL SLEEP

For children with positioning difficulties and excessive drooling, the side-lying positioning is recommended, i.e., cerebral palsy, Pierre Robin syndrome

Establishment of regular bedtime and awake time

Daily exercise in the morning may strengthen sleep

Avoid exercise late in day, because it may create difficulty with calming and restful sleep

Night-time routine to enhance calming, i.e., warm bath, shower

Avoidance of caffeinated beverages

Decrease daytime naps

Successful management of pain

Teach relaxation techniques

Support verbalization of fears and concerns that delay successful sleep

For chidren with painful joints, use of an electric blanket or other warm bedding may assist in enhancing restful sleep

Use of water beds may be effective for some children if they are safe

Management of medications needed for attention deficit disorders to avoid side effect of disturbed sleep pattern

Swaddling, rocking, self-calming activities

and family determine there is a sleep pattern disturbance, but the family does not see it as a priority for intervention. For example, Joe, a small boy with cerebral palsy and severe seizures, not well controlled, would go to sleep after much work to get him settled in his parents' bed. His father would check on him periodically until he was ready to retire. Then he would sleep with Joe, and Joe's mother would sleep by herself in another room. The family was happy with this arrangement and did not want to make changes. As the nurse began to establish a close relationship with the family, it was learned that Joe's parents were staying married just because of Joe and that the father took the night-time responsibility for Joe and the mother took the daytime responsibility.

Of course, there may be times when the successful sleep routine that the family has establish does not seem possible at the hospital. If, however, the family has worked for months to get a 6- to 8-hour block of continuous sleep, the staff may need to diligently work toward keeping the same schedule, if safe for the child. Sleep retraining must be an intervention that is planned and may take a interdisciplinary team approach to be successful. Changing of sleep routines and locations should be made when the child's life has been stable for a period of time and not disrupted by illness, hospitalization, or other stressors. Table 12–13 gives suggested methods of supporting successful sleep that can be incorporated into the plan of care.

SUMMARY

Sleep, rest, and relaxation are valuable for successful growth, development, and wellness. For the child with a disability or chronic condition and the family, having the pleasure of a healthy balance in all components may not be consistently possible. The pediatric rehabilitation nurse's role is to assess and identify problems and facilitate interventions including teaching, to treat and prevent problems in the area of sleep and rest.

CONCLUSION

The pediatric rehabilitation nurse uses the nursing process to identify needs and problems in the areas of nutrition, elimination, activity, sleep, and skin integrity. Appropriate interventions are selected that contribute to health and development, and the nurse provides ongoing support, teaching, and consul-

tation for the child or adolescent and family in these vital areas. Assisting the child or adolescent with a disability or chronic condition to be as independent as possible in self-care activities enables him or her to participate more fully in all aspects of life at home, in school, and in the community.

REFERENCES

American Academy of Pediatrics Task Force on Infant Positioning and SIDS (1992). Positioning and SIDS. *Pediatrics*, 89, 1120–1126.

Anderson, J. (1994). Tips when considering the diagnosis of food allergy. *Topics in Clinical Nutrition*, 9(3), 11–21.

Bailey, J., & Gilbert, E. (1989). Mr. Crenna couldn't rest—and neither could we. *Nursing*, 19(11) 50–51.

Bandini, L., Patterson, B., & Ekvall, S.W. (1993). Cerebral palsy. In Ekvall, S.W. (Ed.). *Pediatric nutrition in chronic disease and developmental disorders*. New York: Oxford University Press, pp. 93–99.

Barber, N. (1996). Dermatological diseases. In Burns C.E., Barber N., Brady M.A., & Dunn A.M. (Eds.). *Pediatric primary care*. Philadelphia: W. B. Saunders, pp. 717–737.

Betz, C., Hunsberger, M., & Wright, W. (1994). *Family-centered nursing care of children* (2nd ed.). Philadelphia: W.B. Saunders.

Braden, B., & Bergstrom, N. (1989). A conceptual schema for the study of the etiology of pressure sore. *Rehabilitation Nursing*, 12(1), 8–16.

Burns, C. (1996). Activities and sports for children and adolescents. In Burns C.E., Barber N., Brady M.A. & Dunn A.M. (Eds.). *Pediatric primary care*. Philadelphia: W. B. Saunders, pp. 289–311.

Buss, I., Halfens, R., & Abu-Saad, H. (1997). The effectiveness of massage in prevention of pressure sores: A literature review. *Rehabilitation Nursing*, 22(5), 229–234.

Chumlea, W. (1993). Growth and development. In Queen, P., & Lang, C. (Eds.) *Handbook of pediatric nutrition*. Gaithersburg, MD: Aspen, pp. 3–25.

Chwals, W. (1994). Overfeeding the critically ill child: Fact or fantasy? *New Horizons*, 2(2), 147–155.

Cochran, E., Phelps, S., & Helms, R. (1988). Parenteral nutrition in pediatric patients. *Clinician Pharmacy*, 7(5), 351–368.

Deloian, B. (1996). Developmental management of infants. In Burns C.E., Barber N., Brady M.A., & Dunn A.M. (Eds.) *Pediatric primary care*. Philadelphia: W. B. Saunders, pp. 81–101.

Deloian, B. (1996). Developmental management of toddlers and preschoolers. In Burns C.E., Barber N., Brady M.A., & Dunn A.M. (Eds.). *Pediatric primary care*. Philadelphia: W. B. Saunders, pp. 101–123.

Deitz, W.H. (1987). Nutrition and obesity. In Grand, R.J., Sutphen, J.L., & Dietz, W.H. (Eds.).

Pediatric nutrition: Theory & practice. Boston: Butterworths.

Dorsey, L., & Diehl, B. (1992). Fostering improved nutritional status for the pediatric burn patient. *Rehabilitation Nursing*, 17(6), 338–339.

Dunn, A. (1996). Elimination pattern. In Burns C.E., Barber N., Brady M.A., & Dunn A.M. (Eds.). *Pediatric primary care*. Philadelphia: W. B. Saunders, pp. 277–289.

Dunn, A., & Evers, C. (1996). Nutrition. In Burns C.E., Barber N., Brady M.A., & Dunn A.M. (Eds.). *Pediatric primary care*. Philadelphia: W. B. Saunders, pp. 205–258.

Edwards-Beckett, J., & King, I. (1996). Bowel control in children. *Rehabilitation Nursing*, 21(6), 292–297.

Ekvall, S. (Ed.) (1993). *Pediatric nutrition in chronic diseases and developmental disorders*. New York: Oxford University Press.

Ekvall, S., Bandini, L., & Ekvall, V. (1993). Obesity. In Ekvall, S. (Ed.). *Pediatric nutrition in chronic diseases and developmental disorders*. New York: Oxford University Press, pp. 165–172.

Ekvall, S., Ekvall, V., & Frazier, T. (1993). Dealing with nutrition problems of children with developmental disorders. *Topics in Clinical Nutrition*, 8(4), 50–57.

Feber, R., & Kryger, M. (1995). *Principles and practice of sleep medicine in the child*. Philadelphia: W.B. Saunders.

Gender, A. (1996). Bowel regulation and elimination. In Hoeman, S. (Ed.) *Rehabilitation nursing: Process and application* (2nd ed.). St. Louis: C.V. Mosby, pp. 452–475.

Gibbons, S. (1990). Care of epidermolysis bullosa patients: A nursing challenge. *Dermatology Nursing*, 2(4), 195–200.

Glass. R.P. & Lucas, B. (1990). *Making the transition from tube feeding to oral feeding. Nutrition focus for children with special health care needs*. Seattle: University of Washington, pp. 1–6.

Gordon, M. (1994). *Nursing diagnosis, process and application*. St. Louis: Mosby.

Gorski, P. (1988) Fostering family development after preterm hospitalization. In Ballare, R. (Ed.). *Pediatric care of the ICN graduate*. Philadelphia: W. B. Saunders, pp 27–32.

Gray, M. (1996). Atraumatic urethral catheterization of children. *Pediatric Nursing*, 22(4), 306–310.

Harvey K. (1996). Bronchopulmonary dysplasia. In Jackson, P., & Vessey J. (Eds.). *Primary care of the child with a chronic condition*. St. Louis: Mosby, pp. 172–192.

Hurwitz, S. (1993). *Clinical pediatric dermatology*. Philadelphia: W.B. Saunders.

Huston, C., & Boelman, R. (1995). Autonomic dysreflexia. *American Journal of Nursing*, 95(7), 55.

Hutsler, D. (1991). Nutritional monitoring of a pediatric burn patient. *Nutrition in Clinical Practice*, 2(6), 11–17.

Kenny, D., & Judd, P. (1988). Oral care for developmentally disabled children: The primary denti-

tion stage. *Infants and Young Children*, 1(2), 11–19.

Kramer, S., & Eicher P. (1993). The evaluation of pediatric feeding abnormalities. *Dysphagia*, 8(3), 215–224.

Kuntzleman, C. (1993). Childhood fitness: What is happening? What needs to be done? *Preventive Medicine*, 22(4), 520–532.

Kunz, K. (1996). Management of pressure sores. In Kurtz L.A, Dowrick, P.W, Levy S.E., & Batshaw M.L. (Eds.). *Handbook of developmental disabilities. Resources for interdisciplinary care*. Gaithersberg, MD: Aspen, pp. 361–369.

Kurtz, M., VanZandt, K., & Sapp, L. (1996). A new technique in independent intermittent catheterization: The Mitrofanoff catheterizable channel. *Rehabilitation Nursing*, 21(6), 311–314.

La Mantia, J.S., Hirschwald, J.T., Goodman, C.L., Wooden, V.M., Relisser, O., & Stass W.E. (1987). A program to reduce chronic readmissions for pressure sores. *Rehabilitation Nursing*, 12, 22–25.

Lobo, M., Barnard, K., & Coombs, L. (1992). Failure to thrive: A parent–infant interaction perspective. *Journal of Pediatric Nursing*, 7(4), 251–161.

Liptak, S. (1997). Neural tube defects. In Batskow, M. (Ed) *Children with disabilities*, (4th ed.). Baltimore: Paul H. Brookes, pp. 529–552.

Miller, K. (1996). Urinary tract infections: Children are not little adults. *Pediatric Nursing*, 22(6), 473–479, 544.

Morris, S.E. & Klein, M.D. (1987). *Prefeeding skills: A comprehensive resource for feeding development*. Tucson: Therapy Skill Builders.

National Pressure Ulcer Advisory Panel (1989). Pressure ulcers prevalence, cost and risk assessment. Concensus development conference statement. *Decubitus*, 2, 24–28.

Nickel, R. (1996). Controversial therapies for young children with developmental disabilities. *Infants and Young Children*, 8(4), 29–40.

Nicol N., & Hill. M. (1994). Altered skin integrity. In Betz C., Hunsberger M., & Wright S. (Eds.). *Family centered nursing care of children*. Philadelphia: W. B. Saunders, pp. 1678–1717.

Orenstein, S. (1994). Gastroesophageal reflux. In Hyman, P. (Ed.). *Pediatric gastrointestinal motility disorders*. New York: Academy Professional Information Services, pp. 55–88.

Ott, C. (1994). Healthy dietary practices. In Betz, C., Hunsberger, M., & Wright, S. (Eds) *Family centered nursing care of children*. Philadelphia: W.B. Saunders, pp. 546–601.

Pires, M. (1995). Bladder elimination and continence. In Hoeman S.P. (Ed.). *Rehabilitation nursing: process and application* (2nd ed.). St. Louis: Mosby, pp. 417–451.

Quine, L. (1991). Sleep problems in children with mental handicap. *Journal of Mental Deficiency Research*, 35(4), 269–290.

Rallison, M. (1986). *Growth disorders in infants, children and adolescents*. New York: John Wiley & Sons.

Rudy, S. (1991). From conception to birth: The development of skin and nursing care implications. *Dermatology Nursing*, 3(6), 381–389.

Satter, E. (1987). *How to get your kid to eat, but not too much*. Palo Alto: Bull.

Schmitt, B., & Mauro, R. (1992). 20 common errors in treating encopresis. *Contemporary Pediatrics*, 9, 47–52, 65.

Spiers, P., & Guntheroth, W. (1994). Recommendations to avoid the prone sleeping position and recent statistics for sudden infant death syndrome in the United States. *Archives of Pediatric and Adolescent Medicine*, 148(2), 141–146.

Thorn, K. (1995). The Harris-Benedict equation: A simple plan for nutrition intervention in HIV/AIDS. *The Journal of Care Management*, 1(2), 10–18.

Trefler, E., Hobson, D., Taylor, S., Monahan, L., & Shaw, C. (1993). *Seating and mobility*. Tucson: Therapy Skill Builders.

U.S. Department of Health and Human Services (1990). *Healthy people 2000: National health promotion and disease prevention objectives for the year 2000*. DHHS Pub. No. (PHS) 91–50212. Washington, DC: U.S. Government Printing Office.

Vaughan, V., & Litt, I. (1990). *Child and adolescent development: Clinical implications*. Philadelphia: W.B. Saunders.

ADDITIONAL RESOURCES

Adair, R.H., & Bauchner, H. (1993). Sleep problems in childhood. *Current Problems in Pediatrics*, 23(4) 147–70.

Bach, C. (1992). Traveling with technology. *Rehabilitation Nursing*, 17(3), 141–146.

Baggerly, J., & DeBlasi, M. (1996). Pressure sore prevention in a rehabilitation setting: Implementing a programmatic approach. *Rehabilitation Nursing*, 21(5), 234–238.

Balsmeyer, B. (1990). Sleep disturbances of the infant and toddler. *Pediatric Nursing*, 16(5), 447–449.

Baumann, D. (1992). Coping behavior of children experiencing loss of mobility. In Miller, J. (Ed.). *Coping with chronic illness: Overcoming powerlessness*. Philadelphia: F.A. Davis, pp. 85–109.

Christiansen, C. (Ed.) (1994). *Ways of living: Self-care strategies for special needs*. Albuquerque: American Occupational Therapy Association.

Dunbar, S. (1991). The transition from nonoral to oral feeding in children. *The American Journal of Occupational Therapy*, 45(5), 402–408.

Glass, R., & Wolf, L. (1993) Feeding and oral-motor skills. In Case-Smith. *Pediatric occupational therapy and early intervention*. Boston: Andover Medical pp. 225–289.

Jimmerson, K. (1991). Maternal, environmental, and temperamental characteristics of toddlers with and toddlers without sleep problems. *Journal of Pediatric Health Care*, 5(2), 71–77.

Joyce, P., & Clark, C. (1996). The use of craniosacral therapy to treat gastroesophageal reflux in infants. *Infants and Young Children*, 9(2), 51–59.

Kitzinger, S., & Kitzinger, C. (1991). Food as metaphor. *Mothering*, 91(61), 42–47.

Klein, M., & Delany, T. (1994). *Feeding and nutrition for the child with special needs*. Tucson: Therapy Skill Builders.

Macht, J. (1990). *Poor eaters: Helping children who refuse to eat*. New York: Plenum Press.

Mast, M. (1994). Facilitating employment opportunities for people with spina bifida or cerebral palsy: The importance of individualization. In Lollar D.S. (Ed.). *Preventing secondary conditions*. Washington, DC: Spina Bifida Association of America, pp. 34–42.

Minde, K., Popiel, K., Leos, N., Falkner, S., Parker, K., & Handley-Derry, M. (1993). The evaluation and treatment of sleep disturbances in young children. *Journal of Child Psychology and Psychiatry*, 34(4), 521–533.

Nelson, C., & Halgren, R. (1989). Gastrostomies: Indications, management and weaning. *Infants and Young Children*, 2(1), 66–74.

O'Rorke, C. (1995). Helping children overcome fecal incontinence. *American Journal of Nursing*, 95(4), 16A–D.

Padgett, D. (1992). Behavior management of feeding problems. *Nutrition Focus*, 7(1), 1–6.

Palmer, M., & Heyman, M. (1993). Assessment and treatment of sensory-versus motor-based feeding problems in very young children. *Infants and Young Children*, 6(2), 67–73.

Rosenbaum, P., & Law, M. (1996). Craniosacral therapy and gastroesophageal reflux: A commentary. *Infants and Young Children*, 9(2), 69–74.

Schmidtt, B. (1992). The 'two step' approach to infant sleep problems. *Contemporary Pediatrics*, 9(11), 37–38.

Skewes, S. (1996). Skin care rituals that do more harm than good. *American Journal of Nursing*, 96(10), 33–35.

White, M. (1990). Sleep onset latency and distress in hospitalized children. *Nursing Research*, 39(3), 134–139.

Wolf, L., & Glass, R. (1992). *Feeding and swallowing disorders in infancy: Assessment and management*. Tucson: Therapy Skill Builders.

Wolff, R., & Lierman, C. (1994). Management of behavioral feeding problems in young children. *Infants and Young Children*, 7(1), 14–23.

Organizations

American Camping Association
5000 State Rd
Martinsville, IN 46151
800-428-2267
Disabled Sports USA
1145 19th Street, #717
Washington, D.C. 20036
202-393-7505
Special Recreation, Inc.
362 Koser Ave.
Iowa City, IA 52246-3038
319-337-7578

Wheelchair Sports, USA
3595 East Fountain Blvd, Suite L1Y
Colorado Springs, CO 80910
719-574-1150

Videotapes

Hays, S. R. (1993). *Potty Learning for Children Who Experience Delays*. From Clinician's View Catalog, Albuquerque.

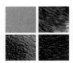

Chapter 13

Psychosocial Health Care Patterns and Nursing Interventions

Susanne R. Hays

This chapter covers six psychosocial health patterns initially discussed in Chapter 8 and the interventions associated with specific nursing diagnoses. The following patterns are included: cognitive-perceptual, self-perception, role-relationship, coping—stress tolerance, value-belief, and sexuality-reproductive. It is important for the pediatric rehabilitation nurse to have a strong foundation of knowledge regarding each of these patterns to enhance skills and nursing interventions and promote a holistic view of the child and family. Each functional pattern is briefly discussed in relation to the child's normal development, specific alterations related to that pattern, and pediatric rehabilitation nursing management. The pediatric rehabilitation nurse can use this information to enhance critical-thinking skills used in the decision-making process when providing care to the child or adolescent and family in the hospital, clinic, school, and community.

COGNITIVE-PERCEPTUAL PATTERN

The cognitive-perceptual functional health pattern includes cognitive processing, use of language, memory, judgment, problem solving and decision making, and sensory-perceptual activities such as hearing, vision, touch, smell, and taste. Additionally, comfort and pain sensation are included in this pattern because they have a significant effect on how the child or adolescent perceives and interacts with the world (Gordon, 1994). The pediatric rehabilitation nurse plays a vital role in teaching the child or adolescent and family about

specific health care problems, related treatments, and ongoing management and adaptation to a disability or chronic condition. Helping a child or adolescent learn and adapt depends on understanding how the child perceives information based on his or her cognitive developmental level and sensory-perceptual processing, as well as specific alterations in development. Table 13–1 is a summary of the important developmental tasks in these areas as the child grows from infant or toddler through adolescence.

Expected Development and Alterations

Thought Processes

Learning requires that the child be able to perceive and process information from a variety of external and internal sources. This process is very complex, and learning changes with each new piece of data. Cognitive functioning is only one part of the thought process. More in-depth information regarding cognitive development is provided in Chapter 10. Sensory-perceptual components of learning are also very important and add information to the total learning process.

As children mature cognitively, they theoretically will possess more skills and can be involved in higher levels of decision making. Allowing the child to be involved in decision making starts right after birth. When the baby cries, the mother adds her thought about the interpretation of the cry to the baby's sounds and actions and decides what to do in response to the cry. If the cues are not very clear, then the mother must decide which ac-

Table 13–1 AGES AND STAGES: EXPECTED DEVELOPMENT—COGNITIVE, SENSORY, AND PERCEPTUAL LEARNING

Infant/Toddler

First, reflex-directed activity; later, able to organize activities
Learns through senses and movement
Understands objects only as they are associated with a need (e.g., nipple for comfort)
Develops hand/eye coordination
Moves from actions being separate events to actions related to objects and in patterns that are novel
Understands that objects exist even if out of sight, sound, smell, feel, or taste
Can imitate actions
Uses trial and error to develop many ways to achieve a goal, then moves to thinking about solutions and consequences before taking action toward the goal
Uses make-believe play for learning and takes pleasure in that activity
Can retain mental images
Believes inanimate objects have a life of their own
Uses language

Preschooler

Attention span of 10–15 minutes develops to 30 minutes at 5 years
Image of the world is bound by their experiences
Judges people by one activity they did for the child
Views experiences in one direction; may not believe pain will go away because they cannot reverse their experience and remember when the pain was not there
Believes that if something moves it is alive (e.g., x-ray machine) and fears it will hurt them
Believes that two events that happen close in time are related, and may think that the first event caused the second
Believes events occur by magic
May have imaginary friends
May judge the nurse as mean if the nurse does a painful procedure

School-Aged Child

Able to share in discussion of health care with ability to take more responsibility for own care
Period of concrete operations; able to deal with objects as perceived or imagined

Adolescent

Period of formal-operational thought
Able to understand effects of proposed treatments

Data from Vaughn, V., & Litt, I. (1990). *Child and adolescent development: clinical implications.* Philadelphia: WB Saunders; and Rosen, L. (1985). *Piagetian dimensions of clinical relevance.* New York: Columbia University Press.

tion to take and may have to try several alternatives before the baby is satisfied. As the child develops the ability to understand consequences, even greater decision-making skills are needed. For example, a child may really want to explore the books up on a high shelf, which is off-limits, and must decide if the "time out," which may be the consequence, is worth the climb.

Sometimes children, because of their learning, want to be more self-directed and do tasks that are not always safe for them because they lack maturity. It is up to the adults in the family to decide which decisions the child can safely make, and therefore which tasks they can do for themselves. For example, a school-aged child may want to ride a bicycle in the street, and acknowledges the need to watch for the cars. The parent knows that the child is sincere about the request, but when the child is really busy riding and playing, the fact that a car is coming may not get the child's attention until the car is too close for safety. For the adolescent, the ability to make responsible decisions may be affected by peer pressure.

Children can experience difficulty with thought processes as a result of congenital or genetic disorders, trauma, or many unknown causes. They may have generalized thought-processing impairments, such as those present with mental retardation or developmental delays, or more specific impairments, such as those occurring with learning problems or difficulties related to brain trauma.

Children with sensory deficits may also

have impaired thought processes because of the absence or disorganization of data coming from their various sensory systems. The infant mentioned previously may become calm when hearing the mother prepare food, or if sensory deficits are present, he may not be able to interpret the sounds, sights, smells, and voice in an organized manner and may not even be able to read his own body cues about hunger until he is very hungry. Children with sensory-perceptual difficulties can also display impairments in their thought processes based on difficulty interpreting the sensory messages they receive. Some children display impaired thought processes as a result of multiple factors. This is often the situation for children diagnosed with autism.

These types of problems are the most complex, and a very skilled team of professionals is required to assist in the diagnostic and treatment processes. These children present multiple challenges; they have the most frustrating school experiences, and the family must become the child's advocate for success to take place. These children are unique in their style of learning, and the school system may not have the expertise to adequately educate them. Skilled pediatric rehabilitation nurses can help the family in understanding the problem and help them find the necessary information and resources to assist their child.

Children with attention deficit–hyperactivity disorder (ADHD) have difficulty with thought processes because of lack of attention, hyperactivity, and impulsiveness. ADHD is a complex and not well understood disorder, but it affects every aspect of a child and family's life. Boys are more commonly diagnosed with ADHD (Murphy & Hagerman, 1992), and often the diagnosis is not made until the early school years. The nurse can be instrumental in the diagnostic process and an integral member of the team in the educational setting.

Sensory Integration

The ability to perceive sensations from the environment and the body and to learn from them, thus accomplishing a self-directed activity in the environment, is basically the process of sensory integration. When an infant or developing child succeeds at integrating all the messages that come from their senses, including tactile, vestibular, visual, auditory, and proprioceptive, the child is able to take the parts and make them into a whole

response (Ayers, 1973). For example, when an older infant feels hungry and starts to cry for food, the mother can talk to the infant, providing a calming effect for a short time as the food is prepared. The infant has learned the calming sound of the mother's voice, has remembered the sound of food preparation, and can calm himself to wait in anticipation of feeding. This is a very complex nervous system process, and as the infant matures, so does the skill of integrating and making sense of the stimuli from the environment.

The senses—sight, sound, smell, taste, and touch—enable the child or adolescent to take in information and respond to stimuli, and assist in forming their perception of themselves and the environment. Alterations in any of these areas need to be detected early and corrected or treated to support optimal development.

Visual problems may result from retinopathy of prematurity, ophthalmia neonatorum, eye injuries, genetic diseases, maternal infections, refractive errors or unknown causes. Vision screening should be a part of the nursing assessment and the appropriate techniques used depending on the child's age, developmental level, and specific disability or condition. The nurse should also teach parents how to detect visual problems in the child and discuss eye care, safety issues, and prevention of injuries and damage to the eyes.

Impairment of hearing may have a significant impact on the development of speech and expected educational progress. Early detection is extremely important because it is thought that 80% of language growth has taken place by 3 years of age. Hearing loss may result from genetic disorders, pre-natal and perinatal factors (e.g., infection, ototoxic medications, metabolic disorders), and postnatal conditions (e.g., infection, trauma, neoplastic disorders). They may be classified as central (i.e., within the central nervous system), peripheral (i.e., within the auditory system), or functional (i.e., non-organic). The hearing level is measured in decibels (dB) and is used to describe the impairment. Children with normal hearing are in the 0- to 20-dB range. When assessing the child, the pediatric rehabilitation nurse should consider the following:

- degree of hearing loss
- cause and age of onset
- type of impairment
- other conditions (e.g., physical, psychosocial)

- family relationships and interactions (Scudder, 1994)

Sensory-Perceptual Difficulties

Children with developmental delays, disabilities, or other chronic conditions are at high risk for sensory-perceptual difficulties. This is thought to reflect a sensory processing disorder in the central neural system. That, combined with the fact that an infant born with problems often does not have the opportunities for early holding and handling, sets the stage for early sensory integration problems. This basic disorder leads to a cyclic situation in which interactions with the environment are misinterpreted by the central nervous system resulting in maladaptive responses (Ayers, 1973). For example, Johnnie was born 6 weeks premature and was small for gestational age. Because of his size, he stayed in the hospital for a few weeks until he gained some weight and was medically stable enough for his family to care for him at home. When he got home, his mother noticed that he nursed more effectively if he was held very tightly during feedings, often did not look at her during feedings, needed to be wrapped tightly to sleep, and hated being bathed in a tub of water. She adapted to his behavior by bathing him in a tub of water only infrequently, holding him tightly to feed him, and wrapping him well for sleep. As he grew, he did not develop head control at the expected time. Finally, he was referred by the home care nurse for a developmental evaluation, and the family learned that Johnnie had motor delays as well as a sensory-perceptual processing disorder. His sensory-system interpretation of the messages that he had gotten from his environment had told him that light touch was not very pleasant. As he got less touch, he was not trained to learn to process this touch in a way that was positive for him. The evaluation team referred Johnnie for developmental and sensory integration therapy provided by an occupational therapist on a regular basis. Johnnie finally became more comfortable with light touch, making his bath fun, developed head control, continued to develop his motor skills, and started to crawl.

Children born with central nervous system problems such as spina bifida or cerebral palsy or those who have an infection-, trauma-, or malformation-related brain injury are at high risk for sensory integration disorders. Children who are later diagnosed with ADHD also may have sensory integration problems. The expressions of these disorders are varied and complex. These infants and children require a highly skilled team of pediatric rehabilitation specialists for assessment and treatment of these conditions; however, many times it is the nurse who first identifies that a developmental concern exists.

Children born with spina bifida and other conditions that result in asensate skin also have sensory perceptual problems related to loss of sensation. They may totally ignore the part of their body that does not give them feedback. For example, a child does not assume responsibility for protecting their asensate feet from trauma while playing in the sandbox. It is as though they do not realize their feet are a part of them. Some children actually do drawings of themselves that omit the parts of their bodies that are asensate.

Comfort and Pain

The ability to perceive cutaneous sensations starts developing as early as the 7th week of gestation. By the 30th week, synaptic and neurotransmitter mechanisms within the dorsal horn and the conducting pathways to the brain stem and thalamus are complete (Foster & Stevens, 1994). Therefore, even though the central nervous system is still immature at birth, the infant can feel pain and respond to it. Pain has been classified as acute, which is of sudden onset and limited duration, and chronic, which is pain that lasts longer than 6 months.

The ability to talk about painful experiences is based on cognitive learning and maturity. Pre–school-aged children often talk about pain in terms of location and events. They may think they had pain because they were bad. Older children are able to understand the causes of pain. Adolescents can understand pain and its related physiologic link. The ability to cope with pain is also related to the child's developmental level; the younger child has fewer skills needed for coping with painful experiences.

Pain is a subjective experience that is complex and difficult to define. McCaffery (1972) emphasizes this fact and stresses that the nurse must listen carefully to the child for information regarding pain. Acute pain is usually described as pain with a sudden onset. For children, anxiety, fear, and sadness may increase the perception of pain because of previous experiences. Chronic pain, as defined by McGrath and Unruh (1987), is pain that has a long duration and interferes with the activities of daily living. This definition certainly best represents the experiences of children with juvenile arthritis.

Children who are fearful of shots or are culturally conditioned not to express pain may deny that they are having it; therefore, other signs and symptoms of pain must be assessed. Unusual motor behaviors such as limping, facial expressions that may indicate pain, or posturing an extremity to protect it from harm may be indicators of pain. Physiologic signs such as increased heart and respiration rates, elevated blood pressure, and sweating may also indicate pain.

Decisional Conflict

Decisional conflict is "the state in which an individual/group experiences uncertainty about a course of action when the choice involves risk, loss or challenge" (Carpenito, 1995, p. 103). It may arise when the child or family has a choice to make that involves care, treatment, or education. Delay in making a decision, talking about the possible negative result of the decision, and experiencing feelings of stress are all signs of a decisional conflict. Families may experience this type of conflict when trying to deal with finances and obtaining the most appropriate care for their child with a disability or chronic condition, and some may say they just cannot decide what is best when they look at all the issues. See the following Case Study for an example.

CASE STUDY

Susie, age 12 years, had a severe traumatic brain injury from a car accident. She was recently considered for discharge but had not recovered to the point at which she was able to care for herself. The family had heard about a specialized subacute pediatric program that was 300 miles from their home. The insurance company case manager indicated that there is medical coverage for this program, and the rehabilitation team felt it would be an appropriate placement for Susie. The admissions team from the subacute program has evaluated Susie and indicated that they feel she would benefit from their program and urged her mother to come with her for specific teaching regarding Susie's program. The family was in a decisional conflict because Susie's father has a well-paying job

for which he has to travel away from home many days per month, and her mother is a homemaker. They have 3 younger children who are very active in school and community programs. The family does not have the support of extended family and cannot pay for someone to come into the home to take over if Susie's mother goes with her. In this type of situation, the family may experience making this decision as a no-win situation.

The pediatric rehabilitation nurse communicated with the parents that the social worker, the psychologist, and the rehabilitation team could meet with them to assist in resolving the conflict. During the meeting, the team assisted the parents in deciding what the choices would be for Susie's discharge. It was evident that the parents wanted to take Susie home, but they would need a rehabilitation home care program. The nurse called the insurance company case manager and explained the family's needs, seeking approval for funding to cover the home care program. After much discussion, it was determined that a home care program provided by a home health agency in the family's community would be less costly per day than the subacute program. Approval for the discharge plan was given, and Susie was transferred home after the home care team had time to collaborate with Susie's inpatient staff and the family had a successful rooming-in overnight stay.

▬▬▬

Decisional conflicts often arise in the teenage years when the adolescent with a chronic condition or disability is becoming more involved in making decisions regarding their own treatment or is able to assume more responsibility for their daily care regimen. Adolescents have the ability to analyze problems and understand information, but peer pressure may encourage them to take an approach that is not in keeping with what is recommended. This situation occurs more frequently when there is a daily management regimen that may not allow for much deviation without consequences. One example is when the adolescent is taking a medication and should not consume alcohol, yet friends are drinking at a party. Perhaps the most difficult situation for parents is when their child does not have an obvious condition, yet has delays in the ability to make safe decisions. The parent may not get much support from family and friends regarding restrictions they feel they must impose on the child for safety, so support and encouragement from the nurse are very important.

Decisional conflict can also be related to altered compliance if the family or child is not completely committed to the treatment team's recommendations. The conflict or lack of compliance may come from confusion or lack of understanding about the treatment regimen; lack of willingness to follow through because of verbalized or non-verbalized reasons; difficulty following through because of other forces in the family's life, such as transportation problems, finances, and difficulty performing the tasks and regimens; or delayed maturity, among others. For example, therapy staff recommended that Judy, a 6-year-old girl recovering from a traumatic brain injury, receive specific therapy, requiring about 10 minutes for each session, three times per day. The family had been taught the therapeutic technique, and nodded in agreement that they had no questions regarding the recommendations. When Judy and her family returned to the clinic 1 month later, it was obvious to the staff that the family had not followed through with the recommended home program. The staff felt the family had been noncompliant, when in fact the family had tried to do the program but slacked off because Judy became ill with a severe cold. In this situation, the issue of noncompliance is a judgmental one on the part of the staff. The family had all the best intentions in following through with the program, but were unable to do so because of the complications. The family felt guilty, and thought about changing Judy's care to another agency. With clarification by the nurse and social worker, the therapy staff decided to show the family which exercises were of top priority and how to better integrate the therapy into the Judy's daily play as well as self-care activities. The family's priority was sequencing of activities. The team suggested having Judy, with her mother's assistance, make a picture chart of the sequence for the morning self-care routine so Judy could use it and start becoming responsible for her own care. Another sequence chart was made for setting the table in the evening to assist Judy in learning how to set the table without forgetting any of the items. With these activities, the family felt they could see changes in Judy's ability to provide her own care and assist with the dinner preparation. They also felt that they were more a part of the rehabilitation process, and felt proud that Judy had made progress.

Rehabilitation Nursing Management

Assessment

The pediatric rehabilitation nurse must have a thorough knowledge of appropriate assessments and interventions in the areas of cognition and perception to formulate an appropriate plan of care. The child's age, developmental level, and specific disability or chronic condition, as well as the child-family inter-relationships, must be incorporated into the assessment. In many instances a pain experience history obtained from the parent or a verbal child can also provide information on their relationship to past experiences, the child's behaviors during painful experiences, and the treatments that were effective in the past.

Suggested questions and observations for the child and family include:

Does the infant or child have very specific problems with transitions in movement, bathing, or certain types of touch? Do they require a pacifier or fingers in their mouth excessively for calming and organization?

Does the infant or child use excessive rocking behaviors for calming?

Does the infant or child become very upset with loud noise, bright lights, riding in the car, or being strapped in the car seat, or does the child hate public places with multiple types of stimulation?

Is the child very picky about the textures, colors, and temperatures of foods they eat?

Does the child have a sensory-perceptual deficit? Describe the deficit.

Is the family verbalizing confusion or concern about recommendations from the treatment team?

Is the child having problems learning in school? Describe the child's grade level and problems.

Observe for motor and physiologic signs that may indicate pain.

Has the family been consistent in following through with therapy and medical care?

Pain measurement scales can allow the child or adolescent to self-report pain or provide the nurse with a tool for behavioral observation. Table 13–2 provides information about some of the pain measurement scales more commonly used for children.

Nursing Diagnoses

In the cognitive-perceptual area, several nursing diagnoses should be considered. These include:

Table 13–2 PAIN MEASUREMENT SCALES FOR CHILDREN

Scale	Age or Developmental Level	Self-Report or Observation	Description
Faces Scale	3–7 years	Self-report	Seven faces—smily face (no pain) to very pained face (worst pain)
Washington, D.C., Comfort Scale	Pre-verbal and non-verbal	Observation	Points assigned for blood pressure, crying, movement, agitation, and verbal evaluation
Numeric/Visual Analog Scale	≥5 years*	Self-report	Line with points from 0–10 (no pain to worst pain)
Color Tool	≥4 years†	Self-report	Front and back body outlines—color location of pain
Poker Chip Tool	≥4 years*	Self-report	Four red poker chips to measure intensity of pain—little bit of hurt to most hurt you ever could have
Oucher	≥3 years	Self-report	Photos of children and numeric scale from 0 to 100 (by 10s), no hurt to biggest hurt
Adolescent/Pediatric Pain Tool	8 years through adolescence	Self-report	Front and back body outlines—word graphic rating scale
Verbal 0 to 10 Rating Scale	≥8 years	Self-report	Respond to 0 = no pain to 10 = worst possible pain
Children's Hospital of Eastern Ontario Pain Scale	All ages	Observation	Behavioral observation of cry, facial expression, verbal communication, torso motion, touch, and leg motion; numeric rating

*Provided they have some concept of numbers and can count.
†Provided they have the concept of colors.
Data from Children's Hospital Pain Treatment Staff. (1997). *Pain measurement scales.* Boston: Children's Hospital; Wong, D. (1995). *Whaley and Wong's nursing care of infants and children* (5th ed.). St. Louis: CV Mosby; and Foster, R., & Stevens B. (1994). Nursing management of pain in children. In C. Betz, M. Hunsberger, & S. Wright (Eds.). *Family-centered nursing care of children,* pp. 856–881. Philadelphia: WB Saunders.

- Altered thought processes
- Decisional conflict
- Impaired memory
- Sensory-perceptual alterations: visual, auditory, kinesthetic, gustatory, tactile, olfactory
- Pain and Chronic pain
- Unilateral neglect

If a diagnosis of "Pain" or "Chronic pain" is identified, the nursing plan of care found in Table 13–3 can be used after it is individualized to meet the child's needs.

Expected Outcomes

The overall expected outcomes for the child and family include:

Identify the cause of pain and activities that increase or decrease pain.

Use appropriate relief measures for pain management.

Identify activities or situations that increase anxiety and appropriate coping strategies.

Cognitive and perceptual problems are decreased, and the child or adolescent increases self-care activities.

Intervention and Teaching

Interventions for cognitive learning must always be at the child's level of understanding. Infants learn by sensorimotor pathways. Position, touch, sight, sound, smell, and a parent's responses to their distress cues are all very important parts of the infant's learning. The infant learns that the world can be trusted when their needs are met in a gentle manner. The infant learns that the world may not be a comfortable place to be if their needs are ignored or attention is very delayed. Positive reinforcement is necessary for positive learning at this age.

Interventions for the cognitive-perceptual area are:

Refer children for evaluation if they consistently show abnormal patterns of behavior or express suicidal thoughts.

Allow children and adolescents to become a part of the decision-making processes as they mature and can assume decision-making skills regarding their own needs and care.

Reduce factors that contribute to pain experiences.

Use pharmacologic management of pain as necessary.

For chronic pain, teach alternative methods of management such as relaxation, distraction, and activities.

Refer for complementary treatment of chronic pain such as acupuncture, hypnosis, biofeedback, and counseling.

Use assistive devices and systems that will help compensate for deficits as necessary.

Encourage child to become as independent as possible.

Children of all ages are always in need of positive reinforcement for their actions and learning. The nurse must be able to understand the child's level of development related to their responses, interact with the child, and reinforce the child's behavior. For example, Alice, age 4 years, was born with a chromosome abnormality, had difficulties with growth, and is now in the classroom for the first time. She is starting to shake her head "no" and refuse to eat. The staff are frustrated because she needs to eat and she is refusing. They want to force her to eat by holding her hands in front of her and holding her head and forcing food into her mouth. Alice is simply learning to control her world in another way with the powerful use of "no." To not respond to that behavior and in fact negate the behavior by forcing her, she will get the message that her wishes are not important and that she is not respected for her attempts to become an individual in this world. A solution to the situation is to weigh her weekly and encourage the family and the school to keep a diet intake record. However, although she is learning to control her world and needs to be reinforced for that learning experience to support her self-esteem and independence, it is still important to maintain adequate nutrition and hydration. As her efforts to control her environment were honored, Alice did not shake her head "no" as often. She began gaining weight and her food intake, even with refusing to eat at times, had increased.

Mary, a very active 3½-year-old born with spina bifida, uses many words and has just started a classroom experience. She crawls for ambulation and is pulling to stand. The nurse in the school is interested is setting some goals for teaching her independence in toileting skills. Mary is starting to imitate the other students in the classroom with movements to a song. Using this new skill of imitation, the nurse starts by placing Mary on the toilet each time they have bathroom time to imitate the other children and start a pattern for

Table 13-3 NURSING PLAN OF CARE

Nursing Diagnosis: Pain

Related to: Reflex or smooth muscle spasms   Effects of cancer
Tissue trauma   Surgery
Inflammation   Diagnostic tests

Goals	Nursing Interventions/Teaching
Fear and anxiety are reduced and child or adolescent can more effectively cope with the pain experience	Form a trusting relationship with the child or adolescent, share concern about their reports of pain, and allow participation in decision making Prepare for procedures that may be painful, use honest explanations, and remain with the child Encourage discussion of pain experiences and provide opportunities for choice when possible Determine the effect of pain on the child and family Provide information to correct misconceptions about pain experiences and treatment strategies Teach child and parents several strategies prior to the pain experience and assist them in using an intervention during the pain experience Provide opportunity for rest during the day and uninterrupted sleep at night if possible
Effective pain management: pharmacologic	Collaborate with other health care team members in the selection of the right medication, dose, route, and time to optimize pain control Provide pharmacologic interventions that promote optimal pain relief and evaluate their effectiveness at regular intervals Observe for side effects of medications: respiratory depression, constipation, pruritus, tolerance, or dependence Use supportive statements when administering medications to enhance effectiveness Teach child and family about the expected effects of medications and the possible adverse reactions
Effective pain management: non-pharmacologic	Experiment with a number of non-pharmacologic strategies to discover the most effective approach. Consider the developmental level of the child when making the selection Distraction: assist to identify strong distractors, involve in play, use humor, music, tell stories Relaxation: positioning, rocking, massage, rhythmic breathing, progressive muscle relaxation Guided imagery: use imagination in creating pleasant images Coping skills training and positive self-talk Cutaneous stimulation: rubbing, pressure, heat or cold application Behavioral contracting: rewards, written contracts

Expected Outcomes

Identify source of pain and activities that increase or decrease pain
Describe measures that provide relief
Use pharmacologic and non-pharmacologic strategies as appropriate
Expresses less pain and increases participation in activities of daily living

timed toileting. If her interest in imitation at this level is ignored because of beliefs that she will not be able to be continent because of her diagnosis, the opportunity to start a toileting routine may be lost. When she is ready for her specific toilet training program, she may not be interested in participating because she has other developmental tasks that are of more importance to her. Mary became very interested in imitating the other children when they went to the bathroom and always wanted to sit on the toilet at the regular times. With this new skill, the nurse contacted Mary's mother and encouraged her to take Mary to the spina bifida clinic where she could get specific information regarding a continence program. Over a few months, Mary was taught to do intermittent self-catheterization at home and at school. Her bowel program was also established.

Summary

Cognitive and sensory-perceptual functioning is very complex, and alterations in this functional health pattern will affect many aspects of the child and family's life. The pediatric rehabilitation nurse's role is to assist with early identification, intervention, and ongoing management, as well as teaching the family and child successful adaptive techniques for management of the alterations resulting from the underlying condition.

SELF-PERCEPTION PATTERN

The self-perception functional health pattern includes the child and family's perceptions of attitudes about self, body image, identity, self-worth, ability to perform, and general emotional pattern. It also includes information about the child's nonverbal patterns of posture, movement, and communication (Gordon, 1994).

Expected Development and Alterations

Reality for the developing infant and child is based on how experiences in the world are perceived. That reality is shaped and changed as life experience expands. Each person therefore has their own unique reality based on how life is perceived and experienced. The richness of each person's reality may never be fully verbalized or understood by another person. Table 13–4 is a summary of the developmental areas of self-perception as the child grows from infant or toddler through adolescence.

Temperament

The infant's expression of individuality is thought to be affected by constitutional factors. The term temperament is often used to describe these behaviors. A study of temperament by Chess and Thomas (1986), resulted in clustering of traits into three groups thought to represent an infant's temperament.

> The "easy" infant adapts well to change, has generally a positive mood, and has regularity of behaviors.
> The "difficult" infant adapts slowly to change, often after a negative first response; has an intense mood; and is more irregular in behaviors.
> The "slow-to-warm-up" infant is slow to adapt to change and usually does so only after a somewhat negative initial response, has a low intense mood, and has generally regular behaviors.

Understanding the infant's usual temperament assists in understanding the infant's view of the world. The infant's temperament plays a major role in self-perception and self-concept development. Adjustment and change is less difficult for a child with an "easy" temperament than for the child with a more "difficult" temperament. Being aware of a child's temperament will assist care providers in developing an effective plan of care.

Fear and Anxiety

As the infant or child begins to learn about the world and gather knowledge from experiences, fear and anxiety are possible. Fear is a focused feeling of dread arising from a sense of threat or danger to oneself, whereas anxiety is a nonspecific feeling with a recognized focus (Gordon, 1994). According to Vaughn and Litt (1990), there are three basic fears that are a result of early psychologic development: fear of abandonment, fear of the loss of love, and fear of bodily mutilation. Fear from within that does not have any external component and has no basis in reality is usually defined as anxiety. Because of the child's blossoming understanding but limited experience in the world, the door is wide open for rich fantasies that develop into false realities, fears, and anxieties. This same blossoming of understanding can also lead to the development of "true" realities. The infant and child's

Table 13-4 AGES AND STAGES: EXPECTED DEVELOPMENT—SELF-PERCEPTION

Infant/Toddler

Experiences feelings of separation anxiety/abandonment
Experiences feelings of loss of love
Has physiologic changes associated with fear
Has the ability to say "no" with feeling and to have temper tantrums
Has sense of self as separate

Preschooler

Fears bodily mutilation
Fears changes in personal environment, darkness, and masks
Has rich fantasy play during the day, nightmares and night terrors at night
Uses role models (usually adults in the environment) for learning how to act as they are growing up
Needs discipline to learn how to conform to standards and rules
Develops ability to feel pride and shame
Uses initiative to choose activities
Struggles for control
Uses "I" to refer to self
Recognizes differences between self and others

School-Aged Child

Fears separation with entry into school
Fears failure, reacting with anxiety, depression, or hostility
Gains sense of industry, duty, and accomplishment
May develop antisocial behavior to get attention
May feel failure for the first time
Evaluates self by using external evidence

Adolescent

Fears rejection
May have periods of low self-perception
Depends on peer approval
Late in the stage, has established clearer sense of self

Data from Deloian, B. (1996). Developmental management of infants. In C. Burns, N. Barber, M. Brady, & A. Dunn (Eds.). *Pediatric primary care* (3rd ed.), pp. 81–101. Philadelphia: WB Saunders; Murphy, M.A. (1996). Developmental management of toddlers and preschoolers. In C. Burns, N. Barber, M. Brady, & A. Dunn (Eds.). *Pediatric primary care* (3rd ed.), pp. 101–123. Philadelphia: WB Saunders; Billings, P., & Burns, C. (1996). Developmental management of school-age children. In C. Burns, N. Barber, M. Brady, & A. Dunn (Eds.). *Pediatric primary care* (3rd ed.), pp. 123–139. Philadelphia: WB Saunders; Wildey, L.S. (1996). Developmental management of adolescents. In C. Burns, N. Barber, M. Brady, & A. Dunn (Eds.). *Pediatric primary care* (3rd ed.), pp. 139–159. Philadelphia: WB Saunders; and Vaughn, V., & Litt, I. (1990). *Child and adolescent development: clinical implications*. Philadelphia: WB Saunders.

world of experiences and perceptions can easily be a rich blend of the "true" reality and their own fantasies, or it may be a "false" reality. Phobias are fears that keep a person from participating in normal activities. Children who have developed phobias allow those fears to prevent them from exploring and learning.

Anxiety and fear are understandable in the infant or developing child who has already experienced hospitalizations; painful procedures; a strange, uncomfortable environment; restricted mobility and activities; and hearing, seeing, and feeling sensations that are not familiar. It is not uncommon for a mother to swaddle her baby to assist with calming and sleep. For children who were swaddled dur-

ing painful procedures while in the hospital, the repressed memory of the sensations of the swaddling may be lasting and cause the child to cry unexplainably when later swaddled or touched, even when the environment and circumstances are positive.

With the school-aged child's sense of industry, the opportunity to experience failure also occurs. Many children with disabilities or chronic conditions experience for the first time that sense of failure when they realize they are not able to perform at the same level as their peers. For some children, this experience comes later chronologically because of their delays in the ability to process information. With the inability to meet expectations and standards, the child may react to feelings of failure by becoming withdrawn, depressed, hostile, and anxious. This also is a time when inappropriate behavior may develop as the child makes an effort to gain attention and feel recognized (Vaughn & Litt, 1990).

It is the young child who challenges the family's skills, especially in the area of discipline. The family's need to mold the child after their pre-conceived ideas of how the child should act and behave may affect the child's spirit and independence. Being careful not to "break the child's spirit" is important. When the child has a developmental delay or chronic condition, the parents may not have worked through their own grief and thus may have difficulty allowing the child to be a unique person and disciplining them, thus inhibiting the child's psychosocial development. Self-perception, self-concept, self-esteem, and self-image are words that are often used interchangeably. The sense of self develops from interaction with others as well as from one's sense of significance, worth, and competence. Children who experience difficulty with these areas of development often look externally for their identity (Barber, 1996).

Hopelessness and Powerlessness

According to Hymovich and Hagopian (1992), "Hopelessness occurs when a person believes that nothing can be done to change a situation, does not feel worthy of help, and has feelings of giving up" (p. 157). Powerlessness, which includes hopelessness, is the sense that an outcome will not be affected by an individual's actions or that personal control is lacking in relation to a situation or event. Characteristics of hopelessness include passivity, non-participation in activities, dependence, verbal expressions of lack of control, crying, failure to seek or provide relevant information, or expressions of depression. Hopelessness and powerlessness are closely aligned. Powerlessness may be a short-term or a long-term perception for children with disabilities or chronic conditions and their families. This perception that there is no control over what is happening, and thus no control over the outcome, can easily immobilize a family. Because there are no simple quick cures or surgical procedures that will "fix" the problem, and there are ongoing situations and issues that need to be managed continuously, family members can easily be overcome with feelings of powerlessness (Miller, 1992).

Self-Esteem, Body Image, and Personal Identity Disturbance

Self-esteem, a major part of the concept of self, develops from the evaluation of worth in relation to both the ideal and the performance of others. Children with disabilities or chronic conditions have been reported to have lower self-esteem than other children. Another part of self-concept, body image, can also be significantly affected by a disability or a chronic condition (Hymovich & Hagopian, 1992). The child's overall sense of his or her body and ability to function is taken from the verbal and nonverbal input received from the family, other persons in the environment, and personal experiences. Children with a negative sense of self may feel they are a failure at everything, may feel like victims, and focus on their own needs and self-worth (Berne & Savary, 1992). Difficulties with self-perception are often intertwined with complaints about one's body, and although the bodily complaints are assessed, the difficulties with self-perception may not be identified (Barber, 1996).

Children with developmental delays, disabilities, chronic conditions, and disruptive environments are at high risk for alterations in self-perception, body image, and personal identity. This can be related to their physical appearance, which may be different from the norm. But even those without outward physical variations may experience low self-perception because of how they feel about themselves. Children who have difficulty learning or who do not grow at the expected rate are also at risk for negative self-perception. Unresolved family problems can also affect the child's sense of self. Having unrealistic hopes and dreams for their child, unmanaged family stress, inconsistent discipline guidelines, and previous negative experiences that have not been resolved can all affect the child's development of self-esteem.

Rehabilitation Nursing Management

Assessment

The young child may not be able to verbalize feelings and information about self-perception and self-concept, so the family must be the focus of the assessment. The nurse must also assess nonverbal cues about the child's self-perception and self-concept and integrate this information into the complete assessment; however, these observations must be validated and clarified with the family.

Suggested questions and observations for the child and family include:

General mood state: is the child or family irritable, depressed, fearful, or anxious?

How does the child describe himself or herself, his or her body, and his or her accomplishments?

What does the family say about the child's identity and body?

Are the child and family able to explore their capabilities and limitations?

Is achievement of new skills and feelings supported in a positive manner?

Are the child's peer interactions productive or problematic?

Can the child try learning new skills within limits and experience success without adult interference?

Is family discipline clear, consistent, and supportive?

Does the child or family have multiple somatic concerns without significant diagnostic findings?

Are feelings of powerlessness or hopelessness, fears, and anxieties verbalized by the child and family?

Nursing Diagnoses

In the area of self-perception, several nursing diagnoses must be considered. These include:

- Fear
- Anxiety
- Hopelessness
- Powerlessness
- Self-esteem disturbance
- Body image disturbance
- Personal identity disturbance

If a diagnosis of "Powerlessness" is identified, the nursing plan of care found in Table 13–5 can be used after the assessment is complete and the plan is individualized for the child and family.

Expected Outcomes

The overall expected outcomes for the child and family include:

Experiences self-identity in a positive way.
Shows and talks about feelings.
Shows competence and feels good about it.
Has productive peer relationships.

Interventions and Teaching

Specific areas of intervention and teaching related to self-perception and alterations include:

Teach effective parenting skills, including respecting their own feelings, caring for themselves, accepting their own skills, being available to care for the child by understanding their own uniqueness and value and avoiding shame or critical attitudes, and allowing the child to be an individual without comparison to others.

Teach effective discipline that guides and directs the child, respecting the need to seek effective techniques for accomplishing new tasks and resolving frustrating situations. See Teaching Topic: Discipline for additional information.

Demonstrate effective communication with the child by modeling problem-solving techniques, listening, respecting feelings, and assisting the child to express feelings without judgment, while avoiding "you should" by using "I" statements.

Provide unconditional love, security, support, self-respect, and value.

Refer family for counseling and assistance in learning effective parenting skills.

Refer child for individual counseling if necessary.

Teaching Topic: Discipline

Age-appropriate discipline techniques (see Tables 13–1, 13–4, 13–6, 13–7, and 13–8)

Use discipline as an activity to teach the child how to live in a society that has rules and regulations

Use clearly identified limit setting with consequences that are used if the child does not control negative behavior themselves

Realize that the young child needs external control and gradually learns to internalize control as they get older

---

Summary

Development of a sense of self is complex for all children and adolescents, and a child with differences is set apart from his or her peers, no matter how large or small the difference. The challenge for the family and the pediatric rehabilitation nurse caring for the child is to acknowledge and respect the person within, envisioning hope, accomplishments, and successes that are specific to the child and with-

Table 13–5   NURSING PLAN OF CARE

Nursing Diagnosis: Powerlessness

Related to: Health care environment   Inability to communicate
                Interpersonal interaction/lifestyle   Progressive disease
                Illness-related regimen

Goals	Nursing Interventions/Teaching
Express thoughts and feelings about present situation	Show concern for individual and develop a trusting relationship Take time to listen and encourage questions Teach to communicate needs and feelings
Identify areas that can be controlled and increase sense of power	Assist to recognize own limits and set realistic goals Encourage choices and participation in decision making Provide positive reinforcement for desired behaviors and opportunities to be successful Gradually increase expectations of self-care performance Allow manipulation of surroundings (e.g., location of personal articles or furniture in room) Assist to identify areas that cannot be controlled and ways to deal with feelings
Learn assertive and effective communication skills	Assist to set realistic goals Demonstrate appropriate communication of needs and feelings Encourage use of support systems Refer to counseling and support groups if indicated

Expected Outcomes

Expresses sense of control over current situation
Makes choices related to plan of care and future
Involved in therapeutic activities

---

out limits. The child who has experienced non-judgmental guidance and respect and unconditional love for their individuality will be able to meet any challenge in the world when venturing out from the protection of home.

ROLE-RELATIONSHIP PATTERN

Gordon (1994) describes the role-relationship pattern as one that includes both formal and informal role engagement and relationships, including the child and family's perception of their current life roles and responsibilities. This pattern also focuses on the child and family's ability to communicate their needs and desires. The child first experiences relationships with their family, then as they get older, with siblings, friends, and the larger community. The quality and the child's perceptions of their early relationships affect the rest of their lives as they interact with themselves and others. Just as the child is growing and developing, so is the family, and role relationships and ability to communicate are

a dynamic process. Table 13–6 provides an outline of these areas as the child grows from infant or toddler through adolescence.

Expected Development and Alterations

Interactions in Relationships

Bonding and attachment are critical for the infant's development. Those persons that the infant forms an attachment to will be sought out in the future for nurturing, protection, and love (Vaughn & Litt, 1990). Bonding and attachment are of major importance for all infants and children and sets the stage for their later interactions and relationships.

The infant is capable of initiating interaction and is thought to do so more than half of the time. It is thought that the mother's or caretaker's responsiveness to that initiation is of great importance to the behavioral development of the infant. That interaction serves as a basis for the development of a sense of trust, knowing that their needs will be met physically and emotionally, and mistrust,

Table 13–6 AGES AND STAGES: EXPECTED DEVELOPMENT—ROLE RELATIONSHIPS

Infant/Toddler

By first week, can distinguish between voice of mother and others
By second week, can associate voice of mother and her face
Able to use steady gaze into mother's eyes to facilitate attachment
Able to move in rhythm with the voice of an engaging person
Able to initiate interactions by movement, crying, and fussing
Produces social smile at 3–5 weeks of age
Development of basic trust
Laughs at pleasurable social interactions
Language production of 0–50 words by 18 months
Use of language in egocentric focus
Uses dawdling and "no" to control others
Enjoys wide range of relationships
Responds to death by regression, sleep and eating disturbances, and irritability
Expresses grief and mourning by clinging, screaming, and exaggerated separation behaviors

Preschooler

Has social language and can carry on short conversations
Able to relate to siblings
Responds to death with regression in continence, having nightmares, temper tantrums, and crying spells
Views death as reversible, a sleep-like state
May feel responsible for the death

School-Aged Child

Increased ability to self-regulate and self-control
Sense of duty and accomplishment
Communicates with logical thought processes
Responds to death by poor concentration, school problems, somatic complaints, crying spells, and fears
 of imagined diseases
Views death as natural, irreversible, and likely to happen to themselves as well as others

Adolescent

Increased expressions of individuality and independence
Peer group is a great influence and they tend to conform to peer group standards
Interpersonal and heterosexual relationships are very important
Can communicate regarding hypothetical situations
Understands death at an adult level
Reacts to death with poor school performance, depression, somatic complaints, acting-out behaviors,
 and suicide attempts

Data from Green, M. (1986). Helping children and parents deal with grief. *Contemporary Pediatrics* 3(10), 84–89;
Vaughn, V., & Litt, I. (1990). *Child and adolescent development: clinical implications.* Philadelphia: WB Saunders; and
C. Betz, M. Hunsberger, & S. Wright (Eds.). *Family-centered nursing care of children.* Philadelphia: WB Saunders.

when needs are not being met (Vaughn & Litt, 1990). If there is a perceived "mismatch" between the mother and child, parenting skills may be altered. This can happen more easily when the child has a disability or chronic condition and therefore does not fit the expectations of the family (Barnes, Beardslee, Schafer, & Shannon, 1986).

During the first year of life, the infant thrives at the highest level emotionally, spiritually, and physically if needs are met consistently, promptly, and in a loving manner. This is not, as some people think, a time for letting the infant cry or for harsh handling to com-municate disapproval. Unless the family is extremely overindulgent or overprotective, spoiling the infant is not thought to be possible.

For families who experience the birth of a child with a disability or chronic condition or one who is medically fragile, the loss of the opportunity for early interaction that leads to bonding and attachment may affect their relationship (Vaughn & Litt, 1990). Infants who have experienced a lack of nurturing when they cry may learn that they cannot affect their world by action, and they there-fore become withdrawn, depressed, and anxious and develop mistrust toward the world (Vaughn & Litt, 1990).

Children who are very irritable prove the greatest challenge to caregivers, because they may change quickly from irritable to asleep or from asleep to irritable. Because of the lack of alert periods and opportunities for joyful interaction, they are at high risk for attachment disorders during infancy. Irritability can also affect caregiver-child interaction when the child is older. For example, Emily had been shaken as an infant and then had a non-accidental skull fracture as a toddler. Because of the trauma, she had a severe visual impairment, among other deficits. She was extremely irritable and did not want to be touched. This made it very difficult for the nurses and her foster mother to care for her. Caregivers who provide care for children with high levels of irritability are also at high risk for caregiver stress and role strain.

Caregiver role strain can also be caused by children who are active and need constant attention because they are not safe alone in the environment. For example Joe, who at 3 years of age has just learned how to open doors, is interested in going outside to play but does not have the motor skills to safely go down the stairs. Perhaps the most stressful experience for caregivers is when the child requires constant care day and night.

Relationships and Communication

The immediate social structure and roles of a family and its members are altered when there is a child with a disability or chronic condition. More information on family structure and relationships is provided in Chapter 9. Communication patterns may change because of hostility, role changes, exclusion of some members from conversations, silence, difficulty in discussing the child's condition, and lack of knowledge. Sensitivity to the importance of both verbal and nonverbal communication is an important part of enhancing relationships and increasing trust within the family. Open and honest communication sends the message that thoughts and opinions are valued and results in an increased sense of self-worth and trust.

Response to Loss or Change

Grieving the loss of a child or the child's ability to perform is a normal, healthy response. Unresolved grief is unhealthy and may interfere with continued psychosocial development. Chronic sorrow is a concept that describes the family's psychologic reaction to their child with a disability or chronic condition as a prolonged sadness that persists throughout life. This reaction was first suggested by Olshansky (1962), and research has begun to determine specific components of chronic sorrow (Clubb, 1991). The intensity of the feelings are "determined by parental perceptions of the severity of their child's limitations and parents' characteristics, e.g. personality, religious beliefs, social class and ethnic background" (Hymovich & Hagopian, 1992, p. 155). Four particularly stressful periods occur when the child:

- begins to walk
- enters school
- celebrates a 21st birthday
- is surpassed in development by a sibling

The family may respond to the loss of their dream of the perfect infant or the loss of the child's ability to function normally after a traumatic injury or the onset of a chronic condition by changing their parenting skills and allowing the child to have more control over their lives than is healthy or overprotecting the child more than is necessary. This may lead to the "vulnerable child syndrome," which results in a problematic relationship and poor psychosocial development (Culley, Perrin, & Jordan-Chaberski, 1989). Hospitalizations and long separations from the child, not being able to care for the child, and not knowing what is going to happen to the child can also disrupt previously successful parenting skills. For example, a mother who was a nurse gave birth to an infant with spina bifida. The baby needed several surgeries and, because the mother was a nurse, she had many of the skills needed to provide the infant's care. She performed the nursing care but realized that she was not having the opportunity to attach to the infant as a mother.

Depression usually occurs in the adolescent who experiences the onset of a fatal illness. Boys often become depressed because of the loss of the ability to prove themselves in an activity in which they had previously planned to participate. Girls may become depressed if they feel the illness was caused by the loss of a loved one, such as in breaking up with a friend (Vaughn & Litt, 1990).

Rehabilitation Nursing Management

Assessment

The Neonatal Behavioral Assessment Scale developed by Brazelton (1973) is often used to assess the infant's ability to relate to the world. The seven clusters of the 28 items in the assessment scale are:

- habituation—response to stimuli while awake and inhibition while asleep
- orientation—response to visual and auditory stimuli when alert
- motor performance—movement and tone
- general arousal level
- response when aroused
- autonomic stability
- reflexes (Wong, 1995)

One of the categories of items assesses interaction processes, specifically the neonate's ability for orientation, alertness, consolability, and cuddliness. Deficits in neurobehavioral function can be identified early in an infant's life by an experienced assessor.

Role relationships are often defined by cultural expectations. There are those who believe that having a child with a disability is a real adversity for the family, whereas others believe that this is part of the diversity of life. To thoroughly assess the issues surrounding roles and relationships, the pediatric rehabilitation nurse must understand what beliefs are held by each child and family. For many, it is the relationship that dictates the behaviors rather than the child's ability. With today's role diversification, fathers may be home providing the child's care while mothers are out earning the family income, so the nurse must be sensitive to these factors and be aware of who affects the child's relationships with his or her family. Adults in many cultures believe that it is possible to spoil infants, and if so, such beliefs must be explored as a component of their role and relationships.

The following are suggested areas of assessment of the child and family:

Observe family-child interactions to evaluate relationships and signs of "vulnerable child syndrome."
Determine the family composition: household members, culture, roles, patterns of decision making, and concerns.
Are the child's peer relationships developmentally appropriate? Does the child associate with gangs? Are there family concerns regarding child's peer relationships?
Assess the child or family's recent experiences with loss: Are they able to discuss feelings and experiences?
Explore the family's expectations of their child with a chronic condition or disability.

Evaluate caregiver stress, including number of hours spent caring for child day and night, availability of relief caregivers such as respite or baby sitters, and caregiver returning to work outside of home.
Assess family and child's experiences of social isolation, including number of meaningful activities in the community that they attend regularly and last time adults in family had a night out together or with friends.
Observe for signs of violence, subtle or obvious, toward the child or adults within the home or community.

Nursing Diagnoses

In the area of role relationships, several nursing diagnoses must be considered. These include:

- Impaired communication
- Altered family processes
- Altered parenting
- Altered role performance
- Impaired social interactions
- Social isolation
- Grieving: anticipatory or dysfunctional

Expected Outcomes

The overall expected outcomes for the child and family include:

Attachment behaviors, interaction skills, and role relationships that are developmentally appropriate.
A family and social environment that promotes development of roles and relationships.

Intervention and Teaching

General areas of intervention used to strengthen attachment and bonding include teaching the family how to observe specific cues from their child that indicate that the child is ready for interaction, and then support positive responsiveness. Additionally, understanding the cues for the child's desire to be left alone is necessary, for there are times when the child does not want to engage in interaction (Vaughn & Litt, 1990). For example, the child who has his arms extended out away from the adult and is squirming as if he wants to be put down may be saying "leave me alone for now."

Cues from the child regarding interaction may also come in the form of sounds. To encourage development of reciprocal interaction skills, the child needs to have the adult respond to his sounds and then wait for the child to "answer" back. This behavior of turn-taking and rhythmic interaction assists children in learning that they are separate individuals with importance. For the family who has a child with a disability or chronic condition, the opportunities for this type of interaction may be few, so it is the nurse's role to demonstrate this behavior to them.

Teaching the family how to support the child developing a quiet alert state, especially when the child is either very irritable or asleep, is also a much needed intervention. After making certain the child's physical needs are met, techniques for supporting the child in coming to an alert state include:

- decreasing stimuli in the environment
- allowing the child to suck on a pacifier
- providing the child with rhythmic movements
- swaddling the child or holding the child to snuggle
- positioning the child to support flexion
- vocalizing gently to the child

Additional intervention strategies include routines that encompass nurturing activities such as singing or reading to the child, playing games with the child, or nighttime rituals for calming. Teaching the adults in the home to massage the infant or child with a disability or chronic condition is one way of encouraging reciprocal interaction, attachment and bonding, relaxation, and increasing growth and development. Touch has very powerful messages (Schneider, 1996).

When families express a concern about "spoiling" the child who is developmentally functioning at a level under 1 year of age by always being responsive to their cries, the nurse must thoroughly assess the family's concern. The family may be expressing a desire to have their child be more independent, or they may be in conflict as to how to interpret the child's needs in terms of which ones to try to allow the child to meet and which ones to meet themselves.

For example, one mother said she could not tolerate listening to her child cry because it forced her to feel her own pain regarding the loss of a "perfect child," and if she started to feel that pain she would become so depressed that she would not be able to care for her child, herself, or her family. She went on to say that she did not want to spoil her child, but she also did not know how to encourage her child to be more independent and how to meet her own needs. Further discussion with the nurse gave her the opportunity to verbalize her feelings and find positive ways to deal with them and interact effectively with her child.

Summary

The interplay among the various family members' roles and their formal and informal relationships is very complex, and alterations in this functional health pattern will affect many aspects of the child and family's life. The pediatric rehabilitation nurse's role is to assist with early identification, intervention, and ongoing management, as well as teaching the family and child successful adaptive techniques for management of the alterations resulting from the underlying condition.

COPING–STRESS TOLERANCE PATTERN

This pattern includes styles of coping, how an individual manages stress, and the tolerance for stressful events. Specific information about how children and adolescents manage stress, what they perceive as stressful and the resources for the management of stress are described (Gordon, 1994). Table 13–7 provides an outline of the areas related to stress and coping experienced by the child at each level of development.

Expected Development and Alterations

Stress

A stressor is defined as an event that a person experiences as a threat or challenge. In the production of a psycho-physiologic response, the person can either use the stressor as a challenge for growth or allow it to cause further disorganization (Gordon, 1994). Children's responses to stress are affected by the their cognitive, psychosocial, and physical development. Illness and disability can easily be defined as a stressor.

The stress of having a child with a disability or chronic condition may be experienced differently by each adult in the family. One study looking at differences between fathers' and mothers' perceived stress found that fathers and mothers did differ in their perception of the stress of having a child with a severe disability (Rousey, Best, & Blacher, 1992). Another study found that the fathers

Table 13-7 AGES AND STAGES: EXPECTED DEVELOPMENT—COPING AND STRESS TOLERANCE

Infant/Toddler

Indicates stress with physiologic changes (e.g., heart rate, breathing)
Copes by using sensorimotor behaviors such as crying; sucking; staring; clutching at toy, blanket, or familiar person; rejecting being held; increased or decreased motor activity; or anorexia
Able to distinguish between friendly and angry voices
Babbles with intricate inflection
Can say "no" meaningfully
Toddler may regress to infant coping behaviors or have temper tantrums, withdraw, or use control- or ritual-type behaviors
Able to ask simple questions
Uses make-believe play

Preschooler

Copes by asking questions, aggression, regression, denial, withdrawal or leaving the situation
Tries again with reassurance and reasons when unable to accomplish task
Can tolerate "friendly" teasing
Verbalizes feelings to another without hitting
May see treatment as punishment for bad behavior
May cope by grinding teeth, banging head, or use other self-stimulation behaviors

School-Aged Child

Difficulties with coping may affect school performance and social interactions
Experiences social isolation if coping difficulties occur
Begins to understand that treatment is not punishment for bad behavior
Uses physical activity and academics as outlet and means of coping with stress

Adolescent

Challenges reality as coping strategy
May use denial or inconsistent care as coping technique
Uses social isolation and withdrawal from peers
Experiences peer group shunning if different
Understands treatments are necessary and not punishment for bad behavior
Verbalizes concerns and stresses

Data from Mott, S., James, S., & Sperhac, A. (1990). *Nursing care of children and families.* Redwood City, CA: Addison-Wesley Nursing; and Vaughn, V., & Litt, I. (1990). *Child and adolescent development: clinical implications.* Philadelphia: WB Saunders.

are more affected by the gender of the child and have more difficulty adjusting their expectations if the affected child is a son. The mother's role was more likely to be one of daily caretaking, which necessitated being able to cope with stress on a moment-by-moment basis. The father, on the other hand, may be able to avoid daily care and develop a pattern of avoidance, which can be associated with greater stress. Another factor affecting successful coping is a support system. Families also have different perceptions about the child's disability or chronic condition, depending on their frame of reference in relation to other possible situations, other persons, and other times. The ability of the family to be able to control their lives also affects their coping ability. Families are able to have a more positive coping style if they feel they are still in control of their lives (Frey, Greenberg, & Fewell, 1989).

Sometimes families choose a style of coping that may seem to the nurse to interfere with the child's well-being. For example, a child with muscular dystrophy was being hospitalized for back surgery. The mother chose not to make daily visits to the hospital to see her son, but she did maintain phone contact with him and the staff. When asked why she had chosen not to come, she said she knew her son was being well cared for and she needed rest to be able to care for him when he came home. This mother had already told her son her plans, and he understood, but he still missed seeing her.

For some families and children, moving from one environment to another can cause stress. This is especially the situation when a child has had a severe traumatic brain injury, has been cared for in an acute hospital, and is moved to a rehabilitation center for therapy. Even though the child has not recovered sufficiently, is dependent for self-care, and has a feeding tube because of poor swallowing, the doctors decide the child should be moved home or to a long-term care center. The family desperately wants the child home but wants the child to be able to run and play as before the accident. The family experiences stress surrounding the relocation and becomes angry toward the rehabilitation staff for "not working hard enough" with their son. Post-traumatic responses are sustained crisis reactions to an overwhelming event. These responses, as well as responses to relocation stress, can easily impair adjustment to an illness or disability (Nypaver, Titus, & Brugler, 1996).

Coping

Coping, or the response to a stressor, is multidimensional. As the child develops, a coping style based on temperament and life experiences is also developed. Very early in the infant's life, the beginning of their individuality and coping style becomes evident. Coping skills are learned through trial and error. As successful skills are developed, the child can effectively cope and experiences mastery with self-improvement. If maladaptive skills are learned, the child develops a sense of failure and incompetence (Williamson, Zeitlin, & Szczepanski, 1989).

Lazarus (1977) identified two major styles of coping: problem-focused and emotion-focused. Problem-focused coping occurs when a person takes action using problem-solving methods, believing the stressors can be changed. One family used problem-focused coping when faced with their child's sudden undiagnosable illness by seeking out resources from the medical community to assist in finding a diagnosis and treatment. Emotion-focused coping occurs when one feels the stressors cannot be changed, so the emotions surrounding the stressors will have to change. Use of denial (a healthy coping mechanism), use of avoidance, and engaging in physical activity to vent anger and self-blame are all examples of emotion-focused coping. At times, both styles may be used. Each person in the family has his or her own style of coping. When confronted with a crisis, each member will use skills from past experiences or develop new skills if those styles are not

effective. People will usually attempt to use familiar skills before attempting to develop new ones.

Research in the area of children's coping strategies has identified a number of emotional and behavioral categories.

- aggressive activities
- behavioral or cognitive avoidance
- behavioral or cognitive distraction
- cognitive problem-solving and restructuring
- emotional expression
- information seeking
- isolation
- self-control activities
- social or spiritual support
- stressor modification (Byrne & Hunsberger, 1994)

Some strategies may be more frequently used by different age groups, and it is important that the nurse identifies the typical strategies used by the child or adolescent to deal with stressful situations. Some typical strategies used by each age group are:

Infant

- movement or rocking
- crying
- sleeping
- sucking

Toddler/Preschooler

- asking "Why?"
- motor activities
- temper tantrums
- withdrawal or regression

School-Aged Child

- talkative and questioning
- play or fantasy
- withdrawal or regression
- projection

Adolescent

- problem solving or reasoning
- acting out
- conformity with peers
- rationalization or projection

Rehabilitation Nursing Management

The measurement of current stressors requires an assessment of both life events and daily encounters, including precipitating events, child and family perceptions, situational supports, coping strategies, and defense mechanisms.

Assessment

Suggested questions and observations for the child and/or family include:

What is the child and family's reaction to new situations or experiences?

What are sources of stress for the child and the family?

Identify current and past methods of handling stress.

Identify strengths and resources for coping with stress.

How do you manage your daily life during stress?

Nursing Diagnoses

In the area of coping and stress tolerance, several nursing diagnoses must be considered. These include:

- Ineffective coping (individual, family, and community)
- Caregiver role strain
- Impaired adjustment
- Post-trauma response
- Relocation stress syndrome
- Risk for violence

Expected Outcomes

The overall expected outcomes for the child and family include:

Each person is able to cope with and tolerate stress in a manner that continually promotes his or her growth and health.

Internal and external stress is managed in an age-appropriate manner.

Individual coping skills are recognized and supported.

Intervention and Teaching

Some specific areas of intervention and teaching related to coping-stress tolerance and alterations include:

Support family and child in learning effective behavioral and cognitive coping skills that meet their needs and goals.

Teach child- and family-specific care, involving the child as much as possible to allow control over the situation and opportunity to learn self-care.

Use rituals and play to facilitate coping for the young child.

Understand that boys and girls may use different coping techniques.

Encourage peer activities for older children.

Seek activities that the child can participate in with peers.

Support the family system and encourage communication among the members.

Refer child and family to support groups for assistance with coping.

Educate neighborhood children, families, and school staff regarding the child's disability or chronic condition.

According to Hymovich & Hagopian (1992), there are five categories of coping strategies:

Seeking information. type and amount may vary depending on the context of the situation; may use personal or impersonal sources; also includes using the information

Performing skills: those needed for management and adaptation to the environment; self-care endeavors for the child; parental management including nutrition, medications, treatments, and preventing complications

Seeking resources: parental coping strategy; includes using resources such as family and friends and support services (e.g., health care, financial assistance, material resources, organizations)

Monitoring/self-monitoring: assessment methods; may increase compliance with treatment plans

Incorporating into family lifestyle: vary in degree and form; involves entire family system; may include "obtaining knowledge and skill for continuing care; maintaining sense of normalcy by trying to preserve usual patterns or taking a chance and letting the child participate in family activities; hiding or minimizing the condition; living normally despite therapy and symptoms; giving up activities; and modifying the routine" (p. 184)

Summary

Coping with a disability or chronic condition requires energy, time, and resources. Often the family and child feel isolated and set apart because of the condition or disability. If the condition is obvious to the public and peers, the child will feel different and separate from the necessary social group. Coping with differences is a continual learning process. The pediatric rehabilitation nurse can assist with the coping process by active listening, education, resource development, and recognizing that having a disability or chronic condition can be very stressful at times.

VALUE-BELIEF PATTERN

Value-belief patterns are the philosophic basis for life. They provide guidance for health management, care decisions, and how a family relates to their child with a disability or chronic condition. Values assist in deciding what is right and wrong, whereas beliefs are what the person holds to be true based on their philosophic and theologic understandings (Gordon, 1994). Some families value *who* the child is, so autonomy and dignity serve as the framework for them; others value *what* the child has, so individualism and competition guides them in their goals and expectations for the child.

Expected Development and Alterations

The child's own values and beliefs expand as they mature in their cognitive, moral, and spiritual development. Early in the child's life it is the family's values and beliefs that establish the norms for them and direct their patterns of decisions, goals, and life commitments. As the child becomes older, the process of establishing a personal sense about what is correct, meaningful, and proper begins. This, combined with the social and cultural norms that are usually part of the personal norms, integrates with the individual's values and beliefs (Gordon, 1994). Table 13–8 provides an outline of these areas for each developmental level.

Values and Beliefs

Values have been variously described as standards of worth or assertions of importance and are said to develop in the process of making choices about behavior and thoughts. They can be categorized as personal, social, professional, and overlapping; can be both unique to the individual and common to a family; and vary by culture and ethnic group. Values are determined through experience, and the presence of a child with a disability or chronic condition within the family challenges the existing system. Children customarily learn values through moralizing, modeling, being allowed to do what they desire, and values clarification. The pediatric rehabilitation nurse should be sensitive to value indicators such as feelings, worries, goals, and

interests when assessing the child and family and incorporate this knowledge into the plan of care and decision-making aspects of management (Hymovich & Hagopian, 1992).

Beliefs are personal ideas about the environment that influence how the child and family assess a situation. Beliefs about health and illness influence understanding of a child's disability or chronic condition, expectations of interactions with health care providers, and decisions regarding care and treatment. The pediatric rehabilitation nurse who is sensitive to the extent to which beliefs influence attitudes about health and the decision to seek care can effect positive outcomes in the areas of prevention, regimen compliance, and participation in health-related actions.

Spirituality

Spirituality is identified by Reed (1992) as intra-personal, inter-personal, and trans-personal relationships with a higher power, self, and others. Belief in higher powers that influence one's life can provide meaning and direction to life. It is that relationship that often assists the child and family in their ability to cope with stress and even overcome it, emerging with a heightened sense of self.

Often the birth of a child with a disability, the child's development of a chronic condition, or changes in a child due to trauma motivate the family to reassess their life goals and determine again what is important for them. They may ask such questions as "Why me, God?," "What did I do to cause this punishment?," or "What am I to learn from this?" The child, depending on his or her cognitive awareness and understanding, may also go through this same assessment and reassessment. According to Myss (1996), human stress corresponds to a spiritual crisis, and with maturation of the spirit there is an opportunity for increased spiritual well-being.

Major themes occur with the integration of chronic illness into one's life; these are confronting loss, fluctuating emotions, implementing changes, and gaining control of an altered life direction. Understanding the complexity of this process is just beginning to occur through research.

Rehabilitation Nursing Management

The pediatric rehabilitation nurse must be sensitive to the family and child's values and

Table 13–8   AGES AND STAGES: EXPECTED DEVELOPMENT—VALUES AND BELIEFS

Infant/Toddler

Vocalizes pleasure and distress
Enjoys being the center of attention
Values own property—says "mine"
Takes pride in own accomplishments—may resist assistance
Demonstrates independence—may refuse to hold the hand of an adult when out in public
Develops sense of trust, attachment, and being nurtured
Primal faith experienced in relationships

Preschooler

Participates in family religious activities and rituals
Intuitive-projected faith—uses images, feelings, and symbols
Develops sense of self as separate from others
Needs positive role models for development of values and beliefs

School-Aged Child

Has sense that rules are for keeping order
Develops sense of industry and takes pride in self-competence
Has mythic-literal faith
Asks questions regarding life
Begins to understand own 'meaning in life'

Adolescent

Develops ideas about spirituality from peers and family
Expands on information about life's meaning
Develops sense of identity

Data from Erikson, E. (1963). *Childhood and society* (2nd ed.). New York: Norton Fowler, J. (1980). Moral stages and the development of faith. In B. Munsey (Ed.). *Moral development, moral education*, pp. 130–160. Birmingham, AL: Religious Education Press; and Vaughn, V., & Litt, I. (1990). *Child and adolescent development: clinical implications.* Philadelphia: WB Saunders.

beliefs, as well as the process of working through the distress and moving toward increased spiritual well-being. This process usually happens deep within the person. The nurse must intuitively sense this for discussion regarding spiritual beliefs to take place. The nurse must also have a clear understanding of personal values, beliefs, and spirituality and the ability to openly and honestly discuss these issues and ensure that the values of the child and family are central to the planning and decision-making process.

Assessment

In interacting with the family during a crisis in their child's life, the nurse must assess each person's beliefs and values and integrate the information with data from all other functional health patterns. Suggested areas to explore and questions to ask are:

What religious practices are important?
Who does the family or child turn to for support during a crisis?

How has the child's condition changed or tested existing value and belief systems?
What health care practices interfere with or invalidate existing beliefs and values?
How has this experience changed the child or family's spirituality?

Nursing Diagnoses

In the area of values and beliefs, two nursing diagnoses must be considered:

- Spiritual distress
- Potential for enhanced spiritual well-being

Expected Outcomes

The overall expected outcomes for the child and family include:

Values and beliefs will be useful in promoting strength and hope.
A healthy body, mind, and spiritual connection is developed and used as a framework for actions in life.
Value and belief patterns will become a

source of guidance for life as well as health management and care decisions.

Child will have opportunities to become aware of right and wrong.

Child will experience the environment as providing a sense of strength and hope (Dunn, 1996).

Intervention and Teaching

Specific areas of intervention and teaching related to values and belief alterations include:

Create a non-judgmental environment that allows the child and family to feel understood; communicate acceptance of spiritual practices.

Acknowledge the importance of spiritual needs and initiate discussion of spiritual welfare if necessary.

Referral to supportive counseling staff when appropriate.

View sorrow as a normal response to disability or chronic condition.

Listen to the family and child's stories as a means of validating their importance and complexity.

Encourage the family and child to be in contact with important spiritual or religious support persons.

Encourage the family and child to maintain spiritual or religious rituals that have meaning to them.

Use the child's ability for self-expression in play and drawings to assess spirituality.

Summary

All humans have a spiritual dimension. It is often with distress, such as disability or chronic condition, that the family and child seek out their spiritual dimension in an effort to find meaning and value and to reaffirm their beliefs. This search for new meaning should be supported by the pediatric rehabilitation nurse and the rehabilitation team.

SEXUALITY-REPRODUCTIVE PATTERN

Sexuality is a crucial aspect of the total person and expresses the essence of one's feelings and behaviors as male or female. Sexuality goes beyond genital response to the depth of intimate relationships between human beings (Smith, 1993; Selekman & McIlvain-Simpson, 1991). Sexuality is influenced by cultural, so-cial, psychologic, and biologic factors (Andrist, 1988). Sexual identity is regulated by cultural norms and mediates the expression of sexuality (Gordon, 1994). Sexual identity develops from information obtained from the psychosocial, cultural, and environmental background of the child and family. Sexuality is a natural part of life, and children are sexual beings. The child's gender is an important part of their sexual identity. In the past, society has tended to view the child or individual with a disability as asexual or sexually threatening. As a result, children with disabilities rarely received sexuality education and frequently lacked any specific information about the interaction between their disability and sexual potential.

Expected Development and Alterations

Human sexuality and identity formation starts at conception and develops throughout the life span. At birth, the infant's gender is based on the appearance of the genitals. If there are questions due to ambiguous genitalia, gender identity may be in doubt until further diagnostic information is obtained. This delays the process of formation of sexual identity and may cause some confusion if diagnosis is delayed. Parental expectations greatly influence the child's early sexual identity and gender identity by naming the child with a masculine or feminine name, dressing the child in feminine or masculine clothing, or providing feminine or masculine types of toys. Developmental gender differences between boys and girls are well recognized. See Chapter 10 for more information on physiologic changes based on gender and the development of secondary sex characteristics.

Parental behavior regarding sexuality creates the model for the child that determines, in large part, the child's attitude toward sex and sexual behavior. Development of healthy sexual attitudes in children is based on the message that sex is a good and natural part of all people, sexual curiosity is natural, and sexual response is a natural part of body functioning (Smith, 1993) Modeling healthy, respectful relationships between men and women is a key part of parents' sexuality teaching.

Infants need touch and body contact to support development and a sense of trust, as well as to recognize affection and learn about body boundaries. Toddlers begin to develop interest and curiosity about their bodies and begin to explore their genitals. At this age, outside influences such as television, media, and peers begin to have a profound effect on emerging gender and sexual identity. Research suggests that television and other media portrayals of sex and violence influence the attitudes and behaviors of children (Smith, 1993; Murray, 1989). Pre-school children frequently engage in exploratory sex play and need to have limits set with regard to behaviors that should occur in private, such as masturbation. Children of this age also identify with a same-sex role model and learn about appropriate sexual identity and role behavior from them. School-aged children tend to be less focused on their own bodies and more focused on the world around them. Modesty begins to become more important, and it is essential that this is respected. At about age 9 or 10 years, discussion about the changes of puberty may be initiated using simple, concrete representations. Parents often need guidance at this point, and the nurse can suggest books about body changes and sexuality. Books that can be read by the child and parent together are especially helpful (Smith, 1993).

Adolescence is a time of rapid physiologic and emotional changes that present challenges to the child and family. Personal and sexual identity formation is in its final stages, and adolescents test their limits and those of society. Sexual experimentation begins with most adolescents becoming sexually active during the middle or late period of adolescence. Smith (1993) states that "A primary goal of the encounter with an adolescent is to guide the teen in making healthy choices that are positive, and exposing choices that may have a detrimental effect. Discussing sex and sexuality help flush out those positive and negative choices" (p. 43). More information on psycho-sexual development can be found in Chapter 10. Assisting the child to develop good interpersonal skills and the ability to maintain communication within a close relationship is critical.

Effect of Disability or Chronic Condition

Chronic conditions and disabilities affect the child's identity and self-concept as well as the ability to engage in sexual activity and to reproduce. Children and adolescents with disabilities have sexual drives and express interest in dating, marriage, procreation, and raising children, the same as other children (Morse & Ross, 1994). Although most adolescents with a disability or chronic condition

express a desire to marry and have children, few of them seek out information about their sexual or reproductive functioning (Cromer et al., 1990). The majority of children with disabilities and chronic conditions fail to receive sexuality education through schools, health care providers, or home due to discomfort with the subject, lack of knowledge about the effect of the disability or chronic condition on sexual functioning, or negative attitudes toward sexuality and disability. Instruction to prevent sexual exploitation and abuse is frequently neglected. Information on sexuality may be presented in ways that are inaccessible to the child with a disability or chronic condition due to the child's sensory deficits, learning disabilities, or intellectual level (National Information Center for Children and Youth With Disabilities [NICHCY], 1992).

Disabilities and chronic conditions may affect sexuality in a variety of ways. Despite these effects, it is usually possible for individuals with even very severe disabilities to achieve satisfactory, intimate relationships with a chosen partner. One very significant challenge that many children and adolescents with disabilities face is that of forming friendships and developing intimate relationships. Often, children with disabilities are very isolated from their peers due to segregated schooling, difficulties with mobility, or lack of accessible public facilities for recreation. Forming friendships that could develop into intimate relationships becomes extremely difficult. Another potential barrier is the development of social skills. Often this problem, rather than the disability itself, is the greatest barrier to developing friendships that lead to intimate relationships. Social skills development begins early in childhood, when the infant first learns how to relate to others. A variety of experiences with peers and adults reinforces unfolding inter-personal social skills. Inclusion in child care, pre-schools and school programs with peers who are not disabled as well as others with disabilities is one of the best vehicles for supporting the development of social skills, friendships, and relationships for children with disabilities and chronic conditions.

Common Concerns

Common concerns of children and adolescents with disabilities and chronic conditions that affect sexual development and sexuality include pain, fatigue, motor control, offensive odors, contractures, sensory changes, and altered body image (Selekman & McIlvain-Simpson, 1991). The presence of these physiologic or psychologic alterations may create barriers to forming and maintaining intimate relationships.

Pain can result from joint stiffness such as that which occurs with juvenile arthritis; back pain from scoliosis or sensitivity of the skin around the spinal lesion in spina bifida; or uncomfortable positioning during sexual activity. Autoimmune conditions contribute to fatigue as well as cardiovascular conditions. Motor control, or lack of motor control and coordination, interfere with the physical performance of sexual and intimate activities. Speech difficulties may interfere with communication and establishment of relationships. Adolescents with bowel and bladder dysfunction may experience odors of feces and urine which are unpleasant to others and interfere with formation of relationships. Bowel and bladder dysfunction may also interfere with sexual activity if the individual fears having an accident during intimacy. Joint contractures may contribute to pain as well as difficulties with positioning and physical touching of one another. Sensory changes, such as vision and hearing impairment, may complicate communication and formation of relationships. Lack of or alterations in skin and genital sensation have the potential to alter sexual response. Body image may be altered by physical factors, such as the scarring that results from burns, or by psychosocial factors, such as low self-esteem, self-consciousness, or embarrassment. Altered body image may also result from the effects of medications (e.g., steroids) that can cause changes in body shape or delay or accelerate sexual maturation (Selekman & McIlvain-Simpson, 1991).

Delays in sexual maturation may also result from causes such as nutritional deprivation, which may occur in children with severe cerebral palsy who are unable to take in enough calories to support development; or chronic hypoxia, such as that which occurs in those with congenital heart disease or cystic fibrosis. Any condition that results in growth retardation may also delay sexual maturation. Accelerated sexual maturation, or precocious puberty, has been associated with obesity, acquired hypothyroidism, some types of visual impairment, spina bifida, some genetic syndromes (e.g., Prader-Willi syndrome), and pituitary tumors. Because of these effects, some authors recommend that physical examination of children with disabilities or chronic conditions always include estimation of Tanner stages (Selekman & McIlvain-Simpson, 1991).

Children and adolescents with spinal cord dysfunction—for example, spinal cord injury, spina bifida, or neuromuscular diseases—experience limitations in mobility and sensory function and neurogenic bowel and bladder, which may complicate accomplishment of physical intimacy. Girls and women with these conditions may become pregnant, but they generally experience a high-risk pregnancy with some increased risk to the fetus. Women with spina bifida are capable of normal fertility. Boys and men, on the other hand, have varying functional sexual ability, such as fertility and erectile capacity, which may be difficult to determine (Sloan, 1993). Orgasmic capabilities vary based on genital sensation. However, with good medical planning, pregnancy in women with disabilities may be carried out safely. Individuals whose condition has a genetic basis should undergo genetic counseling to determine risk of occurrence of the affected gene in offspring.

Young men and women with cerebral palsy are capable of normal sexual functioning but may need assistance because of motor difficulties. Women with cerebral palsy have normal fertility and are able to maintain a pregnancy; 90% of pregnancies in this population are normal, with only a slightly higher risk of abnormal births (Winch et al., 1993).

CASE STUDY

Sherree was a 19-year-old young woman who came to the rehabilitation clinic for the first time. Her family had just moved to the area from a small town in another state. She started taking classes at the local community college last fall. Sherree was diagnosed with cerebral palsy when she was an infant. She uses a wheelchair most of the time, is able to perform activities of daily living independently with adaptive equipment, and can walk short distances with a walker. She was accompanied to clinic by her parents and her boyfriend David.

At the beginning of the clinic evaluation, Sherree asked to talk to someone privately about "personal things." Her parents agreed to leave the room, but her boyfriend stayed. Sherree tentatively asked about sexuality education. She stated that she and David were thinking about getting married but were not sure if they would be able to have a "normal relationship" or have children. When asked about the type of sexuality education she already had, Sherree replied that she had attended some classes at school but they didn't say anything about someone with her condition.

Before making recommendations, the nurse obtained a thorough sexual and health history from Sherree and David, which included evaluating their level of comfort discussing sexuality. After taking the history, the nurse shared the following information with Sherree and David:

- There is no reason why they should not enjoy a normal sexual relationship. Although cerebral palsy affects muscle strength and coordination, it does not affect sensation, and women with cerebral palsy should be normally orgasmic. Positioning for sexual intercourse is best accomplished by experimenting with different positions. Side-lying, side-by-side positions often are most comfortable for individuals with weak musculature and tightness at the hip and knee. Sexuality counseling for Sherree and David includes information on other sexual practices such as manual stimulation, oral-genital stimulation, and the use of appliances such as vibrators.
- Sherree faces the same risk of getting pregnant with unprotected intercourse as any other woman. There is no data to suggest that her fertility will be affected by her condition. However, her choice of birth control will be affected by her condition. Due to her reduced level of activity and muscle tone, she has a greater risk of developing blood clots with birth control pills. Instead, she should consider other forms of birth control. Voluntary sterilization is a possible option for either partner, but should be a mutual decision by both partners.
- If they do decide to have a child, Sherree's condition would make her pregnancy high risk. She would be at greater risk than a non-disabled woman for complications of immobility with pregnancy such as urinary tract infections, blood clots, hypertension, and constipation. Women with disabilities in general are at higher risk for cesarean section due to deformities of the spine and hips. Fatigue would be increased and could decrease her functional abilities. The fetus may be at greater risk due to maternal complications.
- An important consideration with regard to

pregnancy is the care of the child after the birth. Although women with disabilities are capable of providing competent mothering and care for a child, the tasks of caring for the child will need to be integrated into both parents' daily routines and may be affected by Sherree's own self-care needs.

Children with cognitive disabilities such as traumatic brain injury may exhibit socially inappropriate sexual behaviors, which can be a management challenge. Behaviors such as inappropriate touching of other people, use of profanity, masturbation in public places, or making unwelcome sexual advances are threatening to other children and adults and further isolate the child. A comprehensive, consistent program of behavioral support and reinforcement of appropriate behaviors may be required.

Adolescent and Young Adult

Adolescents with specific disabilities or chronic conditions can benefit from counseling in the areas of alleviation of uncomfortable symptoms such as pain prior to sexual activity. Information about different or altered sexual practices may be necessary. Adolescents who are unable to participate in sexual intercourse require instruction in different methods of giving and receiving sexual pleasure, such as oral-genital sex, manual stimulation, masturbation, and use of vibrators. Guidance regarding the use of different positions for sexual intercourse may be necessary. At times, adolescents with disabilities may engage in same-sex activities simply because partners of the opposite sex are not available to them. This occurs more often in institutional settings or group homes.

Adolescents with disabilities or chronic conditions are just as susceptible to peer pressure with regard to high-risk behaviors as other adolescents, perhaps more so due to a desire for social acceptance. Development of an open, trusting relationship with the adolescent with a disability or chronic condition will aid in providing guidance about healthy decision making with regard to high-risk activities. The importance of counseling about birth control, risk of sexually transmitted diseases such as human immunodeficiency virus (HIV), and sexual exploitation cannot be emphasized enough.

For young women, choice of birth control methods must take into consideration the underlying medical condition as well as the young woman's needs. Young women with disabilities or chronic conditions may have never received a pelvic examination or a Papanicolaou (Pap) smear, particularly those with significant physical challenges, such as cerebral palsy, or those with cognitive disabilities who do not understand and fear the process of the pelvic examination. Oral contraceptives or implanted hormonal devices are contraindicated for women who use a wheelchair, have circulatory difficulties, or have immune conditions because of the risk of thrombophlebitis (Selekman & McIlvain-Simpson, 1991; Rogers, 1989). Women with spinal cord dysfunction may face increased risk with an intrauterine device due to absent sensation and the associated difficulty in determining whether the device has become dislodged. Although voluntary sterilization or vasectomy of male partners is an option, it is very important for this decision to be made by the woman and her partner; too often sterilization is forced on young women with disabilities by parents or health care providers. In most states, involuntary sterilization of a child or woman with a disability is illegal.

Young men with disabilities or chronic conditions may have difficulty with erections, retrograde ejaculations, and sterility. Hand function may be a limiting factor both when engaging in sexual activity with another person and when using male contraceptives. Men with spinal cord injuries who lack genital sensation claim they experience orgasm that is "in their heads" rather than in their genitals.

It is probably most important when discussing sexuality issues to emphasize the emotional aspect of loving and caring for another person—of meeting the emotional needs of intimate partners as well as the physical needs. Establishing and maintaining trust and open lines of communication with one other person is as important, if not more so, than physical activities.

Rehabilitation Nursing Management

Assessment

Suggested areas of observation for the child or adolescent and family include:

Child and Family

- child's developmental level and level of psychosocial development

- family attitudes and perceptions about sexuality
- knowledge about the child's disability and it's effect on sexual development
- sexual behavior on the part of the child, such as masturbation or sex play
- Tanner stage of the child, signs of precocious puberty, or delay of secondary sex characteristics
- child's self-concept and self-esteem

Adolescent

- female—age of menarche, length and characteristics of menstrual cycle
- female—breast self-examination, Pap smear history
- female—pregnancy history
- male—age at first nocturnal emissions, erectile capacity (presence of spontaneous erection)
- breast self-examination, testicular examination
- Tanner stage
- disability and its effect on sexuality
- adolescent's knowledge of sexuality and of the disability or condition
- sexual activity, frequency, number of partners
- sexual preference—if homosexual, at higher risk for substance abuse, runaway history, prostitution, physical and sexual abuse, depression, or suicide ideation
- knowledge and use of birth control
- knowledge of sexually transmitted disease and prevention

Nursing Diagnoses

In the sexuality-reproductive area, two nursing diagnoses should be considered:

- Altered sexuality patterns
- Sexual dysfunction

Expected Outcomes

The child and family will develop understanding of sexuality and reproduction necessary for maximizing the potential of the child's gender, sexual development, and reproduction.

Child with a disability or chronic condition will be able to fulfill their role as a sexual human.

Adolescent with a disability or chronic condition will discuss concerns about body image, sex role, and desirability as a sexual partner.

Intervention and Teaching

Teach information regarding sexuality, sexual anatomy, and function at the child's cognitive developmental level.

Support development of positive self-esteem and self-concept and comfort with own body.

Teach appropriate areas and situations for intimate physical contact, prevention of sexual exploitation, and alternative means of sexual expression.

Present information using the child's questions as a guide; never ignore child's questions.

Support family in the development of positive sexual identity in the child with a disability or chronic condition.

Identify verbal and nonverbal cues indicating the need or desire to discuss sexual concerns and give permission for discussion.

Provide an atmosphere of acceptance and privacy when discussing sexuality.

Encourage and accept expressions and concerns and assist to deal with stages of grieving if appropriate.

Summary

Provision of sexuality education to children and adolescents with disabilities and chronic conditions is crucial to their human development and quality of life. These children have unique needs and often lack the opportunity to gain information from their peers or knowledgeable, approachable adults. Children and adolescents with disabilities and chronic conditions often are less likely to observe, develop, and practice the interpersonal skills and sexual behavior necessary to develop intimate relationships. Limitations in intellectual ability, learning, or reading restrict their access to the usual educational materials; additionally, information must be explained in ways that meet each adolescent's unique needs. Pediatric rehabilitation nurses provide a valuable resource of sexuality information and counseling to these children and families.

CASE STUDY

During Micah's yearly visit to the spina bifida clinic, his mother, Fay, asked the nurse for help. "Micah is almost 12 years old now, and he is starting to become interested in girls. His father and I have tried to talk to him about sexuality, but we aren't doing a very good job and he doesn't seem very interested in what we have to say. Neither one of us is very comfortable talking about sex, and we just don't know what to say to him. Can you help, or send me to someone who can help us with this?"

Micah's spina bifida is at the L5-S1 level. He walks with braces most of the time but is increasingly interested in using a wheelchair, especially for sports activities. He manages his bladder with clean intermittent catheterization and his bowels with rectal suppositories every other night.

When she interviewed Micah by himself, with his mother out of the room, the nurse found that he had a lot of questions about his body. He had been having nocturnal ejaculations, did not know what they were, and was worried about them. He also had concerns about his body and how it was different from those of other boys his age. He had never had any sexuality education in school and depended on street talk with peers and the occasional "girlie" magazine furtively passed around on the bus for his information. Micah was very shy around girls, but had met one girl in the sports program that he was particularly interested in.

The nurse assured Micah that the nocturnal ejaculations were normal and indicated that he was developing typically in this area. She stated that even though he was capable of getting an erection, it didn't necessarily mean that he could father children, but that when he was more interested in that aspect, the urologist could perform a test to determine his fertility. She cautioned him not to depend on being sterile, however, and to avoid unprotected sexual intercourse. Micah was more concerned at this point in what to say to a girl, and he and the nurse talked about social skills and becoming friends with members of the opposite sex.

Following their private discussion, the nurse recommended that Fay sign Micah up for a sexuality education class the clinic was offering. The class was to be attended by parents and children. While the nurse and one of the male physical therapists talked to the children, the social worker discussed socialization, sexuality, and transition issues with the parents. The class was open to children with disabilities aged 10 to 14 years. The nurse also shared some resources with Fay for teaching sexuality to children, including books that described the human body and basic sexuality education. She assured Fay that most parents are not comfortable discussing sex with their children, whether the child has a disability or not. She stated that the best thing that Fay and her husband could do for Micah is to help him feel more comfortable with his body and support positive self-esteem.

CONCLUSION

The pediatric rehabilitation nurse uses the nursing process to identify needs and problems in the psychosocial areas. Appropriate interventions are selected that contribute to health and development, and the nurse provides ongoing support, teaching, and consultation for the child or adolescent and his or her family in these vital areas. Assisting the child or adolescent with a disability or chronic condition to be as independent as possible in all activities, but especially self-care, enables them to participate more fully in all aspects of life at home, in school, and in the community.

REFERENCES

Andrist, L. (1988). Taking a sexual history and educating clients about safe sex. *Nursing Clinics of North America,* 23(4), 959–973.

Ayers, A. (1973). *Sensory integration and the child.* Los Angeles: Western Psychological Services.

Barber, N. (1996). Dermatological diseases. In C. Burns, N. Barber, M. Brady, & A. Dunn, (Eds.). *Pediatric primary care* (3rd ed.), pp. 717–737. Philadelphia: WB Saunders.

Barnes, C., Beardslee, C., Schafer, P., & Shannon, R. (1986). The child with failure to thrive. *Pediatric Nursing Forum,* 1(1), 3–11.

Berne, P., & Savary, L. (1992). Building self-esteem in children, New York: Continuum Publishing.

Brazelton, T. (1973) *Clinics in developmental medicine series,* No. 50: Neonatal behavior assessment scale. London: Willian Heinemann.

Byrne, C., & Hunsberger, M. (1994). Stress, crisis and coping. In C. Betz, M. Hunsberger, & S. Wright (Eds.). *Family-centered nursing care of children,* pp. 629–650. Philadelphia: WB Saunders.

Carpenito, L. (1995). *Handbook of nursing diagnosis* (6th ed.). Philadelphia: JB Lippincott.

Chess, S., & Thomas, A. (1986). *Temperament in clinical practice.* New York: Guilford Press.

Clubb, R. (1991). Chronic sorrow: adaptation patterns of parents with chronically ill children. *Pediatric Nursing,* 17(5), 461–467.

Cromer, J., Enrile, B., McCoy, K., Gerhardstein, M., Fitzpatrick, M., & Judis, J. (1990). Knowledge, attitude and behavior related to sexuality in adolescents with chronic disability. *Developmental Medicine and Child Neurology,* 32, 602–610.

Culley, B., Perrin, E., & Jordan-Chaberski, M. (1989). Parental perceptions of vulnerability of formerly premature infants. *Journal of Pediatric Health Care,* 3(5), 237–243.

Dunn, A. (1996). Values and beliefs. In C. Burns, N. Barber, M. Brady, & A. Dunn (Eds.). *Pediatric primary care,* pp. 423–435. Philadelphia: WB Saunders.

Foster, R., & Stevens, B. (1994). Nursing management of pain in children. In C. Betz, M. Hunsberger, & S. Wright (Eds.). *Family-centered nursing care of children,* pp. 856–881. Philadelphia: WB Saunders.

Frey, K., Greenberg, M., & Fewell, R. (1989). Stress and coping among parents of handicapped children: a multidimensional approach. *American Journal on Mental Retardation,* 94(3), 240–249.

Gordon, M. (1994). *Nursing diagnosis—process and application.* St. Louis: CV Mosby.

Hymovich, D., & Hagopian, G. (1992). *Chronic illness in children and adults: a psychosocial approach.* Philadelphia: WB Saunders.

Lazarus, R. (1977). Cognitive and coping processes in emotion. In A. Monat & R.S. Lazarus (Eds.). *Stress and coping,* pp. 145–158. New York: Columbia University Press.

McCaffery, M. (1972). *Nursing management of the patient with pain.* Philadelphia: JB Lippincott.

McGrath, P., & Unruh, A. (1987). *Pain in children and adolescents.* New York: Elsevier.

Miller, J. (1992). *Coping with chronic illness—overcoming powerlessness.* Philadelphia: FA Davis.

Morse, J., & Roth, S. (1994). Sexuality. In S. Roth & J. Morse (Eds.). *A life span approach to nursing care for individuals with disabilities.* Baltimore: Paul H. Brookes.

Murphy, M., & Hagerman, R. (1992). Attention deficit activity disorder in children: diagnosis, treatment and follow-up. *Journal of Pediatric Health Care* 6(1), 2–11.

Murray, J. (1989). Helping your child use TV sensibly [letter]. *Child and Adolescent Behavior,* 5(9), 1, 4–5.

Myss, C. (1996). *Anatomy of the spirit.* New York: Harmony Books.

National Information Center for Children and Youth with Disabilities (NICHCY) (1992). Sexuality education for children and youth with disabilities. *NICHCY News Digest,* 1(3), 1–27.

Nypaver, J., Titus, M., & Brugler, C. (1996). Patient transfer to rehabilitation: just another move? *Rehabilitation Nursing,* 21(2), 94–97.

Olshansky, S. (1962). Chronic sorrow: a response to having a mentally defective child. *Social Casework,* 43, 190–193.

Reed, P. (1992). An emerging paradigm for the investigation of spirituality in nursing. *Research in Nursing & Health,* 15(5), 349–357.

Rogers, M. (1989). Psychologic aspects of pregnancy in patients with rheumatic diseases. *Rheumatic Disease Clinics of North America,* 15(2), 361–375.

Rousey, A., Best, S., & Blacher, J. (1992). Mother's and father's perceptions of stress and coping with children who have severe disabilities. *American Journal on Mental Retardation,* 97(1), 99–109.

Schneider, E. (1996). The power of touch: massage for infants. *Infants & Young Children,* (3), 40–55.

Scudder, L. (1994). Sensory and communication alterations. In C. Betz, M. Hunsberger, & S. Wright (Eds.). *Family-centered nursing care of children,* pp. 2042–2079. Philadelphia: WB Saunders.

Selekman, J., & McIlvain-Simpson, G. (1991). Sex and sexuality for the adolescent with a chronic condition, *Pediatric Nursing,* 17(6), 535–538.

Sloan, S. (1993). *Sexuality issues in spina bifida: spina bifida spotlight,* pp. 1—3. Washington DC: Spina Bifida Association of America.

Smith, M. (1993). Pediatric sexuality: promoting normal sexual development in children. *Nurse Practitioner,* 18(8), 37–44.

Vaughn, V., & Litt, I. (1990) *Child and adolescent development: clinical implications.* Philadelphia: WB Saunders.

Williamson, G., Zeitlin, S., & Szczepanski, M. (1989). Coping behavior: implications for disabled infants and toddlers. *Infant Mental Health Journal,* 10(1), 3–13.

Winch, R., Bengtson, L., McLaughlin, J., Fitzsimmons, J., & Bridden, S. (1993). Women with cerebral palsy: obstetric experiences and neonatal outcome, *Developmental Medicine and Child Neurolology,* 35 (11), 974–982.

Wong, D. (1995). *Whaley and Wong's nursing care of infants and children* (5th ed.). St. Louis: CV Mosby.

ADDITIONAL RESOURCES

Bernstein, A. (1996). How children learn about sex and birth. *Psychology Today,* Jan., 73–78.

Brandt, P. (1993). Negotiation and problem-solving strategies: collaboration between families and professionals. *Infants & Young Children,* 5(4), 78–84.

Carmen, S. (1994). Attachment intervention. *Infants & Young Children,* 7(1), 34–41.

Case-Smith, J. (1993). *Pediatric occupational therapy and early intervention.* Boston: Andover Medical Publishers.

Hauck, M. (1991). Cognitive abilities of preschool children: implications for nurses working with young children. *Journal of Pediatric Nursing,* 6(4), 230–235.

Johnson-Martin, N., Jens, K., Altermeier, S., & Hacker, B. (1991). *The Carolina curriculum for infants and toddlers with special needs.* Baltimore: Paul H. Brookes.

Keller, M., Duerst, B., & Zimmerman, J. (1996). Adolescents' views of sexual decision-making. *IMAGE: Journal of Nursing Scholarship,* 28(2), 125–130.

Krajicek, M. & Cassidy, E. (1997). Sexuality. In H.M. Wallace, R.F. Biehl, J.C. MacQueen, & J.A. Blackman (Eds.). *Mosby's resource guide to children with disabilities and chronic illness.* St. Louis: CV Mosby.

Nosek, M., Rintala, D., Young, M., Howland, C., Foley, C., Rossi, I., & Chanpong, G. (1996). Sexual functioning among women with physical disabilities. *Archives of Physical Medicine and Rehabilitation,* 77(2), 107–155.

Revell, G., & Liptak, G. (1991). Understanding the child with special health care needs: a developmental perspective. *Journal of Pediatric Nursing,* 6(4), 258–263.

Wright, B. (1983). *Physical disability—a psychosocial approach* (2nd ed.). New York: Harper Collins.

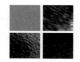

Chapter 14

The Home, School, and Community Environments

Patricia A. Edwards

The health, development, and well-being of children and their families is fostered by interaction with positive environments. These include the home in which they reside, the schools and day care programs they attend, and their neighborhood and the larger community, where they interact socially, culturally, spiritually, and recreationally. In the current world in which children with disabilities and chronic conditions live, there are forces and influences moving the need for and provision of health care services beyond the office or hospital door and into the larger community.

Pediatric rehabilitation nurses have unique and important contributions to make to ensure that a successful collaborative model of care in the home, school, and community can become a reality. A developmental perspective allows the nurse to make a sensitive matching of intervention strategies to the bio-psycho-social issues of each age group and provide others with understanding of age-appropriate child health concerns. Knowledge of all of the potential factors that contribute to a child's health (e.g., genetics, family, environment) and the ability to recognize physical, developmental, social, and emotional disorders allow the nurse to institute interventions that are appropriate to individual needs. The nurse is prevention oriented; promotes healthy lifestyles; stresses immunization, nutrition, and injury prevention; emphasizes meeting individual needs and valuing differences; and understands the normality of variations and how to tailor a unique response to each child or adolescent

and his or her family. The provision of continuity for families and the nurse's ability to establish the trust and openness that promote a long-term relationship are essential as the complex care of the child is managed while growth and development takes place.

The environments of home, school, and community are explored in this chapter in regard to their impact on children and their families. The types of children who are dependent on technology to live at home, to attend school, and to have specialized care and services provided for them are included in each section.

HOME ENVIRONMENT

Children with disabilities and chronic conditions have the right to live at home with their family and receive all the necessary love and care to grow and develop to their fullest potential. Caring for these children can be a difficult endeavor that requires a coordinated effort to meet their complex medical, physical, and psychosocial needs. Pediatric rehabilitation nurses can be instrumental in the development of a realistic, coordinated home care plan that ensures that a comprehensive continuum of services is available to the family in the home and community.

Discharge to Home

As the coordinator of care, the nurse assists the family in obtaining information and making responsible decisions to enable a safe transition to home. The long-term success of

289

the child's experience at home is greatly influenced by the hospital discharge plan, which must be tailored to the child and family, and the quality of the services provided to the family. "Children currently cared for at home generally have to meet hospital discharge criteria such as capacity for self- or family care; supportive, stable home environments; and funding for necessary equipment, supplies and professional nursing services" (Samuel, 1991, p. 5).

The planning process must be comprehensive and should include a variety of factors:

- care needs and medical stability of the child or adolescent
- available family members who are willing to have the child at home and cope with the intrusions on their lives resulting from the child's care needs
- professional caregivers trained in the necessary skills
- appropriate home environment
- medical, social, psychological, educational, and community supports
- appropriate equipment and supplies
- financial support systems

An educational plan for family learning must also be formulated so that they have adequate training and preparation. The plan must address topics such as daily routines and treatments, care of equipment, safety, medications, and nutrition. Family members should be aware of the developmental issues that might arise and the availability of community resources (including transportation), local medical supervision, emergency facilities, and alternative methods of care (including respite care services), should they be required.

Current data indicate significant savings when a child receives care at home, but the greatest benefit is not monetary. Having the child at home promotes the integrity and well-being of the family and fulfills the child's right to receive love and affection from parents, siblings, and extended family members. The child's recuperative functions are supported in the home environment, and the nurturing received increases the child's long-term productive capabilities (Caring Institute of the Foundation for Hospice and Homecare, 1987). These children frequently have decreased experiences because of their hospitalization, their condition, or the limits of technology and can exhibit delays because their movement opportunities are limited by tubing, lines, and intravenous therapy. The pediatric rehabilitation nurse with a strong foundation in childhood growth and development and skill acquisition, an understanding of family systems, and a knowledge of community resources can assist the family through the various stages from discharge to the ultimate goal of full integration into the larger community. The home is the least disruptive environment for the child and a place where the child explores and learns. This facilitates growth, improvement, and change in a child's development.

A variety of technologies are employed for the care of a child with a disability or chronic condition in the home environment. Technological aids may be therapeutic, diagnostic, rehabilitative, or palliative and are distinguished by a rapid pace of innovation. Children or adolescents with disabilities or chronic conditions may leave the hospital with central lines for medications and gastrostomy tubes or buttons in place. The use of enteral and parenteral treatments in the home has increased as a result of improvements in materials and formulas for nutrition therapy, and many children now also receive intravenous antibiotic therapy at home. Children may require home oxygen therapy, have tracheostomies for breathing, or be supported on ventilators. The use of monitors (e.g., apnea, emergency response, cardiac) is also commonplace. Other issues related to assistive technology are presented later in this chapter.

Adaptive Equipment and Housing

Prior to discharge, two important areas must be considered: an assessment of the home/living environment and the physical challenges of everyday life. A visit to the home and community by members of the rehabilitation team can provide an evaluation of the existing environment and recommendations for adaptations to enhance a child's potential for independence. Table 14–1 lists areas to consider in the home, school, and community as well as those that will contribute to independence in activities of daily living.

If it is determined that modifications in the home environment are needed, the accessibility guidelines should be followed.

- doors should provide an opening of at least 2 feet, 8 inches
- maximum wheelchair ramp slope of 1 inch of rise to every 12 inches of length
- kitchen sink and bathroom vanity maxi-

Table 14–1   AREAS OF ENVIRONMENTAL EVALUATION

In the Home	Activities of Daily Living	School/Community
Ramping	Adaptive seating	Site modifications
Adaptations for safety	Eating aids	Special learning tools
Room modifications	Bathroom safety	Page turner system
Environmental control systems	Kitchen adaptations	Computer system
Furniture modifications	Communication system	Adaptations for safety
Wheelchair lifts	Emergency system	Communication system
Stair chairs	Wheelchair modifications	Emergency system

mum height 34 inches, knee space beneath, pipes insulated
- carpeting should be close-knit low pile (RehabNET, 1997)

Other areas to consider would be eliminating hallways with angles and curves and providing an outside exit from the bedroom. Back-up generators may be a necessity if special electrical equipment is in use.

Many hospitals and rehabilitation facilities have special areas within the facility that provide real-life settings that can be used by the child or adolescent and family prior to discharge. These settings bring the real world into focus and help the child to learn or relearn skills, gain independence in a controlled setting, and face the physical challenges of everyday life before actually moving to the home. One type of setting that might be found is called *Easy Street Environments*. These are a variety of modules connected by a realistic "Main Street" that simulate driving experiences (e.g., getting in and out of an automobile), shopping in a grocery or department store, going to the bank, and eating at a café or restaurant. After practicing in the hospital environment, home visits are scheduled to allow the family to experience the care activities and make modifications prior to the final discharge. This also allows for a planned transition for the child and might include a visit to the school to assess specific needs in that setting.

As accessibility in all areas of life has been increasingly emphasized, one group has recently developed a universal design concept to simplify life for everyone by making more housing usable by more people at little or no extra cost. This approach incorporates products as well as building features that, to the greatest extent, can be used by everyone. Although accessible design requirements are presently specified by codes for some buildings and are aimed at benefiting people with mobility limitations, the universal design con-

cept applies to all people and all buildings. Universal features can be used by everyone, regardless of their level of ability, and include:

- electric receptacles placed higher than usual above the floor
- standard but wider doors
- louver or loop handles for doors
- stair landings big enough to accept lifts
- audible and visual alarm systems
- low and high storage space (Pastalan, 1996)

If this concept is incorporated during the construction of housing, fewer modifications may be required in the future to accommodate individuals with special needs.

Rehabilitation and Habilitation Technology

No other single area causes more frustration for children, adolescents, and their families than equipment that is not tailored to the child's needs. A wonderful new wheelchair can become a constant aggravation without critical adjustments. A misplaced switch not only causes frustration but also reduces functional ability. Activities of daily living, whether at home, school, or play, can be frustrating and uncomfortable for a child who has limited mobility or who lacks the ability to communicate or control the environment. It is important to have assistive technology that is designed, fabricated, and fit for the child, to allow communication, movement, and interaction with the environment. This may include wheelchair controls, protective head gear, computer access equipment, independent living tools, recreational equipment, and devices to increase mobility and independence.

The multidisciplinary rehabilitation team seeks to address these problems, assess needs, and find solutions for children and adolescents with disabilities and chronic conditions that require integrated technologies and special designs. The team assesses the child's capabilities and makes recommendations for appropriate technologies and assistive devices and helps with ordering, fittings, and finding funding sources. This can include custom-made, modified, or commercially available equipment and technical devices needed for personal care, mobility, seating, communication, and other activities of daily living, including recreation.

The assessment includes:

Evaluating physical ability—muscle strength, ambulation capabilities, stamina, and energy level

Determining the activities in which the person currently participates and where he or she takes part in them, as well as other activities in which he or she wants to be involved and other places he or she wants to go but cannot without assistance

Identifying the accessibility of the environment in which the person wants to function—entrances and exits to buildings, floor coverings, hallways and doorways, location of bathrooms, climate and

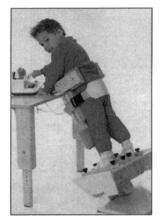

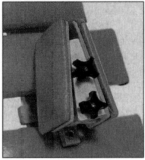

Figure 14–2 Prone-stander designed to attach to a sturdy table or counter allows for positioning at different distances. (From *Flaghouse special populations fall 1996 catalog.* Hasbrouch Heights, NJ: Flaghouse, Inc., p. 185.)

expected weather patterns, outdoor and recreational areas

The age of the individual and the stability of his or her condition, which may have an impact on future needs (Bader, Gilson, & Huss, 1995, p. 88)

Recommendations can be made in the following areas:

- adaptive seating and postural support systems
- mobility devices
- augmentative and alternative communication
- environmental control units, control interfaces, and computer applications
- adaptive devices
- orthotics

Keep in mind that, although these devices may be very useful, they should only be recommended after considering the child's unique needs and motivations to use the de-

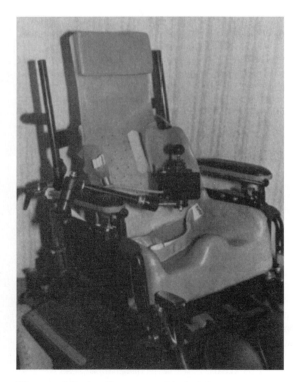

Figure 14–1 Custom-molded sitting-support. (From Campbell, S. K. [1994]. *Physical therapy for children.* Philadelphia: WB Saunders, p. 316.)

vice, as well as the cost, cosmesis, and safety of the device.

Adaptive Seating and Postural Support Systems

Examine each child and adolescent and their specific needs to create a seating system that improves daily living skills, considers the caretakers needs, and does not interfere with other function. Growth, weight changes, progressive conditions, neuromuscular and skeletal status, and use of tubes or devices must all be considered when selecting a seating system. Seats can be molded for the child's unique requirements, have modular components, and incorporate body orthoses. Custom wheelchair seating includes contoured seating shells that fit and support the hips, back, and upper body; position the pelvis and trunk upright to improve function; increase

circulation; assist in balance; and free the hands for other activities such as propelling the wheelchair, eating, or using a communication device (Fig. 14–1). This contributes to increased self-esteem and independence. Other types of positioning devices are "sidelyers" and standers. These can be used to promote alignment and normal posture and enhance upper extremity use (Figs. 14–2 and 14–3).

Mobility Devices

Mobility devices that provide support during ambulation, such as canes, crutches, and walkers, and wheeled devices, such as wheelchairs, scooters, and adapted tricycles, provide the child or adolescent with the opportunity to move independently in the environment, expanding their interactions and ac-

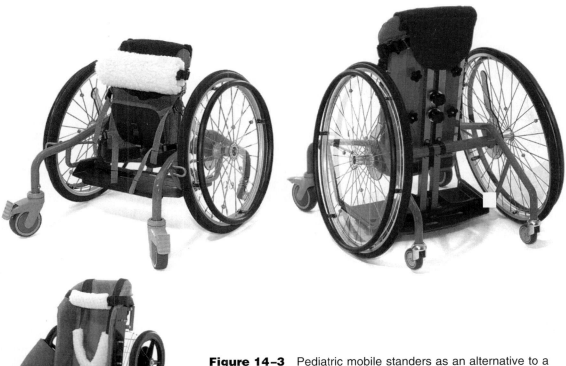

Figure 14–3   Pediatric mobile standers as an alternative to a wheelchair. The three sizes are based upon the height of the user. (From *Rifton equipment 1997–98 catalog.* Rifton, NY: Bruderhof Communities in NY, Inc., p. 18. © Rifton Equipment. Used by permission.)

cess to learning experiences. To identify which mobility device is appropriate for the child, the following areas need to be considered:

- the child's cognitive ability and awareness of surroundings and safety
- the environment for use (home, school, community)
- the child's physical ability to use or operate the device
- financial issues and availability of funding
- transportability of large devices
- motivation to use the device
- adjustment for growth
- aesthetics
- maintenance considerations

A wide range of wheelchairs are available to match the child or adolescent's abilities and needs. Improvements in weight and design enable even smaller children with strength limitations to use manual devices. If powered mobility is indicated, the child's voluntary movement must be assessed so that the appropriate controls can be provided to accommodate their ability. Tricycles that are specially adapted can provide extra support and allow the child to join in the fun of play while providing exercise, mobility, and practice in balance and coordination (Fig. 14–4). When the device is obtained, the child or adolescent, family, and other caregivers should receive training in its use, care, and maintenance so it can be used safely and correctly. When the family needs a chair for transporting the child, there are a number of possibilities, such as travel chairs, strollers, and modified manual wheelchairs (Fig. 14–5).

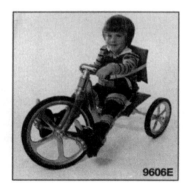

Figure 14–4 Pedal Trike provides both active and passive exercise for both younger and older children because it has an adjustable seat. (From *Flaghouse special populations fall 1996 catalog.* Hasbrouch Heights, NJ: Flaghouse, Inc., p. 32.)

Augmentative and Alternative Communication

Silence is not golden for the child or adolescent who is unable to speak, because the ability to communicate opens many doors. The inability to speak may be the result of physical limitations caused by neurologic impairments but the child or adolescent can hear and understand the speech of others. Whatever the cause of the deficit, some form of augmentative or alternative communication is needed to provide the child with a functional and effective means of communication and aid in his or her social, emotional, and cognitive development. Augmentative communication is an approach that supports and enhances the child's existing speech skills. Alternative communication is an approach that provides the child with functional, effective communication and replaces critical functions normally fulfilled by writing or speaking (Tanchak & Sawyer, 1995). Augmentative communication systems range from simple manual aids to sophisticated electronic devices, including computers. Their purpose is to provide children or adolescents with an appropriate method of communication so they can gain control over their lives and environment and have greater access to educational and social opportunities. When a communication system is being considered, gather the following information about the child:

- communication needs across all environments
- skills and abilities—cognitive and educational performance; motor skills; seating and positioning; sensory and perceptual skills; socio-emotional development; and speech, language, and literacy skills.

After a device is selected, a trial period can provide time for instruction of the child and family, ongoing evaluation of the intervention program, and follow-up supports and reassessments as required. The following is a case example of the use of augmentative and alternative communication.

CASE STUDY

Eight-year-old Becky had a neurologic infection that left her severely physically impaired. Her communication was limited to making simple sounds and looking at something she wanted. Because the pediatric rehabilitation nurse realized that Becky's communication

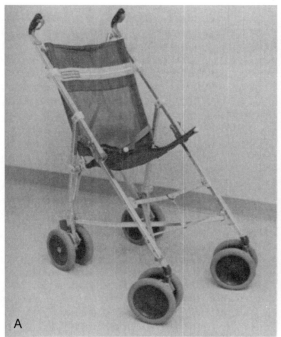

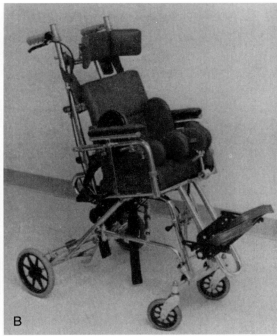

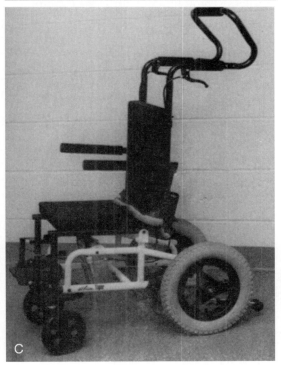

Figure 14–5   *A,* Transporter chair with a stroller base. *B,* Transporter chair with a travel chair. *C,* Transporter chair with manual wheelchair-style base with smaller rear wheels, stroller handles, and tilt mechanism to 45 degrees. (From Campbell, S.K. [1994]. *Physical therapy for children.* Philadelphia: WB Saunders, p. 643.)

needs far surpassed her physical abilities, she was referred to a technology resource center where the team assessed her capabilities and needs and determined that her most reliable motion was head movement. They found that Becky could identify pictures and, with training, could eventually learn to use phrases and sentences. The team recommended and arranged for an appropriate communication device. Now Becky wears a headpiece with a long-range optical pointer that activates a computerized light board, which cues a voice synthesizer. By moving her head to focus the light beam on a particular spot on the board,

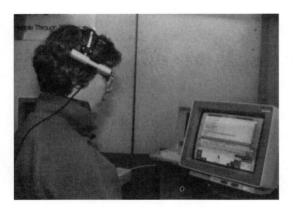

Figure 14–6 Computer-based communication system with visual keyboard on computer screen and head pointer acting as controller. (From Campbell, S. K. [1994]. *Physical therapy for children.* Philadelphia: WB Saunders, p. 510.)

Becky is able to "talk" to those around her (Fig. 14–6). The team worked with the personnel at Becky's school to incorporate the communication system into her Individualized Education Plan (IEP). Her teacher and the school nurse report that she has learned to use her device well, is much less frustrated, participates eagerly in school, and is enjoying life more fully.

Environmental Control Units

Environmental control units provide children with a degree of independence and freedom as they develop and allow them to operate equipment in a number of ways and places. The unit may consist of a control switch, a visual display, and a central processing unit and be used to operate devices such as emergency bells, telephones, televisions, lights, computers, and mechanically activated toys (Alexander et al., 1991). Systems may be as simple as activating a pressure switch to operate a toy (Fig. 14–7) or as complex as operating a computer workstation. A variety of switches and controls may be used and these vary in size, shape, cost, performance capabilities, and method of activation. Other important considerations are the location of the switch or control device and how to mount it so that it is secure and stable while being used.

Adaptive Devices

Other adaptive devices can provide greater independence in feeding, dressing, and hygiene, and the possibilities for adapting are endless. The following are some examples:

Eating—spoons, forks, knives with special handles; food bumpers or scoop plates; special cups; long straws; or other feeding aids (Fig. 14–8)

Dressing—dressing stick, sock aids; button hookers; Velcro fasteners; and loops in the clothes

Grooming—long-handled sponges and bath mitts; special handles for toothbrushes, combs, razors, and hairbrushes; and long-handled mirrors

Other—prism glasses; mouthsticks; telephone holders or a speaker phone; spe-

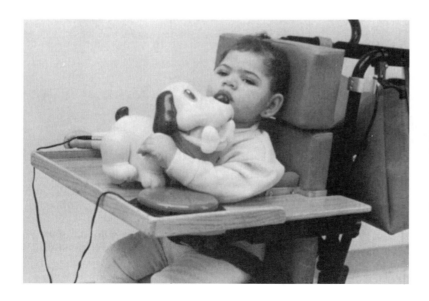

Figure 14–7 A large pressure switch can be used to activate a battery-operated toy placed on a lap tray. (From Campbell, S.K. [1994]. *Physical therapy for children.* Philadelphia: WB Saunders, p. 653.)

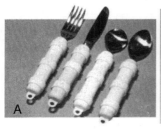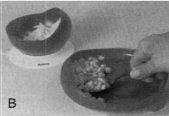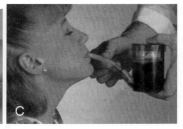

Figure 14–8   Living aids. *A*, Adapted eating utensils. *B*, Scooper plate. *C*, Drinking aids. (From *Flaghouse special populations fall 1996 catalog.* Hasbrouch Heights, NJ: Flaghouse, Inc., p. 80.)

cialized car seats; and advancement chairs (Fig. 14–9)

Orthotics

For children with certain orthopedic conditions or spine disorders, spinal or limb orthotics may be required. Orthoses provide supportive and corrective forces to the spine or limbs to prevent progression of a curved spine or to minimize orthopedic conditions. Spinal orthotics correct a curved spine and protect and stabilize a healing spine after surgery. Upper limb orthotics are splints to hold

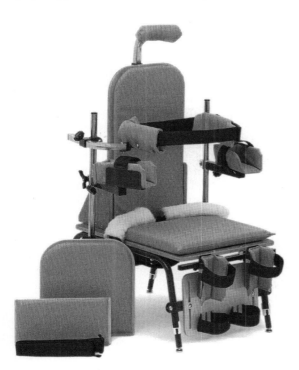

Figure 14–9   Advancement chair that adjusts for growth. (From *Rifton equipment 1997–98 catalog.* Rifton, NY: Bruderhof Communities in NY, Inc., p. 50. © Rifton Equipment. Used by permission.)

hands or arms in a corrected position; improve the child's range of motion; or support a weak wrist to allow the child to eat, write, or use a keyboard. Lower limb orthotics are braces for the hip, knee, ankle, and foot to prevent and minimize orthopedic problems, improve body posture, and increase mobility. The nurse working with children or adolescents who use spine or limb orthotics must understand their correct application and use and teach and reinforce information essential to their proper care and maintenance. The orthotic device should be as comfortable and attractive as possible, and the child and family should be aware of its proper application and the need for inspection of the skin under the device to prevent areas of redness or breakdown.

Other Resources

Many rehabilitation facilities have special programs and services to help children and families with assistive technology needs and questions. These may include an equipment demonstration program with a variety of devices available for evaluation; a used equipment registry with information and referral sources for mobility devices, environmental control units, augmentative or alternative communication devices, and other devices for independent living; or an adapted toy lending library.

A computerized resource library could be used to help children and families locate commercially available adaptive devices and services such as wheelchairs, classroom equipment, personal care devices, computer programs, mobility devices, or augmentative or alternative communication devices. Another computerized service (RehabNET, 1997) provides current information on vendors, consultants, sources for fabrication of customized equipment, repair sites, organizations, and facilities. An electronic database called

ABLEDATA (see Resources) lists assistive technology and rehabilitation equipment available in the United States, including adaptive clothing, low vision reading systems, and voice output programs. A complete description of each product and contacts for information are provided.

Canine Companions

Many children and adolescents benefit from the use of animal aids such as dogs trained specifically for a purpose and who fill the role of a dependable personal assistant. These include service dogs that perform tasks such as turning lights on and off, retrieving items, carrying parcels, helping pull clothes on, pushing buttons, or pulling a wheelchair. Hearing dogs alert people to the sounds of a telephone, alarm, or baby's cry, and social dogs can be provided for situations in which supervision is required.

Hazards and Safety Precautions

Children and adolescents with disabilities or chronic conditions may be at risk for injury in and around the home because of decreased safety awareness or environmental hazards. The pediatric rehabilitation nurse should educate the child and family about potential hazards and help the family evaluate the home situation and make necessary modifications or changes. Some hazards found in the environment and the appropriate safety precautions are as follows:

Falls during transfers or when reaching from the wheelchair. Keep wheelchair in good working order; be sure the child or adolescent knows how to transfer safely and realizes his or her limitations when stretching or reaching. Use properly installed grab rails.

Burns from applications of heat or cold (e.g., if metal wheelchair parts become hot or cold, hot water in the bath, dishwasher or washing machine, sink pipes, cooking liquids, and electrical appliances and heaters). Stress safe use of applications of heat or cold; be cautious around fireplaces, heaters, and wood stoves; adjust water temperature before bathing; insulate exposed pipes under sink; be cautious when handling hot liquids, food, or cookware.

Bruises, abrasions, lacerations, pressure areas from transfers, clothing seams, or

bulky clothing; items in pockets; or braces or assistive devices. Care should be taken during transfers; appropriately fitting clothing is essential; skin should be checked frequently; and preventive measures should be incorporated into daily activities.

LEARNING ENVIRONMENT

Learning begins in infancy as part of intellectual development and mastery of tasks. Much of the child's early learning and acquisition of skills comes through imitation of parents, caregivers, and siblings. As the child grows older, a variety of other factors influence learning, such as extended family members, peers, pre-school and school personnel, community members, and the media. The school environment provides skill training, cultural exposures, models for children to imitate, and opportunities for self-actualization, intellectual growth, and participation in social functions (Betz, Hunsberger & Wright, 1994).

Transitions

Just as all children are different in their growth and development and mastery of tasks, they also differ in their readiness for school experiences. Table 14–2 lists the characteristics that indicate maturity for the experiences of school and activities that can prepare children to participate in the more structured school setting.

From a health perspective, the first 5 years of life are a time of immense change in growth and development. It is important that an optimum state of wellness be maintained so as to promote neurologic and musculoskeletal growth and the later development of psychomotor, cognitive, and speech and language abilities. Accessible primary care with a community-based "medical home" may be the gateway to the health care system for the child and family. This concept is discussed later in the chapter. If minor or major health issues are identified, steps must be taken to eliminate the problem or reduce its impact. Special equipment, therapy, surgery, or a combination of these may be required (Urbano, 1992).

At the time of entry into an infant or child care program or pre-school, clear information must be available about the child's disability or chronic condition. A plan for learning should be formulated that supports the child's individual needs and includes practi-

Table 14–2   CHECKLIST FOR SCHOOL READINESS

Characteristic	Preparatory Experiences
Physically healthy and strong	Balanced diet Adequate rest and sleep Opportunities for exercise Positive reinforcement for skill mastery
Capable of separating from parent	Experiences with substitute caregivers in caregiver's home Day care or nursery school a few hours a day or a couple of days a week Social activities away from home (e.g., play at a friend's home)
Has sufficiently long attention span	Listening to rather long stories Experiences working through activities that take time, such as large puzzles Sitting through a full-length TV program, movie, or circus show
Able to tolerate frustration	Parents should not always respond to requests immediately; help child learn to wait If siblings, enforce rules about taking turns Experiences with small groups of children and a single caregiver
Has some basic hand-eye skills	Practice with child and provide toys that stimulate recognizing shapes and colors Books in which child has to turn pages Experiences with a pencil and crayons Craft experiences; cutting with blunt-ended scissors, pasting, painting, molding clay Exposure to simple computer games and to TV shows that reinforce learning word sounds, alphabet letters, shapes, and colors

From Betz, C.L., Hunsberger, M., & Wright, S. (1994). *Family-centered nursing care of children* (2nd ed.), p. 269. Philadelphia: WB Saunders.

cal recommendations for activities and therapeutic techniques. The pediatric rehabilitation nurse, in coordination with the caregivers and teachers, can help develop a plan that includes goals and specific tasks for achieving these goals (Donlin-Shore, 1993).

It is also important for the family, health care professionals, and all individuals in learning environments to be aware of the developmental transitions that children go through in relation to school. These tasks, which are intended to foster the child's intellectual and social development, are shown in Table 14–3. At each transition point, conflicts may arise when the child's abilities do not match expectations. Children and adolescents with disabilities and chronic conditions go through these transitional stages while also managing the changes that occur because of their specific needs or problems. For example, a boy with muscular dystrophy entering high school has the task of becoming familiar with a new building and new personnel and must also deal with a decline in mobility necessitating the use of a wheelchair for distances. He will require support and assistance to become comfortable in the new environment and ad-

just to the changes. Some important factors that foster adjustment are:

- respect for the child's or adolescent's individuality
- responsiveness of support groups to an identified need
- a learning environment that is conductive to growth
- availability of support systems that are effective

A successful transition requires planning and should include the following key components:

- commitment by administrators to the provision of quality services
- an awareness and understanding of the needs of students with disabilities or chronic conditions, the implications of their altered health status, and its impact on learning and psychosocial development
- preparing the school environment by removing architectural barriers, providing emergency protocols, and adjusting school scheduling if necessary; also providing appropriate transportation
- a strong school nursing component, includ-

Table 14–3 DEVELOPMENTAL TRANSITIONS OF THE SCHOOL MILIEU

School-Critical Developmental Tasks	Potential Conflicts
School Entry (Age 3–5 Years*)	
Peer interactions—sharing, taking turns Social development—basic self-care skills Following directions Developing language skills	Demands do not match motor or mental abilities No previous exposure to other children No previous experience with separation from parent(s)
Academic Reading Instruction (Age 5–7 Years)	
Learning fundamentals of reading	Neurologic or cognitive unreadiness; success interferences such as moving, family upsets, poor self-concept
Reading to Learn (Second–Third Grade)	
Content of reading becomes important	Poor mastery of reading fundamentals results in poor reading skills, with resultant behavior or attendance problems Learning deficits associated with neurologic immaturity or experiential naiveté
Start Middle School (Junior High)	
Subject-oriented emphasis Change to multi-teacher and multi-class experience Often change in school building and administrative personnel	Output failure is greatest potential problem because of difficulty for child in having a relationship with a single caring adult, risk of losing sight of child's specific or special needs, troublesome nature of organizational structure for child with more rigid personality
Start High School (Ninth or Tenth Grade)	
Change in building and administrative personnel Student selection of courses to coincide with career goals Student responsible for balancing academic and social obligations	Removes familiar supportive adults and records/information about child's specific or special needs Student may not yet have identified any career goals Diminished special-education focus and special education resources Vocational education now available but too late for failure-prone child whose academic problems began at junior high level or earlier Serious mismatch of developmental rate and school expectations has greatest likelihood in this transition

*Earlier if disabled.
From Betz, C., Hunsberger, M., & Wright, S. (1994). *Family-centered nursing care of children,* Second Edition, Philadelphia, W.B. Saunders p. 96

ing a process to monitor changes in health status

- a written Individualized Healthcare Plan (IHP) developed by a team prior to attendance
- a good working relationship with parents, which includes respect for their needs and values; getting permission before doing evaluations is essential (Hertel, 1991)

A child or adolescent who has been developing normally and is hospitalized with an injury or illness faces challenges when returning to home and community and re-entering the school environment, especially if a disability has resulted. Re-entry programs have been developed for diverse medical conditions to facilitate the child's transition from the protected hospital environment into the normal routines of the typical classroom setting. One program for burned children includes the following:

- telephone contacts with the school soon after admission and before discharge; also during hospitalization as needed
- in-hospital school program
- video with visual portrayal of the child's

injuries and a description of the rehabilitation process, whether commercially produced or individualized

- school visit by the burn team, whether individually or together
- written materials (Blakeney et al., 1995)

Whether the child is facing a transition to or re-entry into the school, it is important that all personnel involved understand how the disease process or disability impacts the child's or adolescent's day, recognize when to decrease or change participation in an activity, and understand the need for adaptive equipment and tools.

Educational Issues

As mentioned in Chapter 4, a variety of legislative initiatives have mandated provision of special education and related services for school-aged children. The document that guides the program of education, resources, and services for children and adolescents is called the Individualized Education Plan (IEP). This IEP is developed by members of the education team and parents and must include:

- statement of present level of educational performance
- statement of annual goals, including short-term instructional objectives
- statement of specific education and related services to be provided and the extent of participation in the regular education program
- projected dates for initiation of services and anticipated duration
- appropriate objective criteria and evaluation procedures and schedules for determining, on at least an annual basis, whether the short-term instructional objectives are being achieved

This document is also used as a management tool, to evaluate compliance, and for monitoring.

The Individuals With Disabilities Education Act (IDEA) has extended educational services to infants and toddlers and required that services be provided in a family-centered context. For infants and toddlers and their families, an Individualized Family Service Plan (IFSP) is developed. The IFSP differs from the IEP in its focus on infant development and family functioning. The IFSP must be a written document formulated by the multidisciplinary team, including the parent or guardian. Family guidance in its development is one of the IFSP's strengths, and it includes statements about:

- present developmental level—physical, cognitive, communication, social, emotional, adaptive
- family resources, concerns, priorities
- expected outcomes and how achievement will be measured
- specific services, including frequency, intensity, and delivery method, and environment in which the services will take place
- steps to support transitions and name of the service coordinator

These legislative initiatives include protections against discrimination in testing and the concept of providing educational services in the least restrictive environment. This concept of inclusion means grouping all students, with and without disabilities, in the same classroom to allow opportunity for the child with a disability to become as independent and productive as possible and interact with his or her peers on a daily basis. An important aspect of inclusion is the collaborative relationship between the teacher and the school nurse and the provision of adequate support in the classroom. Pediatric rehabilitation nurses can support this collaboration by assisting the school nurse in understanding the medical aspects and procedures necessary for the child as well as any accommodations that must be made to improve the child's function and quality of life. "Teachers have primary responsibility for children in the classroom. Working together, teachers and nurses can provide a supportive environment for managing special health needs within the general education system" (Becker, Johnson, & Greek, 1996, p. 79).

Through the development of a document called the Individualized Healthcare Plan (IHP), health personnel and the education team can establish what health services the student requires to maximize learning and provide a safe environment. The written plan, using the nursing process, includes:

Assessment data—information pertinent to current health status with a focus on what affects learning and safety in the school environment

Nursing diagnosis—to identify the problem areas and determine appropriate goals and interventions

Student goals or desired outcomes—stated as a student response, it should be measurable and realistic

Interventions—actions of the staff or school nurse to help the student reach identified goals

Evaluation of outcomes—IHP is reviewed and the plan modified as necessary

There should also be an emergency plan, a separate document that includes interventions in an emergency situation. The basic components are:

- student identification information
- signs of an emergency
- action to initiate
- emergency phone numbers

Table 14–4 is a sample of an IHP for a child with multiple medical diagnoses and the nursing diagnosis of Impaired Swallowing (Poulton, 1996). If paraprofessionals are providing services as part of the IHP, they must be appropriately trained, the educational component documented, and their performance supervised and evaluated through a written monitoring plan.

A set of guidelines for schools and communities to use in providing educational services that enhance learning and functioning for the child or adolescent with a disability or chronic condition can be found in the Project School Care manual (Haynie, Palfrey, & Porter, 1989). This text contains information and suggested procedures to help families and schools develop individualized programs that address children's needs in the context of available community resources. This information can be used for teaching and training staff; performing specific technical procedures; writing procedures, policies, and emergency plans; and developing forms, checklists, and other necessary documents. Major sections of this document include:

1. Procedure for Entrance into an Educational Setting for the Child Assisted by Medical Technology
2. Universal Precautions and Infection Control
3. Procedural Guidelines for areas such as tube feeding, catheterization, ostomy care, intravenous lines, and respiratory care
4. Skills Checklists to review and document caregiver training
5. Bibliography, General References, and a list of manuals and resources (Haynie, Palfrey, & Porter, 1989)

Injuries in the School Environment

The school contains many potential hazards, and the risk of injury changes as students move through their school day from supervised, structured classroom environments to science laboratories, outdoor playgrounds, industrial arts shops, and gymnasiums. Transportation may include walking, bicycling, or taking the school bus. Because one of the most frequent conditions cared for by school nurses is injury, it is important to gain an understanding of the patterns and causes of injuries. An examination by Gallagher and DiScala (1994) reported causes of injuries in school from 1988 through 1993.

Boys were injured at school twice as often as girls.

Almost half of the injuries occurred among 10- to 14-year-olds.

Pre-existing medical conditions were reported in 18% of children.

Recreational areas were the site of 41% of the injuries.

Violence accounted for 10% of the injuries.

Falls were the most frequent cause of injury, followed by sports activities and assaults.

Schools must begin to understand the importance of preventing unintentional injuries and create a safe environment for learning. Methods to accomplish this include:

Make changes to improve physical surroundings and maintain equipment and facilities. perform annual safety checklist for school premises; and remove hazards.

Develop protocols for staff in the event of an injury and collect injury data; have school-wide safety policies and regulations and enforce them.

Educate everyone about potential hazards and preventive measures to change behaviors; train school staff in emergency first aid.

Learning at Home

Everyone learns and teaches at home. Many families supplement the education received in pubic and private schools, and some families choose to provide their children's education within a home-based school setting. If the pediatric rehabilitation nurse is working with families who select this option, it is important to understand the expectations from students, government, and the community, as well as the legal issues and costs. Information on home schooling can be obtained from local and state support groups as well as organizations such as the Home School Legal Defense Association (see Resources). Discuss with the child and family how home schooling has an impact on their home life, how they are scheduling the educational activities, the type of curriculum devised, other resources used, and how they provide for after-school play and socialization with other children, as this is important for the child's development.

Transition Services

The transition to adulthood and the world of work is a difficult process for the most mature young persons and an especially critical time for the adolescent with a disability or chronic condition. Adolescents potentially encounter a number of major transitions during this period:

- anxiety over finding employment and financial independence
- community and home living arrangements
- post-secondary educational opportunities
- independent mobility and self-care
- changing peer relationships
- sexuality and self-esteem

Within the past decade there has been a heightened interest on the part of youths with disabilities or chronic conditions, their parents, and their families in planning for the transition from school to adulthood. IDEA's new definition of "transition services" requires that these be included in the students' IEPs beginning not later than age 16 years and then annually. The definition states:

> Transition services means a coordinated set of activities for a student, designed with an outcome oriented process, which promotes movement from school to postschool activities, including postsecondary education, vocational training, integrated employment, including supported employment, continuing adult education, adult services, independent living or community participation. The coordinated set of activities shall be based upon the individual student's needs taking into account the student's preferences and interests and shall include instruction, community experiences, development employment and other postschool adult living objectives, and when appropriate acquisition of daily living skills and functional vocational evaluation. [Individuals With Disabilities Education Act of 1990. Public Law Number 101-476,20, U.S. Congress, Chapter 33, Section 1401 (a)(19)]

Ideally, a process within the school setting should identify young persons with disabilities or chronic conditions that put them at risk for unsuccessful transition to adulthood as early as age 10 years. This early identification would provide adequate planning time for education, training, and preparation to meet post-secondary or vocational requirements, learn to manage health issues, establish linkages with agencies to address specific needs, and locate sources of financial assistance. It may be necessary for schools to critically evaluate their curricula to significantly emphasize vocational preparation, work opportunities, needed competencies, essential experiences, and self-directed learning. The following are some areas identified as important competencies:

- allocating time, money, and material resources
- working on teams, teaching others, serving customers
- knowing how to acquire information and process data
- understanding social, organizational, and technologic systems
- selecting appropriate equipment, tools, and technology
- social skills

Pediatric rehabilitation nurses must be cognizant of the issues of transition, especially in the area of health care needs and services. In the role of advocate, the nurse can greatly influence the implementation of transition services by promoting self-determination in students with disabilities and chronic conditions, encouraging curriculum reform, anticipating service needs of students on graduation, having an impact on legislative policy to ensure funding and access, encouraging public–private cooperation in provision of services, and making information available to health care providers to enhance awareness and increase skills.

To assist in the transition to adult health services, the nurse should help the individual find a "medical home." This concept includes the critical components of geographic and financial accessibility, linkages to community services, continuity of care, and comprehensive care. Sia (1992) conceptualized the "medical home" as the center of a circle in which the primary care provider addresses the needs of the whole child and family while integrating all other services. Services essential to provide a continuum of care include:

- prevention
- recognition of emergency needs
- access to emergency services

Table 14–4 INDIVIDUALIZED HEALTHCARE PLAN

Student name: _____ Birth date: _____

School: _____ Effective date: _____

Nurse: _____ Physician: _____

Medical diagnosis: Congenital cytomegalovirus; extensive/pervasive mental disability; microcephaly; spastic quadriplegia; seizure disorder; decreased visual acuity; dysphagia with silent aspiration; delayed gastric emptying; Nissen fundoplication; gastrostomy button; left elbow radial head dislocation; severe scoliosis.

Assessment data: Aspirates solids and liquids taken by mouth directly into lungs, as evidenced by swallow studies done at UIHC. Patient is, therefore, susceptible to aspiration pneumonia. Patient must not take anything by mouth.

Nursing diagnosis: *Impaired swallowing* (NANDA 6.5.1) characterized by history of aspiration related to neuromuscular impairment.

Student Goals	Interventions/Person Responsible	Evaluation of Actual Outcomes
1. _____ will remain free of aspiration pneumonia this school year.	*Medication Administration* (NIC 2300) • Give Reglan _____ 1/2 hour before tube feeding (approx. 11:30 am) (Associate)	
2. _____ will maintain weight at 50th percentile during this school year.	*Nutritional Therapy* (NIC 1120) • Administer tube feeding at noon over 30–40 min in lunchroom (Certified associate)	
3. _____ will remain hydrated evidenced by 3 wet diapers/day during this school year.	• Monitor for side effects during and after feeding (Certified associate) • Change diapers q 2 hr; note if wet or dry on log (Associate) • Weigh each semester (Nurse)	
	Emergency Care (NIC 6200) • Discontinue tube feeding if side effects noted; notify nurse immediately (Certified associate) a. *Nausea/Cramping/Discomfort/Abdominal distension*—This occurs when the feeding is too fast or too cold, or the student is overfull. If this occurs stop the procedure, check the rate of the feeding and the temperature of the feeding. If all the above are okay and the problem continues, stop feeding and call school nurse. b. *Feeding won't go in/Blocked tube*—The tube may have been clogged with dry or thick feeding. If this occurs do not try to flush tube or squeeze tube. Contact school nurse.	
4. _____ will cooperate with oral stimulation program during this school year.	*Oral Health Maintenance* (NIC 1710) • Brush teeth after tube feeding (Associate) • Implement oral stimulation program daily (Associate)	

Table 14–4   INDIVIDUALIZED HEALTHCARE PLAN *Continued*

Student Goals	Interventions/Person Responsible	Evaluation of Actual Outcomes
5. _____ will tolerate toothbrushing during this school year.	*Delegation* (NIC 7650) • Teach associate to give medications and tube feedings (Nurse) • Review side effects and emergency procedures for tube feeding with staff (Nurse) • Review with staff monthly that _____ should receive *Nothing by Mouth* (Nurse) • Teach associate oral stimulation program (OT) *Documentation* (NIC 7920) • Record medication and tube feedings as administered (Associate) • Record wet/dry diapers (Associate) • Record weight each semester and compare with growth chart (Nurse) *Health Care Information Exchange* (NIC 7960) • Report to IHP and IEP teams at scheduled meetings (Nurse) • Report any changes or problems to team members as appropriate (Nurse) • Report to parents, health care providers regularly (Nurse) • Review progress toward or attainment of goals regularly (Nurse)	

I have read and approve of the above plan for school health care:

Parent signature: _____

Nurse signature: _____

Physician signature (optional): _____

Date reviewed by the education team: _____

[Gastrostomy-vertical]

Developed by Susan Poulton, R.N.

- transportation to primary care provider, hospital, or both
- hospital care services
- rehabilitation

Making a transition is easier when continuity of care and coordination, maximizing existing resources and avoiding duplication, occurs. A team approach is essential in planning, implementation, and evaluation, and the pediatric rehabilitation nurse must remember to build on the strong points and minimize the disability. One unknown author said it best:

ON FAITH
When you have walked to the edge
Of all of the light that you know,

And are about to step into the
Darkness of the unknown
. . . Faith is believing
That one of two things will happen . . .
That there will be something solid
To stand on or
You will be taught
HOW TO FLY

COMMUNITY ENVIRONMENT

Community-Based Care

In 1982, recognition of the plight of children dependent on technology came about when Surgeon General Koop emphasized the importance of community-based, family-centered care. "To make this a reality, communities must be able to plan realistically" and "determine where and how many services will be needed to make care available at the community level" (Palfrey et al., 1991, p. 618). In Chapter 3, community-based service delivery systems are described, and it is emphasized that the care should be family-centered and the system should include primary, secondary, and tertiary health services as well as specialized programs. This community system includes the neighborhood in which the family lives and the health, educational, social, and recreational institutions in the larger environment. Services should be provided in or near the family's home and should be comprehensive, flexible, accessible, coordinated, family-centered, and culturally sensitive.

As mentioned previously, it is commonplace for children to be discharged to home with tracheostomies, gastrostomies, and central venous lines. This growing population of children challenges pediatric rehabilitation nurses and society to create appropriate health, social, and educational systems that fully meet their needs. The child's first and most impressionable exposure is to the neighborhood, or the world right around the home. This environment can either promote the health and development of the child or become an impediment to the attainment of full potential. To foster healthy development, the neighborhood should be friendly and familiar, and the child should experience it as accepting, supportive of his or her physical and psychosocial needs, reinforcing of self-confidence, and safe. When the neighborhood is perceived negatively, it inhibits learning and socialization and disturbs the development of trust and confidence.

These external factors can be viewed as macro-influences, forces impacting the nature and scope of the larger society, or micro-influences, the day-to-day interactions in the family and the neighborhood that are the child's immediate world context. Some macro-influences identified by Palfrey (1994) are:

- child-centeredness of the society—how visible and important are children
- racial and cultural tolerance
- gender role stereotyping
- societal attitudes toward individuals with disabilities
- how society spends its money—for social care and health
- presence of violence in the society
- public attitudes on sexuality
- impact of public health policies
- rights, entitlement, and access to services

Micro-influences exert measurable effects because they are conditions close to the child and family. These include:

- family structure, supports, and priorities
- living and child care arrangements
- employment status
- physical and mental health of family members

Recently there has been strong support for the African proverb "it takes a village to raise a child," and this is even more significant when the child or adolescent has a disability or chronic condition. Pediatric rehabilitation nurses must begin to address these issues and direct energy toward solving problems within the context of family and community influences.

Access

Access to the community environment includes the resources necessary to support the child's or adolescent's physical movement from the home and school into the larger community. The following areas must be considered:

- transportation
- health care and social services
- recreation, social, and leisure activities
- architectural barriers

The pediatric rehabilitation nurse must be concerned with assisting the child or adolescent and family to eliminate obstacles to access so they can develop confidence in their ability to be participants in the activities of the community.

Transportation

Transportation is a crucial service for children and adolescents with disabilities and chronic conditions, to enhance the quality of their lives and enable them to access health care, education, and other services. In many large metropolitan areas, various resources are readily available and mass transportation has adapted equipment to allow access to trains, buses, and airplanes. In rural areas, transportation may be less available, and families will need to rely on their own automobiles or vans. If the child needs a special wheelchair, the family's car or van may need to be modified to allow for the child or adolescent to be transported in the wheelchair.

For adolescents, independence comes with a driver's license and is often the difference between being homebound or enjoying full integration in the community, but adolescents with a disability or chronic condition may need extra testing to determine their specific needs and whether they meet established criteria. Not all persons with disabilities can or should learn to drive. Changes may also need to be made in the vehicle to accommodate their disability. Many rehabilitation facilities have driver education services for adolescents who drove prior to the disability as well as those who are learning and driving for the first time. Adolescents are expected to attain the same level of proficiency in driving skills as other people, regardless of their disabilities or conditions.

Students who can adequately transfer into a standard-sized automobile are taught in this environment, where they encounter typical problem-solving situations of everyday driving. A van equipped with wheelchair access by a power lift enables the adolescent to operate from either a standard seat or the wheelchair. Changes can be made to a vehicle to allow an adolescent to drive with his or her hands:

- hand controls to use arms and hands to control the brake and gas
- custom attachments fitted to the steering wheel, including spinner knobs and special handles
- shoulder harness to provide balance
- power locks, power windows, and power seats

Recreational, Social, and Leisure Activities

Recreational, social, and leisure activities are activities or programs in which a child or adolescent with a disability or chronic condition participates for the purposes of fun, relaxation, or amusement and can include almost anything. Typically, these programs may be classified in one or more of the following ways:

- physical, cultural, or social
- indoor or outdoor
- spectator or participant
- formal or informal
- independent, cooperative, or competitive
- sports, games, hobbies, or toy play

Age-appropriate activities in school, community, and home environments are included, as are community-based integrated recreation programs. Pediatric rehabilitation nurses should be sure that every child or adolescent has equal opportunity to participate in recreation activities. This can be accomplished by looking at specific activities currently offered by recreation agencies, schools, and the community and determining what skills and capabilities are required to successfully participate. Then the capabilities of the child or adolescent who wants to participate are assessed to see if he or she has the kinds and levels of skills necessary for participation. If the child or adolescent does, the activity is considered programmatically accessible. If the child or adolescent does not, the activity may still be made accessible through some type of adaptation, either by compensating for the skill deficit or by adapting the activity itself without significantly affecting the enjoyment and participation of others. "The primary reason for making recreation programs fully accessible is the basic right of all people to be judged according to their capabilities, not their disabilities; their right to be included in all aspects of public life; their right to have fun like everybody else" (Cipriano, 1995, p. 456). Adaptation strategies can include various additions or modifications to a building or facility, provision of additional or alternative equipment including assistive technology, or modifications in the rules or program procedures.

Adolescents with a disability or chronic condition can benefit from participation in a planned exercise and fitness program, and this will also have a positive effect on their health. Exercise has been shown to improve strength and endurance, improve appearance and the ability to relax, and provide certain physiologic benefits. An individualized plan should be developed that includes a health appraisal, including physiologic areas such as flexibility, muscle strength, and activity to maximize oxygen transport; the psychosocial areas of body image and self-esteem; and a fitness assessment, including evaluation of aerobic capacity, endurance, flexibility, body measurements, and body composition. A prescription outlining a specific type and amount of exercise that maximizes benefits and minimizes risks is developed after determining the goals, interests, and limitations of the adolescent. Matching the activities to the adolescent's ability and interest is essential, and the more personalized the exercise prescription, the more effective it will be for the adolescent. A program can include weight training, arm and leg exercises using specialized or adapted equipment, wheelchair-accessible exercise courses and wheelchair sports, or a combination of fitness and sports. Children of all ages can participate in wheelchair sports and enjoy the interaction with peers and the spirit of cooperation and competition (Edwards, 1996).

For children and adults, travel is equated with freedom, fun, and adventure, and a disability or chronic condition should not limit choices of destinations or modes of transportation. For the child or adolescent, travel is a fantastic therapeutic learning experience and provides exposures to new and different people, environments, and activities. Mobility limitations should not pose a barrier to vacations and travel, because most places are accessible and wheelchair travel gets easier every year. The most important ingredients to insure a safe and enjoyable trip are pre-planning, stamina, patience, and the ability to laugh at minor problems—the family should pack a sense of humor along with the clothing.

All modes of transportation are available to the child or adolescent and family, including trains, buses, and airplanes. The pediatric rehabilitation nurse should suggest planning with a travel agent and mention specific information that they should provide about individual needs. The family should be sure to obtain written confirmations for mode of travel, hotel, and car rental. Special arrangements may also be made through "travel clubs" that obtain group rates and plan an itinerary to include many accessible attractions. One children's rehabilitation hospital has taken children with chaperones to many major cities and Walt Disney World, and after that trip one young person commented that being able to travel such a long distance, make new friends, and participate in varied experiences showed that it is truly a small world after all.

School-Based Clinics

Communities have begun to develop new and innovative approaches to the delivery of health care to children and adolescents. School-based clinics (SBCs) functioning as primary health care centers located at junior and senior high schools represent one approach. They offer a wide range of services including:

- general health assessments
- sports physicals
- laboratory tests
- diagnostic screenings
- immunizations
- first aid treatment
- health education
- family planning counseling and services
- counseling and related mental health services

> Additional services SBCs may provide include dental care, prenatal and postpartum care, day care and medical care for children of students, drug and alcohol abuse counseling, nutrition counseling, job and career counseling, family counseling and other services needed by students and accepted by the community and school. (Lovick, 1991, p. 45)

School Health Programs as Family Health Center

A plan for using family health centers located at or near schools to address the health care needs of America's families is part of nursing's agenda for health care reform. The plan calls for:

> A basic "core" of essential health care services to be available to everyone
> A restructured health care system that fosters consumer participation and responsibility, with services delivered in familiar and convenient sites such as schools, workplaces, and homes
> A shift from the predominant focus on illness and cure to an orientation toward wellness and care (Igoe & Giordano, 1992, p. ix)

These centers could deliver family-focused primary health care that is accessible and linked with the other components of a community's health care system. These centers reflect the growing belief that society bears at least some responsibility for helping parents and families meet the needs of their children and elders. Family health centers will become the neighborhood source of primary health care, where consumers will find providers ready to:

Diagnose and treat common illnesses on site, early in the course of a disease

Screen and refer more complex health problems, which require additional diagnostic and therapeutic interventions

Prepare consumers to become their own case managers

Monitor stable chronic disease

Provide guidance and counseling to individuals and groups about personal health practices and the use of disease prevention and health promotion strategies to stay well (Igoe & Giordano, 1992, p. viii)

HIGH-TECHNOLOGY CARE

The need for new technologies depends on a variety of factors, including preventive strategies that are implemented, size of the potential population of clients, attitudes about quality of life, and reimbursement policies (Samuel, 1991). The use of assistive technology has increased tremendously in the United States and has had dramatic impact on the quality of life of children and adolescents with disabilities and chronic conditions. Assistive technologies include both the tools for enabling the child's future development and important compensatory and instructional implements for providing a wide range of options that allow even the most disabled children maximum opportunity to participate fully in the home, school, and community. These technologies correct or remediate a specific disability and assist in learning specific tasks (Parette & VanBiervliet, 1991).

Because each individual is unique, with different points of view and ways to solve problems, when assistive technology is used the focus must be on how it will enable an individual in the performance of essential activities and tasks. As mentioned previously, if the child or adolescent has a reason for not applying himself or herself or the technology, it may be useless. Pediatric rehabilitation nurses who help recommend the use of assistive technology should plan in a collaborative environment with the child or adolescent and family's unique and focused input (Bazinet, 1995).

Definitions

Public Law 100-407, the Technology-Related Assistance for Individuals Act of 1988, defines assistive technology in a broad sense, as "any item, piece of equipment, or product system (whether acquired commercially off the shelf, modified, or customized) that is used to increase, maintain, or improve functional capabilities of individuals with disabilities." [29 U.S. Congress, 2202, Section 3(1)]. A 1994 amendment, Public Law 103-218, strengthened and expanded the original act, emphasizing systems change and advocacy (see Chap. 4).

Assistive technology devices are any items, equipment, or product systems that help make life easier for a person who has a disability, deafness, or chronic illness, or who is elderly. The devices may range in complexity from a simple strip of Velcro purchased in a department store to highly specialized mechanical, electronic, and computerized tools. These include positioning and mobility devices, augmentative communication aids, customized computer applications, adaptive toys and games, electronic interfaces, and adaptive environments, as described previously in this chapter.

Medical Issues

Medical expertise continues to expand, with greater understanding of the basic physiologic demands placed on the body by injury and illness, and biomedical and rehabilitation engineering developments such as more durable and flexible materials and miniaturization. Furthermore, many procedures previously done in health care institutions are now handled in the home, early intervention programs, and schools. Increased comfort with the procedures has moved them into mainstream pediatric care. The aggressive use of medical technology in prolonging lives is contributing to an increased prevalence of children and adolescents with disabilities and chronic conditions.

> The use of high technology appears to be improving the outcome for some children who may be able to 'outgrow' their conditions. The use of gastrostomy feedings for children with Pierre Robin syndrome and home oxygen for children with bronchopulmonary dysplasia has resulted in the survival of many of these children to the point where their physical growth allows them to function without these supports. (Palfrey et al., 1991, p. 617)

Financing and Costs

Dependence on medical technology must include the issue of costs, both for inpatient medical care and community-based care. Because many technologies are new and changing, training, retraining, and monitoring of caregivers is also a need with an attached cost. Additional discussion of financing issues can be found in Chapter 5.

Although the technology exists to allow children and adolescents with disabilities and chronic conditions to attend school, live independently, and participate in community life, for many the technology and devices are not available because of lack of family finances, complexity of third-party payment regulations, rigid federal and state regulations, or lack of health care coverage. Assistive technology (AT) has been shown to be cost-effective and beneficial to children or adolescents and their families and increases their capacity to function independently in the home, school, and community. In a comprehensive study by O'Day and Corcoran (1994) on the financing of AT, it was reported that about

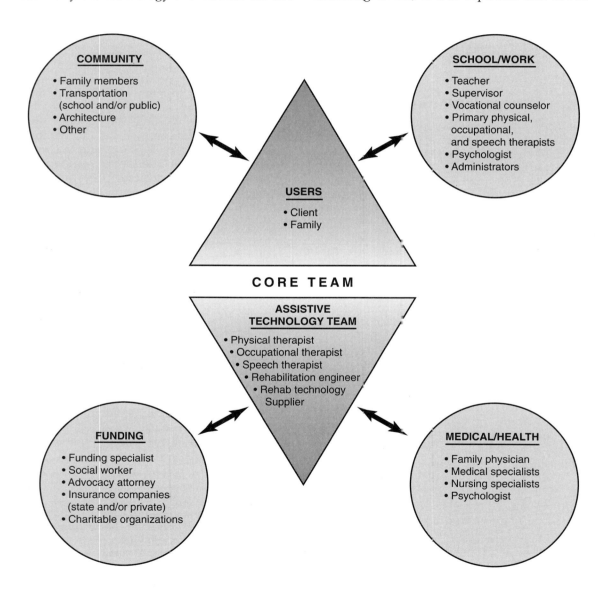

Core team interactions important in selecting and procuring assistive technology.
Members and roles of each component may fluctuate depending on specific client problems and settings.

Figure 14–10 Core team interactions. (Adapted from Carlson, S., & Ramsey, C. [1994]. Assistive technology. In Campbell, S.K. [Ed.]. *Physical therapy for children.* Philadelphia: WB Saunders, p. 622.)

75% of children who received AT were able to remain in a regular classroom, and about 45% were able to have a reduction in school-related services. It is essential for the pediatric rehabilitation nurse to understand how federal and state programs for rehabilitation and other services help children or adolescents and families attain or retain capabilities for independence or self-care. During the past decade, Medicaid has been used on behalf of individuals with disabilities to gain access to AT equipment and services. The definitions of the various therapies include statements that ATs include any necessary supplies and equipment; therefore all health care professionals should advocate for these necessary items to be available to children under Medicaid (Bergman, 1994).

Prescribing Assistive Technology

Because of the complexity and expense of most AT devices and equipment required by children and adolescents with disabilities and chronic conditions, it is essential that a thorough and careful process of selection and construction be undertaken. Many professionals and others should bring to bear their particular area of knowledge and expertise, and individuals interacting with the child or adolescent on a regular basis should be involved (Fig. 14–10). The configuration of the team varies with the type of AT needed and the setting in which it will be used, but the core role is shared by the users of the equipment and the team members who prescribe and obtain the devices (Carlson & Ramsey, 1994).

SUMMARY

The child or adolescent with a disability or chronic condition needs guidance and assistance to maximize his or her potential and prepare for the world of adulthood and independent living. To live and thrive in an environment that requires access and manipulation and control of information, these children and adolescents need strong support from family, health care providers, school personnel, and the community. Pediatric rehabilitation nurses in their role as advocates can act in a variety of settings to help the child or adolescent receive necessary technology and services and successfully make the transition into the challenging world of the twenty-first century.

REFERENCES

Alexander, M., Demasco, P., Gilbert, M., Miller, L., Nelson, M., & Shah, A. (1991). Rehabilitation technology for disabled children. *Physical Medicine and Rehabilitation: State of the Art Reviews*, 5(2), 365–387.

Bader Gilson, B., & Huss, D. (1995). Mobility: getting to where you want to go. In K. Flippo, K. Inge, & J. Barcus (Eds.). *Assistive technology: a resource for school, work and community*, p. 87. Baltimore: Paul H, Brookes.

Bazinet, G. (1995). Assistive technology. In O. Karam & S. Greenspan (Eds.). *Community rehabilitation services for people with disabilities*, pp. 437–458. Boston: Butterworth-Heinemann.

Becker, H., Johnson, M., & Greek, L. (1996). Assessing teachers' knowledge about healthcare procedures for children with special needs. *Rehabilitation Nursing Research*, 5(3), 71–79.

Bergman, A. (1994). Funding for assistive technologies. *Rehabilitation Management*, June/July, 26–31.

Betz, C.L., Hunsberger, M., & Wright, S. (1994). *Family-centered nursing care of children* (2nd ed.). Philadelphia: WB Saunders.

Blakeney, P., Moore, P., Meyer, W., Bishop, B., Murphy, L. Robson, M., & Herndon, D. (1995). Efficacy of school reentry programs. *Journal of Burn Care and Rehabilitation*, 16(4), 469–472.

Caring Institute of the Foundation for Hospice and Homecare (1987). *The crisis of chronically ill children in America: triumph of technology—failure of public policy.* Washington, DC: Foundation for Hospice and Homecare.

Carlson, S., & Ramsey, C. (1994). *Assistive technology.* In S. Campbell (Ed.). *Physical therapy for children*, pp. 621–659. Philadelphia: WB Saunders.

Cipriano, R. (1995). Therapeutic recreation: historical paradigms and a conundrum for use in the future. In O. Karam & S. Greenspan (Eds.). *Community rehabilitation services for people with disabilities*, pp. 437–458. Boston: Butterworth-Heinemann.

Donlin-Shore, K. (1993). The hospital to pre-school transition new guidelines for clinicians. *Headlines*, Sept/Oct, 25–28.

Edwards, P. (1996). Health promotion through fitness for adolescents and young adults following spinal cord injury. *SCI Nursing*, 13(3), 69–73.

Gallagher, S., & DiScala, C. (1994). Injuries in the school environment. *Rehabilitation Update*, 6–7.

Haynie, M., Palfrey, J., & Procter, S. (1989). *Children assisted by medical technology in educational settings: guidelines for care.* Boston: Project School Care, The Children's Hospital.

Hertel, V. (1991). Transitioning students with special health needs. In A. Snyder (Ed.). *Implementation guide for the standards of school nursing practice*, pp. 41–43. Kent, OH: American School Health Association.

Igoe, J., & Giordano, B. (1992). *Expanding school*

health services to serve families in the 21st century. Washington, DC: American Nurses Publishing.

Lovick, S. (1991). School-based clinics: meeting teens' health care needs. In A. Snyder (Ed.). *Implementation Guide for the Standards of School Nursing Practice*, pp. 45–46. Kent, OH: American School Health Association.

O'Day, B., & Corcoran, P. (1994). Assistive technology problems and policy alternatives. *Archives of Physical Medicine and Rehabilitation*, 75(10), 1165–1169.

Palfrey, J. (1994). *Community child health: an action plan for today.* Westport, CT: Praeger.

Palfrey, J., Walker, D., Haynie, M., Singer, J., Porter, S., Bushey, B., & Cooperman, P. (1991). Technology's children: report of a statewide census of children dependent on medical supports. *Pediatrics*, 87(5), 611–618.

Parette, H., & VanBiervliet, A. (1991). Rehabilitation assistive technology issues for infants and young children with disabilities: a preliminary examination. *Journal of Rehabilitation*, July/Aug/Sept, 27–36.

Pastalan, L. (1996). *Universal design: a definition* [On-line]. Available: http://www2.ncsu.edu

Poulton, S. (1996). *Guidelines to writing individualized healthcare plans* [On-line]. Available: http://www.nursing.uiowa.edu/www/nursing/...2/students/sp1996/96-222we/guidelines

RehabNET. (1997). Accessibility and modifications to the living space. [On-line]. *Rehabilitation Monographs*, Available: http://www.rehabnet.com/monographs/access.htm

Samuel, F. (1991). High technology home care: an overview. In M. Mehlman & S. Youngner (Eds.). *Delivering high technology home care*, pp. 1–22. New York: Springer.

Sia, C. (1992). The medical home: pediatric practice and child advocacy in the 1990s. *Pediatrics*, 90(3), 419–423.

Tanchak, T., & Sawyer, C. (1995). Augmentative communication. In K. Flippo, K. Inge, & J. Barcus (Eds.). *Assistive technology: a resource for school, work and community*, pp. 57–86. Baltimore: Paul H. Brookes.

Urbano, M. (1992). *Pre-school children with special health care needs.* San Diego, CA: Singular Publishing Group, Inc.

ADDITIONAL RESOURCES

Browning, P., Dunn, C., & Brown, C. (1993). School to community transition for youth with disabilities. In R. Eaves & P. McLaughlin. *Recent advances in special education and rehabilitation*, pp. 193–206. Boston: Andover Medical.

Campbell, S. (1994). *Physical therapy for children.* Philadelphia: WB Saunders.

DelVecchio, J. (1992). Home pediatric rehabilitation. *Journal of Home Health Care Practice*, 5(11), 12–15.

Driving. (1997). [On-line]. Available: http://www.charweb.org/health/rehab/scin/driving

Eaves, R., & McLaughlin, P. (1993). *Recent advances in special education and rehabilitation.* Boston: Andover Medical.

Effgen, S. (1994). The educational environment. In S. Campbel (Ed.). *Physical therapy for children*, pp. 847–872 Philadelphia: WB Saunders.

Flippo, K., Inge, K., & Barcus, J. (Eds.). (1995). *Assistive technology: a resource for school, work and community.* Baltimore: Paul H. Brookes.

Halloran, W. (1993). Transition services requirement: issues, implications, challenges. In R. Eaves & P. McLaughlin (Eds.). *Recent advances in special education and rehabilitation*, pp. 210–223. Boston: Andover Medical.

Kurtz, L., & Scull, S. (1993). Rehabilitation for developmental disabilities. *Pediatric Clinics of North America*, 40(3), 629–643.

Mehlman, M., & Youngner, S. (Eds.). (1991). *Delivering high technology home care.* New York: Springer.

Nimec, D. (1997). Personal communication. January 23.

Proctor, S., Lordi, S., & Zarger, D. (1993). *School nursing practice: roles and standards.* Scarborough, ME: National Association of School Nurses.

Robotics and rehabilitation. (1988). *REHAB Brief*, 10(2), 1–4.

Selekman, J. (1995). Children in the community. In C. Smith & F. Maurer (Eds.). *Community health nursing*, pp. 693–718. Philadelphia: WB Saunders.

Smith, C., & Maurer, F. (1995). *Community health nursing.* Philadelphia: WB Saunders.

Snyder, A. (Ed.). (1991). *Implementation guide for the standards of school nursing practice.* Kent, OH: American School Health Association.

Wehman, P. (1993). Transition from school to adulthood for young people with disabilities: critical issues and policies. In R. Eaves & P. McLaughlin (Eds.). *Recent advances in special education and rehabilitation*, pp. 178–192. Boston: Andover Medical.

RESOURCES

ABLEDATA
8455 Colesville Rd., Suite 935
Silver Spring, MD 20910
800-227-0216
http://www.abledata.com/faq.htm

Canine Companions for Independence National Headquarters
P.O. Box 446
Santa Rosa, CA 95402-0446
1-800-572-2275

The Center for Universal Design
School of Design
North Carolina State University, Box 8613
Raleigh, NC 27695-8613
800-647-6777
http://www2.ncsu.edu/ncsu/design/cud

Home School Legal Defense Association
http://www.learnathome.com/hslda.htm

Injuries in the School Environment: A Resource
   Packet
Children's Safety Network
National Injury and Violence Prevention Resource
   Center
Education Development Center Inc.
55 Chapel St.
Newton, MA 02158-1060
617-969-7100

LEARN@Home Web Site
http://www.learnathome.com:80/howto1.htm

MATP Update
Massachusetts Assistive Technology Partnership
   Center
Children's Hospital
1295 Boylston St., Suite 310
Boston, MA 02115
617-335-7820 or 800-848-8867

National Spinal Cord Injury Association
Fact Sheet 12: Medical Facilities and Resources for
   Ventilator Use
8300 Colesville Road, Suite 551
Silver Spring, MD 20910
301-588-6959 or 800-962-9629
E-mail: NSCIA2@aol.com

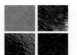

Part II

Perspectives on Children and Families and Their Environment

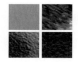

Chapter 15

Management of Central Nervous System Impairment

Susanne R. Hays

Children with the diagnoses of spina bifida and cerebral palsy are often seen in the pediatric rehabilitation population. It is essential for the nurse to have an in-depth understanding of the multi-faceted care required by children with these conditions across their life span. An individualized assessment of the needs of these children and their families will enable the nurse to plan appropriate care and provide the necessary nursing services and referrals to other medical and community resources.

SPINA BIFIDA

The most common congenital conditions affecting the central nervous system are neural tube defects (NTDs). NTDs result from failure of spontaneous closure of the neural tube during the 3rd and 4th weeks of fetal development. If the failure to close is in the area of the head, anencephaly or encephalocele is the result; anencephaly is incompatible with life, and such children usually do not live after birth. When the spinal column fails to close, spina bifida results. Spina bifida cystica, also referred to as myelodysplasia or spinal dysraphism, refers to an abnormal embryologic development of the spinal cord. Spina bifida cystica may manifest itself in varying degrees of severity, with the opening extending to the skin and including nervous tissue. Categories of spina bifida cystica include myelomeningocele and meningocele (Disabato & Wulf, 1994). Throughout this text, the term spina bifida is used to describe the various types of spina bifida cystica.

The types of spina bifida include:

Myelomeningocele: the spinal column is open and the sac contains neural tissue from the spinal cord and possibly spinal nerves, meninges, and spinal fluid

Meningocele: the spinal column is open, covered only by a thin tissue sac which contains meninges

Myeloschisis: the spinal cord is flattened without meninges and often without any skin or other covering (Dahl et al., 1995)

Myeloschisis is one of the most severe forms of myelodysplasia, and myelomeningocele is the most common. All of these forms of spina bifida are accompanied by central nervous system, neuromuscular, and skeletal dysfunction and deformity.

Spina bifida occulta, a less severe form of meningocele, results from incomplete fusion of a vertebral body. The defect is covered by skin and is not readily visible. The skin over the site may show a dimple, a tuft of hair, discolored skin, or a dermoid sinus. Spina bifida occulta is not usually accompanied by symptoms and, if symptoms occur, they are mild. The condition is usually diagnosed incidentally during evaluation for an unrelated complaint, whereas spina bifida is diagnosed pre-natally or at birth.

Failure of closure of the neural tube is accompanied by malformations of the vertebral column, which develops spontaneously with the neural tube. The neural tube forms not only the spinal cord but the brain as well. Other conditions such as hydrocephalus, Chiari II malformation of the brain and brain stem, defects of cellular migration, and other brain abnormalities often occur with spina bifida and are related to the anomalous development of the neural tube (Disabato & Wulf, 1994; Reigel, 1989).

An array of typical deficits accompanies spina bifida due to the spinal cord damage resulting from the failure of neural tube closure. Depending on the vertebral level of the lesion, innervation to various areas of skin, muscles, and internal organs is interrupted. Typically, bowel and bladder function, skin sensation, muscular control, and the central nervous system are affected. The higher the level of the lesion, the greater the neuromuscular damage. The last area of the neural tube to close is the lumbosacral area; therefore, the majority of individuals with spina bifida (approximately 85%) have a lumbar-level lesion (Disabato & Wulf, 1994).

Etiology and Incidence

The cause of spina bifida is unknown. There are many genetic, environmental, and nutritional factors that are thought to contribute to a multi-factorial etiology. Chapter 10 contains more information on multi-factorial genetic patterns. Maternal nutrition, especially a diet poor in zinc, folate, and other vitamins, is also thought to place the developing fetus at high risk for NTDs (Milunsky et al., 1989). Folate supplementation is recommended for all women who are considering becoming pregnant to prevent the occurrence of NTDs.

Perhaps as a result of poor nutrition, NTDs are more common in lower socioeconomic groups. The incidence is approximately 1 to 2 per 1000 live births in the United States (Disabato & Wulf, 1994) and is currently thought to be decreasing somewhat due to prevention efforts. Incidence is higher in individuals of English and Irish backgrounds, is less frequent in African-American and black populations, and is extremely rare in Asian populations. However, the effects of poverty on maternal health, nutrition, and health care access may mediate ethnic occurrence rates. Genetic counseling is important for families with one affected member, because future offspring have an increased risk of being affected (Molnar, 1992). After one child in a family is born with spina bifida, the risk of recurrence goes up to 3% to 4% (Haslam, 1996a).

Pathophysiology

Spina bifida causes dysfunction of skin sensation and neuromuscular control to those or-gans and structures that are innervated at or below the level of the lesion. Resulting conditions include neurogenic bowel and bladder, complete or partial paralysis of the lower extremities, complete or partial loss of sensory function below the level of the lesion, and skeletal deformities resulting from altered muscular function. Examples of common skeletal deformities include talipes equinovarus (clubfoot); congenitally dislocated hips; congenital hip, knee, and ankle contractures; kyphosis; and scoliosis. In some cases, associated defects of the kidneys or urinary tract may occur and complicate the clinical picture. Associated central nervous system conditions include Chiari II malformation, which is a kinking of the medulla and elongation of the brain stem that slows the flow of cerebrospinal fluid and can result in hydrocephalus. Chiari II malformation occurs in virtually all children with spina bifida (Dahl et al., 1995). Hydrocephalus may develop pre-natally and be detected on ultrasonography, or it may develop post-natally, following surgical closure of the spinal lesion.

Complications that compromise the child's functional abilities may occur. One of the most devastating complications occurs when the Chiari II malformation becomes symptomatic, resulting in displacement of the cerebellar tonsils and medulla downward through the foramen magnum. The fourth ventricle is thereby blocked, causing hydrocephalus, and cranial nerves may be stretched, resulting in potentially life-threatening neurologic degeneration. Common symptoms seen in young children include apnea, changes in sucking and swallowing, vomiting, weak or absent cry, and inspiratory stridor during agitation. Older children may show signs of changes in deep tendon reflexes or decreased strength and function in the upper extremities (Disabato & Wulf, 1994). Estimates of the number of children with Chiari II malformation–related symptoms range from 5% to 20%, and are reported to be up to 85% in one study (Dahl et al., 1995).

Other associated central nervous system dysfunctions that may contribute to the complications of Chiari II malformation include compression of the medulla in the foramen magnum; hemorrhage of the brain stem with infarction and dysgenesis of the brain stem; spinal cord cysts; tethered spinal cord; syringomyelia, or cavitation within the spinal cord; diastematomyelia, or bone spurs that impinge on the spinal cord; and lipoma involving the conus medullaris (Disabato & Wulf, 1994;

Dahl et al., 1995). Many of these conditions may exist concurrently with spina bifida and are thought to be related to the general central nervous system dysfunction.

Tethered cord is a common neurologic complication that may compromise the child's functional ability. As the child grows, the spinal cord moves upward in the spinal column. (See Chapter 10 for additional information on growth and development.) If the cord becomes tethered or caught due to adhesions or bony abnormalities, the resulting tension causes changes in neurologic function such as an increase in scoliosis, change in bowel and bladder function, or change in muscle control in the lower extremities. Some children develop spasticity not previously seen as a result of tethered cord.

Changes due to growth may also complicate the child's functional abilities. Elongation of limbs may increase tightness of tendons. Decreased range of motion results in contractures that may contribute to bony deformity, such as dislocated hips. Muscle imbalance in the spine results in progression of scoliosis. Any child with a lesion above the lumbar area is at increased risk for the development of scoliosis. Scoliosis may also result from vertebral abnormalities. Kyphosis is generally congenital, resulting from vertebral abnormalities, but worsens with growth if not treated. Rib and cranial vault abnormalities may also exist (Molnar, 1992).

Clinical Aspects and Functional Limitations

Children born with spina bifida have physical and functional limitations which are dependent upon the location and extent of the lesion. These limitations are usually in the form of paralysis of the lower extremities, absence or alterations of bowel and bladder control, sensory deficits, orthopedic deformities, hydrocephalus, and intellectual and personality variations (Farley & Dunleavy, 1996).

The range of paralysis is related to the location of the spinal defect. However, sometimes there is upper extremity involvement in children who have lumbar lesions, and there is also the possibility of asymmetry of the motor and sensory deficits. If the lesion is in the upper thoracic area, the child has paralysis of the lower extremities with motor and sensory loss, absence of bowel and bladder control, weakness of the abdominal trunk musculature, and possible respiratory compromise. If it is in the lumbosacral area, the child has some hip, knee, and ankle flexion which, with braces, crutches, and other assistive devices, will support some degree of functional ambulation. There will still be absence of total bowel and bladder control and sensory loss. If the lesion is in the sacral area, there is usually no motor function deficit but the child may have hammer toes. There may, however, be some sensory deficits and bowel and bladder dysfunction in these children (Farley & Dunleavy, 1996).

Other problems associated with myelodysplasia are seizures, visual perceptual problems, cognitive deficits, and possibly latex allergic reactions (Farley & Dunleavy, 1996). As a result of the vertebral and rib deformities, as well as asymmetric muscle imbalance caused by asymmetric kyphosis (which is evident at birth) and scoliosis (which develops in 100% of children with thoracic lesions), deformities become more evident as the child grows. If no intervention is provided, cardiopulmonary functioning may be severely compromised. Fractures due to osteoporosis resulting from paralysis, immobility, lack of weight-bearing, and inactivity are common. Because of the lack of pain sensation, fractures are sometimes overlooked until swelling and redness or crepitus and angulation at the site are noted (Molnar, 1992).

Neurogenic bowel and bladder dysfunction of varied complexity is almost always present in children with myelodysplasia. This occurs because of a lack of or incomplete motor and sensory innervation from the spinal cord to the bowel and bladder. Obesity may become a problem for children born with spina bifida. Feeding problems may also be of concern with children who have the Chiari malformation.

Functional limitations are also evident. Depending on the level of motor deficit, the child may be able to ambulate without equipment but usually needs braces for support and often a wheelchair to become mobile. Delays in development of self-care skills are also common. This is related to motor deficits and central nervous system conditions such as hydrocephalus. With delays in development and functional limitations, social interactions, peer relationships, academic achievement, and transition into independence may also become problems.

Children with spina bifida may have some cognitive involvement. Usually, the higher the lesion, the more likely it is that cognitive involvement will exist. Intelligence quotient (IQ) scores tend to vary in performance and verbal ability. Although the presence of shunting is not thought to adversely affect intelligence, the presence of central nervous system infection does have an adverse effect on intelligence. Children with spina bifida and hydrocephalus who also have seizures are more likely to have an intellectual deficit. Children with spontaneously arrested hydrocephalus, which is not shunted, may show intellectual deficits, as well as "cocktail party syndrome" (CPS), which is evidenced by good verbal skills but little meaningful content in their talk. There is some evidence to suggest that CPS indicates subtle function deficits similar to those found in adults with frontal lobe damage (Tew, 1991). These deficits may account for poor school performance, difficulty in learning sequenced tasks, and low motivation seen in many children with spina bifida.

Diagnostic Assessment

If the myelodysplastic sac is open, the amniotic fluid can be tested pre-natally, between 16 and 18 weeks' gestation. Elevated alpha-fetoprotein and acetylcholinesterase levels plus the use of ultrasonographic studies are necessary for a definitive intra-uterine diagnosis. If the infant is not diagnosed with spina bifida pre-natally, the lesion is recognized at birth, and treatment begins immediately. Once the lesion is covered to prevent infection and to protect the delicate neural structures, the child is frequently transferred to a tertiary care hospital for further diagnostic workup and treatment.

Initial workup consists of close monitoring for signs of hydrocephalus and cranial ultrasonography or computed tomography (CT) if the signs are positive. Usually, a CT scan of the spine is obtained to determine the extent of spinal cord and spinal nerve involvement. The infant is examined for signs of urinary retention, and a urologic workup is initiated to assess for bladder, ureteral, and kidney abnormalities, usually using ultrasonography. It is important to diagnose ureteral reflux if it is present to prevent infection and preserve kidney function. An orthopedic assessment is performed, including radiographs of the spine, hip, knees, and feet, as necessary, to determine the extent of skeletal involvement. A thorough neonatal examination is also performed to identify any associated congenital malformations that may be less obvious, such as cardiac or gastro-intestinal anomalies. After a complete assessment, the results are shared with the family, and the immediate treatment options and long-term prognosis are discussed.

Therapeutic Management

Interdisciplinary

Children with myelodysplasia must be cared for by a team of knowledgeable professionals in concert with the family. The core of most professional spina bifida rehabilitation teams consists of the following members: a pediatrician, orthopedist, physiatrist, urologist, neurosurgeon, nurse specialist, physical therapist, occupational therapist, speech pathologist, dietitian, and psychologist. Other professionals are consulted as necessary to meet the child and family's care needs. The goals of maximizing the child's ability to function and the effective management and supervision of the many facets and intertwined aspects of the child's care are paramount. One person on the team must take on the responsibility of coordinator and advocate, and this could be the role of the pediatric rehabilitation nurse.

Medical

Monitoring of the child's growth and development, including periodic assessment of visual, perceptual, sensory, motor, and cognitive skills, is necessary. Frequent monitoring of the genito-urinary system with management of urinary infections is necessary. Prevention of further complications of renal function may necessitate medications for improvement of bladder muscle tone and complete emptying of the bladder. The importance of primary care, as well as specialty medical services, cannot be emphasized enough. Children with spina bifida need regular well-child care, immunizations, and minor acute illness treatment just like any other child. Neglecting primary care for children with disabilities may lead to an increase in secondary disability due to overlooked health problems.

Surgical

Surgical management of the infant and child with spina bifida is complex and continues throughout the life span. However, frequency of surgical procedures is greatest in the early years of life and during the periods of most rapid growth. At birth, the open lesion on the back is surgically closed, and the spinal cord, meninges, and spinal nerves repaired to the greatest extent possible. Early and comprehensive closure and repair of the defect can improve the child's functional potential. Prevention of infection at this time is a paramount concern, because central nervous system infection is associated with cognitive deficits.

The neonate is closely monitored for signs of hydrocephalus. If positive signs are noted, cranial ultrasonography or CT is performed to determine the extent of hydrocephalus. Placement of a ventriculo-peritoneal (VP) shunt is performed to drain the excess cerebral spinal fluid from the ventricles and into the peritoneal space, where it is absorbed. Some children may receive a ventriculo-atrial (VA) shunt, particularly later in life if there have been many complications and difficulties with a VP shunt. The VA shunt is associated with a higher rate of complications than the VP shunt, including that of sudden death. During the child's life, many shunt revisions may be performed to lengthen the shunt, to repair or replace the device itself if it has malfunctioned, or to repair blockage. The frequency of shunt revisions lessens as the child reaches adolescence, and revisions are rare during adulthood. Shunt infection is of particular concern due to its association with negative cognitive outcome and requires rapid and thorough treatment, sometimes to the extent of removing the shunt, treating the infection, and replacing the shunt.

Surgical procedures may be performed for the complications of spina bifida or for accompanying neural anomalies. If the Chiari II malformation becomes symptomatic, the child may require surgical decompression of the brain stem. Spinal cord cysts, or syringomyelia, may require drainage and repair and possibly shunting of cerebral spinal fluid. Development of a tethered spinal cord can result in significant loss of function if the condition is left untreated. The spinal cord is surgically released so that it can move easily in the spinal canal and traction and symptoms are relieved.

Orthopedic surgery is also a frequent occurrence for most children with spina bifida. Surgical correction of clubfoot, release of contractures, repair of hip dislocations, and correction of scoliosis and kyphosis may be necessary to maintain and improve the child's functional abilities. Scoliosis, and especially kyphosis, often cause restrictive lung disease and may result in cardio-respiratory failure if untreated (Gold, 1993).

Management of the child's urologic system may also necessitate surgery. Ureteral re-implantation may be required if the child experiences frequent reflux and urinary tract infection. Bladder augmentation is used to correct a small, spastic bladder that makes continence difficult and increases reflux. Implantation of artificial urinary sphincters can aid in development of continence (Light, 1991). The construction of a continent urostomy is also an option for children with significant bladder and kidney problems. Clean intermittent catheterization of the urostomy is much easier for many children to manage than urethral catheterization.

Therapy

Mobility technology, plus positioning and seating systems, are of utmost importance for the child who is unable to ambulate and must rely on wheeled devices for movement. These devices should be used in conjunction with other therapeutic interventions. The goal is to provide independence in mobility, prevent pressure sore development, provide trunk stability to allow for upper extremity functioning, and prevent further deformity. Further discussion of assistive technology is found in Chapter 14.

Controversy continues to surround the use of augmentative mobility for children with a high-level neurologic lesion. For children with lesions in the thoracic or upper lumbar level and limited muscle power, some rehabilitation teams believe that it is best for the child to learn to walk exclusively using braces, crutches, walkers, or other standing devices while they are young. The benefits include increased bone density and thus fewer fractures, decreased contractures and back deformities; reduction of skin breakdown; facilitation of better bowel and bladder functioning; increased cardio-vascular fitness; decreased obesity; and better social interaction. Other teams believe that for children with high-level lesions, the benefits of supporting walking without the use of a wheelchair are not that significant. The child in a wheelchair often becomes more independent in self-care skills, including management of bowel and bladder programs. Both groups acknowledge that children with high-level lesions will eventually use wheelchairs for mobility. Research does not provide a clear direction to assist in developing a treatment plan for the use of wheelchairs or walking with devices to facilitate overall developmental, psycho-social, or medical outcomes (Butler, 1991).

It is important for physical and occupational therapists involved in the child's care to provide therapy for muscle strengthening and stretching, facilitate developmental progress, improve coordination and self-care skills acquisition, and assist with the child's mobility. The speech pathologist provides therapy in the areas of language development, communication, and management of oral motor disorders.

Management of Bowel Dysfunction

Specific bowel and bladder programs are necessary for effective management of incontinence in the child with spina bifida. Often the program is performed by a parent, and the child is essentially left out of the learning. Because these children do not have sensation, they can easily ignore that part of their body and the process of the bowel and bladder program, experiencing it as something that takes them away from their play and is an inconvenience.

Bowel training for the child with myelodysplasia must start at the time of birth. Education of the family and prevention of constipation is important. Individualized bowel programs must be developed. Use of rectal suppositories for lubricant or stimulation on a regular or periodic basis may be necessary, as well as use of medications to increase or decrease the firmness of the stool. Dietary management for the prevention and treatment of constipation is important, as is encouraging the child to drink adequate amounts of liquid.

Many children who are totally dependent on their families to provide bowel and bladder care are reluctant to learn. They are already past the developmental time when toilet learning should take place, and other developmental tasks distract from learning. The use of peer modeling with older children, plus camps specifically designed for children with spina bifida and integration with adults in wheelchairs who are independent, is of value when teaching children to become independent in bowel and bladder care.

Important interventions for bowel care for the child with spina bifida include encouraging the development of an effective bowel program; teaching the importance of key elements of a bowel program such as timing, diet, exercise, positioning, and stimulation of the rectum; and demonstrating the use of exercise and positioning to aid evacuation of the bowel. Adequate lower body exercise stimulates movement of stool through the colon, and positioning, such as the knee-chest position, enhances evacuation. In addition, use of medications and supplements such as bulk formers, stool softeners, and laxatives can aid in maintaining proper stool consistency. Use of suppositories and enemas is often necessary.

One study by King, Currie, and Wright (1994), regarding bowel training and management for children with spina bifida and intact bulbocavernosus or anocutaneous reflex functioning, used a protocol for bowel clean-out. If hard stool was present, the program included manipulation of diet and bulk agents to support soft stool consistency. The researchers then used a reflex-triggered program that included the use of glycerine suppositories, bisacodyl (Dulcolax) suppositories, or both to initiate an evacuation at a regular time; use of digital stimulation 20 minutes post-suppository; and oral medications to stimulate evacuation if none occurred with the first stages of the protocol.

King, Currie, and Wright (1994) found that initiation of the program at least every day between 2 and 5 years of age increased compliance as well as maintained functioning of the anal reflexes. If the child did not have functioning anal reflexes, the ability to be socially continent was more difficult but not impossible. Socially acceptable bowel continence was defined as less than one incontinent stool per month. There are also other programs which use biofeedback and behavior modification to effectively establish socially acceptable bowel continence (Whitehead et al., 1986). Additional information regarding bowel programs can be found in Chapter 12.

Bladder Program

The development of a bladder program must start with specific bladder function evaluations to determine the condition of the upper urologic tracts and the type of bladder and sphincter tone present. Children with spina bifida may have spastic bladder and sphincter tone, an atonic bladder and sphincter, or a mixed picture, which is most common. The bladder program prescribed depends on the type of neurogenic bladder function and the presence or absence of reflux, hydronephrosis, and kidney damage.

If the child has neurogenic bladder functioning, continence can be maintained by use of medications to relax the bladder and tighten the urinary sphincter and clean intermittent catheterization on a regular basis. The child must be encouraged as early as possible to become involved in the process. Further information regarding bladder programs can be found in Chapter 12. Other methods are used as well; surgical procedures such as vesicostomy and continent ileostomy and implantation of artificial sphincters are used in some areas.

Important interventions for bladder care for the child with spina bifida include providing an effective, socially appropriate management of the neurogenic bladder; teaching the program to the child and family and reinforcing the information as needed; teaching the child and family how to monitor for urinary tract infection and what to do if an infection is suspected; and encouraging adequate fluid intake and timing of fluid intake to prevent nighttime incontinence.

A typical situation illustrating bladder care for the child with spina bifida is that of a boy born with a sacral-level lesion who has partial bladder control. Early in life, the child experienced periods of dryness with sudden onset of wetness from voiding and could stay dry with a timed voiding program initiated by his mother. The program was integrated into the daily routine, with voiding on the toilet at specific intervals during the day. These intervals were: first thing in the morning after arising, after regular meals, after going out to play, before watching favorite television programs, and just before bed. By around 7 years of age, the child had more awareness of bladder sensations and began to depend more on the bladder sensations than the timed program. If the child needed to void and ran, incontinence would occur, so the child had to stop, think about holding the urine in, and walk slowly to the bathroom.

This child's program was successful because the parent was knowledgeable about bladder care and was in close contact with a nurse specialist who believed that the child could stay dry and was able to teach the parents how to direct the program. In this case, the child had minimal neurogenic bladder, stayed infection free, and had age-appropriate developmental skills.

Skin Programs

Children with spina bifida are at high risk for skin breakdown due to inattention to areas of the body that lack sensation. Pressure from braces, sitting in one position for long periods without shifting weight or changing position, or exposure to extreme heat or cold may result in skin breakdown. Skin breakdown is difficult to treat, may cause the child to miss school, and may require frequent clinic visits or even surgery; therefore, prevention is the best treatment. For younger children, parents must provide good skin care and monitoring, and for older children and adolescents, parents should reinforce good skin care habits. The goals are for the child and family to be aware of high-risk situations and practice prevention and good skin care. Further information on skin care programs can be found in Chapter 12.

Severe allergic reactions to latex and products containing latex have recently become a problem. It is postulated that chronic exposure predisposes a child to the allergic reaction. The reaction is particularly of concern for children with myelodysplasia and can even cause death if not properly managed. Every effort should be made to provide a safe environment free of products containing latex (Romanczuk, 1993).

Self-Esteem and Socialization

Children born with spina bifida often have cognitive and mobility problems. In the process of getting the child's body functioning at its highest potential, the team should always remember that in that body there is a real, unique person who has a very special family. Socialization with peers and having the ability to learn from them is very important and must be encouraged. Too often, the child's life is focused around the clinic, hospital, and therapy, with little time left for normal family activity and socialization.

Cognitive Issues

Children born with spina bifida have IQs in the average range. Those who have hydrocephalus and shunts have IQs in the low-average to below-average range. Infections and frequent shunt revisions further affect the child's ability to perform cognitively. Many children have verbal strengths but memory, integrated functioning, and acquired knowledge deficits (Lollar, 1993). Therefore, it is important for the nurse to assess the child's abilities when preparing to teach about care and focus the information so the child is able to understand and use it.

Additionally, many children with spina bifida, although within norms on standardized tests of intelligence, experience learning disabilities that affect retention of sequenced tasks, problem solving, memory, and motivation. As a result, frequent repetitions and reinforcement of teaching is critical to maintain consistent performance on the part of the child or adolescent.

Dietary Issues

For the child with spina bifida, failure to thrive or obesity can be problems; obesity is more common. Prevention is best accomplished by early education regarding the necessary calories for growth of a child with spina bifida, promotion of activity, and parent education. Early in the child's life and periodically as they grow, specific information should be given to the child and family regarding necessary calories for growth. As the pediatric rehabilitation nurse develops the plan of care, the registered dietitian on the team is the most appropriate person for consultation regarding this issue.

Impact on Child and Family

The birth of a child with spina bifida may be devastating to the family. In addition to the initial grief and anger, the family must learn about the defect, the associated complications, recommended surgical and non-surgical procedures, and a variety of treatment options. Many times the shock of the diagnosis and need to make immediate decisions about surgery and early treatment prevents the family from allowing themselves to grieve for the loss of the dream for a normal newborn. Because of the necessary life-saving focus on the medical condition, the family does not have an opportunity to focus on normal issues and get to know their infant. This can be even a greater problem when the infant has to be transported to a center away from the family's community, delaying crucial bonding, attachment, skin-to-skin contact, and holding.

When the infant's life is not at risk, some centers choose to delay the necessary surgery to repair the lesion. This allows the family more time to work through their feelings and be able to prepare for necessary early treatments. It also allows them time to get to know their infant as a special person. Allowing a family whose child has a similar condition to provide support is often most helpful in assisting the family in making decisions, expressing feelings, and getting questions answered. One study by Van Cleve (1989), regarding parents' coping skills in response to a child with spina bifida, suggests that successful coping can be supported by increased use of groups for families and children to discuss their feelings, resources, and management techniques. The pediatric rehabilitation nurse can encourage participation in family- and child-focused groups for support, learning, and advocacy. Clarifying misconceptions, providing information, and assisting in identifying resources promote confidence, increase self-advocacy, and foster coping and adapting to the disability or chronic condition.

Application of the Nursing Process

Coordination of care for the child with spina bifida and his or her family is one of the major roles of the pediatric rehabilitation nurse, in addition to parent/child education and nursing intervention. Because of the child's multiplicity of needs, the nurse must use critical-thinking skills to design and implement interventions to obtain the best possible functional outcomes. The level or type of spinal defect, the age and developmental level of the child, cognitive functioning, associated problems, and the setting in which the pediatric rehabilitation nurse interacts with the child and family directly affect the process of nursing assessment. As the child grows, periodic reassessment is important to facilitate increased learning and to perfect the skills necessary for independence. The assessment should include determining the condition or conditions that affect self-care abilities and barriers to participation in the regimen, determining existing skills and strengths, and assessing what self-care is usually performed at home. Chapter 11 provides information on functional assessment.

Children with spina bifida have complex care needs in all the functional health patterns. Chapters 12 and 13 describe assessment and nursing management of specific functional health patterns. The major concerns for children with spina bifida are elimination, skin care, mobility, nutrition, and psycho-social adjustment. Nursing diagnoses that may be identified in this population include:

- Risk for infection
- Nutrition altered: more/less than body requirements

- Altered bowel elimination
- Altered urinary elimination
- Impaired physical mobility
- Risk for injury
- Ineffective coping: child and/or family
- Self-care deficit
- Risk for impaired skin integrity

The child with spina bifida can be at risk for infection because of the number of surgeries and invasive procedures he or she must undergo. It is extremely important for the pediatric rehabilitation nurse, in interactions with the child and family, to assess for predictors of infection risks, confounding factors, and clinical manifestations of infection. The nurse and other caregivers should reduce the possibility of entry of organisms by meticulous hand washing and use of appropriate aseptic techniques when providing care and performing procedures. The child and family should be instructed about specific risk areas and precautions that should be taken to prevent infection as well as the steps to take if an infection is suspected.

The child with spina bifida may have impairments in cognitive and motor function and have difficulty in performing self-care activities, which are those tasks necessary for daily living. Carpenito (1995) identifies five self-care deficits: feeding, bathing, dressing, toileting, and instrumental self-care deficits.

Feeding self-care deficit is defined as "a state in which an individual experiences ·an impaired ability to perform or complete feeding activities for oneself" (p. 690).

Bathing/hygiene self-care deficit includes difficulty with "washing entire body, combing hair, brushing teeth, attending to skin and nail care and applying makeup" (p. 694).

Dressing/grooming self-care deficit includes the impaired ability to don, fasten, and take off clothing and to perform grooming activities.

Toileting self-care deficit includes problems with getting to and from the toilet, handling clothing and carrying out hygienic activities.

Instrumental self-care deficit is defined as "a state in which the individual experiences an impaired ability to perform certain activities or access certain services" essential to living in the community (p. 703).

Instrumental self-care deficit may include one or more of the following: taking medications, telephone usage, managing money, using transportation, and obtaining food or clothing. In this area the pediatric rehabilitation nurse can be most helpful to the child and family by determining transportation sources and social supports and promoting self-care and adherence to a medication schedule. If self-care deficit is identified as a problem, specific interventions and teaching found in Table 15–1 can be individualized and used as the child's nursing plan of care. Additionally, the nurse should provide opportunities for and encourage self-care whenever possible to facilitate coping, thereby increasing the child's self-esteem and sense of control. Promoting prevention of secondary complications by education, regular monitoring, and referrals for specific care is important, as is promoting positive self-esteem and self-concept development with social and psychologic skill development. Healthy eating habits also contribute to positive self-image, and participation in outdoor activities and sports should be encouraged.

Expected Outcomes—Child and Family

The overall expected outcomes for the child and family include:

Child will develop and maintain abilities to be as independent as possible.

Family will use resources to facilitate the child's learning of functional independence and academic skills.

Child and family will adapt to the disability at as high a level as possible.

Child is free of preventable complications and secondary disabilities.

In many rehabilitation settings, both inpatient and outpatient, the nurse specialist manages the bowel, bladder, and skin care programs as well as provides information and emotional support to the child and family, using multiple available resources. The nurse works with other team members in the development of self-care and independence and in the use of assistive devices. The nurse also acts as a consultant for other nurses in the community or hospital setting and maintains contact with the family and child.

Long-Term Outlook

The future of children born with spina bifida is brightest when the pathway from infancy to adulthood is supported by effective health

Table 15–1 NURSING PLAN OF CARE

Nursing Diagnosis: Self-Care Deficit: Feeding, Bathing/Hygiene, Dressing/Grooming, Toileting

Related to: Decreased strength   Pain
Neuromuscular impairment   Cognitive impairment
Mobility limitation

Goals	Nursing Interventions/Teaching
Participate in activities related to self-care	Encourage participation in self-care as soon as child shows interest, even if child is clumsy and needs more time to accomplish task Promote participation in decision making and flexibility in modes of care Provide privacy during activities of daily living Allow time to accomplish activities and structure routine Teach energy conservation strategies with activity Reinforce positive coping patterns Reinforce teaching of self-care activities as needed Encourage performance of self-care activity and teach modifications as needed Consider appropriate setting for task, free from distractions and with equipment within easy reach Encourage communication between child and caregivers about specific needs and activities Suggest bathroom adaptations for toileting and bathing that improve independence (e.g., grab bars and rails, height of toilet paper and soap holders, adapted handles, nonskid mats)
Feeding	Allow child to be as independent as possible Provide food items according to preference and assist with positioning and set-up as needed Provide pain relief if needed Encourage oral hygiene after meals
Bathing	Encourage use of shower or tub if physically able Instruct in use of mirror to inspect skin while bathing
Dressing	Help to select clothing that is comfortable and easy to put on: loose fitting, wide sleeves and pant legs, Velcro closures Allow sufficient time for unaided practice to promote independence Sequence learning of activities Establish consistent routine for dressing—use picture board if necessary
Toileting	Assist with selection of toilet sitting device that promotes sitting balance Start toileting activities and child's participation early when child first shows interest
Use adaptive equipment	Assist with needed adaptations to home environment Collaborate with therapists to provide appropriate equipment, utensils, and cues (e.g., plate guards, wrist splints with clamps, utensils and secure grips) Use appropriate seating to provide proper support; should enable head, trunk, and pelvis to be in midline Instruct in use of assistive technology and adaptive equipment Assist with selection and use of an appropriate mobility device and orthotics
Achieve tasks in a safe manner	Identify safety concerns Provide safe environment with necessary supervision and/or assistance Allow rest periods between activities as needed Supervise activity until it can be safely performed

Expected Outcome

Perform self-care activities and techniques appropriate for age and level of ability to the highest degree possible care management and increasing independence in self-care, mobility, education and vocation, psychosocial development, and all other aspects of life. Today, increasingly more children with spina bifida live longer, and the comprehensive care they receive as children determines their success as adults.

Summary

Children born with spina bifida require constant attention to prevent complications and manage their primary disability. As the child grows and develops, 6- to 12-month complete rehabilitation team evaluations are necessary for reassessment and establishment of new goals. When the child reaches adolescence, annual team evaluations are most appropriate. The child or adolescent and family often need continued support and education to foster maximum independence. It is often the pediatric rehabilitation nurse who is the consistent member of the team and develops a long-lasting therapeutic relationship with the child and family. It is important for the nurse to have a thorough knowledge of the condition and its management as well as an idea of how the child will move from dependence to independence (Peterson, Rauen, Brown, & Cole, 1994).

CASE STUDY

Judy is an 11-year-old girl with spina bifida. She walks with crutches and braces but has come to the clinic because she is having problems with her bowel program. Judy has been independent in her clean intermittent catheterization program for several years and it has allowed her to be almost accident-free. Her bowel program has also been almost accident-free until recently. She has also started to have problems with constipation.

The nurse performed a thorough assessment of Judy's bowel and bladder history, physical activities, diet, and fluid intake. Judy recently started a physical fitness program and was working with a personal fitness trainer twice a week. Although an increase of activity may cause more frequent stooling, in Judy's case it caused the opposite to occur. The nurse concluded from the data gathered that, due to the delicate balance between fluid intake and use of medications for bladder incontinence management that can cause some dehydration, the stool consistency had

changed, resulting in constipation and poor control. Judy's increased activity without any increase in fluid intake may have been a factor.

To rule out impaction and to determine the amount of retained stool in the abdomen, the nurse asked the physiatrist to order a flat plate radiograph of Judy's abdomen. There was a large amount of stool and gas present in the lower intestine, and the rectal vault was enlarged with stool.

After discussing the findings with Judy and her mother, the nurse decided to take the following steps to remedy the problem:

- Judy was to keep a record of fluid intake and output for 3 days to determine how much to increase her fluid intake to make up for the insensible loss from exercise. Once the record was complete, Judy was to call the clinic, and the nurse would recommend how much more fluid to add.
- Judy was also asked to increase the amount of high-fiber foods in her diet. In addition to her daily bran cereal with fruit and the salad she usually ate for lunch, Judy was to add two tablespoons of a psyllium-based fiber supplement to her diet.
- The nurse instructed Judy to use an enema to clean out the retained stool and then resume her usual bowel program.

The nurse assured Judy and her mother that the problem could be solved and that she should continue with her activities. Also, the nurse made sure to praise Judy for her increase in physical activities and her fitness program.

Two months later, Judy came into the clinic while she was having her braces adjusted in physical therapy to visit the nurse. The bowel problem had been resolved, and Judy was very happy.

CEREBRAL PALSY

Cerebral palsy (CP), a major childhood disability, is a non-progressive disorder that results from damage to parts of the immature brain that affect purposeful movement and coordination. Although the damage to the brain is non-progressive, abnormal muscle tone may result in orthopedic problems and progressive functional limitations and physical deformities as the child grows.

The term "cerebral palsy" is used to describe many posture and movement disorders ranging from mild to severe and from low to high muscle tone. All of the body may be involved or only one extremity may be affected. Many children with CP also have seizure disorders, mild to severe global developmental delay, and varying expressions of functional limitations and physical disability.

CP is usually classified by a description of the motor dysfunction in terms of the physiologic and topographic data. The most common physiologic types are spastic, ataxic, mixed, and athetoid, with topography of monoplegia, hemiplegia, diplegia, or quadriplegia (Haslam, 1996b). Table 15–2 provides a summary of the types of CP and associated characteristic motor dysfunctions.

Etiology and Incidence

The cause of CP is an insult to the central nervous system, specifically the pyramidal tract of the brain, extra-pyramidal tract of the brain, or both. The insult can occur as a result of pre-natal factors such as trauma, infection, poor maternal health and diet, and blood incompatibilities; complications at birth due to prolonged labor, anoxia, or trauma; or childhood infections, trauma (e.g., falls, accidents, child abuse), poisonings, or cerebral vascular accidents (Betz, Hunsberger, & Wright, 1994). Many times the cause of CP is not well understood or easily identified. Prevention is a key aspect in avoiding CP, and measures include preventive women's health and obstetrical management, adequate balanced nutrition, immunizations, teaching safety and injury prevention, and avoidance of drugs, alcohol, medications, and excessive x-ray procedures.

The incidence of CP varies depending on the country of birth. The incidence of all types of CP ranges from 1 to 4 per 1000 live births in the United States, although additional cases are acquired in early childhood. Even

Table 15–2 TYPES OF CEREBRAL PALSY

1. Spastic

Hyperactive reflexes, increased muscle tone, muscle clonus/spasms, persistent infantile reflexes, motor weakness

Hemiplegia: most frequent type, involves one side of the body, usually arm is weaker and leg is more spastic, affected side is smaller, fine motor movement of the hand has mild to severe involvement with posturing of the hand and flexion of the elbow and wrist, child can walk but has gait changes with knee flexion and plantar flexion of the foot, sensory deficits or cortical neglect of affected side; often seen from early head trauma or stroke

Diplegia: involvement of all four extremities, lower more involved than upper, with weakness and varying levels of increased tone; upper extremities more mildly involved; often seen with prematurity

Quadriplegia: involvement of total body, increased muscle tone, rigid in flexion and extension of all four extremities, usually severe impairment of postural and motor control, hip adductor spasticity causing "scissoring" of the legs, plantar flexion of the feet, hands fisted with thumb inside, feeding and speech difficulty with oral motor involvement, exaggerated startle reflex, highest incidence of associated conditions and severe impairments; impairment of cognitive functioning often caused by some type of anoxia

2. Athetoid

Characterized by abnormal involuntary movements of all extremities that disappear during sleep, resulting in "worm-like" writhing and flailing of extremities and trunk, facial grimacing, dystonic movements of the tongue and mouth, poorly articulated speech, forced movements of hand and feet, distorted posturing; often caused by newborn kernicterus

3. Ataxic

Hypotonia, "floppy" muscle tone with balance and coordination impairment; walk with wide-based, unsteady gait; uncoordinated upper extremity function; least common type

4. Mixed

Combination of several types of cerebral palsy; severe delayed cognitive ability and other conditions common with this type

Data from Logigian, M. K., & J. D. Ward, (Eds.). *Pediatric rehabilitation, a team approach for therapists.* Boston: Little, Brown & Company; and Gold, J. (1993). Pediatric disorders: cerebral palsy and spina bifida. In M. S. Eisenberg, R. L. Glueckauf, & H. H. Zaretsky (Eds.). *Medical aspects of disability,* pp. 231–306. Philadelphia: WB Saunders.

with the recent improvement in management and survival of premature infants, the incidence of CP has not changed. Athetoid CP has become rare with aggressive management of hyperbilirubinemia, which is a major cause of this type of CP (Haslam, 1996b).

Pathophysiology

Damage to or maldevelopment of the motor centers of the immature brain causes CP. Three types of lesions have been identified: subependymal (hemorrhage below the ventricle lining, more common in low-birth-weight infants); encephalopathy with lesions of the white or gray matter due to anoxia; and neuropathy from central nervous system malformations leading to anoxic or hemorrhagic lesions (Olney & Wright, 1994). Different clinical signs reflect the area of brain damage. Often there are other neurologic signs that accompany the motor damage and are a result of damage to other areas of the brain (Haslam, 1996b).

Clinical Manifestations

Motor dysfunction, especially in the areas of coordination, balance, muscle tone, and purposeful movement, is the main clinical manifestation. Tone changes are classified as spasticity, athetosis, ataxia, or a mixture of these and can affect one extremity (monoplegia), one side upper and lower (hemiplegia), or all extremities (quadriplegia) including the trunk. Spasticity or hypertonicity with predominant flexor or extensor tone and ataxia with hypotonicity or floppiness can exist together in the same child. The tone quality is often dependent on the child's position. For example, in spastic quadriplegia, the extremities have increased tone and the trunk has decreased tone. Children with athetosis have fluctuating tone, whereas children with ataxia have difficulty with coordination, especially when attempting a task.

There is great variety in degrees of motor involvement and in combinations of types. Spastic CP accounts for 60% to 70% of all the types. Athetoid CP, which usually becomes obvious later as the child develops motor skills, is often diagnosed as diffuse hypotonia before the athetoid movements are recognized. Children with ataxic CP show hypotonia and delay of motor milestones.

CP is characterized by brisk deep tendon reflexes, is always central versus peripheral in cause, and has a non-progressive pattern.

Sometimes it is difficult to determine whether the condition is truly non-progressive and what the signs and symptoms are, because the clinical manifestations change as the child grows and their condition deteriorates without intervention. For some, the spastic tone quality does not become obvious until after 2 years of age. These children show motor delays and a decrease in muscle tone, or appear floppy early in life and rigid later in life. Table 15–3 provides a summary of the early signs of CP.

Other Associated Conditions

Cerebral palsy is a multi-disabling condition. It may include cognitive delays along with seizures; sensory impairments, such as visual and hearing difficulties; growth delays and speech and feeding difficulties; bowel and bladder incontinence related to cognitive delays and constipation; increased respiratory infections; skin breakdown issues; dental problems; and orthopedic problems such as joint contractures, scoliosis, and hip dislocations. Vision impairment in the form of strabismus, refraction errors, and hemianopsia is often seen in children with CP. Spasticity management includes treatment aimed at facilitation of normal movement and inhibition of abnormal reflex activity. Nutritional deficits are common because the child expends large amounts of energy to participate in daily activities but may have difficulty eating and swallowing food. Many children with CP have normal intelligence but appear retarded because of difficulty in communication.

Seizures occur in almost one half of children with CP, and medications may be neces-

Table 15–3   EARLY SIGNS OF CEREBRAL PALSY

Feeding difficulties: poor suck, tongue thrusting, regurgitation, poor lip closure, abnormal gag reflex, poorly organized swallow

Hypotonia, 'floppy', absent or abnormal grasp, Moro or stepping reflexes, poor head control, low general activity level

Hypertonic or increased muscle tone with arching of the head and back, leg extension, scissoring of the legs, hands fisted after 4 to 5 months of age, early hand preference before 18 to 24 months of age, asymmetric movement patterns

Retention of infant reflexes past 6 months of age, seizures

Failure to reach early motor milestones

sary to control the seizure activity. The type of seizure activity and its clinical manifestations dictate the treatment. For example, in a child who has petit mal seizures, medications such as valproate (Depakene) and clonazepam (Klonopin) may be prescribed to control the seizure activity. Safety precautions should be in place for the child with a history of seizures, the child who is having a seizure should be protected from injury, and both family and child should be provided with reassurance and support. Safety considerations include:

- helmets
- chairs with arms
- environmental evaluation for harmful objects
- supervision with activities of daily living
- emergency plan if breathing does not resume or there is a serious injury

Functional limitations are usually related to the severity of the motor difficulties plus the other developmental delays, including cognitive delays. Children with spastic quadriplegia most often are also severely developmentally delayed and totally dependent for all of their care. Many of these children never develop functional communication skills, and the caregivers need to rely on nonverbal cues or specific consistent sounds for recognition of the child's needs or requests. Some of these non-verbal cues include restlessness when they need to be fed, have their position changed, or have their diaper changed. Children with severely affected communication should be evaluated for augmentative communication. Chapter 14 provides information on adaptive equipment and technology.

Diagnostic Assessment

Signs of possible CP that occur early in an infant's life include concerns about sucking ability and feeding skills with inadequate weight gain; irritability; muscle tone changes, either very floppy or very stiff, with tendency to arch and extend out; and showing little interest in their environment. By 3 months of age, if the infant has not developed head control and has tightly clenched fists, there is reason for concern and a need for multi-disciplinary team evaluation and therapeutic management. Often the family brings their child to the primary care provider expressing concern about delays in accomplishing motor skills (Molnar, 1992).

Diagnosis is based on a history of risk factors, physical signs and symptoms, and delayed development. The child with CP usually has retention of early reflex patterns plus muscle tone changes and therefore has difficulty with the development of coordinated movement patterns. The retained abnormal reflex patterns most often seen include:

- asymmetric tonic neck reflex
- symmetric tonic neck reflex
- tonic labyrinthine reflex in supine and prone positions
- positive supporting reflex
- extensor thrust reaction and crossed extension reflex
- rooting reaction

These are all normal reflexes that infants display early in life but, because of the brain damage, the motor skills of a child with CP do not progress past the time when these reflexes would normally fade and coordinated motor movements would appear (between 6–12 months).

Early diagnosis and intervention is important to prevent or treat complications. The diagnostic assessment must include a complete history and physical examination by the primary care provider. Orthopedic evaluations, neurologic evaluations, chromosomal and metabolic studies, vision and hearing evaluations, and determination of a developmental level are also important for an accurate diagnosis. The neurologic evaluation should include thorough examination of posture and reflexes and the grouping of clinical findings into six categories for diagnosis:

1. Postures and movement patterns
2. Oral motor patterns
3. Strabismus
4. Tone of muscles
5. Evaluation of postural reactions and landmarks
6. Deep tendon, plantar, and infantile reflexes (Logigian, 1989, p. 30)

Developmental assessment is an important component of evaluation and should include all areas of gross and fine motor function, self-care skills, and psycho-social activities. A number of assessment tools may be used by the interdisciplinary team to obtain a complete picture of the functional ability of the child. The pediatric rehabilitation nurse can use the Pediatric Evaluation of Disability Inventory (PEDI) or Functional Independence Measure for Children (WeeFIM) as part of the assessment process. These and other tools are described in Chapter 11. Following these assessments, the team may refer the child for additional evaluation in specific problem areas.

A computer tomographic (CT) scan or magnetic resonance (MR) imaging of the brain can often be helpful in determining areas of infarction, hypoxic ischemia, atrophy of the brain with dilated ventricles, or areas of abnormal myelination associated with developmental delay. Single-photon emission computed tomography and positive emission tomography, which show brain metabolism and perfusion, are useful in diagnosis but currently available only in select situations (Molnar, 1992).

Therapeutic Management

Early intervention is important, especially for management of feeding problems; teaching of positioning, handling, and exercise techniques; and teaching of methods of early sensorimotor stimulation. Ongoing therapy goals for the child with CP should be individualized and directed toward maximizing functional skills in areas of mobility, self-care, and communication.

Interdisciplinary Team

Children with CP are best managed by a team of professionals who work together with the family and periodically evaluate the child to establish goals for treatment as the child grows and develops. The core of the team should be made up of specialists from neurology, rehabilitation medicine, orthopedics, pediatrics, rehabilitation nursing, physical therapy, occupational therapy, speech pathology, psychology, social work, education, and other disciplines (e.g., nutrition, orthotics, dental, vision) as necessary to improve the child's health and wellness.

Therapy for children with CP is usually neurodevelopmental and sensory integrative in focus (Logigian, 1989). Therapeutic management should include psychologic and vocational assessments and treatment. The goal must be for these children to be as functional as possible and be able to live as independently as possible. Physical and occupational therapists should be actively involved in the planning and implementation of the therapy program to promote normal movement and tone. This includes evaluation of the child or adolescent's ability to perform activities of daily living, teaching skills to increase the child's independence, and recommending

mobility aids and adaptive equipment. In some instances, casting, braces, and splints may be used to control involved movements, treat or prevent contractures, and maintain range of motion.

For the child who has CP and is unable to move normally, positioning is of great benefit to assist in normalizing muscle tone and allowing the child to be as functional as possible. For those who are not able to ambulate, seating systems with a mobility base are important. The use of custom-molded seating systems for children who are the most severely involved may be of benefit to support a higher level of functioning (Colbert, Doyle, & Webb, 1986). Chapter 14 provides information on assistive technology.

Other pieces of adaptive equipment may be necessary to facilitate the child's independence and to assist adults caring for the child in the home. Equipment for positioning to allow the child to play is important, equipment for support in the bath is useful, and positioning equipment for feeding is often necessary. When the child becomes older, a specialized toilet seating system may be beneficial to support continence. Adaptive and augmentative communication systems may be necessary to facilitate interaction with family and peers as well as communication in the educational process, and adapted toys allow the child to participate in play activities.

Medical and Surgical

Medical management of conditions such as seizure disorders, vision and hearing impairments, and growth and developmental problems, including growth failure due to oral motor problems, is required. Referrals to a center where children with CP can receive care by an interdisciplinary team working in conjunction with the family and primary care provider is very beneficial.

Surgical management may include methods used to improve the child's functional ability such as tendon transfers and releases, heel cord lengthening, osteotomies, and local nerve blocks to decrease spasticity. The risks and benefits of such surgeries must be carefully evaluated by a team of professionals and the family before decisions are made and treatments initiated.

In some select situations, botulinum toxin is used to decrease spasticity and improve functioning for children with spasticity and athetosis (Gooch & Sandell, 1996). In other situations, neurosurgical procedures such as posterior rhizotomy is used to decrease spasticity at the spinal cord nerve root level and improve functioning. Children with spastic diplegia have the best results with this procedure, which results in increased functioning. The selection process for the surgical procedure is very important and must be completed by a highly trained group of specialists, including the neurosurgeon, the orthopedic surgeon, and physical and occupational therapists (McDonald, 1991; Staudt & Chandler, 1990).

Impact on Child and Family

Tremendous family involvement is necessary for children with CP. Early in the child's life, the family worries and feels that something is wrong. It is usually family members who see differences between their infant and others and wonder what is wrong long before the professionals are clear regarding the diagnosis. Early feeding problems can physically and emotionally affect the family. For example, an infant who had poor oral skills with low muscle tone and poor lip closure was small for gestational age at birth. The physician told the mother that the child might need to have a feeding tube for growth and adequate nutrition. The mother was determined to avoid the feeding tube and fed her baby every hour during both night and day. Years afterward, those early weeks were a blur for the mother, and she continued to feel guilty about ignoring the rest of her family. Her child did avoid a feeding tube but remains small for her age.

As the child starts to show increased motor tone and misses motor milestones, the family becomes involved in establishing the diagnosis and therapy programs. Many of the programs require family involvement in daily regular exercise and handling programs; parents, siblings (if old enough), and other caregivers will need to participate. Because of the hypertonicity of the muscles, children with CP are difficult for the family to handle. Holding, cuddling, and diapering may be difficult because the infant has difficulty with flexion movements and may be very stiff. Often, the child with CP does not get held, cuddled, and played with as much as other children. These children are sometimes irritable because they cannot calm themselves for sleep. Families learn certain ways to handle their child to assist them in meeting their needs, but it is time consuming and there is potential for caregiver burn-out. The nurse must understand these issues and intervene to provide support and referral to appropriate resources.

Because of the ongoing controversy regarding the benefits of therapy and its cost, some children with CP do not get individual therapy past 4 or 5 years of age. Therefore, unless there are annual evaluations of need by a team of professionals at a pediatric rehabilitation center that includes evaluation of home management and the child's functional care skills, the child may continue to be dependent on the family for care. For many children, learning self-care skills away from the actual home environment may be ineffective, and transferring those skills into the actual home setting is difficult without coordination of care and work with the family to integrate the new skills into the self-care routine.

Even when children with CP learn new self-care skills, it may be easier for the family to do the task because it is faster and the child depends on it. The child may be emotionally dependent on the family, and the one-on-one attention during care is rewarding. Without it, the child may feel as if they are not getting as much attention and may be either very slow at completing tasks or start acting out in other ways to get attention. For example, one child learned to stay dry with a scheduled toileting program at school but because he did not have the same toilet chair at home and his family felt it was quicker to diaper him, he was not continent at home.

More than 50% of adolescents with CP live at home with their families and are dependent on them for care. They may experience lack of responsibility for self-care and lack of information about their sexuality, with limited exposure to social activities and sexual relationships (Hirst, 1989). As they mature, adolescents with CP can lead normal, productive lives, and the pediatric rehabilitation nurse can encourage their independence and assist with transitions to adulthood. Coordination of services continues to be a key element as the young person moves to independent living in the community, further education at the secondary level and beyond, or a meaningful work environment. More information on assisting with transitions can be found in Chapter 14.

Application of the Nursing Process

The pediatric rehabilitation nurse functions as the coordinator of care in many settings and must have a thorough knowledge of the appropriate assessments and interventions for the child or adolescent with CP and his or her family. Because of the child's multiplicity of needs, the nurse must use critical-thinking skills to design and implement interventions to obtain the best possible functional outcomes. The type of CP, the age and developmental level of the child, the child's cognitive functioning, associated problems, and the setting in which the pediatric rehabilitation nurse interacts with the child and family directly affect the process of nursing assessment. As the child grows, periodic reassessment is important to facilitate increased learning and perfecting of skills necessary for independence.

Assessment

Pediatric rehabilitation nursing assessment of a child with CP must include information from all of the functional health patterns. Chapters 11, 12, and 13 provide information that can be applied to the nursing and functional assessment with particular attention given to the areas of mobility, feeding and nutrition, communication, and body image and self-esteem. Age, severity of the disability, and developmental level must all be incorporated into the individualized assessment and care plan for each child or adolescent and his or her family. The developmental history is an important component and should include:

- family, genetic, and pregnancy/delivery history
- developmental milestones
- social and emotional areas
- self-care abilities
- school involvement
- past medical information
- parental involvement

Nursing diagnoses can be identified in any of these primary areas and may include:

- Impaired physical mobility
- Alteration in nutrition: less or more than body requirements
- Impaired swallowing
- Impaired communication
- Body image disturbance
- Self-esteem disturbance

Other nursing diagnoses that should be considered are:

- Altered growth and development
- Self-care deficits

- Ineffective coping: child and/or family
- Diversional activity deficit
- Disuse syndrome

If a nursing diagnosis of Impaired physical mobility is identified, the plan of care should include:

- promotion of activity and mobility, especially correct positioning and therapeutic handling
- safety needs and equipment
- adaptive and assistive devices
- recreation activities
- information about complications
- exercise and activity plan, including activities of daily living

The diagnosis of Risk for impaired physical mobility is also included in the cluster of diagnoses that is a part of Disuse syndrome. This is defined as "the state in which an individual is at risk for a deterioration of body systems or altered functioning as a result of prescribed or unavoidable musculoskeletal activity" (Carpenito, 1995, p. 106) and includes 11 diagnoses related to inactivity. Specific areas are skin integrity, constipation, respiratory function, tissue perfusion, infection, injury, activity, sensation and perception, body image, and powerlessness. The plan of care must include interventions that:

- maintain skin integrity and full range of motion
- promote bowel and bladder function
- maximize pulmonary function and peripheral blood flow
- integrate social activities and contacts

Nurses working with children with the diagnosis of CP often have the benefit of being involved with a multi-disciplinary team and can learn therapeutic handling techniques and corrective positioning from other team members. When the nurse does not have this opportunity and needs to know some of the basic handling techniques to decrease the reflex pattern and allow the child to be more functional, it is important to seek out educational opportunities and appropriate consultation or be able to differentiate the abnormal movement patterns from movements seen in seizure activity, and to be aware that significant physical involvement does not always correlate with cognitive impairment.

The pediatric rehabilitation nurse must also have knowledge of the child's method of communication as well as the expected developmental level and appropriate behaviors. When working with a child or adolescent who has impaired communication, the nurse should:

Use appropriate language for the child's developmental level, contact a translator if needed, and integrate language into the plan of care.

Use techniques that promote understanding: talk distinctly, minimize distractions, use gestures, make eye contact, and teach these techniques that improve communication to child, family, and other caregivers.

Consult with therapists if a communication system is needed, assist the family in selecting and using the child's communication system, and allow time for the child to use the system.

Encourage the child and family to discuss feelings about communication difficulties.

If alterations in growth and development are identified, the nurse should discuss this with the family and provide information about the expected age-related tasks. Self-care activities should be encouraged, and time and opportunity should be provided for the child to participate in appropriate play and recreational activities with periods of interaction with other children.

Expected Outcomes—Child and Family

The overall expected outcomes for the child and family include:

Child will develop and maintain abilities to be as independent as possible in mobility, self-care, and communication.

Child will experience minimal associated conditions and complications.

Child will have a supportive environment, especially related to learning and social systems and resources.

Additionally, the nurse should encourage the collaboration of family, therapists, and health care providers and teach the use of safe and effective techniques for feeding to avoid aspiration. Development of cognitive skills can be promoted by referral to early intervention programs, pediatric rehabilitation teams, and school programs; socialization, healthy parenting, and communication skills can be provided by referral to play groups, family support groups, respite programs, and sports and recreation programs. The nurse can assist with practical home management skill learning by being a member of the home evaluation team and working collaboratively with the child and family to propose solutions to identified problems.

Long-Term Outlook

The future of children with CP is always expanding as new technology and information about management techniques, resources, and procedures are developed. One of the newer techniques for management of severe spasticity is intrathecal baclofen therapy. This involves administration of baclofen from a small pump into the spinal fluid to block nerve impulses that lead to spasticity (Albright, 1997). Other recent developments have been made in the area of therapy; these include a total daily program to encourage the child in developing successful patterns of functional and self-care skills.

Summary

Cerebral palsy is a disability with varying degrees of involvement. As the degree of severity increases, the child's care is more complex. The family must devote increasingly more time to care with children who have more severe and complex global developmental delays. The pediatric rehabilitation nurse's role in caring for children with CP and their families is long term and encompasses acute care in the hospital, community care, and home care.

REFERENCES

Albright, L. (1997). Intrathecal baclofen therapy for severe spasticity. *Exceptional Parent*, 27(9), 79–82.

Betz, C., Hunsberger, M., & Wright, S. (1994). Understanding altered development. In C. Betz, M. Hunsberger, & S. Wright (Eds.). *Family-centered nursing care of children*, pp. 953–1001. Philadelphia: WB Saunders.

Butler, C. (1991). Augmentative mobility: why do it? *Physical Medicine and Rehabilitation Clinics of North America*, 2(4), 801–815.

Carpenito, L. (1995). Handbook of nursing diagnosis (6th ed.). Philadelphia: JB Lippincott.

Colbert, A., Doyle, K., & Webb, W. (1986). DESEMO seats for young children with cerebral palsy. *Archives of Physical and Rehabilitation Medicine*, 67(7), 484–486.

Dahl, M., Ahlsten, G., Carlson, H., Ronne-Engstrom, E., Lagerkvist, B., Magnusson, G., Norrlin, S., Olsen, L., Stromberg, B., & Thomas, K. (1995). Neurological dysfunction above cele level in children with spina bifida cystica: a prospective study to three years. *Developmental Medicine and Child Neurology*, 37(1), 30–40.

Disabato, J., & Wulf, J. (1994). Altered neurologic function. In C. Betz, M. Hunsberger, & S. Wright, (Eds.). Family-centered nursing care of children (2nd ed.), pp. 1717–1814. Philadelphia: WB Saunders.

Farley, J., & Dunleavy, M. (1996). Myelodysplasia. In P.L. Jackson & J.A. Vessey (Eds.). *Primary care of the child with a chronic condition*, pp. 580–598. St. Louis, CV Mosby.

Gold, J. (1993). Pediatric disorders: cerebral palsy and spina bifida. In M.S. Eisenberg, R.L. Glueckauf, & H.H. Zaretsky (Eds.). *Medical aspects of disability*, pp. 281—306. Philadelphia: WB Saunders.

Gooch, J., & Sandell, T. (1996). Botulinum toxin for spasticity and athetosis in children with cerebral palsy. *Archives of Physical and Rehabilitation Medicine*, 77(5), 508–511.

Haslam, R. (1996a). Congenital anomalies of the central nervous system. In W.E. Nelson (Ed.). *Textbook of pediatrics* (15th ed.), pp. 1677–1685. Philadelphia: WB Saunders.

Haslam, R. (1996b). Encephalopathies. In W.E. Nelson (Ed.). *Textbook of pediatrics* (15th ed.), pp. 1713–1714. Philadelphia: WB Saunders.

Hirst, M. (1989). Patterns of impairment and disability related to social handicap in young people with cerebral palsy and spina bifida. *Journal of Biosocial Science*, 21, 1–12.

King, J., Currie, D., & Wright, E. (1994). Bowel training in spina bifida: importance of education, patient compliance, age, and reflexes. *Archives of Physical Therapy Rehabilitation*, 75(3), 243–247.

Light, J. (1991). Surgical correction of incontinence: artificial sphincter. In E.T. Gonzales & D. Roth (Eds.). *Common problems in pediatric urology*, pp. 181–186. St. Louis: CV Mosby.

Logigian, M. (1989). *Cerebral palsy*. In M.K. Logigian & J.D. Ward, (Eds.). *Pediatric rehabilitation, a team approach for therapists*, pp. 23–61. Boston: Little, Brown & Company.

Lollar, D. (1993). *Spina bifida spotlight: learning among children with spina bifida*, pp. 1–6. Washington, DC: Spina Bifida Association of America.

McDonald, C. (1991). Selective dorsal rhizotomy: a critical review. *Physical Medicine and Rehabilitation Clinics of North America*, 2(4), 891–917.

Milunsky, A., Jick, H., Jick, S., Bruell, C., MacLaughlin, D., Willett, W., & Rothman, K. (1989). Multivitamin/folic acid supplementation in early pregnancy reduces the prevalence of neural tube defects. *Journal of American Medical Association*, 262(20), 2847–2852.

Molnar, G. (1992). Cerebral palsy. In G. Molnar (Ed.). *Pediatric rehabilitation*, pp. 481–535. Baltimore: Williams & Wilkins.

Olney, S., & Wright, M. (1994). Cerebral palsy. In S. Campbell (Ed.). *Physical therapy for children*, pp. 489–523. Philadelphia: WB Saunders.

Peterson, P., Rauen, K., Brown, J., & Cole, J. (1994). Spina bifida: the transition into adulthood begins in infancy. *Rehabilitation Nursing*, 19(4), 229–238.

Reigel, D. (1989) Spina bifida. In R.L. McLaurin, L. Schut, J.L. Venes, & Epstein, F. (Eds.). *Surgery of the developing nervous system* (2nd ed.), pp. 35–52. Philadelphia: WB Saunders.

Romanczuk, A. (1993). Latex use with infants and children: it can cause problems. *Maternal Child Nursing*, 18(4), 208–212.

Staudt, L., & Chandler, L. (1990). The role of selective posterior rhizotomy in the management of cerebral palsy. *Infants and Young Children*, 2(3), 48–58.

Tew, B. (1991). The effects of spina bifida and hydrocephalus on learning and behavior. In Bannister & Tew (Eds.). *Current concepts in spina bifida and hydrocephalus, clinics in developmental medicine no. 122*, pp. 158–179. New York: Cambridge University Press.

Van Cleve, L. (1989). Parental coping in response to their child's spina bifida. *Journal of Pediatric Nursing*, 4(3), 172–176.

Whitehead, W., Parker, L., Bosmajian, L., Morrill-Corbin, E., Middaugh, S., Garwood, M., Cataldo, M., & Freeman, J. (1986). Treatment of fecal incontinence in children with spina bifida: comparison of biofeedback and behavior modification. *Archives of Physical Medicine and Rehabilitation*, 67, 218–224.

ADDITIONAL RESOURCES

Anderson, S. (1989). Secondary neurologic disability in myelomeningocele. *Infants and Young Children*, 1(4), 9–21.

Bauer, S. (1991). Evaluation and management of the newborn with myelomeningocele. In E.T. Gonzales Jr. & D. Roth (Eds.). *Common problems in pediatric urology*, pp. 169–180. St. Louis: CV Mosby.

Darrah, J., & Bartlett, D. (1995). Dynamic systems theory and management of children with cerebral palsy: unresolved issues. *Infants and Young Children*, 8(1), 52–59.

Fettes, L., & Kluzik J. (1996). The effects of neurodevelopmental treatment versus practice on the reaching of children with spastic cerebral palsy. *Physical Therapy*, 76(4) 346–358.

Finnie, N. (1975). *Handling the young cerebral palsied child at home*. New York: Dutton.

Fosdal, M. (1992). Living with spina bifida. *Journal of Neuroscience Nursing*, 24(5), 286–289.

Gisel, E., Applegate-Ferrante, T., Benson, J., & Bosma, J. (1996). Oral-motor skills following sensorimotor therapy in two groups of moderate dysphagic children with CP: aspiration vs. nonaspiration. *Dysphagia*, 11(1) 59–71.

Helfrich-Miller, K., Rector, K., & Straka, J. (1986). Dysphagia: its treatment in the profoundly retarded patient with CP. *Archives of Physical Medicine and Rehabilitation*, 67(8), 520–525.

Laurent, J. (1991). Tethering of the spinal cord. In E.T. Gonzales Jr. & D. Roth (Eds.). *Common problems in pediatric urology,* pp. 205–209. St. Louis: CV Mosby.

McGrath, S., Splaingard, M., Alba, H., Kaufman, B., & Glicklick, M. (1992). Survival and functional outcome of children with severe cerebral palsy following gastrostomy. *Archives of Physical Medicine and Rehabilitation,* 73(2), 133–137.

Peterson, P. (1992). Spina bifida—nursing challenges. *RN,* 55(3), 40–46.

Reyes, A., Cash, A., Green, S., & Booth, I. (1993). Gastroesophageal reflux in children with cerebral palsy. *Child: Care, Health and Development,* 19(2), 109–118.

Samuelson, J., Foltz, J., & Foxall, M. (1992). Stress and coping in families of children with myelomeningocele. *Archives of Psychiatric Nursing,* 6(5), 287–295.

Segal, E., Deatrick, J., & Hagelgans, N. (1995). The determinants of successful self-catheterization programs in children with myelomeningocele. *Journal of Pediatric Nursing: Nursing Care of Children & Families,* 10(2), 82–88.

Sochaniwskyj, A.E., Koheil, R.M., Bablich, K., Milner, M., & Kenny, D.J. (1986). Oral motor functioning, frequency of swallowing and drooling in normal children and in children with cerebral palsy. *Archives of Physical Medicine and Rehabilitation,* 67(12), 866–874.

Taylor, S., & Shelton, J. (1985). Caloric requirements of a spastic immobile cerebral palsy patient: a case report. *Archives of Physical Medicine and Rehabilitation,* 76(3), 281–283.

Zelle, R., & Coyner, K. (1983). *Developmentally disabled infants and toddlers: assessment and intervention.* Philadelphia: FA Davis.

RESOURCES

American Academy for Cerebral Palsy and Developmental Medicine
6300 North River Road, Suite 727
Rosemont, IL 60018
847-698-1635
http://www.aacpdm.org

National Easter Seal Society
230 West Monroe, Suite 1800
Chicago, IL 60606
800-221-6827 or 312-726-6200
http://www.easter-seals.org

National Hydrocephalus Foundation
12413 Centralia
Lakewood, CA 90715
562-402-3523
http://www.geocities.com/HotSprings/Villa/2300

Spina Bifida Association of America
4590 MacArthur Boulevard NW, Suite 250
Washington, DC 20007
800-621-3141 or 202-944-3285
http://sbaa.org

United Cerebral Palsy Associations, Inc.
1660 L. Street NW, Suite 700
Washington, DC 20036
800-USA-5UCP
http://icupa.org

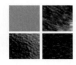

Chapter 16

Musculoskeletal Conditions
Craniofacial Anomalies

Susanne R. Hays

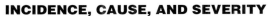

INCIDENCE, CAUSE, AND SEVERITY

Craniofacial anomalies are those which involve the embryonic development of the oro-facial area. The most common group of anomalies in this category are cleft of the lip (with or without cleft of the palate) and cleft of the palate.

Cause and Incidence

The specific cause of cleft lip and palate usually is unknown. Some teratogens, such as alcohol, folic acid antagonists, and retinoic acid, plus a prescription medication for seizures, phenytoin (Dilantin), have been implicated as playing a role in the development of clefting (Gorlin, Cohen, & Levin, 1990).

The cause of cleft lip alone, with or without cleft palate, is thought to be multifactorial. The cause of cleft palate alone is thought to be different genetically from clefting of the lip and palate. The embryonic development for cleft lip with or without palate and isolated cleft palate occurs at different times and has different genetic risks (Robinson and Linden, 1993).

Cleft lip with or without cleft palate occurs on an average of 1 per 1000 births. Cleft palate alone is believed to occur in 1 per 2500 births. Incidence varies by race and sex for cleft lip with or without cleft palate. Boys more commonly have cleft lip with or without cleft palate; if they have both lip and palate clefts, the condition usually is more severe than in girls. Girls tend to have a higher incidence of cleft palate without cleft of the lip or alveolar ridge. There is a higher incidence rate among the Japanese and the Native American populations. There is a lower rate among the black population (Cusson, 1994).

The incidence of clefting combined with a broader pattern of defects is approximately 35%. Some of the syndromes that include clefting are Robin sequence (Pierre Robin syndrome), Treacher Collins syndrome, Stickler syndrome and trisomy 13 (Jones, 1997). For an illustration of the anatomical features of Robin sequence, see Figure 16–1.

Genetic counseling is important for parents who have clefting. If the father has a cleft, the risk factor is 3% for offspring; if the mother has a cleft, the risk factor is 14% for offspring. If one sibling has a cleft, generally, the more severe the cleft, the higher the risk factor for subsequent siblings (Jones, 1997).

Pathophysiology

Embryologically, the fusion of the lip occurs by the 35th day and the palatal shelves completely fuse by the ninth week. In spite of the difference in time of each fusion, there is the possibility of a wide variety of degrees and locations of the cleft. Along with the cleft of the lip, there may be a cleft of the alveolar ridge, creating an opening into the nasal cavity. With clefts of the primary palate, there may also be tooth formation interruption or relocation (Robinson and Linden, 1993).

Depending on the type of cleft and presence or absence of other anomalies, children may experience feeding and growth difficulty, severe middle ear disease, dental problems,

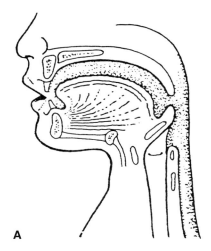 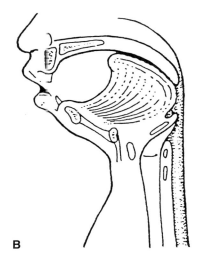

A   B

Figure 16–1 Pierre Robin sequence. Anatomical features of larynx. *A*, Normal. *B*, Mandibular hypoplasia. Note posterior placement of the tongue makes the larynx appear more anteriorly situated than normal. (From Jackson, P. A., & Vessey, J. A. (1996). *Primary Care of the Child with a Chronic Condition.* St. Louis: Mosby, p. 259.)

speech and hearing difficulty, psychosocial and emotional problems, learning problems, cognitive delays, or general developmental delays. Most commonly, children born with clefting do not have developmental delays or other conditions that affect growth unless there have been problems with management, especially of the middle ear disease, or feeding problems early in life. Figure 16–2 shows the various types of cleft lip and cleft palate.

Clinical Aspects and Functional Limitations

Clefting ranges in severity from a small notch in the lip to bilateral clefting of both lip and palate. Supernumerary, deformed, or absent teeth also may be associated with the cleft of the lip and palate, as may nasal distortions (Johnsen, 1996).

Of course, the most obvious clinical signs include clefting of the lip and palate, and these are easily seen as soon as the face appears during the birth process. Cleft of the palate is less obvious and may go undiagnosed at first. Even more easily unnoticed is the submucous cleft, which is a clefting only of the bony part of the palate, with a mucosal covering remaining intact.

Feeding difficulties and verbal communication deficits are related most commonly to the severity of the defect. Infants with clefting of the palate with or without clefting of the lip have a very high incidence of otitis media and therefore may have hearing difficulties.

Other functional limitations include psychosocial concerns related to body image disturbances and ineffective coping either by the family or the child.

Diagnostic Assessment

Prenatal diagnosis is made when the defect is detected with ultrasound in the latter part of the pregnancy. Often the clefting is identified as part of a larger series of anomalies. There is no prenatal test that detects the presence of cleft lip and/or palate (Robinson and Linden, 1993). When parents know about the presence of a cleft condition prenatally, they are able to become informed regarding the condition and prepare for the necessary interventions prior to birth by meeting with the team of specialists. This early information and planning is valuable for the family.

Infants born with craniofacial anomalies must have the benefit of being assessed by a genetics or dysmorphology specialist to determine the specific type of defect and whether the defect is related to a specific syndrome. Based on that information, other diagnostic assessments such as chromosome studies, scans, and consultation with other specialists may be necessary (Robinson and Linden, 1993).

Infrequently, the cleft of the palate or a submucous cleft is missed during the newborn examination after birth. The family then identifies the cleft or "something wrong with the throat" when the newborn cries vigor-

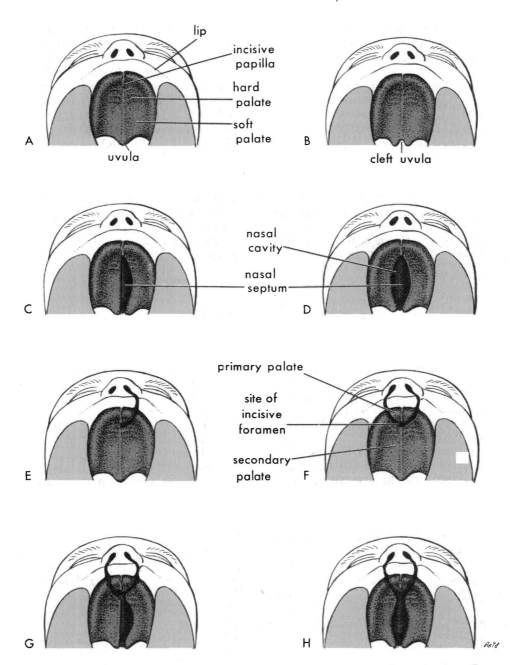

Figure 16–2 Various types of cleft lip and cleft palate. *A,* Normal lip and palate. *B,* Cleft uvula. *C,* Unilateral cleft of the posterior or secondary palate. *D,* Bilateral cleft of the posterior palate. *E,* Complete unilateral cleft of the lip and alveolar process of the maxilla with a unilateral cleft of the anterior or primary palate. *F,* Complete bilateral cleft of the lip and alveolar processes of the maxillae with bilateral cleft of the anterior palate. *G,* Complete bilateral cleft of the lip and alveolar processes of the maxillae with bilateral cleft of the anterior palate and unilateral cleft of the posterior palate. *H,* Complete bilateral cleft of the lip and alveolar processes of the maxillae with complete bilateral cleft of the anterior and posterior palates. (From Cusson, R. (1996). Altered digestive function. In Betz, C. L., Hunsberger, M., & Wright, S. (Eds.) *Family-Centered Nursing Care of Children* (2nd ed.). Philadelphia: W. B. Saunders, p. 1440.)

ously. One such situation occurred in my practice: the mother was distraught and felt the doctor was keeping something from her about her baby. She had not attended to her own care early in the pregnancy and had guilt feelings about that. Therefore, she was afraid something else was wrong with her baby that she had caused. It was only with her infant being able to successfully feed, grow, and meet developmental milestones that she was able to relax. Then, when his speech development was altered related to the cleft, she again became depressed and sought short-term counseling.

THERAPEUTIC MANAGEMENT

Interdisciplinary Approach

Individuals with cleft lip and/or palate are best served by a team of professionals who have experience with management of that particular defect. The team should include specialists in primary care, plastic and oral facial surgery, orthodontics, prosthetic and pediatric dentistry, pediatric otolaryngology, audiology, nursing, speech therapy, growth and development, nutrition, genetics, psychology, and other professionals as needed on a consultation basis. Newborns should be referred to a team as soon as possible after birth. A variety of professionals are necessary at various stages of the child's development and reconstruction.

The family should have the opportunity of receiving information and consultation from each team early in the infant's life and on an ongoing basis throughout the child's growing years (Shprintzen, 1995).

Primary Care

Infants born with clefting must be given close attention regarding the management of the feeding issues until positive weight gain has been demonstrated and the family feels comfortable with the infant's care. Where there is a team available, the nurse specialist, with consultation from other members of the team as necessary, is the most appropriate professional to provide intervention during this phase. See Chapter 12 for information regarding nutrition.

Surgical Care

Surgical management of the cleft lip usually is done within the first 10 weeks of life and sometimes as early as the first month. Weight gain and health are important factors in making the decision to do surgery. Cleft palate usually is repaired before the first year of age and often is done around the ninth month of age in order to support speech development. Based on the decision of the surgeon, sometimes the lip and palate repairs are done in two stages. There is a wide variation in timing of the repairs, depending on the philosophy of the surgeon, the management team, and the family. Revisions of the lip repair are often necessary later in the child's life to provide the optimal appearance. The decision to do revisions usually is based on the appearance and growth of the face, psychosocial concerns, and the desires of the child and family (Bardach and Salyer, 1995).

Repair of the bony alveolar ridge along the gum line usually coincides with dental development, secondary tooth eruption, and orthodontic management. During the late teenage years, after growth of the face is believed to be completed, there may still need to be surgical management of a facial imbalance that cannot be corrected by orthodontics (Vargervik, 1995).

Therapy

Evaluation and intervention by a speech-language pathologist is recommended at 3-month intervals during the first year and as needed after that until speech development has been perfected (Langlois and Nowak, 1990). Successful speech production may depend on surgical revisions of the palate. Surgery and orthodontics also may alter the speech production process, so the child needs to be monitored on a regular basis. Audiologic screening should be done before the infant is discharged from the hospital and on a regular basis thereafter. While the child is developing, screening on a regular basis is recommended, with complete evaluations and interventions when warranted.

APPLICATION OF NURSING PROCESS

Assessment,Reassessment

Health History, Physical/Functional Findings

- Height, weight, head circumference at birth and currently, and any data regarding measurements between birth and currently if possible

- Type and extent of cleft, presence or absence of other anomalies or conditions at birth, respiratory concerns related to micrognathia (as may occur with the Robin sequence)
- Gestational age at birth, type of birth (i.e., vaginal versus cesarian section), family's reactions at birth of child with clefting, knowledge of clefting prior to delivery because of diagnosis from ultrasound, what they expected, and what actually happened
- Other children in the family, other family members, parents, with clefting; their experiences regarding management concerns (surgical and nonsurgical), feeding situations, family reactions, current concerns with that person (i.e., speech and hearing, appearance, dental, growth, psychosocial, emotional)
- Health condition at current assessment, previous health concerns (e.g., ear infections, poor weight gain, parent-child psychosocial problems)
- If a newborn or a child with feeding difficulties or poor weight gain: what are concerns of family or professionals including cultural expectations, current feeding methods and equipment, observation of current feeding by person who does feeding at a time when infant or child usually eats, observation of infant/child. Sensorineurologic organization, current overall developmental level, current oral motor skills: absence of reflexes, ability to establish negative pressure in oral cavity, nasal regurgitation, average daily caloric intake, types and textures of foods consumed, positioning during feedings, usual length of feeding and average volume, family/child interaction during feeding

Diagnostic Tests

- For some infants, a swallowing study may be necessary to assess the swallow process and assist with development of a successful feeding program.

Potential Nursing Diagnosis: Actual or High Risk

- Nutritional deficit: less than body requirement related to sucking, swallowing, or chewing difficulties
- Ineffective breast feeding related to infant anomaly/poor ability to develop negative pressure intraorally
- Oral mucous membrane, altered related to effects of friction from feeding method and/or poor oral hygiene
- Body image disturbance
- Impaired verbal communication
- Caregiver role strain
- Ineffective individual and/or family coping
- Altered parenting related to birth of a child with anomalies

Expected Outcomes: Child and Family

- Child and family will demonstrate and verbalize safe, effective oral and tube feeding (if necessary) with appropriate positioning, caloric intake needs, management of specialized feeding equipment, growth expectations, intraoral skin care management
- Infant/child will demonstrate growth for age
- Child and family will verbalize knowledge regarding cleft condition and medical and surgical management
- Family will demonstrate attachment behaviors, verbalize feeling of competence regarding specialized care, and be able to report positive feeling toward child
- Child will verbalize feelings about facial appearance and speech difficulties (if present), develop confidence to become a part of age-appropriate activities, and verbalize positive focus

Rehabilitation Nursing Intervention

Near-Normal Oral Feeding for Infants with Clefts

The first priority for the family with an infant born with clefting is to establish a safe, effective nurturing/feeding plan. Many mothers choose to breast feed their infant. For the professional, making the most appropriate decision regarding the method of feeding may be difficult, especially if the professional has infrequent experience doing so. For suggestions about decision making in feeding, see Table 16–1. In spite of the fact that there are general types of clefting, it seems from my experience of some 20 years working with these infants that each infant has a slightly different variation and the family has different ideas and nippling choices. These choices must be noted and integrated into the plan; however, the goal should be to support the infant to feed in as near normal a way as possible given the infant's anomalies.

Infants are born with two reflexes that assist them in feeding: the suck reflex and the bite reflex. Remember that nippling requires

Table 16–1 INFANT WITH ORAL-FACIAL CLEFT WITHOUT OTHER ABNORMAL FINDINGS

Infants born with oral-facial clefts may present feeding difficulties related to lack of ability to develop intraoral suction. Intervention specific to the type of cleft needs to be instituted to prevent growth failure.

Does the infant have cleft of the lip only? —Yes→ Breast or bottle feeding? —Yes→ The cleft of the lip only should not create any difficulties with breast or bottle feeding because the infant has normal intraoral suction skills.

| No ↓

Does the infant have notch of the upper alveolar ridge also? —Yes→ Does the mother prefer to breast feed? —Yes→ The cleft of the lip with a notch of the upper alveolar ridge should not create problems with breast feeding. The breast will mold into the lip defect and the hard and soft palate is intact; therefore, intraoral suction can easily be established.

| No →

Does the mother prefer to bottle feed? —Yes→ The cleft of the lip with a notch of the upper alveolar ridge can cause a slight loss of suction in the mouth which can create difficulty with bottle feeding. Modification of the nipple in the form of an enlarged cross-cut will compensate for the loss of intraoral suction related to the upper alveolar notch.

Does the infant have cleft of the lip, hard and/or soft palate, unilateral or bilateral? —Yes→ Does the mother prefer to breast feed? —Yes→ The cleft of the lip, plus hard and soft palate unilateral or bilateral, or cleft of the palate hard and/or soft only, causes a significant loss of intraoral suction that makes it very difficult to effectively breast feed. Therefore, the mother must pump and/or express milk and deliver breast milk to her infant by another method to meet growth demands of her infant.

| No →

Does the mother prefer to bottle feed? —Yes→ Alternate bottle feeding methods that are most effective for feeding are those which allow the infant to use compression for effective delivery of milk into the mouth. Therefore, the use of a soft nipple with an enlarged cross-cut has been found to be most effective.

the infant to be able to demonstrate an organized, effective suck-swallow-breathe pattern and have a structurally intact oral system. To be effective, the suck must have a pulling, suction component that assists the infant in getting milk from the breast or bottle. Even the soft palate has a function: it comes back against the base of the tongue to facilitate this process. If this ability has been changed because of an opening between the mouth and nose that results from a cleft of the hard or soft palate, then the feeding system will have to compensate for the lack of suction, because the opening will not allow the infant to create effective suction. It has been my experience that even with a small notch in the alveolar ridge with cleft of the lip, suction pressure is altered.

In some centers, infants with cleft of the hard and soft palates are fitted with an obturator to facilitate feeding. The obturator covers only the hard palate, and the infant continues to have difficulty in establishing effective suction. Having worked with a center that used obturators and with one that did not, I have found that a safe, effective feeding program can be developed either way.

CASE STUDY

Recently in my practice, I provided intervention for Jackie, an infant born with a cleft of the lip and a notch of the alveolar ridge with an intact palate. When she arrived at the clinic 3 weeks after birth, her mother was breastfeeding her and Jackie had gained just back to her birth weight.

Her mother indicated she felt Jackie could latch on well only on one side and that she preferred not to feed on the other. If the mother encouraged her to do so, Jackie did not seem to empty the breast and lingered at the breast longer, just making lapping tongue movements. Changing positions so the mother held Jackie the same way on each breast was just enough to facilitate successful feeding and appropriate weight gain. The mother's breast was effectively closing off the notch in the alveolar ridge, so Jackie could effectively pull the nipple in and pull milk from each breast. As Jackie's face grew, the cleft became larger, again causing problems with the lack of suction even with proper positioning.

It was at that time that I discussed with the surgeon the possibility of doing surgery earlier than originally scheduled in order to support continued adequate growth and to allow the mother to continue breastfeeding. Because Jackie was growing well and had no health problems, the surgeon completed the lip repair at about 6 weeks of age. After Jackie awakened from the anesthesia, the mother was allowed to return to breast feeding. The mother was delighted to experience Jackie's ability to breast feed effectively just as her other children had done, without any adjustment of position.

Making the choice of breastfeeding for total nutrition when an infant has a cleft that affects the palate is, from my professional experience, not an effective functional option. The infant simply cannot create enough suction to pull the nipple into the mouth or to pull milk from the breast. Many mothers make the decision not to expect their infants with a cleft of the palate to get total nutrition from breastfeeding after they have tried and experienced how frustrating the process is for them both. Some make the decision after seeing pictures of how the palate of a normal infant separates the nose from the mouth and functions to create vacuum in the mouth during feeding.

Mothers should be encouraged to pump breast milk using a bilateral electric system to then provide her milk to her infant in another nippling method. They should also be encouraged to take the infant to the breast during let down so that he or she can receive the milk.

CASE STUDY

One infant born with a wide bilateral cleft of the lip and palate had several days of breast-feeding attempts. His mother did not want to introduce a foreign nipple into her son's mouth, and therefore did not want to consider other methods of nippling. The infant would try to latch on but could not and would become very frustrated, turning away and rooting to try to facilitate the milk coming out.

After he lost nearly 20% of his birth weight and became very lethargic, his mother developed a system of pumping her breasts and feeding him with a spoon and cup. Although this was very time consuming for both of them, his mother was happy with the system that she had developed and he started to gain weight.

▬▬▬

I have found that the most effective and most easily obtained system for supporting the infant with a cleft of the palate to nipple is to use a regular-shaped soft nipple and cut an enlarged **X** or cross-cut to support the infant getting enough milk as he or she bites or munches on the nipple. This system has worked for a vast number of infants with a variety of clefting anomalies. The size of the cross-cut must be adjusted to meet the infant's skill and energy level. Sometimes early in the infant's life, mothers will use nipples with different-sized cross-cuts: one which is larger when the infant is not so hungry, and one that is smaller when the baby is more awake and very hungry. As the infant grows and develops skill, a smaller cross-cut may need to be used. Table 16–2 offers an outline of components of initial teaching for parents of infants with cleft lip and palate.

As the surgeries are completed, the cross-cut may need to be changed. Usually, before infants have the surgeries to close the hard and soft palate, they will be taught to drink from a cup, so nippling is no longer the method of choice. Before that happens, most infants with clefting of the palate will need to use a nipple with a modified cross-cut.

There are many other systems of nipples and bottles with a variety of shapes and prescribed methods of feeding infants with clefting. I personally have tried most of them when they were available. I always go back to the cross-cut method just described for two reasons. First, the materials are always available, and second, the system allows the infant to control the flow of milk, thus supporting near-normal development.

For families in rural areas where transportation of the infant and mother to a center is not available immediately after birth, having to wait for a special feeding system to arrive is not necessary. Often, with written information and phone consultation plus the support of a primary care provider or home nurse, the family can start effective feeding before the opportunity to be seen by the team is available.

The use of a squeeze bottle to facilitate infant feeding is not always safe. It may de-

liver milk into the infant's mouth when he or she is getting ready to breathe, thus choking the infant and not allowing him or her to be in charge of that process the way infants without clefts are.

The use of a supplemental nursing system to deliver milk over the mother's breast nipple during attempts at breastfeeding may not be effective because it also delivers milk to the infant when he or she is trying to swallow and breathe.

For those infants born with micrognathia, undergrowth of the lower jaw, and a cleft of the palate, the tongue, which follows the jaw, will be recessed and may cause difficulty with the feeding process, as well as obstruction of the airway. If that does not occur but the tongue seems to be far back in the mouth, nippling may be difficult unless a longer nipple is used with an enlarged cross-cut. Remember, the nipple must be on top of the tongue at least half-way back for the infant to be able to munch on it and open up the cross-cut to get milk. For these infants, keeping the nipple far enough in the mouth may necessitate using a bent neck bottle and a longer nipple. Sometimes positioning on the side for good alignment is necessary.

For the term infant without other types of anomalies in addition to the clefting, tube feeding is not necessary, although there are occasions when that system of feeding has seemed necessary. If the infant is unable to organize and sustain a successful suck-swallow-breathe pattern that will facilitate nippling, then tube feeding may be necessary until the infant can manage better. For more information, see Table 16–3.

▬▬▬
CASE STUDY

Joe was 3 months old. He had been born with a unilateral cleft of the lip and palate. His parents were young and very concerned: he was their first child. Grandparents were a positive resource in the rural community but had not had any experience with a baby born with a cleft. Joe's family lived about 300 miles from the town where a team of specialists came three times per year to see children with his condition. He had been scheduled for the clinic at birth.

When Joe arrived at the clinic, he weighed just 1 pound above his birth weight. The family had tried everything it knew to feed him, but he continued to grow very slowly and

Table 16–2   FEEDING INFANT WITH A CLEFT OF THE PALATE: INITIAL TEACHING

1. Position of infant
   Hold infant in a relaxed position with head in good alignment with body and chin slightly tucked; avoid arching head back.
   Hold infant at a relaxed 45-degree angle.
   Never leave infant unheld with bottle propped.

2. Use soft nipple with enlarged cross-cut
   Use regular nipple that is soft and slender, such as the "red preemie" nipple made by Ross Laboratories.
   Enlarge cross-cut to provide infant with milk flow that allows bubbles to be seen in bottle during active feeding.
   If infant falls asleep after feeding for at least 20 minutes and has taken less than 30 mL, the cross-cut is not large enough.
   If infant gets more milk than he can handle in his mouth with one short sucking movement, the cross-cut is too big and a nipple with a smaller cut needs to be used.

3. Positioning of the nipple in the mouth
   Nipple should be positioned in the middle of the tongue.
   Allow infant to take nipple in mouth so plastic ring of bottle is very close to the lips.

4. Length of feeding period
   Infant should be able to get enough milk per feeding in 20 to 30 minutes.
   If this does not occur, infant may be too sleepy, or the cross-cut in nipple may not be big enough.

5. Burping
   Infant may need to be burped more frequently to allow for swallowing of extra air during feeding process.

6. Amount of milk necessary for adequate weight gain
   Varies by weight of infant, but roughly the infant should consume at least 50 calories per pound per 24 hours; for an infant whose weight is 7 pounds, that means at least 17 ounces to support growth. Milk contains approximately 20 calories per ounce.
   Example: 50 calories $\times$ 7 pounds = 350 calories, divided by 20 calories per ounce = 17 ounces per 24 hours
   For the first few days, at least until weight gain has started, keep a record of feeding amounts per 24 hours.

7. Care of cleft area
   For cleft of lip and palate, keep cleft area inside and outside of mouth clean by patting with clean, soft cloth moistened with warm water.
   May need to use moisturizing ointment for exposed area of gums to prevent chafing.

Copyright 1993 by Susanne R. Hays.

Table 16–3   GUIDELINES FOR INTERVENTION

Establish effective feeding specific to oral motor developmental skills, reassess and adjust as developmental skills progress and age-appropriate foods are required (see Table 16–1).

Provide family and child with information regarding anomaly, medical, surgical, and team management.

Teach family to recognize subtle signs of middle ear disease such as increased fussiness, decrease desire to nipple, diminished response to sounds, pulling or scratching at ear.

Collaborate with other professionals regarding planning and implementation development, if necessary for success.

Assess for caloric intake and growth regularly.

Refer to support groups or connect with another family whose child has a similar cleft.

Provide the family with pictures of before and after surgery.

Refer for financial resources if necessary and to the interdisciplinary team plus agencies such as Cleft Palate Foundation.

remained irritable. His mother was stressed and anxious. She felt her son was not doing well but could not find resources to assist her with his feeding problem. She was using a flat nipple with a plastic condiment squeeze bottle.

Joe seemed to be developmentally appropriate but did not have the endurance needed for continuous nippling, and the system was not able to support his getting milk from the bottle. His mother also reported that he did not seem to respond to sounds like he had in the past.

Areas to be assessed:

- General health condition, including middle ear functioning
- Intraoral skin condition, checking for any irritations
- Observation of current feeding process

Interventions:

- Modification of the feeding system
- Treatment of middle ear disease if present
- Education and follow-up for assessment of weight gain

Once in the clinic, Joe was immediately changed to nippling with a regular bottle and a nipple with an enlarged cross-cut. He nippled 4 ounces in about 15 minutes and promptly fell asleep. His family said they had never seen him so happy. With medication for treatment of middle ear disease and adequate nutrition, Joe gained 2 pounds over the next 2 weeks.

IMPACT ON CHILD AND FAMILY

Experiencing the shock of learning during the birthing process that the infant has a cleft anomaly or learning that one is going to birth an infant with a cleft is stressful, and families respond in many ways. Mothers especially are concerned about feeding, so immediate intervention to assist with successful feeding experiences is paramount.

As the infant develops, usually the family becomes more adjusted to the infant. I have heard mothers say on the day of surgery that they have become so accustomed to their infant as he or she is that they hesitate to put him or her through surgery to change it.

Perhaps the most powerful experiences occur when the family takes the infant out in public. Everyone loves a baby, and many want to see the new baby. This sets up the family for many questions, stares, and comments. Sometimes mothers carry their babies so the cleft is not exposed and they do not have to explain to anyone. Sometimes they simply do not go out for a long period of time, or go only with another person who can talk to the interested public. The first outing is always stressful, even if it is to see friends and family.

The public is not always very supportive. One mother reported to me that someone in the grocery store, after seeing her baby with a recently repaired lip defect, said, "You should have had your baby taken away from you for hitting him and causing that bad cut on his face."

FUTURE POSSIBILITIES

Fetal surgery for the repair of clefting, if diagnosed by ultrasound, is being proposed and developed. Genetic testing to identify the genes related to the clefting condition is also a real possibility (Oberg, Kirsch, & Hardesty, 1993). Other preventative research is being developed in the way of maternal vitamin deficiencies and environmental factors (Shaw, Lammer, Wasserman, O'Malley, & Tolerova, 1995).

SUMMARY

Children born with clefting of the lip or palate require an interdisciplinary approach for management of their care. Early in life, feeding and growth are the priorities, along with family education and surgical repairs that start during the first year of life. Emerging speech production and management of middle ear disease, if present, are also of concern. When the child becomes older and starts school, there may be concerns regarding psychosocial adjustment to having a physical deformity and having speech that sounds different than that of peers. With treatment and surgery, these children should have an excellent prognosis.

REFERENCES

Bardach, J., & Salyer. K. E. (1995). Cleft classification and cleft lip repair. In Sprintzen, R. J., & Bardach, J. (Eds.) *Cleft Palate Speech Management.* St. Louis: Mosby.

Cusson, R. (1994). Altered digestive function. In Betz, C., Hunsberger, M., & Wright, S. (Eds.) *Family-Centered Nursing Care of Children.* Philadelphia: W. B. Saunders.

Gorlin, R. Y., Cohen, M. M., & Levin, L. S. (1990).

Oralfacial clefting syndromes: General aspects. In Gorlin, R. Y., Cohen, M. M., & Levin, L. S. (Eds.) *Syndromes of the Head and Neck* (3rd ed.). New York: Oxford University Press.

Johnsen, D. (1996). Cleft lip and palate. In Nelson, W. E. (Ed.). *Nelson Textbook of Pediatrics.* Philadelphia: W. B. Saunders, pp. 1041–1042.

Jones, K. L. (1997). *Smith's Recognizable Patterns of Human Malformation* (5th ed.). Philadelphia: W. B. Saunders.

Langlois, A., & Nowak, B. R. (1990). The first year of a child with cleft palate: An approach to facilitate communication development. *Infant and Young Children*, 2(4), 43–50.

Oberg, K. C., Krisch, W., & Hardesty, R. (1993). Perspectives in cleft lip and palate repair. *Clinics in Plastic Surgery*, 20, 815–821.

Robinson, A., & Linden, M. G. (1993). *Clinical Genetics Handbook.* Boston: Blackwell Scientific.

Shaw, G. M., Lammer, R., Wasserman, C., O'Malley, C., & Tolerova, M. (1995). Risks of orofacial clefts in children born to women using multivitamins containing folic acid preconceptionally. *Lancet*, 345, 393–396.

Shprintzen, R. J. (1995). A new perspective on clefting. In Shprintzen, R. J., & Barcach, J. (Eds.) *Cleft Palate Speech Management.* St. Louis: Mosby.

Vargervik, K. (1995). Orthodontic treatment of children with cleft lip and palate. In Shprintzen, R. J., & Barcach, J. (Eds.). *Cleft Palate Speech Management.* St. Louis: Mosby.

ADDITIONAL RESOURCES

Journal Articles

Broen, P. A. (1996). Comparison of the hearing histories of children with and without cleft palate. *Cleft Palate–Craniofacial Journal*, 33(2), 127–133.

Cohen, M., Marshall, M., & Schafer, M. (1992). Immediate unrestricted feeding of infants following cleft lip and palate repair. *Journal of Craniofacial Surgery*, 3(1), 30–32.

Danner, S. C. (1992). Breastfeeding the infant with a cleft defect. *NAACOG's Clinical Issues*, 3(4), 634–639.

Gosain, A. K., Conley, S., Marks, S., & Larson, D. (1996). Submucous cleft palate: diagnostic methods and outcomes of surgical treatment. *Plastic & Reconstructive Surgery*, 97(7), 1497–1509.

Habel, A., Sell, D., & Mars, M. (1996). Management of cleft lip and palate. *Archives of Disease in Childhood*, 74(4), 360–366.

Hinojosa, R. J., & Richard, M. (1996). A research critique: Weight comparisons of infants with complete cleft lip and palate. *Plastic Surgical Nursing*, 15(2), 101–103.

Martin, V. (1995). Helping patients cope [cleft lip, cleft palate, plastic surgery]. *Nursing Times*, 91(31) 38–40.

Richard, M. E. (1994). Weight comparisons of infants with complete cleft lip and palate [the enlarge, stimulate, swallow, rest (ESSR) feeding method]. *Pediatric Nursing*, 20(2), 191–196.

Van Dyke, D. C., & Canady, J. W. (1995). Management of the adopted child in the craniofacial clinic. *Journal of Craniofacial Surgery*, 6(2), 143–146.

Weatherly-White, R. C., Kuehn, D. P., Mirrett, P., Gilman, J., & Weatherly-White, C. C. (1987). Early repair and breast-feeding for infants with cleft lip. *Plastic & Reconstructive Surgery*, 79(6), 879–887.

Videotapes

Hays, S. R. (1993). *Near Normal Feeding for Infants Born with Oral-Facial Anomalies.* From Clinician's View Catalog, 1995, Albuquerque.

Organizations

Cleft Palate Foundation, 1218 Grandview Ave., Pittsburgh, PA 15211, (412) 481–1376, (800) 24–CLEFT, (412) 242–5338.

FACE (Friends for Aid, Correction and Education of Craniofacial Disorders), PO Box 1424, Sarasota, FL 34230, (941) 955–9250.

FACES, The National Association for the Craniofacially Handicapped, Box 11082, Chattanooga, TN 37401, (800) 332–2373.

Federation for Children with Special Needs, 95 Berkeley St., Suite 104, Boston, MA 02116, (800) 331–0688.

Forward Face, Institute for Reconstructive Surgery, H-148, New York University Medical Center, 317 E. 34th, Room 901-A, New York, NY 10016, (800) FWD-FACE.

Foundation for the Faces of Children, PO Box 1361, Bork, MA 02146, (617) 734–7576.

National Foundation for Facial Reconstruction, 317 East 34th St., Room 901, New York, NY 10016, (212) 263–6656.

Support Organization for Trisomy 18, 13, and Related Disorders, c/o Barb Van Herreweghe, 2982 S. Union St., Rochester, NY 14624, (716) 594–4621.

Treacher-Collins Foundation, c/o Hope Charkins-Drazin & David Drazin, PO Box 683, Norwich, VT 05055, (802) 649–3050, (800) TCF–2055.

Limb Deficiencies in Children

Dalice L. Hertzberg

∎

INCIDENCE, CAUSES, AND SEVERITY

Incidence

Rehabilitation nursing care of children with limb deficiencies differs from amputations in adults in several important ways. First, a significant percentage of children have limb deficiencies as a result of congenital conditions. This percentage may represent up to 50% to 57% of the children under the age of 15 years seen at a typical pediatric amputee clinic (Challenor, 1992). Second, the process of growth and development makes frequent follow-up care necessary to adjust prostheses, prevent further complications, and promote function. Children tend to heal more quickly than adults after surgical amputations, and prosthetic fitting can be done earlier than for adults. Bony overgrowth, which occurs most frequently in the humerus, fibula, and tibia, is more common in children with acquired amputations than in adults (Maher, Addamo, & Shabtaie, 1994). Third, children tend to adapt more quickly to an amputation, whether it is congenital or acquired. Although this is a plus in many ways, prosthetics and therapy must be planned carefully and assessments must be performed at regular intervals, because children are less likely to maintain prosthetic use than adults.

Causes and Severity

Congenital limb deficiencies may be caused by environmental factors such as prenatal exposure to industrial chemicals and pollutants, caffeine, aspirin, nicotine, hormones, thalidomide, radiation, contraceptives, and some viral infections (Logigian, 1989; Challenor, 1992). Genetic disorders that cause complete or partial amputations include Holt-Oram and Fanconi syndromes and trisomies 13 and 18 (Challenor, 1992); however, most occurrences of congenital limb deficiency are sporadic (Tachdjian, 1990).

Acquired amputations represent about 40% to 50% of childhood limb deficiency. Of these, about 70% are caused by trauma and 30% are caused by disease or malignancies such as osteogenic sarcoma (Challenor, 1992;

Waskersitz, 1994). Infectious processes such as disseminated intravascular coagulopathy secondary to meningococcemia may cause loss of limbs due to tissue necrosis (Challenor, 1992). Upper extremity limb deficiency represents a more significant threat to overall function than lower extremity deficiency, because of the need for adequate hand function in manipulating objects, feeding, and self-care. The level of amputation or deficiency is also important, because there must be an adequate stump present for fitting of prosthetic devices. Children with amputations or deficiencies of multiple limbs are at a much greater disadvantage with respect to development of appropriate mobility and self-care skills. Also, self-image and self-esteem issues are more common because of the disfiguring nature of the condition, as well as the challenges to function. Conditions that lead to amputation of the limb that affect circulation and sensation or tissue viability, such as osteogenic sarcoma, burns, vascular processes, or infection can make prosthetic fitting and maintenance more difficult because of repeated skin problems on the stump.

Classification

There are several classification systems of congenital limb deficiencies that are used and that are represented in the literature. These systems may follow standard terminology for traumatic amputation, using classifications of above or below the joint and location; others classify limb deficiencies according to congenital occurrence (Challenor, 1992; Logigian, 1989). Common terminology used to refer to limb deficiencies is listed in Table 16–4. One system that categorizes congenital limb deficiencies is included in Table 16–5. Illustrations of the levels of amputation are found in Figures 16–3 and 16–4.

Pathophysiology

Severe congenital limb malformations occur in about 0.5% of births (Scott, 1989). The more severe the deformity, the earlier it occurred in prenatal life. Malformations occur when tissues are formed incorrectly. Deformations such as flexible club foot result from altered

Table 16–4 COMMON TERMINOLOGY USED TO REFER TO LIMB DEFICIENCIES

Amelia—complete absence of one or more limbs
Meromelia—partial absence of a limb
Phocomelia—congenital absence of a limb with the hand or foot attached to the trunk
Terminal deficiency—complete loss of the distal end of the extremity, the hand or foot
Proximal deficiency—partial absence or shortening of a limb at the proximal end, such as complete or partial absence of the femur
Intercalary deficiency—absence of intermediate parts with preserved proximal and distal components of the limb
Don—to put a prosthesis on prior to using it
Doff—to remove a prosthesis
AK—above the knee amputation
BK—below the knee amputation
AE—above the elbow amputation
BE—below the elbow amputation

mechanical forces on the developing fetus (Scott, 1989).

The fetal tissue from which the limbs arise is the ectoderm, which forms the skin, and mesoderm, which forms the bone, muscles, and joints. Limb buds first appear near the end of the fourth week of gestation. The development of the upper limb buds precedes that of the lower limb buds by a few days. Each limb bud is composed of mesenchyme

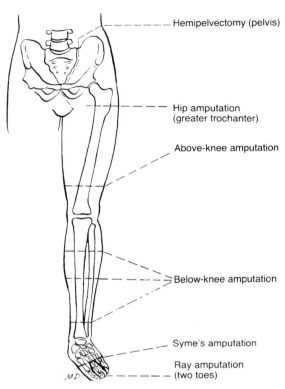

Figure 16–4 Levels of amputation—lower extremity. (From Luckmann, J., & Sorensen, K. D. (1997) *Medical-Surgical Nursing: A Psychophysiologic Approach* (3rd ed.). Philadelphia: W. B. Saunders, p. 1419.)

covered by an ectodermal layer that becomes the skin. Limb buds start out rounded in shape, changing to a paddle shape, and then developing notches between the emerging digits. The digits become more pronounced with webbing in between them before separate fingers and toes emerge. As the limbs grow longer, muscle tissue develops along the limb. Growth in length and width, as well as rotation, occurs (Moore, 1989).

The critical period for limb development is from 24 to 42 days following fertilization. Environmental influences such as teratogens act during this period to cause malformations or deficiencies. Minor limb malformations are relatively common, such as an extra digit, whereas major limb defects are less common. Thalidomide, a medication given for morning sickness, was the cause of numerous limb deficiencies in children born between 1957 and 1962 in the United States. Suppression of limb development during the early part of the fourth week results in amelia, or absence of the limb. Disturbance of differentiation or

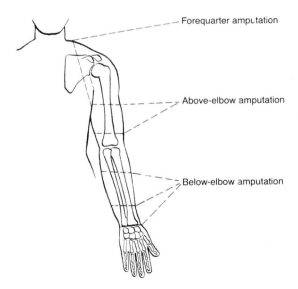

Figure 16–3 Levels of amputation—upper extremity. (From Luckman, J., & Sorensen, K. D. (1997). *Medical-Surgical Nursing: A Psychophysiologic Approach* (3rd ed.). Philadelphia: W. B. Saunders, p. 1419.

Table 16-5 CONGENITAL LIMB DEFICIENCY

Category	Rehabilitation Plan	Nursing Implications
I. Failure of formation of parts		Family teaching about causes of deficiency; preparation for surgery and postop care; proper care of prosthesis; facilitate developmental activities such as object manipulation and midline play for UE deficiency
A. Transverse: all congenital amputation-type conditions, classified by the level at which the existing portion of the limb terminates. All elements distal to that level are absent.		
1. Phalangeal deficiency: one or more digits, any level of digit, hand or foot	1. Mild: no treatment; severe (function impaired); cosmetic prosthesis or surgical reconstruction; if foot, need shoe correction	
2. Transmetacarpal amputation: usually unilateral, hand short and wide with skin nubbins	2. Prosthesis	Family teaching, care of prosthesis, developmental activities as above
3. Transcarpal amputation: total absence of phalanges and metacarpals; may have skin nubbins and fusion of carpal bones	3. Prosthesis	Family teaching, care of prosthesis, developmental activities as above
4. Transtarsal amputation: absence of phalanges, metatarsals, cuneiform and cuboid bones missing in forefoot; muscle in lower leg	4. Supportive shoe with ankle support	Family teaching, support of therapeutic exercise to prevent contracture; proper care of shoes
5. Wrist disarticulation a. Unilateral: long stump, skin nubbins, no skeletal elements distal to radius and ulna b. Bilateral	5. Single or bilateral prosthesis	Family teaching about cause and care of prosthesis; encourage developmental UE activities; developmental activities to improve strength, coordination, and antigravity control of trunk; adapted toys; promote self-esteem
6. Forearm amputation: below-elbow deficiency	6. Below-elbow prosthesis	Family teaching about cause and care of prosthesis; encourage developmental UE activities; developmental activities to improve strength, coordination, and antigravity control of trunk; adapted toys; promote self-esteem
7. Elbow disarticulation: absence of bone distal to distal humeral epiphysis	7. Elbow prosthesis	Family teaching about cause and care of prosthesis; encourage developmental UE activities; developmental activities to improve strength, coordination, and antigravity control of trunk; adapted toys; promote self-esteem

Table 16-5   CONGENITAL LIMB DEFICIENCY *Continued*

Category	Rehabilitation Plan	Nursing Implications
8. Above-elbow amputation: absence of distal epiphysis	8. Above-elbow prosthesis	Family teaching about cause and care of prosthesis; encourage developmental UE activities; developmental activities to improve strength, coordination, and antigravity control of trunk; adapted toys; promote self-esteem
9. Shoulder disarticulation: complete absence of upper limb, may be unilateral or bilateral	9. Shoulder disarticulation prosthesis	Family teaching about cause; care of prosthesis; encourage adaptive self care activities; encourage developmental UE activities; developmental activities to improve strength, coordination and antigravity control of trunk; adapted toys; promote self-esteem
10. Ankle disarticulation: ankle and foot bones absent distal tibial and fibula epiphyses present	10. Below-knee socket with foot	Family teaching about cause; anticipatory guidance; care of prosthesis including skin care; developmental activities; upper body and LE strengthening; encourage self-esteem
11. Below-knee amputation: proximal tibia present, fibula slightly shorter; stump may be turned in	11. Below-knee prosthesis with foot	Family teaching about cause; anticipatory guidance; care of prosthesis including skin care; developmental activities; upper body and LE strengthening; encourage self-esteem
12. Knee disarticulation with symmetrical stump	12. Knee disarticulation prosthesis with foot	Same as above
13. Above-knee amputation	13. Knee disarticulation prosthesis with foot	Same as above
14. Hip disarticulation: femur absent, no acetabular development	14. Hip disarticulation prosthesis	Same as above
B. Longitudinal: all nonformation of limbs other than transverse		
1. Radial deficiency: radius and thumb missing, radius only missing, thumb only missing	1. Casting, surgery	Family teaching about causes of deficiency; preparation for surgery and postop care; facilitate developmental activities of UE and trunk

Table continued on following page

Table 16–5 CONGENITAL LIMB DEFICIENCY *Continued*

Category	Rehabilitation Plan	Nursing Implications
2. Tibial deficiency a. Complete: leg short, varus foot, great toe absent, knee unstable, tibia absent, fibula bowed b. Incomplete: partial tibia, fibula positioned abnormally	2. a. Knee disarticulation amputation and prosthesis b. Below-knee amputation and prosthesis	Family teaching about causes of deficiency; support family with decision making about surgery; preparation for surgery and postop care; anticipatory guidance; care of prosthesis including skin care; developmental activities; upper body and LE strengthening; encourage self-esteem; proper care of prosthesis developmental activities
3. Ulnar deficiency: may occur with radial defects and shoulder girdle/proximal humerus defects; anomalies of elbow, wrist, hand, and digits	3. Above-elbow prosthesis	Family teaching about cause and care of prosthesis; encourage developmental UE and trunk activities; adapted toys; promote self-esteem
4. Central ray deficiency (carpal or digital or both); affecting 2nd–4th rays (lobster or claw hand)	4. Surgical reconstruction to improve function/cosmesis	Family teaching about causes of deficiency; preparation for surgery and postop care; encourage developmental UE and trunk activities; adapted toys facilitate developmental activities and self-esteem
5. Phocomelia: proximodistal failure of limb development a. Upper limbs: complete, proximal and distal	5. a. Complete: use lower extremities for function, or may use shoulder disarticulation prosthesis. Proximal/distal: reconstructive surgery	Family teaching about cause and care of prosthesis; presurgical teaching and postop care; encourage adaptive self-care activities using lower extremities and mouth; encourage developmental UE activities; developmental activities to improve strength, coordination and antigravity control of trunk; adapted toys; promote self-esteem Family teaching about cause; care and use of prosthesis or other mobility device; encourage mobility and exploration; promote self-esteem
b. Lower limbs: complete proximal and distal	b. Complete: hip disarticular prosthesis Proximal: electric wheelchair Distal: prosthesis	

LE, lower extremity; UE, upper extremity.
Adapted from Logigian, M. (1989). Physical disorders. In Logigian, M., & Ward, J. (Eds.) *A Team Approach for Therapists, Pediatric Rehabilitation.* Boston: Little, Brown & Company, p. 234.

growth arrest of the limb during the fifth and sixth weeks causes meromelia, or partial absence of the limb. Absence or deformation of the terminal part of the limb would affect the hand or foot. Causes of limb deficiencies and malformations in children are partially genetic, due to environmental causes, or may result from multifactorial causes (Moore, 1989).

Shortening, or incomplete longitudinal development, of the bone results in limb deficiencies. Other associated deficits include absence or malformation of joints and malrotation of the limb. These deficits contribute to shortening of the limb or structural abnormalities of the hand or foot. (Tachdjian, 1990; Rosenblith, 1992). Absence deficits such as proximal focal femoral deficiency (congenital shortening of the femur) or absence of the fibula are usually unilateral, partial (affecting part of the limb), and likely to be accompanied by other unusual physical characteristics (Scott, 1989). Many other congenital limb defects that do not directly cause amputation result in such dysfunction of the limb that amputation and subsequent fitting with a prosthesis is the best option for a functional limb. Examples of congenital limb defects for which surgical amputation often is recommended include absence of the tibia and fibula. Congenital limb deficits generally are noted at birth, but may be recognized before birth using ultrasonography.

Neoplasms are a significant cause of amputation in children. Osteogenic sarcoma is a tumor of the bone that generally is diagnosed during the adolescent growth spurt. It occurs mostly in long bone areas that demonstrate rapid growth, such as the distal femur, the proximal tibia, and the proximal humerus. Osteogenic sarcoma has a guarded prognosis, influenced by the presence or absence of metastatic disease at the time of diagnosis. When the condition is diagnosed early and the child is treated with a combined modality approach, survival rates at 5 years may be as high as 50% (Waskersitz, 1994).

Trauma combined with other acquired conditions accounts for approximately 40% to 50% of limb deficiencies in children. Traumatic amputation or injury leading to amputation occurs most frequently from auto accidents or accidents with farm equipment, power tools, explosions from firecrackers, chemical experimentation, or gunshot wounds (Challenor, 1992). Other types of accidents such as electrical injuries or burns may lead to amputations in children. Improved safety practices can dramatically reduce the number of these injuries.

Vascular processes that lead to amputation of limbs are less common in children than in adults. Compartment syndrome, a rare complication of casting, surgery, or trauma to a limb, results in very high pressure in the muscle compartment in the closed fascial space, causing poor perfusion and extensive tissue damage (Pellino & Polacek, 1994). In extreme cases, compartment syndrome may lead to amputation. Infections or diseases that lead to disseminated intravascular coagulation or microvascular thrombosis can cause tissue damage and sloughing in limbs and digits that necessitate amputation. Infection is also an infrequent cause of amputation in children. Rarely, severe osteomyelitis may result in surgical amputation of a limb, usually in children with some other medical condition or disability that affects circulation and healing, such as spina bifida.

Secondary Processes

Secondary processes that may occur with limb deficiency and amputation in children are (1) developmental delay and lack of mobility; (2) muscle imbalance resulting in further disability or need for treatment, such as scoliosis; (3) overgrowth or angulation of the stump; (4) contractures; (5) disturbance of self-concept; (6) poor compliance with prosthetic use; and, (7) less commonly than in adults, skin problems and phantom limb pain (Maher, Addamo, & Shabtaie, 1994; Challenor 1992). Early and timely diagnosis and treatment of the limb deficiency is crucial in order to promote appropriate development. Encouragement and facilitation of normal motor activities as well as therapeutic exercise will assist the child in developing and maintaining strength, range of motion, balance, and coordination. The child with upper extremity limb deficiency should participate in developmentally appropriate play through the use of adapted toys and methods to accommodate typical play activities for individuals and groups of children. Children who have lower extremity limb deficiencies may use toys such as a hand-powered tricycle for gross motor play, as well as taking part in active play with or without the prosthesis. Swimming and water play are good forms of exercise for the child with a limb deficiency (Challenor, 1992).

With surgical amputations for any reason, care is taken to preserve the growth plate to maintain the length of the limb as much as possible to prevent the complications of leg-length discrepancy following maximal growth, to prevent postural imbalances, and to facilitate prosthetic fit. Preservation of range of motion and strength in the remainder of the limb is crucial to the child's ability to manipulate the prosthesis and to maintain proper body alignment. Maintenance of strength, range of motion, and developmentally appropriate function in the child's remaining limbs is also of utmost importance

(Challenor, 1992; Thompson & Leimkuehler, 1989).

For those children who are undergoing surgical amputation for any reason, stump care is critical to promoting a good prosthesis fit. Children tend to exhibit more bony overgrowth of the stump than adults because of appositional bone growth and therefore require regular monitoring of the stump and prosthesis to determine the need for stump revisions (Lancet, 1991; Maher, Addamo, & Shabtaie, 1994). Proper positioning to prevent contractures is essential after surgical amputation.

As is the case with any child with a disability or chronic condition, family involvement is extremely important to the child's success with prosthetic use and to the overall positive outcome for the child with limb deficiency. Parents of children with congenital limb deficiency often experience grief or a sense of loss initially. Facilitating the family's view of the child as a child first of all, and the limb deficiency second, is helpful to promote family adjustment. The attitude of family members toward the child with a limb deficiency and their love and support are crucial to the child's eventual acceptance of self and of the disability, as well as of the adaptations that are needed to develop and maintain independence and life skills. Children who are valued for themselves and are not devalued for their disability adjust to the disability better and are less likely to experience low self-esteem and disturbed self-concept. Children and adolescents whose amputation is the result of trauma or disease have more difficulty adjusting to the change in body image. Body image disturbances occur most frequently in older children for whom amputation is necessitated by trauma or neoplasm. Early ambulation and rapid provision of a cosmetically pleasing prosthesis, combined with meeting other children or adolescents who have amputations, can aid in adjustment. One hospital program promotes development of mobility, independence, and adjustment to the amputation by encouraging participation in a long-distance bicycle ride as well as other adaptive sports programs (Challenor, 1992; Pizzutillo 1989).

Timing of therapy and prosthetic fitting influences family and child compliance with prosthetic use. Prostheses that are difficult to use or maintain or are difficult to fit, as in the case of hip disarticulations or shoulder disarticulations, are less likely to be used appropriately and consistently. The importance of regular follow-up with the pediatric rehabilitation team cannot be emphasized enough. Children who have bilateral lower extremity amputations from any cause are more likely to use a wheelchair, especially as they grow older and heavier, because of the greater energy requirment needed to use two prostheses. Children and adolescents who are overweight tend to have more difficulty, especially with lower extremity prostheses.

Good skin care of the stump is important in order to prepare the skin surface for weight bearing in the lower extremity, and for contact with and friction from the prosthesis in both the upper and lower limbs. Phantom pain, neuroma, and skin breakdown are seen less frequently in children than in adults. Some sources have reported phantom limb sensations in young children with surgical amputation as well as congenital limb deficiencies, but most sources describe phantom limb sensations as occurring primarily in individuals older than 6 years of age who have had surgical or traumatic amputation (Maher, Addamo, & Shabtaie, 1994). Skin breakdown becomes more of a problem as the child grows older and heavier and when the prosthetic cup is too small due to growth.

Treatment

Treatment for the child with limb deficiency differs depending on the cause of the deficiency. The overall goals of treatment are to render the limb as functional as possible and promote development and adaptive skills in the child. The prosthesis should promote optimum function, comfort, and cosmesis (Thompson & Leimkuehler, 1989). Those children who require a surgical procedure to ready the limb for a prosthesis, as a result of trauma, or who have been diagnosed with a malignant bone tumor, are referred to an orthopedic surgeon. With children who have congenital limb deficiency, anomalous structures such as incompletely formed digits or other appendages may be retained to maintain tactile exploration of the environment and sensory feedback, as well as potential control of switches on externally powered prostheses (Challenor, 1992). An interdisciplinary team consisting of the pediatric physiatrist, pediatric orthopedic surgeon, physical or occupational therapist, prosthetist, pediatric rehabilitation nurse, and the family provides the core of care and services for the child and family. Additional consultations with a genetic counselor in the case of a genetic cause for a congenital limb deficiency, a social worker for family support and to aid with funding, a psychologist for diagnosis and treatment of emotional problems, or another medical specialist, such as an oncologist, may also be necessary, depending on the cause of the limb deficiency and the circumstances surrounding the child and family.

General rehabilitation treatment includes (1) stump care, (2) promotion of development, (3) timely prosthetic fitting and maintenance, (4) prosthetic training by the occupational or physical therapist, and (5) maintenance of positive body image and self-esteem. Information must be obtained about the strength of the limb and the range of motion of any joints involved, at least those just above and below the amputation. The status of the child's other limbs with regard to strength, range of motion, and presence or absence of congenital malformations or injury, as well as the child's general health, developmental level, age, and size also are important. The child and family's perception of the situation and the child's psychologic status also are important factors (Borgman-Gainer, 1996).

Surgical Treatment

The child with a congenital limb deficiency may receive one of several general types of surgery to prepare the limb for a prosthesis and to render the limb more functional with regard to size, shape, and length. Principles followed when deciding whether or not surgical intervention is the best course for a child with a congenital limb deficiency are (1) maintenance of strength and muscular control of the residual limb, (2) prevention of progressive deformity with growth, (3) protection of the long bone growth plates, and (4) preservation and stabilization, when necessary, of the proximal joints (Kruger, 1981; Thompson & Leimkuehler, 1989). When choosing the site for amputation of a congenitally deficient limb, the decision to amputate above or below the joint, knee, or elbow is based on the functionality of the joint, the presence of an intact alternate limb, the placement on the limb of the deficiency, and the status of the hip or shoulder joint (Tachdjian, 1990). Care must be taken to preserve the correct proportions of the upper and lower parts of the limb and prevent over- or undergrowth of the bone, making for a less functional and less cosmetically pleasing limb when the child's full growth is reached. Two common types of amputations done for chil-

dren with congenital deficiencies such as fibular hemimelia, or deficiencies of the foot, are the Boyd and Symes amputations. Both of these surgeries maintain as much length of the limb as is possible for the specific child and create a good, weight-bearing surface that tolerates a prosthesis well. The Symes amputation is essentially a disarticulation of the ankle joint, leaving the full tibia and the heel pad to create a stump at the level of the ankle. The retention of the heel pad makes a good, tough weight-bearing surface with proprioceptive sense. The Boyd amputation retains the calcaneus and fuses it to the tibia. In both procedures, the distal tibial growth plate is preserved to maintain maximal growth of the lower leg (Kumar, 1989; Maher, Addamo, & Shabtaie, 1994).

In children with a lower limb deficiency but an intact foot, surgery may not be necessary and the limb may be fitted with a special type of prosthesis that is fit over the foot and leg, or an extension orthosis, which is fit over the short leg. In some cases, a surgical procedure known as the Van Ness rotation may be performed in which the foot is rotated on the leg, using the ankle to produce a functional joint where the knee would be. Following the procedure, a prosthesis is fitted with the foot providing the weight-bearing surface. However, there are more complications to this procedure than with an amputation and, without the prosthesis, the leg has an unusual appearance and may be cosmetically unacceptable.

With the upper extremity, the presence of a functional hand may be more important that the length of the limb and may obviate amputation in the case of a congenital limb deficiency. Operative techniques to improve the function of the existing hand or residual structures more commonly are performed than amputation because of the difficulty of replacing hand function with a prosthesis. After congenital deficiencies, upper extremity amputations are most likely the result of trauma, bone tumor or, more rarely, an infectious or vascular process.

Following surgical amputation, a cast or other pressure dressing is placed immediately postoperatively to assist with stump shrinkage and shaping. In many cases, the mold for the prosthesis is made at the time of surgery in order to promote early ambulation. In other cases, the prosthetic fitting is not done until the site is healed and the stump has shrunk to its final size. If a pin is used to stabilize the skin flap over the end of the bone, the pin is removed after about 6 weeks.

Weight bearing is not allowed while the pin is in place. Once the pin has been removed and the stump is healed, a pylon is placed onto the stump cast so the child can begin ambulation and weight bearing. Once the incision is healed and the swelling is reduced, the plaster cast or pressure dressing is removed and the stump is wrapped with elastic bandages to further reduce swelling and to continue the process of shaping the stump to better fit into the prosthesis. During this recuperative period, as later, proper positioning of the stump is critical to maintaining range of motion and preventing joint contractures that would affect prosthetic fit and functional ambulation.

Osteogenic Sarcoma Treatment

When a bone neoplasm is the cause of the amputation, additional treatment of the cancer is necessary. Localized pain that becomes more and more severe and frequent is the first symptom of osteogenic sarcoma. Swelling or a mass associated with the pain is a late finding. The history often reveals a fall or an accident that preceded the pain, but this is only the incident that elicited pain from the tumor that was already present (Waskersitz, 1994). A plain x-ray of the painful region is used to identify a bony lesions that shows destructive changes and indistinct margins. Once osteogenic sarcoma is recognized, tests are necessary to define the lesion and determine the extent of the disease, including metastases. A surgical biopsy is done to confirm the diagnosis. Metastases occur most commonly in the lungs, but may also be seen in other bones, the lymphatic system, and the liver. Lung metastases account for the greatest number of metastatic recurrences following osteogenic sarcoma. A combined approach to treatment that includes chemotherapy (to shrink the tumor and treat micrometastases) with resection of the tumor and amputation of the limb after several weeks is the usual approach. Some small and intercompartmental tumors with no spread to other tissues may be treated by limb salvage procedures instead of amputation. Following surgery, a prosthetic replacement or cadaver bone is placed. Limb salvage procedures are preferable for upper extremity lesions. A limb salvage procedure is one where the cancerous part of the bone is resected and replaced by an autograft (bone from another part of the body) or an internal prosthesis or rod. With limb salvage procedures, there is still a risk

of problems such as infection or recurrence of the tumor (Waskersitz, 1994; Tachdjian, 1990).

Chemotherapy usually is continued after healing of the stump or surgical site. The exact regimen is based on the child's response to the preoperative chemotherapy. Radiation therapy is used only for palliation for pain in tumors that do not respond well to treatment (Waskersitz, 1994). Postoperative stump care does not differ essentially from the care of the stump following any other surgical amputation.

Prosthetic Management

Children tend to do best with simple, comfortable, functional prostheses that are durable and have an acceptable cosmetic design. For younger children, the parents choose the type of prosthesis based on the information given to them by the rehabilitation team and the prostetist. It is important that parents have the opportunity to see the different types of prosthetic devices demonstrated and understand the advantages and disadvantages of each before making an informed choice for their child. The older child should have the same advantage, along with the advice and support of parents (Thompson & Leimkuehler, 1989; Challenor, 1992).

Basic principles of choosing and fitting a prosthesis for the child amputee are based on the different body contours, movement patterns, and functional requirements of children, which differ from those of adults. The child is constantly changing in size, shape, coordination, and functional demand because of the processes of growth and development. The size and weight of the child, in comparison to the weight of the prosthesis, which affects its ease of use, is an important factor. The child with a lower extremity limb deficiency generally is fitted for a prosthesis at about the time pulling to stand and independent ambulation begins to occur. In most children, this is between 9 and 15 months of age. The leg-length discrepancy resulting from limb deficiency, especially when fitted too late for standing, can lead to scoliosis (Logigian, 1989).

Factors that may influence timing of prosthetic fitting in addition to attainment of this developmental milestone include the level of the limb deficiency, the involvement of the other leg, associated upper extremity deficiencies, and the child's general health or presence of other disability or disease (Thompson & Leimkuehler, 1989). Above-the-knee deficiency may cause delays in sitting or affect posture. With this situation, it may be necessary to apply a lightweight limb extension before the child pulls to stand (Challenor, 1992). A knee joint usually is not added to the prosthesis until 2½ to 3 years of age, in order to maintain stability in the younger child, and due to the added energy expenditure of walking with an unlocked knee joint (Challenor, 1992; Thompson & Leimkuehler, 1989). Below-the-knee prostheses on young children usually require additional means of suspension, such as a thigh corset or belt to maintain stability for the very active child who runs, jumps, and climbs. A suction prosthesis, such as is used for adults, is not realistic for a child until 6 or 7 years of age, because of difficulty with accurately fitting the socket in a growing child, and because the prosthesis is more difficult to don and doff (see Table 16–4). Usually, lower extremity prostheses are made with a solid ankle cushion heel (SACH) foot, which are available in many pediatric sizes and can be changed to accommodate shoes with different heel heights, an important consideration for adolescents. Other types of prosthetic designs that make for more natural movement are hydraulic knee units and energy-storing foot units such as the Flex-foot. These designs are available for adolescents as well as adults. Children with below-the-knee amputation receive a prosthesis with a modified patellar tendon weight-bearing socket of the type commonly used for adults.

Children who have deficiencies of the foot receive a shoe insert that may or may not have a socket and suspension device to keep the insert in place, depending on the extent of the amputation. Children who have absence of both lower limbs and no real stumps on which to fit a traditional prosthesis may have a bucket prosthesis made, which fits over the lower part of the body and is attached to bilateral lower extremity prostheses. The child uses crutches to ambulate with a swing-through gait (Challenor, 1992). For children with bilateral lower extremity amputations, ambulation with prostheses is more likely during early life, whereas increasing age and weight often necessitate wheelchair use.

Children with upper limb deficiency generally are fitted with a passive prosthesis at around 3 to 4 months of age, to aid in achievement of sitting balance and development of eye-hand coordination. Encouragement of manipulation of objects at the midline is important developmentally, as well as to develop and maintain muscle strength and coordination in the upper arms, shoulders, and trunk. Bilateral upper limb deficiency places development of posture and balance at risk and necessitates extensive therapeutic intervention for this purpose, as well as for sensory development and manipulation of objects. A prosthesis with a terminal device activated by the child, such as a pincer or hook, is indicated at 14 to 18 months of age.

Criteria for readiness to learn how to manage a prosthesis includes an attention span of at least 10 minutes, ability to follow two-step directions, interest in bimanual activities, and the strength and coordination to perform the movements needed to control the prosthesis (Challenor, 1992). Both preprosthetic training and ongoing therapy for use of the prosthesis are necessary for the young child. As soon as the limb deficiency is recognized, therapeutic interventions by the occupational therapist begin in order to promote development and provide sensory stimuli for the child. Stimulating awareness of textures and sensations helps the child develop the sensorimotor system and is important for general development, as well as for the child's eventual need to respond to and manipulate the prosthesis. Timing of prosthetic training is important, because once the child develops a preference for gross motor activities, the degree of attention needed to develop manual dexterity with a prosthesis may wane (Challenor, 1992).

Most upper limb prostheses prescribed for children with a below-elbow deficiency are composed of a socket fitted to the end of the limb and a terminal device that substitutes for a hand. The prosthesis is held in place by a harness that fits over the opposite shoulder and under the arm. The terminal device is linked by a cable attached to the proximal section of the suspension, and responds to flexion and relaxation of the humerus. Above-elbow prostheses that contain an elbow joint have an additional cable that flexes the elbow in response to movement of the upper arm. For older children and adolescents, myoelectrically controlled prostheses are available that are less energy consuming to manipulate but are heavier in weight. This type of prosthesis appears more natural during use, but costs more initially and is more expensive to maintain that the traditional muscle-and-cable operated devices. Terminal devices come in many shapes and sizes, but function essentially as either a hook or a pincer device, with or without a cosmetically pleasing molded hand.

Nursing Interventions

Pediatric rehabilitation nursing interventions for the child with limb deficiency are focused on (1) the care of the stump following surgery; (2) prevention of complications such as skin breakdown and early detection of complications; (3) pain management following surgery and if phantom limb sensations are present; (4) promotion and maintenance of child development, development of independence, and positive self-concept; (5) family support; and (6) child and family teaching. The pediatric rehabilitation nurse's role spans the continuum of care from diagnosis through community life for the child and family.

Assessment

The nursing history includes prenatal events as well as any potential exposure to teratogens. The presence of any genetic disorders in the family may suggest a genetic link for congenital limb deficiency, especially when it is associated with other manifestations such as deficiency or deformity of more than one limb or cardiac or kidney problems. For children with a traumatic amputation, a description of the circumstances of the accident may suggest safety precautions that should be put into place to prevent other injuries. Children who lose a limb as a result of disease have additional health problems that may jeopardize skin integrity, prosthetic fit and use, and child and family adjustment to the limb loss. The family should be interviewed with regard to its cultural and personal attitudes toward amputation and disability and the need for additional social support evaluated.

Physical assessment should include inspection of the limb for skin integrity, general strength, range of motion, circulation and sensation, presence or absence of residual appendages, and assessment of other limbs for abnormalities. For children who have had a surgical amputation, examination of the surgical scar should reveal a healing or healed incision without skin breakdown or sign of infection. Children who wear prostheses should be examined for any sign of redness, callus, or skin breakdown that might suggest an ill-fitting prosthesis. Bony or hard protuberances on the stump suggest overgrowth of the bone and may lead to development of pressure ulcers or bursae.

Diagnostic tests for the child with a congenital limb deficiency include radiographs to determine the bony structures underlying the short limb, and may include a leg-length scanogram, a type of radiograph that accurately measures leg length, as well as computed tomography (CT). Analysis of the child's gait for lower limb deficiency and upper extremity function are performed by the physician and therapist. Thorough evaluation of strength, including muscle testing, coordination, and range of motion is performed by the physical or occupational therapist. Functional assessment of the child's mobility and age-appropriate self-care ability is also done, as well as a general developmental assessment.

Nursing Diagnoses

Nursing diagnoses that are appropriate for the child with a limb deficiency include (1) impaired adjustment; (2) diversional activity deficit; (3) altered growth and development; (4) impaired mobility; (5) knowledge deficit; (6) self-care deficit; (7) high risk for impaired skin integrity; and (8) alteration in participating: noncompliance. For the child who has undergone a surgical procedure, additional nursing diagnoses include (1) high risk for infection, (2) pain, (3) high risk for altered nutrition, and (4) grieving related to loss (Maher, Addamo, & Shabtaie, 1994).

Stump Care

Stump care is composed of skin care and examination, maintenance of stump socks and elastic wraps, and maintenance of the prosthetic socket. The skin of the stump should be cleaned with soap and water daily. Thorough drying of the skin before the sock or elastic bandage is applied is critical in order to prevent skin breakdown. Children who have had a surgical amputation should have the stump massaged by their parents to desensitize the area, or should do it themselves if they are old enough. If scar tissue is present, techniques of friction massage may be used to break up the adhesions so that the skin does not adhere to the underlying tissues and cause irritation and infection under the prosthesis. Areas of skin breakdown should be kept clean and dry and exposed to air frequently. A deep or large area of skin breakdown precludes wearing the prosthesis until the skin is healed. Stump socks are changed daily and kept clean, and always allowed to dry thoroughly before wearing. The socket of the prosthesis should also be washed regularly with soap and water and dried before wearing (Maher, Addamo, & Shabtaie, 1994).

Stump shrinkage devices are applied following amputation, before the prosthesis is fit, and at any time when the prosthesis is not worn. Elastic bandages are the most commonly used device to decrease swelling and to shape the stump for prosthetic wear. They must be applied properly to be effective, however, and are difficult for a child to apply independently. The size of the elastic bandage depends on the age and size of the child, but adequate width is necessary to provide the needed compression. Elastic bandages are applied in a figure-of-eight pattern. The end of the bandage is started at the end of the stump, with the most pressure distally, progressing to the proximal part of the limb in order to prevent dependent edema and to give the stump the proper shape. The bandage is wrapped to the thigh for a below-the-knee amputation, or around the waist for an above-the-knee amputation. Elastic bandages

are inexpensive and may be fit to a variety of sizes of limb (Maher, Addamo, & Shabtaie, 1994). Illustration of the technique for wrapping a stump above and below the knee is shown in Figure 16–5.

Other stump shrinkage devices include shrinker socks and rigid dressings. Shrinker socks are relatively easy to apply and provide uniform compression of the stump. They are more expensive than elastic bandages and are not as adjustable to the shrinking stump. Rigid dressings most commonly are used in children who have surgical amputations. A plaster cast is placed over the stump at the time of surgery, and suspended by stockinette, straps, or a harness. Rigid dressings do not have to be rewrapped and are very efficient in reduction of swelling, prevention of trauma to the stump, and promotion of more rapid maturation of the stump. When the rigid dressing begins to appear loose, it is removed and another cast is applied. With a rigid dressing, hematomas are less likely to

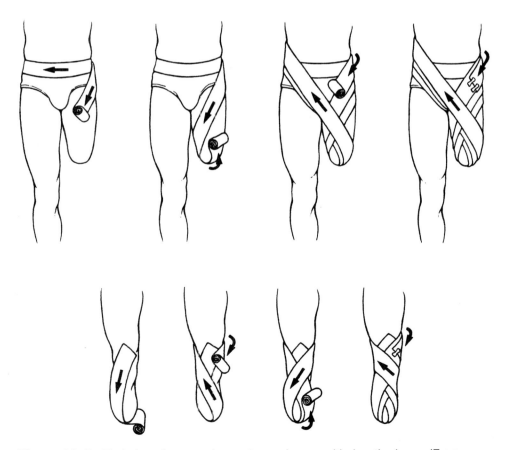

Figure 16–5   Technique for wrapping a stump above and below the knee. (From Maher, A. B., Salmond, S. W., & Pellino, T. A. (1988). *Orthopaedic Nursing* (2nd ed.). Philadelphia: W. B. Saunders, p. 732.)

develop postoperatively, and earlier weight bearing on the stump is possible (Maher, Addamo, & Shabtaie, 1994).

Pain Management

Management of postoperative pain is critical to the child's eventual acceptance of the amputation. Adequate levels of pain medications should be administered to maintain the child's comfort, according to pediatric guidelines. Elevating the affected limb to reduce swelling for the first 24 hours aids in reducing pain (Waskersitz, 1994).

Phantom limb sensations are experienced by most individuals with an acquired amputation who are older than 6 years of age. The sensation may be self-limiting or may last indefinitely. The sensation may fade with time, giving the impression to the individual that the hand or foot is floating in midair, before the sensation disappears completely. Often, the last sensation is that of the great toe or thumb or index finger (Maher, Addamo, & Shabtae, 1994).

Phantom limb pain is a painful or unpleasant sensation that can occur soon after surgery or develop as late as 2 to 3 months after surgery. The phenomenon is most severe in trauma patients who experienced severe pain before surgery, individuals who had poor pain control after surgery, and in people with above-the-knee amputations. In children, phantom limb pain is more likely to occur in adolescents, in older children who lost a limb through trauma, and in children who have cancer (Waskersitz, 1994; Maher, Addamo, & Shabtaie, 1994). Other physiologic risk factors include multiple past surgeries or illnesses, acute osteomyelitis, peripheral vascular disease, and poor wound healing. Psychologic factors include altered body image and depression, and lack of emotional support and feelings of insecurity (Maher, Addamo, & Shabtaie, 1994). There is no definitive theory that explains the cause of phantom limb pain. Theories that have been proposed involve excitation of nerve endings in the stump, the loss of inhibitory influences in the stump, and interruption of a sensorineural matrix (Maher, Addamo, & Shabtaie, 1994).

Phantom limb pain may take the form of cramping; electric, shock-like sensations; burning; or stabbing sensations. It may be triggered by contact with the stump or by contact with trigger points on the trunk, the other limb, or the head or by activities such

as urinating or defecating (Friedman, 1990; Maher, Addamo, & Shabtaie, 1994).

Treatment for phantom limb pain includes medications such as beta blockers, anticonvulsants such as carbamazepine, phenytoin, or baclofen; antidepressants such as amitryptyline, imipramine, or trazodone; and benzodiazepines. Stump desensitization methods such as massage, tapping the stump, and spraying the stump with ethyl chloride can also help to treat the pain. Other measures include transcutaneous electric nerve stimulation (TENS), biofeedback, hypnosis, and, as a last resort, surgery to eliminate sensory pathways (Maher, Addamo, & Shabtaie, 1994).

Prosthetic Care

Prosthetic training primarily is performed by the occupational therapist for upper limb deficiencies; gait and prosthetic training is performed by the physical therapist for lower limb deficiencies. The pediatric rehabilitation nurse works closely with these therapists to reinforce proper prosthetic wear and use with the child and family. Children who are 6 years of age or older should participate in monitoring of prosthetic fit and stump care. The child should be independent in donning and doffing the prosthesis by about 8 to 10 years of age, depending on general health and presence of other disabilities, with the consideration that upper extremity prostheses may be somewhat more difficult to don than lower extremity prostheses.

Psychosocial Care

Promotion of positive self-esteem and a healthy self-concept is crucial to the child's ability to be independent, no matter what the severity of limb deficiency. The child with a congenital limb deficiency who receives positive feedback and experiences mastery of developmental tasks is more likely to develop positive self-esteem, independence, and achieve success in social and academic settings. Adolescents who experience loss of a limb through disease or trauma are at a greater risk for poor adjustment and often require support to work through issues of developing self-concept and body consciousness. Encouraging the adolescent to participate in care of the stump and prosthesis as soon as possible can help to promote integration of the stump into the body schema. Positive role models who have succeeded in life despite loss of a limb are most helpful in assisting the adolescent to accept the disability. Adults and other children or adolescents of similar ages provide the kind of support and encouragement that can only come from one who has gone through a similar experience. Once the prosthesis is fit and the child or adolescent is proficient in its use, sports participation contributes to good muscle tone and strength, general health, and positive self-concept. Sports that may be particularly well adapted for children with limb deficiency include skiing, swimming, and bicycling, but most other sports can be adapted as well by using special equipment (Pizzutillo, 1989).

Family support is a particularly important role of the nurse. Families cope with grief and loss in different ways, and it is important for the nurse to respect the family's coping strategies and support them whenever possible. Many families do not seem to undergo a period of adjustment after a child with a congenital limb deficiency is born and are able to accept the child for him- or herself along with or in spite of the disability. Occasionally, parents, siblings, or other family members have more difficulty adjusting to the changes in expectations and life style occasioned by a child with a limb deficiency, and these individuals may require additional counseling and therapy by a social worker or psychologist. Children who are diagnosed with life-threatening disease that causes amputation present the most difficulty for families and benefit from the intensity and specificity of support available from specialty organizations such as those for families of children with cancer.

Financial stresses may influence the family's ability to adjust to the disability and to the child's additional needs. Specialty care and prosthetic devices are expensive, and less and less likely to be covered by managed care organizations. The frequent monitoring of and adjustments needed for maintaining the prosthesis may be beyond the family's financial reach. State Title V programs generally have some funds available to aid families of children with disabilities who require specialty care and durable medical equipment. Medicaid covers a specified number of outpatient therapy and physician visits, as well as durable medical equipment, in most states. However, as managed care and health care funding systems change, fewer and fewer long-term or rehabilitative services may be covered. For a more detailed discussion of funding issues, see Chapter 5.

Nutrition

Good nutrition is important to promote healing of the surgical site of the amputation, maintenance of skin integrity, as well as to promote proper growth and development. Undernutrition may result from chronic pain, infection, concomitant disease or disability, or depression. Overnutrition results from lack of mobility, overeating in response to loss or depression, or metabolic disorder can make prosthetic fitting more difficult and contribute to skin breakdown and impaired mobility. Families of children with congenital limb deficiencies should be guided toward good nutrition and prevention of obesity. Children who are over their ideal weight for height at the time of an amputation should be placed on a program of good nutrition and adequate exercise that will allow them to slowly regain a more functional weight. The following case study is provided to illustrate the situation.

CASE STUDY

Mary was 14 years old when she was diagnosed with osteogenic sarcoma of the distal femur. Her very supportive family and friends helped her through the process of chemotherapy and surgery. At first after the surgery, she just cried whenever the nurses or therapists referred to her stump, and she refused to look at it or to touch it. After a visit from Alison, who had the same surgery 3 years ago, and has remained cancer free, Mary hesitantly agreed to learn how to care for the stump, and was able to examine it when the prosthetist came to fit her for her prosthesis. Alison continued to visit Mary and they talked a lot about their feelings around the diagnosis and the surgery, and what it was like to have an artificial leg. Alison and the physical therapist, Carol, were training together to ride in a 5-day bicycle trip over the mountains to raise money for the disabled sports program at the hospital. They were both very enthusiastic about it, and encouraged Mary to consider the trip next year. Mary, who at 5 feet, 4 inches weighed 160 pounds, thought they were crazy.

Following her postoperative gait training, Mary was discharged home. Six months later when she returned to the amputee clinic for her prosthetic check, she saw Alison again, who persuaded her to go bicycle riding with her. It was a scary process with the prosthesis, but with Alison's help, as well as guidance from the physical therapist and the clinic nurse, Mary learned how to ride with a prosthesis, and found she enjoyed it. The next summer, she participated in the bicycle trip and finished the entire course, with some help. She resolved to do better the next year, and signed up for the ski program that winter. Mary's sports participation helped her to lose weight and feel more competent and confident after her amputation.

School, Community, and Vocational Issues

Most children and adolescents with limb deficiency experience little or no difficulty with inclusion in school or community. Children with upper extremity limb deficiency may need adaptations to complete school work, such as using a computer for written assignments. Children with congenital limb deficiencies tend to have less difficulty interacting with peers than those children who have experienced a change in their body image following amputation for trauma or disease. Ease of use of the prosthesis and its cosmetic acceptability are key factors in community reentry after amputation.

Adolescents and young adults with lower extremity amputation have few limitations in job choice or life activities. Most individuals who have grown up with an upper limb deficiency have learned methods to adapt activities and accomplish tasks. Especially for those individuals with an intact contralateral limb and hand, there is only moderate limitation of activities. Adolescents and young adults with an acquired amputation can benefit from vocational counseling and services. Prosthetic technology continues to improve, thanks to the development of computerized microprocessors that promise lighter, more efficient prostheses.

In summary, the rehabilitation nursing care of a child with limb deficiency differs in several important ways from that of the adult with an amputation. The influence of developmental changes is an important factor to consider when implementing interventions and assisting with prosthetic management.

REFERENCES

Borgman-Gainer, M. (1996). Independent function: Movement and mobility. In Hoeman, S. (Ed.) *Rehabilitation Nursing: Process and Application*. St. Louis: Mosby, pp. 225–227.

Challenor, Y. (1992). Limb deficiencies in children. In Molnar, G. (Ed.) *Pediatric Rehabilitation* (2nd ed.). Baltimore: Williams & Wilkins.

Friedman, L. (1990). Rehabilitation of the lower extremity amputee. In Kottke, F., & Lehmann, J. (Eds.) *Krusen's Handbook of Physical Medicine and Rehabilitation* (4th ed.). Philadelphia: W. B. Saunders, pp. 1024–1069.

Kruger, L. (1981). Congenital limb deficiencies. Part II: Lower Limb deficiencies. In American Academy of Orthopaedic Surgeons, *Atlas of Limb Prosthetics, Surgical and Prosthetic Principles*. St. Louis: Mosby, pp. 522–552.

Kumar, S. (1989). Syme and Boyd amputations in children. In Kalamachi, A. (Ed.) *Congenital Lower Limb Deficiencies*. New York: Springer-Verlag, pp. 165–179.

Lancet (Editorial). (1991). Stump overgrowth in juvenile amputees. *Lancet, 338*, 417.

Logigian, M. (1989). Physical disorders. In Logigian, M., & Ward, J. (Eds.) *A Team Approach for Therapists, Pediatric Rehabilitation*. Boston: Little, Brown & Company, pp. 229–256.

Maher, A., Adamo, S., & Shabtaie, J. (1994). Amputation and replantation. In Maher, A., Salmond, S., & Pellino, T. (Eds.) *Orthopedic Nursing*. Philadelphia. W. B. Saunders, pp. 761–792.

Moore, K. (1989). *Before We Are Born: Basic Embryology and Birth Defects* (3rd ed.). Philadelphia: W. B. Saunders.

Pizzutillo, P. (1989). Sports medicine in the congenital lower-limb amputee. In Kalamachi, A. (Ed.) *Congenital Lower Limb Deficiencies*. New York: Springer-Verlag, pp. 236–241.

Polacek, L., & Pellino, T. (1994). Complications of orthopaedic disorders and orthopaedic surgery. In Maher, A., Salmond, S., & Pellino, T. (Eds.) *Orthopedic Nursing*. Philadelphia: W. B. Saunders, pp. 195–238.

Rosenblith, J. (1992). *In the Beginning, Development from Conception to Age Two* (2nd ed.). Newbury Park, CA: Sage Publications.

Scott, C., Jr. (1989). Genetic and familial aspects of limb defects with emphasis on the lower extremities. In Kalamachi, A. (Ed.) *Congenital Lower Limb Deficiencies*. New York: Springer-Verlag, pp. 46–57.

Tachdjian, M. (1990). *Pediatric Orthopaedics* (2nd ed.) (Vol. 2) Philadelphia: W. B. Saunders.

Thompson, G., & Leimkuehler, J. (1989). Prosthetic management. In Kalamachi, A. (Ed.) *Congenital Lower Limb Deficiencies*. New York: Springer-Verlag, pp. 221–235.

Waskersitz, M. (1994). Neoplasms/cancer. In Betz, C., Hunsberger, M., & Wright, S. (Eds.) *Family-Centered Nursing Care of Children*. (2nd ed.). Philadelphia: W. B. Saunders, pp. 1874–1937.

Neuromuscular Disorders

Susanne R. Hays

■

MUSCULAR DYSTROPHY

Incidence, Causes, and Severity

Neuromuscular diseases are those that affect components of the motor unit. The major symptom is weakness caused from disease of the anterior horn cell, spinal roots, muscular fiber, peripheral nerves, or neuromuscular junction. The most common of these diseases is Duchenne muscular dystrophy (DMD), a progressive, genetically based primary myopathy that becomes obvious in early childhood. There are a number of other less common muscular dystrophies, each with a different expression, clinical course, and genetic trait (Sarnat, 1996a).

Etiology and Incidence

DMD is an X-linked recessive inherited disorder, caused by mutation in the dystrophin gene on the short arm of the X chromosome. The incidence of DMD is 1 in 3600 live male births, affecting all races and ethnic groups. Approximately 30% are new mutations, which means that the mother is not the carrier. Girls may be carriers and usually are asymptomatic (Sarnat, 1996a). In rare cases, girls may be affected with the disease, but less severely so than the males. Other types of muscular dystrophies are autosomal dominant or recessive, sporadic, or have variable inheritance and are less common. Molecular genetics continues to research the exact causes of these neuromuscular diseases (Sarnat, 1996a).

Pathophysiology

The muscle degeneration that occurs in DMD is caused by absence of dystrophin, a muscle cell protein. Without this protein the cell cannot function properly. Some cells fail to regenerate and some cells generate but at a much smaller, ineffective size. Collagen also is laid down in the muscles, and adipose tissue then replaces the collagen. Therefore, both atrophy and pseudohypertrophy of the muscle occurs. This cell necrosis begins long before the child is symptomatic (Mason & Wright, 1994). Pseudohypertrophy is when the muscle appears unusually large, but the size is due to increased collagen and not to muscle development. This phenomenon accounts for the large, "muscular" looking calves that young boys with DMD exhibit, at odds with their weakness.

Clinical Aspects and Functional Limitations

The male infant with DMD usually does not have symptoms at birth or early life. Some may, however, have mild hypotonia identified during infancy. They often are late to walk and by 3 to 6 years of age begin to fall more frequently and have difficulty with climbing as well as getting up from the floor. They usually have a typical Gower's sign by the age of 3 years. Gower's sign is elicited by instructing the child to stand up from a squatting or sitting position on the floor. Typically, a child comes to a standing position easily using only leg muscles. The child with DMD is too weak in the proximal muscles, so must push on the thighs with both hands in order to stand up. Boys with DMD demonstrate a waddling Trendelenburg gait, toe walking, and have increased lordosis that is caused by gluteal muscle weakness and contractures. Muscle weakness begins in the proximal muscle groups and moves distally, so the first muscles affected usually are the thigh and shoulder muscles.

By 7 years of age, the lower extremity muscle weakness, contractures, and pseudohypertrophy of the calves is obvious. By 9 to 12 years of age, children with DMD usually are unable to ambulate independently for long distances and need a wheelchair. Scoliosis develops as weakness causes muscle imbalance along the spine. Increasing scoliosis contributes to the severity of respiratory and cardiac compromise by compressing the chest cavity. Elbow contractures and obesity also often occur as the disease progresses and the child becomes less active. In the later stages, adolescents' facial and neck muscles become involved as well. Respiratory muscle wasting, excluding the diaphragm, causes a weak, ineffective cough; decreased reserve; and restrictive pulmonary disease with more frequent pulmonary infections. Pharyngeal

363

weakness may create difficulty with phases of swallowing. As the child survives longer, there may be smooth muscle dysfunction that causes intestinal pseudo-obstruction, gastric hypomotility, and urinary retention. Cardiomyopathy also occurs, but the severity is variable. This degenerative condition is usually a painless process, without myalgias or muscle spasms; however, increasing immobility can result in osteoporosis that leads to very painful fractures.

The majority of the children with DMD have learning disabilities but are able to function in a regular classroom with additional assistance. A few children have significant cognitive deficit and about 20% to 30% have intelligence quotients below 70. Most children do not reach their 20s unless artificial ventilation is used. Death occurs from respiratory failure and infection, usually around 18 years of age (Sarnat, 1996a).

Persons with DMD have an increased risk for malignant hyperthermia, which can be a complication of anesthesia. If surgery is planned, special pre- and postoperative monitoring and medications may be necessary (Mason & Wright, 1994).

Spinal Muscular Atrophy

The second most common neuromuscular disease is spinal muscular atrophy (SMA). It also is genetically based and progressive in nature, and hypotonia is the major clinical sign. SMA may be diagnosed at birth because of the early symptoms or may not become obvious until much later (Sarnat, 1996a).

Etiology and Incidence

SMA is an autosomal recessive condition that affects all ethnic groups, with an estimated incidence of one in 25,000 live births. There are believed to be three types of SMA. Type I, known as Werdnig-Hoffmann disease, is an infantile form with an onset before 6 months of age. Motor milestones such as rolling, sitting, and walking are not achieved. Without use of artificial ventilation, death occurs before 4 years of age from cardiopulmonary failure. Most children with type I SMA do not survive past the first year of life. Type II is the chronic form of infantile SMA and is slower in progress, with an onset up to 2 years of age. Children with this type of SMA usually develop motor skills such as walking, but eventually lose the ability to ambulate and regress in motor skills. Many of these

children have respiratory complications before adolescence.

Type III SMA, also called Kugelberg-Welander, has an onset after 2 years of age, and respiratory complications occur usually during adulthood. Children with this form of the disease are often able to ambulate until adolescence when increasing weakness results in wheelchair use. Individuals with Kugelberg-Welander are most likely to live a more normal life span, albeit with significant disability.

Pathophysiology

SMA is caused by a pathologic continuation of programmed cell death of motor neuroblasts (Sarnat, 1996a). It results from selective degeneration of the anterior horn cells in the spinal cord and neurocytes in the motor nuclei. Normally, in embryonic life, an excess of cells that will become motor neuroblasts and neurons is produced. Only about half of these cells survive and go on to become neurons. For those cells that become mature, there is a process that stops the degeneration and death of the cell, allowing it to become a mature motor neuron. In SMA, the gene does not allow the process of programmed cell death to stop, allowing more cells to degenerate and die. Therefore, SMA results from a continuation of the normal programmed cell death in embryonic life. Although this is a progressive, degenerative process, some of the motor neurons will re-enervate, creating giant motor units. These motor units eventually degenerate, causing atrophy of the muscle fibers (Sarnat, 1996a).

Clinical Aspects and Functional Limitations

Infants born with a hypotonia from SMA type I often have a history of poor intrauterine movement. In the first months of life, they may have feeding difficulties, a weak cry, choking episodes, respiratory difficulties, apnea, generalized weakness, and may seem to have diminished facial expressions. These children go on to be delayed in their motor development, especially those movements that require antigravity movement. Infants with Werdnig-Hoffman disease die early in life, usually of respiratory failure.

Children with type II SMA may reach some of the motor milestones: they usually walk with lordosis and weakened muscles, requiring bracing. Because of progressive weakness, they usually need to use an electric wheelchair by school age and go on to develop severe scoliosis if they survive longer. Respiratory and orthopedic problems increase with age.

The type III SMA, Kugelberg-Welander disease, is the least severe form. These children may develop typically early in life and be able to ambulate without equipment for longer periods of time. They have progressive weakness, proximal in distribution, usually involving the shoulder girdle muscles. They live usually into middle adulthood and may survive longer with artificial ventilation support.

With SMA, there is normal intelligence and no cardiac involvement. In fact, the children may seem brighter than their peers. This is attributed to the fact that they have compensated for their inability to be physically active and therefore focused more on learning (Sarnat, 1996a).

Diagnostic Assessment

A thorough history of the onset of weakness, details surrounding the onset, whether the weakness is fluctuating or not, delayed motor milestones, and family history of muscle disease or neurologic disease is important. Clinical assessment should include complete evaluation of the child's motor movements and strength, muscle wasting or hypertrophy, plus observation of the parents. It is possible that the parents may have an unrecognized neuropathy that they have passed on to their child. Questioning the parents about any symptoms of muscle weakness or neurology symptoms is helpful in identifying a familial link for the disease. Recognizing the condition would allow treatment for the parents and provide them with information regarding the risk for future children (Molnar, 1992). Genetic counseling is very important for any family with a child diagnosed with muscle disease.

Laboratory studies are needed to confirm a specific diagnosis of DMD, SMA, or other types of degenerative neuromuscular disease. Elevated serum creatinine phosphokinase (CPK), aldolase, and transaminase indicate a breakdown of the muscle tissue in DMD. Carriers of the DMD gene also may have elevated levels of CPK, but the levels are not as high as in the affected child. In SMA, these studies are only mildly elevated. Electromyography (EMG), nerve conduction velocity, and neuromuscular transmission studies are also of value in the diagnostic process. Motor con-

duction studies are normal in SMA, but EMG studies may show neurogenic changes. EMG studies in DMD show a myopathic condition, but are not specific for DMD. Muscle biopsy to gather data regarding active tissue pathology is the most important component of the diagnostic process and provides the definitive diagnosis for DMD and SMA. There are many disorders that may resemble a neuromuscular disease; therefore, differential diagnosis is very important.

For children with DMD, assessment of the heart by electrocardiogram (ECG) and chest x-ray should be done initially and periodically as the disease progresses. For neuromuscular diseases with known molecular genetic identity, intrauterine diagnosis can be made, as with DMD, and prenatal diagnosis is possible as early as 12 weeks of gestation. Detection of at-risk female carriers for DMD is possible by DNA analysis from blood samples and should be done to determine whether the mother is a carrier or DMD occurred by new mutation (Sarnat, 1996a).

Therapeutic Management

There is no known cure or method of slowing the degenerative process of muscular dystrophies and atrophies. Therefore, these children and adults live a much shorter life than normal and, if the use of artificial ventilation extends their life, they require considerable health and functional support for a long period of time.

Interdisciplinary Team

Children with DMD and SMA and their families are best served by an interdisciplinary team of professionals who specialize in management of these degenerative conditions. In addition to the traditional rehabilitation team members, children with DMD should also be in the care of a cardiologist. Pediatric neurology, pediatric orthopedics, and genetics specialists often are involved in the care of children with neuromuscular diseases, as well as the rehabilitation team. Supportive therapy for the prevention of complications, management of the disabilities as they present, maintenance of independence and function as long as possible, and medical treatment for the cardiopulmonary complications should be the therapeutic focus of the interdisciplinary team.

There are stages in the child's life when the team activity and management increases.

The early diagnostic period is, of course, one of heightened anxiety for the family and the child if he is old enough to realize that he is becoming weak and unable to perform as he did in the past.

The next stage occurs when the child has decreasing energy to walk and needs orthotics and possibly surgery to support continued ambulation. Surgery may consist of heel cord lengthenings or tendon release to counter tightness and contractures. When ambulation takes more energy than the child has, a wheelchair is needed, often a power chair. At this point, the orthotics are no longer used and foot deformities related to contractures increase.

The last stage encompasses management of all the prolonged complications that occur because of progressive weakness and immobility. At this time, scoliosis increases and decisions regarding surgery must be made. Surgery should be done earlier, before scoliosis becomes severe and respiratory compromise increases the risk of the procedure. Another condition that follows the cessation of ambulation is the increased problem of respiratory illnesses and the risk of pneumonia. This is related to the progressive nature of the disease, with weakened respiratory muscles plus the restrictive function of scoliosis.

By far the most difficult complications of this period are the child's physical dependence on his family for self-care and the child and family's overwhelming need for emotional support. Once again, the anxiety of the early diagnostic stage may reappear for both the child and family. Depression, anger, guilt, and denial may all be mixed together with the active coping process. The child may still be able to do some self-feeding and perform keyboard-type activities, but requires that the environment be set up for him. The environment must be accessible for the use of the electric wheelchair. He will be able to direct his care and request his needs be met, but will no longer have the ability to perform his care independently. He will know when he wants to be turned in bed or have his position changed in his wheelchair, but will not be able to accomplish that task himself. Management of the home environment for care is a tremendous task for families. Many families at first try to do all the care and cope without someone assisting them in the home. This soon becomes difficult, and then the problem of affording dependable care and the invasiveness of hired care givers in the home becomes a major stressor.

Slowed gastrointestinal motility that leads to gastric dilatation, intestinal pseudo-obstruction, and other symptoms may occur with an increase in age of DMD patients. Practitioners must be aware that these conditions may develop and treat them symptomatically to prevent life-threatening situations (Benson, Jaffe, & Tan, 1996).

Therapy

The use of assistive devices and equipment for positioning, mobility, and facilitation of independence in play, communication, and self-care skills is an important part of assisting the child to maintain as much function as possible. Children with DMD and SMA benefit from the use of computers to preserve energy, to enhance learning, and as a means of communicating with peers. Specialized devices for crawling and walking, side-lying positioning devices, and standing frames all support increased movement, independence, and maintenance of upright stance as long as possible in order to prevent complications of immobility. Braces that are lightweight provide support for standing, walking, and increased functional skills, and assist in the prevention of contractures. Complications of sitting with neuromuscular disorders includes curvatures of the spine and restrictive lung disease. Custom-fitted seating systems are important in order to provide external support for the spine. Houston and colleagues (1994) studied children and adults with SMA and found abnormal craniofacial growth patterns that led to malocclusions. Their recommendation was to attend to this condition with dental assessment and management and support optimal nutrition and respiratory functioning. Research by Wong and Wade (1995) used custom dry-floatation cushions for controlling sitting posture and found that this significantly reduced iliotibial band contractures in patients with DMD who sat most of the day.

Mechanical ventilation used for management of the restrictive pulmonary disease related to muscle weakness with DMD and SMA continues to be controversial. Although the use of mechanical ventilation can prolong life, the need for supportive care increases dramatically and quality of life may change. Ideally, the adolescent and family is supported by the rehabilitation team in making a planned decision whether or not to choose prolongation of life using ventilatory support. Too often the child or adolescent enters the hospital in acute respiratory crisis, a tracheostomy is performed, and ventilatory support is initiated without consideration of the pros and cons for the individual and family. Individuals with SMA who continue to have functional bulbar musculature may benefit from noninvasive ventilatory support such as the cuirass or nasal continuous positive airway pressure (CPAP) (Bach, 1995).

Impact on Child and Family

Parents anticipate bringing a perfect child into the world, one who will grow up to become independent. When they learn that their child is not going to be able to fulfill those original expectations and will most likely die early in life, the family has major crises to deal with. Progressive, degenerative, disabling conditions such as DMD and SMA are long-term challenges for the child and family. Both child and family may experience depression at various stages of the shortened life. For the family, the most obvious time for this is during the diagnosis and while coming to an understanding of the degenerative process. For the child, usually depression occurs when he begins to lose the ability to be independent in ambulation and self-care. Caregiver burn-out is frequent, because many families have more than one son with DMD. Even with only one affected child, caregiver stress is common. In a family with DMD, it is often the sisters who assist with the care of their brothers as they become more and more dependent. Thus, the sisters' psychosocial development may be also affected, even more so if they are identified as carriers of the gene. Guilt, anger, depression, exhaustion, and grief are all reactions experienced by families.

CASE STUDY

Joe was 9 years old. He and his family lived in a small rural community and had been coping with the fact that Joe had DMD and was getting weaker. This summer, Joe really wanted to play soccer and had been able to do so the previous summer even with a slowed run and frequent falling. This year, he had gotten weaker and was less able to walk long distances. In fact, his treatment team was considering fitting him for a wheelchair, but the family had postponed making a decision until school was out. Even with the weakness, Joe really wanted to play soccer again. His father wanted him to play, but his mother felt it was going to be difficult and she thought it was better that he did not enroll. In addition,

Joe's younger brother was just starting to get weak and his mother knew he would need more frequent clinic visits for evaluations.

Joe pleaded with his parents to go ahead and sign him up. They decided to do so after talking to the coach. At the first practice Joe fell and could not get up. After that he became so depressed that he refused to leave his room or even play outside at home. He also refused to go to the practice or games. He started crawling more and sometimes was incontinent, seeming not to be able to get to the bathroom in time. All he could verbalize was that he just hated his legs for keeping him from playing soccer.

Joe's family finally talked again with the coach and he and some of the team came to visit Joe. They decided to make a place for Joe even though he would not be able to run. Joe agreed to go but still was not very happy. The day of the next game, the coach and team had decided to give Joe the position of sideline referee. Joe had always known the rules and he could still be a very important part of the game. Joe tried it and, after the first game, he came home saying he was playing soccer again and was happy.

Application of Nursing Process

Assessment/Reassessment

Because of the child's changing functional status, ongoing assessment/reassessment of stress tolerance, coping, and physical care needs is necessary. General assessment criteria as outlined in Chapters 12 and 13 can be used as guidelines. Additional assessment/reassessment includes respiratory status of children with DMD and SMA, cardiac status for child with DMD, and gastrointestinal status for child with DMD.

Potential Nursing Diagnosis

Actual or high risk for

- Family coping—potential for growth
- Ineffective child and family coping
- Distress of the human spirit—child and family
- Hopelessness—powerlessness—fear—anxiety
- Dysfunctional grieving
- Self-care deficits
- Impaired mobility
- Caregiver role strain

Expected Outcomes—Child and Family

- Child and family will be able to use their own coping skills, receive support when necessary

- Child and family will be able to maintain realistic expectations of child's capabilities and allow child to become his own unique individual in spite of the degenerative disease process
- Child and family will continue to function in ways that promote physical health, growth, and development, as well as psychosocial and spiritual

Intervention—Implementation—Teaching

Providing active support and caring is the major role of the pediatric rehabilitation nurse when working with each child and family who experiences the degenerative process of DMD or SMA. The nurse must have a working knowledge of the degenerative process and the specific physical care needs that each brings, as well as methods of supporting independence of the child as long as possible. Independence may constitute the child maintaining the ability to brush his teeth with an electric toothbrush, as well as the ability to direct the care provided by an aide or an attendant. One method of supporting independence for children with muscle disease is the use of service dogs. The dog is specially trained to provide assistance, fetch objects, alert the child to danger or events, and to get help, providing companionship as well as aid.

The nurse must also be alert to the unique emotional dynamics each child and family experiences while coping with this type of disability and be able to provide therapeutic support when needed. Assisting the family to mobilize support and resources is a primary role. Providing support for the child and family in the later stages of SMA or DMD is focused on assisting the child to find meaning in life and face death. Inclusion of the child or adolescent in decision making about treatment is an important part of the process. The nurse is a key advocate for the child's role in treatment decision making. In order to be effective, the nurse must also be self-aware of feelings that might affect care. Involvement with families throughout the life of a child with DMD or SMA can be very demanding and yet rewarding.

Included with the role of emotional support is anticipatory guidance, prevention of further complications, teaching, and resource development. Other components of nursing care include

- Facilitation of maximum level of independence in self-care and mobility—refer for therapy and assistive device consultation as necessary
- Assist the family and child to learn the use of assistive equipment in the home and community
- Establish in-bed turning routine to increase comfort and prevent pulmonary complications
- Evaluate comfort and positioning of the child while in bed and recommend products to relieve discomfort and promote proper positioning; consider use of flotation mattress for comfort
- Teach the family range-of-motion exercises
- Assist the family in establishing routines and setting up the home environment to support providing home care
- Teach and support use of transfer skills, lifting equipment, and safe body mechanics to prevent caregiver injury as the child becomes more dependent for care
- Teach weight shifting and position changing to relieve pressure points and prevent skin breakdown
- Teach techniques to support pulmonary health and management during illness
- Teach respiratory chest percussion, postural drainage, and assistance with cough by supporting the abdominal area (manual cough)
- Encourage adequate fluid intake
- Monitor bowel and bladder elimination—with immobility, urinary stasis and altered bowel functioning may occur
- Implement bowel program if necessary
- Monitor caloric intake and weight—refer for teaching about necessary intake when child becomes immobile or for management of obesity if necessary
- Monitor gastrointestinal functioning for signs of slowed motility and refer when necessary for management—with older patients who have DMD, this can be a problem
- Encourage the family to express feelings of frustration, guilt, anger, depression
- Assist family in getting respite care to relieve them for time to meet their own needs
- Assist family and child in developing support groups provided by specific associations such as Muscular Dystrophy Association
- Encourage counseling as necessary
- Assist family to seek information and help interpret information
- Provide emotional support
- Encourage child and family to make informed decisions regarding therapy and care
- Assist family in learning safe, effective home management

- Refer to other team members for assistance when child's independence changes
- Empower the family and child

Long-Term Outlook

Neither DMD or SMA has cures. There are many hurdles to overcome before gene therapy is feasible in effecting a cure for DMD or SMA. Treatment is essentially supportive (Hauser & Chamberlain, 1996).

SUMMARY

DMD and SMA are progressive, degenerative muscle diseases. With DMD, life expectancy is around 20 years at most, unless artifical ventilation is used, which increases life expectancy. The child is born without deficits and gradually becomes more weak after learning to walk. The condition progresses to complete dependence on others for care. There are three different types of SMA, with the infantile form the most severe. The child with SMA may survive with a milder form of the disease. The third type does not appear until late childhood and has the best hopes for longer survival, into adulthood.

REFERENCES

Bach, J. R. (1995). Noninvasive long-term ventilatory support for individuals with spinal muscular atrophy and functional bulbar musculature. *Archives of Physical Medicine and Rehabilitation, 76*, 213–217.

Benson, E. S., Jaffe, L., & Tan, P. (1996). Acute gastric dilatation in Duchenne muscular dystrophy: A case report and review of literature. *Archives of Physical Medicine and Rehabilitation, 76*, 512–514.

Hauser, M. A., & Chamberlain, J. S. (1996). Progress towards gene therapy for Duchenne muscular dystrophy. *Journal of Endocrinology, 149*(3), 373–378.

Houston, K., Bushang, P., Iannaccone, S., & Seale, N. (1994). Craniofacial morphology of spinal muscular atrophy. *Pediatric Research, 36*(2), 265–269.

Mason, K. J., and Wright, S. (1994). Altered musculoskeletal function. In Betz, C., Hunsberger, M., & Wright, S. (Eds). *Family-Centered Nursing Care of Children* (2nd ed.). Philadelphia: W. B. Saunders.

Molnar, G. (Ed.) (1992). *Pediatric Rehabilitation* (2nd ed.). Baltimore: Williams & Wilkins.

Sarnat, H. (1996). Muscular dystrophies. In Nelson, W. E. (Ed.). *Nelson Textbook of Pediatrics*. Philadelphia: W. B. Saunders, pp. 1745–1752.

Sarnat, H. (1996). Disorders of neuromuscular transmission. In Nelson, W. E. (Ed.). *Nelson Textbook of Pediatrics*. Philadelphia: W. B. Saunders, pp. 1755–1758.

Wong, C. K., & Wade, C. K. (1995). Reducing iliotibial band contractures in patients with muscular dystrophy using custom dry flotation cushions. *Archives of Physical Medicine and Rehabilitation, 76*, 695–700.

Additional Resources: Journals and Books

Bach, C. A. (1992). Traveling with technology. *Rehabilitation Nursing, 17*(3), 141–143.

Bach, J. R., & Barnett, V. (1994). Ethical considerations in the management of individuals with severe neuromuscular disorders. *American Journal of Physical Medicine and Rehabilitation, 73*(2), 134–140.

Call, G., & Zitter, F. A. (1985). Failure to thrive in Duchenne muscular dystrophy. *Journal of Pediatrics, 106*(6), 939–940.

Edwards, P. A., & Posch, C. M. (1990). Impairment of the musculoskeletal system. In McCoy, P., & Votroubek, W. (Eds.) *Pediatric Home Care, A Comprehensive Approach*. Rockville, MD: Aspen Publishers, pp. 182–188.

Harrigan, J. (1996). Nursing practice management: Muscular dystrophy. *Journal of School Nursing, 12*(2), 38–40.

Jaffe, K. M., McDonald, M., Ingman, E., & Haas, J. (1990). Symptoms of upper gastrointestinal dysfunction in Duchenne muscular dystrophy. *Archives of Physical Medicine and Rehabilitation, 71*, 742–744.

Lord, J., Behrman, B., Varzoa, N., Cooper, D., Lieberman, J., & Fowler, W. (1990). Scoliosis associated with Duchenne muscular dystrophy. *Archives of Physical Medicine and Rehabilitation, 71*, 13–17.

McCoy, P. A., & Votroubek, W. L. (1990). *Pediatric Home Care, A Comprehensive Approach*. Rockville, MD: Aspen Publishers.

Parsons, E., Bradley, D., & Clark, A. (1996). Disclosure of Duchenne muscular dystrophy after newborn screening. *Archives of Disease in Childhood, 74*(6), 550–553.

Redding, G. J., Okamoto, G., Guthrie, R., Rollevson, D., & Milstein, J. (1985). Sleep patterns in nonambulatory boys with Duchenne muscular dystrophy. *Archives of Physical Medicine and Rehabilitation, 66*, 818–821.

Rose, V. (1992). Understanding motor neuron disease. *Professional Nurse, 7*(12), 784–786.

Sandler, D. L., Burchfield, D., McCarthy, J., Rojiani, A., & Drummond, W. (1994). Early-onset respiratory failure caused by severe congenital neuromuscular disease. *Journal of Pediatrics, 124*(4), 636–638.

Thomas, S. (1993). Support that prolongs life. Ventilation in motor neuron disease. *Professional Nurse, 8*(10), 656–659.

Additional Resources: Other Sources

Muscular Dystrophy Association, 3300 East Sunrise Drive, Tucson, AZ 85718–3208, (602)–529–2000.

Osteogenesis Imperfecta

Dalice L. Hertzberg

■

INCIDENCE, CAUSES, AND SEVERITY

Osteogenesis imperfecta (OI) is the term for a group of inherited connective tissue disorders that result in brittle bones with an increased susceptibility to fracture, short stature, and significant risk of progressive deformity with growth. In addition to the brittle bone component of OI, other extra-skeletal tissues that contain collagen may be affected in varying degrees. OI is manifested with varying severity according to the type and transmission of the affected genetic material.

OI occurs in one out of every 5000 to 10,000 births. The mildest form, type I, is the most common and occurs in one out of every 3000 births. The most severe form, type II, usually results in death prior to or just following birth. The condition is found in all racial and ethnic groups and does not predominate in either males or females. The different forms of OI may be transmitted genetically by different types of inheritance, including by new mutations (McCullough & Pellino, 1994).

The various types of OI are described in several different systems of classification of the disease. The classification system used by Sillence (1981) is the most commonly used and categorizes four main types of OI. Table 16–6 shows the types, inheritance, and clinical features of each type of OI. Of these categories, types II and III tend to be the most severe, but even within categories, severity varies. Those children with type II who survive have extremely severe disability and major functional limitations. Individuals with type III OI also are significantly affected, but not so much as those with type II. Individuals with type IV OI are moderately affected. Some symptoms, such as dental problems, are found in subtypes of types I and IV.

Pathophysiology

The condition, which is caused by a genetic anomaly, results in alteration of bone density due to impairment of osteoid formation. Unusual modeling of both the diaphysis and metaphysis of the bone occurs. The most dramatic hallmark of OI is the fragility of the bones which, in the most severe forms of the

condition, occur with ordinary handling and movement of the child; the child may be born with multiple fractures from the birth process. After fracture, the bones heal, often with a larger-than-usual callus formation, but leave deformities of the limbs or spinal column and malalignment of bones. Because of the frequent fractures and deformity of the bones, limb length and trunk length are affected. Other characteristics include hypotonia, hypermetabolism with increased seating, fragile skin, dental problems, capillary fragility, and hearing loss due to otosclerosis (Perrin & Saturen, 1992).

The primary pathophysiologic feature of OI is the defect in collagen formation that results in bone with thin, fragile trabeculae. Atypically, there are larger than usual numbers of osteocytes (bone cells), osteoblasts (cell that forms bone cells), and abnormal osteoclasts (resorbs bone tissue). The intracellular matrix of the bone is reduced. The cortex of the bone is thin and eggshell-like. These features result in bone that grows and ossifies slowly, that is very porous, that has a higher rate of bone turnover than is normal, and that is extremely susceptible to fracture. Disturbance of bone growth and maturation occurs at both the ossification centers and at the growth plates. The collagen in the skin is also abnormal (Tachdjian, 1990).

OI is caused by at least four different genetic variations, including autosomal dominant, autosomal recessive, and spontaneous mutation, some of which result from different forms of mosaicism. There is variation in characteristics both among and within groups. The heterogenous nature of the inheritance pattern of OI makes genetic counseling for this disorder extremely challenging. Mosaicism occurs when the parents appear to be physiologically unaffected by the condition and there is no history of the condition in the family. In actuality, one of the parents is mildly affected by the condition and carries the mutation in some somatic cells (general body cells, not reproductive) or in some gonadal cells (reproductive cells). Another variation of mosaicism occurs when the parent is affected by the gene, but with a different genetic variation than the child. The degree to

Table 16-6 CLASSIFICATION OF OSTEOGENESIS IMPERFECTA

OI Type	Inheritance	Clinical Features
I	Autosomal dominant	Mild type Normal or mild to moderate short stature Little or no deformity, bowing and angulation at knees and feet may be due to ligament laxity Fractures occur with moderate trauma, decrease at puberty Blue sclerae Hearing loss common in adolescents and young adults Dentinogenesis rare, present in type IB
II	Autosomal dominant or recessive	Kyphosis may occur Most severe form Lethal in perinatal period due to respiratory or cardiovascular compromise, many are stillborn Numerous fractures present at birth Beaded ribs Compressed femurs Compressed skull Small extremities Marked long bone deformity Can be diagnosed prenatally
III	Autosomal dominant or recessive	Moderately severe form Severe osteoporosis Progressive deformity of bones Frequent fractures associated with minimal trauma Scoliosis and kyphosis common Variable scleral hue Dentinogenesis common Very short stature Often nonambulatory by adolescence Large skull, triangular face shape
IV	Autosomal dominant	Mild type Normal sclera or bluish sclera that lightens with age Fractures may occur at birth or later in life Mild to moderate bone deformity, particularly bowing of the legs Stature variable Dentinogenesis in type IVB Often spontaneously improves at puberty No hearing loss

From McCullough, L., & Pellino, T. (1994). Congenital and developmental disorders. In Maher, A., Salmond, S., & Pellino, T. (Eds.) *Orthopaedic Nursing*. Philadelphia: W. B. Saunders, p. 641.

which the parent is affected depends on the proportion and tissue distribution of the mutation (Raghunath, Mackay, Dalgleish, & Steinmann, 1995). It may be extremely difficult to detect any characteristics of the condition in the parents, or the manifestation of the condition may be obvious but very mild.

Condition and Characteristics

The underlying collagen deficit causes osteopenia, short stature, variable growth plate arrest, and multiple fractures including microfractures. The collagen in the skin and other connective tissues also is atypical, resulting in fragile skin and increased bruising.

Shortened bones and short stature also are caused by frequent fractures and the resulting deformity. Irregular and fragmented growth plates, because of minor trauma and growth arrest, contribute to leg-length discrepancy and deformity of long bones. Dislocation of joints and other joint disorders, especially in weight-bearing joints, may occur. Hip deformities such as limited extension and x-ray findings resembling avascular necrosis may occur. Ligamentous laxity also results from the underlying collagen defect and contributes to joint dysfunction. Pelvic deformity, with acetabular protrusion into the abdominal space, may result in abdominal pain and constipation in individuals who are more significantly affected by OI (Binder, Conway, & Gerber, 1993; Lee, Gamble, Moore, & Rinsky, 1995; Paterson, Burns, & McAllion, 1993; Perrin & Saturen, 1992; Tachdjian, 1990).

Spinal deformity also appears frequently as scoliosis or kyphosis due to compression fractures and vertebral body wedging. Atypical features of the cervical spine include laxity of ligaments and malformed cervical vertebrae that lead to atlanto-axial instability with increased fatigueability as an early sign, leading to spasticity and loss of movement of the trunk and extremities. Thoracolumbar kyphoscoliosis appears early in life, and the short trunk and very rigid curves makes bracing difficult. The lumbar spine may also be affected and cause spinal stenosis (Perrin & Saturen, 1992; Tachdjian, 1990).

The skull also is altered, with a broad forehead with prominent parietal and temporal bones, which contributes to its "helmet-like" appearance. The cranium is out of proportion to the face, giving the child's face a characteristic triangular or "elfin" look. The ears are low set and outwardly displaced. On radiographs of the skull in very severe forms of the condition, wormian bones are present, which are pieces of the primary ossification centers of bones in the skull. This type of unusual bone formation only occurs with some types of bone dysplasias and provides a diagnostic confirmation of the more severe forms of OI (Tachdjian, 1990).

Another characteristic feature of OI is blue-colored sclera. Blue sclerae are generally more pronounced in early life, but may continue into adulthood. Blue sclerae are most common in type I, variable in type II, and may occur with type IV but lighten with age. The variation in occurrence of blue sclera is based on the heterogeneous nature of the genetic inheritance pattern. The blue color results from the thin collagen layer, which lets the intraocular pigment show through. Although vision usually is unaffected, some opacity of the cornea and a higher risk for retinal detachment may be present (Sillence, Butler, Latham, & Barlow, 1993; McCullough & Pellino, 1994; Tachdjian, 1990).

The teeth also are affected in OI. There is a deficiency of dentin, resulting in teeth that break easily, develop cavities easily, and maintain fillings poorly. The teeth usually are discolored and may be termed "opalescent." Dental problems, called dentinogenesis imperfecta, do not occur in all types of OI, but are most common in type II and variations of types I and IV. Most affected are the deciduous teeth (McCullough & Pellino, 1994; Tachdjian, 1990).

Deafness is also a characteristic of some types of OI, appearing in 40% of children with type I and a lower percentage of children with type IV. Hearing loss is caused by one of two mechanisms: otosclerosis or nerve conduction dysfunction. Otosclerosis results from calcification of the large amount of cartilage present in the bones of and adjacent to the inner ear. Nerve conduction loss is caused by pressure on the auditory nerve. Deafness usually is not present at birth, but develops during adolescence or adulthood (Tachdjian, 1990).

Aortic and mitral valve insufficiency is an uncommon feature of OI, usually detected in adolescence or adulthood. Cardiac conditions are thought to result from the underlying collagen defect in the formation of connective tissue (Wong, Follis, Shively, & Wernly, 1995).

A significant complication of OI that may occur in adolescence or adulthood is invagination of the foramen magnum into the posterior cranial fossa, causing brain stem compression and hydrocephalus. Respiratory failure is a frequent complication of this condition, often leaving the individual ventilator-dependent. Quadraplegia also may result, with an accompanying decrease in function and independence. (Tachdjian, 1990; Wang, Yang, & Alba 1994). Other neurologic dysfunction may occur as a result of spinal stenosis or nerve compression from fractures or bony impingement. The most severe types of OI have been associated, although rarely, with cerebral atrophy, hydrocephalus, macrocephaly, problems secondary to skull fracture, seizures and, even more rarely, syringohydromyelia (Charras & Marini, 1993). Children with type II OI may have abnormal microvascular changes in the central nervous system (CNS) secondary to the collagen defect, but these children rarely survive beyond infancy (Verkh, Russell, & Miller, 1995).

OI has not been found to directly affect cognitive function in children with most types of the condition. With less severe types of OI, children fall into the typical range of cognitive function and intellect. Figure 16–6 shows a summary of clinical characteristics of OI.

Diagnosis

Prenatal diagnosis is performed using ultrasound or the more invasive method of chorionic villus sampling (CVS). Ultrasound is

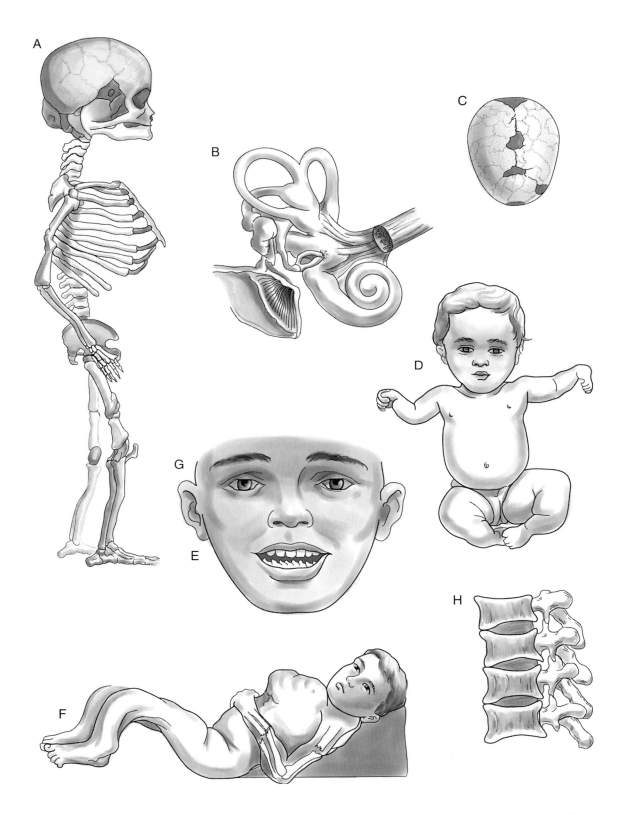

Figure 16–6   Summary of clinical characteristics of osteogenesis imperfecta. *A*, Skeleton. *B*, Ear. *C*, Skull. *D*, Joints. *E*, Teeth. *F*, Bones. *G*, Eyes. *H*, Spine. (Adapted from Tachdjian, M. (1990). *Pediatric Orthopedics* Vol. 2 [2nd ed.]. Philadelphia: W. B. Saunders, p. 742.)

most useful for prenatal diagnosis of the more severe forms of OI, such as type II, which is often lethal in the perinatal period, and types III and IV, which result in early bone deformity. The milder forms of OI, such as types I and some subtypes of IV, usually are missed on ultrasound. The findings that suggest OI on ultrasound include multiple fractures and bowing and angulation of the long bones, the ribs, demineralization of bones, and the thinness of the skull. Limb measurements and size also contribute to the diagnosis. Reduced echogenicity is also a finding. The earliest ultrasound scans that have detected the severe form of OI were done at 15 to 20 weeks of gestation. Routine ultrasound may also pick up the more severe forms of the condition (Thompson, 1993).

CVS is used mostly for families who have a known genetic risk. The tissue taken by CVS is analyzed using DNA linkage studies and biochemical studies. If the actual mutation or variation of collagen abnormality present in a family is known, other types of molecular or biochemical studies may be performed.

If there is an early prenatal diagnosis of one of the more severe forms of OI, the parents are offered the option of termination of the affected fetus. However, prenatal diagnosis is also used to plan the method of delivery, with cesarean section often recommended for the more severe forms of the condition (Thompson 1993).

In the newborn period, the physical features of the child usually lead to the diagnosis of OI. However, there are other types of dwarfism and bone dysplasias that may resemble OI and must be differentiated from it. Characteristic features of the infant with OI are summarized in Figure 16–6. Significant features of the more severe forms include radiographs showing multiple fractures, long bones that are unusually thin, unusually shaped epiphyseal ends of the long bones, wormian bones in the skull, hypoplastic skull with large-appearing head, "popcorn calcifications" in the long bones, and other abnormalities of bone tissue and shape. In milder types of OI, radiographs reveal osteoporosis, impairment of bone modeling, old and new fractures, and joint deformities. Other diagnostic methods that may be helpful include bone densitometry, quantitative analysis of cultured skin fibroblast collagen, a good family history and assessment of parents for subtle signs, and genetic testing that includes DNA testing of the child and family (McCullough & Pellino, 1994; Paterson, Burns, & McAlion, 1993; Tachdjian, 1990).

The frequent fractures and bruising that are characteristic of children with OI may often be mistaken for child abuse, even in those children with moderately severe forms of the condition. Most often, however, it is the child with type I OI or a variant who has few observable symptoms of the condition in early childhood, who is mistakenly diagnosed with child abuse. Even on regular radiographs, the mild osteopenia of the bones of children with very mild forms of the disease may go undetected. Studies have suggested that there is no actual pattern associated with the fractures of OI, and that all types of fractures may occur, including metaphyseal fractures in the absence of clinical data of other bone abnormality (Dent & Paterson, 1991). When differentiating other causes of fracture from child abuse, OI should always be considered (Paterson, Burns, & McAllion, 1993).

Interdisciplinary Management

Interdisciplinary rehabilitative and habilitative management of the child with OI includes coordinated interventions from the entire rehabilitation team, including physical and occupational therapy, speech and language pathology, nursing, genetics, social work, psychology, orthotics, orthopedics, physiatry, and other medical specialties. For children with severe types of OI, specific exercise programs, bracing, and ambulation training is beneficial.

The infant with OI must be handled very carefully and often requires positioning on a padded splint which can be used for feeding and breastfeeding. As the child grows, orthoses that protect the limbs often are necessary. Children with very fragile bones may not be able to weight bear until later childhood or adolescence, when the frequency of fracture is reduced, or they may never be able to tolerate weight bearing. Interventions include positioning, monitoring for fractures, teaching the family how to hold the child, therapy for developmental activities and muscle strengthening, and intermedullary rod placement in the long bones to prevent further fractures and to correct angulation. Rods and bracing may gain time before skeletal maturity, when a more satisfactory correction may be obtained. Bracing for deformities is poorly tolerated. Surgical intervention such as osteotomy must be planned carefully, because any resulting limitation of range of motion can compound disability, interfering with daily activities (Perrin & Saturen, 1992).

Orthopedic treatment of fractures in the newborn period and early infancy is accomplished by splinting. Often fractures may occur in multiple sites, requiring a more extensive splint, or even one that supports the infant's entire body. Healing generally is rapid and is accomplished in 2 weeks. The challenge is to maintain adequate bony and body alignment while permitting as much movement as possible to decrease complications and promote development. For children who have a very severe form of the disease, a full-body orthosis, somewhat like a cradle for the trunk, head, and limbs, is required. Also, pneumatic trouser splints may be used (Cole, W., 1993; Tachdjian, 1990).

Intramedullary rod placement in long bones is used frequently to correct angulation, bowing, and other bony deformity. The indications for this procedure are severe, increasing deformity of long bones that impairs function and fit of orthoses, and frequent fractures. The procedure consists of performing multiple osteotomies in long bones and placing a rod through the center of the bone fragments to straighten and strengthen the bones. Complications of the procedure include migration of the rod, fractures above and below the rod, and damage to the growth plate. This procedure usually is done in the older child, whenever possible, to maintain as much growth in the bones and length of limbs as possible (Cole, W., 1993).

OI is a condition with a great deal of variety in functional potential within the four main types of the disorder, as categorized by Sillence (1981). The majority of children with this condition who require rehabilitation are those whose symptoms fall under types III and IV, because infants born with type II rarely survive, and those with type I have a very mild form of the condition with few fractures and little growth delay. Because functional potential and ability vary so much within the Sillence categories, the system is not very helpful for planning rehabilitation of the child with OI. Therefore, each child must be viewed from the perspective of individual attributes and clinical features, and the rehabilitation approach formulated specifically for each unique child (Binder, Conway, Hason, et al., 1993; Binder, Conway, & Gerber, 1993).

For children with the most severe forms of OI, rehabilitation approaches include prevention of positional contractures and deformities and promotion of as many functional and developmental activities as possible. Some children with severe contractures either at birth or at a very young age may not be able to tolerate the prone position for therapeutic exercise, but may be able to increase the strength of upper extremities and neck muscles by lying across the caregiver's knee or pushing off from the caregiver's shoulder. Positioning in a custom-molded seating or positioning system may include varying degrees of reclining to support limbs, trunk, and spine without causing undue pressure that might lead to fracture. Active range-of-motion (ROM) exercises, strengthening exercises, and water activities serve to increase strength and enhance joint mobility without causing undue stress (Binder, Conway, & Gerber, 1993). Children with this level of severity tend to be mostly or completely dependent for self-care; may or may not be able to feed themselves or assist with dressing, depending on the degree of upper extremity dysfunction; and generally use an electric wheelchair for mobility (Binder, Conway, & Gerber, 1993).

In children and youths with less severe types of OI, ambulatory potential usually is present but complicated by sitting much of the time and by development of hip flexion contractures and deformities and contractures of the feet and lower legs. Leg-length discrepancies that interfere with walking also may occur. Upper extremity involvement such as contractures and malalignment of the bones of the upper limbs and limited forearm supination interferes with many self-care activities. The short trunk and immobile pelvis make moving to standing from sitting more difficult. Rehabilitation interventions include ROM, stretching, and strengthening exercises, some with weights to the child's tolerance, more physical activities such as swimming and bicycling, and exercises leading to standing and ambulation. Most of these children have capacity for self-care and can perform much of their own self-care and activities of daily living (Binder, Conway, & Gerber, 1993).

Within the two types mentioned above, the child with the least-involved condition accordingly has greater functional potential, due to the presence of less malalignment, contractures, and somewhat less fragile bones. This group of children has increased tolerance for antigravity activities, more strength, and usually is capable of more upright physical activity, endurance, and coordination. However, they still experience contractures, joint laxity, and leg-length discrepancy. Long-distance walking is difficult. Children with OI in this functional group tend to be more age-appropriate in their developmental activities and independent for most aspects of self-care (Binder, Conway, & Gerber, 1993).

Orthotics and bracing are used extensively for children with OI, and may range from shoe lifts to ankle-foot orthoses and long-leg braces. Following surgical procedures, short-term bracing can help the child ambulate more rapidly. Durable medical equipment use depends on the degree of functional ability. More involved children require extensive equipment, including positioning devices, bath chairs, adapted potty chairs, as well as molded seating systems, manual wheelchairs that are pushed by others and, more commonly, self-operated electric wheelchairs (Binder, Conway, & Gerber, 1993; Perrin & Saturen, 1992).

Spinal curvature, including scoliosis, kyphosis, and lordosis, is treated first by bracing and positioning with custom seating systems designed to support the child's back in the most optimal position and to prevent further curvature. Due to the frequently atypical shape of the vertebrae, and damage to the vertebrae due to fractures, spinal curvature in children with OI is particularly challenging to treat and to correct, and tends to be very severe. In individuals who are most severely affected, scoliosis occurs in 80% to 90% of adolescents and adults. Surgery to correct spinal curvature is difficult and fraught with complications that range from respiratory problems due to the unusual shape of the chest, an increased risk of hypothermia during surgery, and poor fixation of plates and screws resulting from the soft bone (Tachdjian, 1990; Cole, W., 1993).

Early intervention for the child with OI is very important and aids in promoting typical development in all domains. Intervention can be very difficult, however, because therapeutic exercise may contribute to fractures. The therapists must be very skillful, knowledgeable of treatments for children with OI, and patient. Therapy generally includes physical and occupational therapy, but may also include speech therapy if there are delays or any sign of deafness (Perrin & Saturen, 1992).

Nursing Interventions

Assessment

Nursing assessment of the child with OI begins with a careful family history that focuses on the presence of any genetic condition, history of frequent fractures, unexplained fetal death in the family, or parents who are of shorter stature than same-gender close relatives. A detailed prenatal history, with particular attention to fetal movement and any prenatal diagnostic testing that was done and why it was done, is helpful. Information about labor and delivery, any fractures noted at birth, and any history of frequent fractures of the child in the first 2 years of life after battered child syndrome has been ruled out is very important. A thorough developmental history of the child helps to rule out other disorders and suggests developmental level and functional status. The parent's emotional and psychologic state should be evaluated, as well as that of other family members and siblings. Families who have undergone wrongful accusations of child abuse often are very stressed and may be mistrustful of health care personnel.

Physical assessment of the child includes the usual parameters for age, as well as careful examination for signs of OI, such as bowed and angulated limbs; grayish or blue sclera; opalescent teeth, especially deciduous teeth in the younger child; signs of hearing deficit, particularly in the older child; and a large, out-of-proportion head. Assessment of joint contractures is also very important. Skin condition, including evidence of bruising, should be assessed, as well as any unusual lesions, which may be indicative of physical abuse, such as welts, burns, lacerations, or abdominal or head injuries, to rule out evidence of child abuse. Head circumference, height, and weight for age are very important in light of the short stature typical of children with OI. Physical assessment should be performed very carefully on children who are suspected of having OI, because even gentle manipulation can cause fractures, especially in the young child. Good head support is imperative to prevent cervical fracture (McCullough & Pellino, 1994).

Functional assessment, including developmental assessment for age, is also an important part of the nursing assessment. Use of any splinting, orthotics, positioning devices, or assistive devices for walking or other mobility must be assessed. Motor milestones are particularly important, as is the level of cognitive development. Despite the physical disability, children with OI generally tend to do very well intellectually and should receive interventions that support cognitive development.

Nursing diagnoses for the child include (1)

impaired adjustment, secondary to the disability; (2) diversional activity deficit related to the enforced immobility of the child during the early stages of extreme bone fragility; (3) altered growth and development, resulting both from the condition and from the often long and repeated hospitalizations for surgical procedures that seriously affect school attendance; (4) impaired mobility as a result of the condition and of frequent and long hospitalization; (5) self-care deficit resulting from the disability may occur if independence and self-care skills are not fostered and assistive devices used judiciously; (6) self-esteem disturbance, which depends on the child's self-perception as well as positive and negative social experiences; and (7) pain, resulting from frequent surgeries, invasive procedures, hospitalizations, and frequent or multiple fractures (McCullough & Pellino, 1994).

Nursing diagnoses that may be applied to the family are (1) knowledge deficit, with regard to the cause and treatment of the disorder, as well as the required care; (2) alteration in participating: noncompliance, resulting from the many devices and treatments that are necessary to treat OI, and which may be difficult or painful to use, as well as from parental experience of inaccurate diagnosis, accusations of child abuse, or insensitive treatment by health care providers; differing values and beliefs between the family and the health care provider may also contribute to this nursing diagnosis; (3) parental anxiety and high risk for fracture can be extremely stressful for the family and prevent it from providing appropriate developmental activities and affection to the child. A good understanding of the child's condition, the treatment options, the family's role in guiding the child's care, and sound instruction as to the use of assistive devices can help to reduce parental anxiety (McCullough & Pellino, 1994).

Nursing Interventions

Pediatric rehabilitation nursing care of the child with OI and family includes supportive care, developmental support, pre- and postsurgical care, functional interventions to promote independence and self-care, and child and family psychosocial support. Service coordination also may be necessary to aid the family in obtaining and managing multiple medical and developmental services. Teaching of the child and family about the condi-

tion, about treatments and treatment options, and about how best to promote the child's independence and adjustment to the disability is an extremely important role of the pediatric rehabilitation nurse.

When the neonate is diagnosed with OI, especially in the absence of any family history, the family may experience a variety of emotions such as guilt, loss of the ideal child, grief, as well as fear and apprehension about the future and their ability to care for this very fragile, very complex infant. However, the birth of a child with a disability or chronic condition is not all sadness and grief, and many families are able to adjust fairly quickly to the child's unanticipated condition and to accept the child as a unique and valued family member. Other relatives, such as grandparents, aunts, uncles, and siblings may have mixed feelings or react very differently from parents. Parents in whom there is a known family history, or who may have OI themselves, may have more knowledge of what to expect from the child and be more able to cope, having dealt with the social stigma. Parents who are also affected by the condition themselves may feel secure about helping the child to adapt to the physical and medical implications of the disability, but may have great concern about providing the correct environment for the child (Cole, D., 1993). Emotional support for families who are going through this process, and ensuring that they are knowledgeable about the options of care for their child, is an important role of the pediatric rehabilitation nurse. The nurse's attitude toward the child and the child's possibilities in life can very much influence the family's attitudes both immediately and in the long term.

Developmental support of the child and anticipatory guidance are interventions that aid the child in gaining as many developmental milestones as possible, and that assist the parents in coping with the child's developmental delays as well as planning for the future. Knowledge of the ways in which the child's condition interacts with achievement of typical developmental milestones adds to the families' ability to plan ahead for the child's needs, to optimize potential. An example of planning ahead involves knowledge of surgical procedures that probably are required in the next 2 years. This information aids the family both in planning family activities around these scheduled events, as well as planning for the child's schooling and the adaptations to the educational plan that may be needed during and after hospitalization. Another example of anticipatory guidance is with regard to the child's mobility. Depending on the type of OI with which the child is diagnosed, and the early developmental milestones that are reached, the likelihood of the type of mobility that will be used by the child can be estimated. In this, the nurse supports, reiterates and, in many cases, helps to interpret the information given by other members of the rehabilitation team, such as the physiatrist and geneticist.

Most children with short stature and OI are perceived by others as immature, younger than their chronological age, or cognitively delayed, but in fact intelligence is not affected. Evaluation of each child's level of maturity and capacities and of emotional or adjustment problems that can result from the child's coping with a very visible impairment is necessary. Both children and families can benefit from assistance in coping with devaluing or infantilizing attitudes on the parts of others. Information on potential intellectual function of the child with OI is very important for parents, school nurses, and other school personnel to hear. The pediatric rehabilitation nurse should emphasize this characteristic, as well as provide a careful assessment of the child's cognitive function.

Children with osteogenesis imperfecta may experience hundreds of fractures throughout their childhood and adolescence, as well as a number of surgical procedures to stabilize the spine and to reinforce and straighten deformed long bones. Pre- and postoperative care includes child and family education about procedures, outcomes, postoperative care, and planning for return to school. Following the procedure, discharge planning with the family, any home care providers who may be involved, and the nurse at the child's school is important to ensure optimum healing, as little delay in completion of schoolwork as possible, and prevention of complications or injuries.

Children with disabilities and chronic conditions who require frequent or numerous surgical procedures throughout their childhood often experience academic difficulties because it is difficult for them to keep up with their peers with so many absences. With OI, children who have frequent fractures also may need to stay home from school and remain immobilized, which increases the risk of academic difficulties. It is critical to the child's achievement that these issues and concerns be considered in the Individualized Educational Plan and that a plan for addressing the child's needs during these periods be included. Academics is not the only area that suffers; children who miss school frequently also may have difficulty making and keeping friends and lack in socialization. Teaching other children in the school and the classroom about the child's disability and assisting other children to see the child as one of them instead of as someone different can aid in the process of socialization and reduce bias.

Teaching the child and family about the condition, about various treatments that are available, and about use and care of assistive devices is critical to the child's development and prevention of complications. At birth, the use of various splinting and positioning orthoses to prevent fractures can be confusing and frightening for parents and caregivers. The careful handling the child requires during this period often is intimidating, as is the guilt experienced by parents or others when a fracture does occur. Explanation that fractures happen frequently and that it is not the fault of the parents or caregiver, and careful instruction regarding how to recognize the fracture as soon as possible and which steps to take can help to alleviate anxiety. The pediatric rehabilitation nurse can be an invaluable ally to the family when problems occur with assistive devices, health problems, or school issues, in providing support for problem solving by the family. As the child grows older and is able to understand treatments and therapies, teaching for the child on these same issues, as well as handling negative feelings resulting from bias or prejudice, is necessary to aid the child in developing independence and coping.

Dental care is also very important, both maintenance of good dental hygiene as well as regular evaluations and treatment of frequent caries, especially in deciduous teeth, that occur with dentinogenesis imperfecta. Even those children who do not appear to have dentinogenesis imperfecta may have abnormalities of dental structures (Paterson, Burns, & McAllion, 1993). The pediatric rehabilitation nurse is in an ideal position to support the family in developing good dental hygiene habits with the child early on and in assisting them to prevent further dental problems through anticipatory guidance, such as discouraging bottle feeding at bedtime for the child who can independently hold a bottle and by encouraging good nutrition.

As the child with OI reaches adolescence,

passing the last major growth spurt, fractures decrease, leaving the child with more stable mobility. During this period, however, scoliosis or kyphosis that has been difficult to control may require surgery to stabilize. The risk of later complications for individuals with more severe types of OI increase, such as neurologic complications. For youth with OI who have less disabling types of the condition, this is a period of relative calm, healthwise.

Social issues become even more important as the youth attempts to disengage from the family and establish independence. Independence for the young person with OI may range from occasional assistance with self-care to employment of a full-time aide. Transition from the school system to the world of work can be more difficult if vocational services have not been available during high school.

Perhaps more challenging is the transition from pediatric health services to adult health services. Many adult health care providers lack the knowledge and experience necessary to provide care for adults with disabilities originating in childhood, or limit patients on Medicaid, which many adults with disabilities originating in childhood receive. In addition, many individuals with these chronic conditions have not survived into adulthood in the past, and little is known of how the condition interacts with the general process of adult development and aging. Many health care providers advocate continuation of pediatric services, both primary care and specialty care, for adults with developmental disabilities or chronic conditions originating in childhood, because these providers are more familiar with both the individual and the condition. One problem with this scenario is that those providers are often not familiar with the usual adult conditions, especially those that accompany aging, and may miss health problems. Transition from pediatric to adult health care for individuals with disabilities and chronic conditions continues to be a problem. Nurses can advocate for health transition services for youth with disabilities and chronic conditions and can collaborate in the development of new and better systems of care.

CASE STUDY

Little Daniel was born at 3 a.m. to his mother, Margaret, who was diagnosed with type IV osteogenesis imperfecta from early childhood. Margaret, who was 29 years old, went through three miscarriages before she was able to carry Daniel to term. Daniel was also diagnosed with OI, but his condition was much worse at birth than his mother's was. Daniel was born by cesarean section, which had been planned based on his mother's diagnosis and his prenatal diagnosis. At birth, he had multiple fractures of the scapulae and upper and lower extremities. Both femurs and tibula/fibula were bowed. On x-ray, his bones were thin and osteoporotic and his skull showed significant wormian bones. His head was disproportionately large and showed the typical configuration of broad forehead, overhanging occiput, and elfin face, and his sclera were blue. At birth, he weighed 5 pounds, 2 ounces and was 10 inches long.

Margaret's OI was fairly mild, although she used a walker and braces due to unequal leg length and significant lower extremity bowing. She was relatively short in stature, at 5 feet 1 inch. Her husband, George, was present at Daniel's birth. George used a wheelchair due to cerebral palsy. Both Margaret and George wanted very much to have a child, and felt they were physically able to provide appropriate care for a child. Prior to Margaret's first attempt to conceive, they had sought genetic counseling and had been advised that Margaret's form of OI was autosomal dominant and that any child would have a 50% chance of acquiring the disorder. When Daniel's type of OI was diagnosed as a subtype of type III, both parents were surprised that it was a different type from Margaret's. Further genetic testing showed a spontaneous mutation in some of Margaret's somatic cells that was passed on to Daniel, resulting in parental mosaicism as the genetic cause of the child's condition. Because of the mosaicism, the chance of a second child having a more severe form of the disorder was greatly increased.

Margaret and George lived in a small town in Wyoming, had traveled to Denver for high-risk obstetric care during the pregnancy, and were staying with Margaret's family. Once Daniel was stabilized, fitted with a padded body splint, and his parents and grandparents were taught his care, Daniel was discharged from the hospital. The nurse in the pediatric rehabilitation clinic provided both parents and grandparents with one-to-one instruction and a variety of hand-outs to refer to at home. She also was available to the parents and grandparents by phone if they had any questions. Margaret and George planned to stay with her parents for the next 6 months to receive more intensive care, therapies, and instruction from the pediatric rehabilitation clinic in Denver.

Although both parents were surprised and somewhat overwhelmed by the severity of Daniel's condition, they were also overjoyed to finally have a child after so many failed pregnancies. They were actively planning for the future and how to best provide for this complicated but very much loved child.

Outcome Evaluation

Assessment of rehabilitation outcomes and rehabilitation nursing outcomes are difficult to measure and to quantify. There is a tendency to measure rehabilitation outcomes by the degree of improvement in functional ability, which is particularly difficult with OI. Continuing fractures, surgical procedures, and resulting changes in bony alignment result in changes in strength and flexibility that may have little to do with the rehabilitation process. Standard measurements such as muscle testing and range of motion are difficult to obtain due to malalignment of joints and lack of the usual bony landmarks. Strength testing is difficult because of the fragility of the bones, so standard techniques are not useful (Binder, Conway, & Gerber, 1993).

Nursing outcomes are even more difficult to measure. As discussed earlier in this book, measurement of rehabilitation nursing outcomes is in its infancy, and measurement of pediatric rehabilitation nursing outcomes is even less advanced. Although standard functional and developmental criteria may be applied to children with OI and their families, more attention could be paid to the long-term outcomes of overall independence, management (if not personal accomplishment) of self-care, self-management of health and health care, and overall quality of life.

Conclusion

Pediatric rehabilitation nursing care of the child with OI is multifaceted, addressing the physical, emotional, social, and functional needs of the child as well as the emotional, psychologic, and social needs of the family. Teaching of the child and family is an important role of the pediatric rehabilitation nurse, in all areas of the child's care and development, and provision of anticipatory guidance to help families plan for what to expect in the future. All children live in the community and in their homes more than in the hospital, and children with OI are no different in this aspect. Comprehensive pediatric rehabilitation nursing care of the child with OI covers the range of health and rehabilitative services and supports available in a variety of settings from hospital, to home, to school, and to independence in the community.

REFERENCES

Binder, H., Conway, A., & Gerber, L. (1993). Rehabilitation approaches to children with osteogenesis imperfecta: A ten-year experience. *Archives of Physical Medicine and Rehabilitation*, 74(4), 386–390.

Binder, H., Conway, A., Hason, S., Gerber, L., Marini, F., Berry, R., & Weintraub, J. (1993). Comprehensive rehabilitation of the child with osteogenesis imperfecta. *American Journal of Medical Genetics*, 45(2), 265–269.

Charnas, L., & Marini, J. (1993). Communicating hydrocephalus, basilar invagination, and other neurologic features in osteogenesis imperfecta. *Neurology*, 43(2), 2603–2608.

Cole, D. (1993). Psychosocial aspects of osteogenesis imperfecta: An update. *American Journal of Medical Genetics*, 45(2), 201–211.

Cole, W. (1993). Early surgical management of severe forms of osteogenesis imperfecta. *American Journal of Medical Genetics*, 45(2), 270–274.

Dent, J., & Paterson, C. (1991). Fractures in early childhood: Osteogenesis imperfecta or child abuse? *Journal of Pediatric Orthopedics*, 11, 184–186.

Lee, J., Gamble, J., Moore, R., & Rinsky, L. (1995). Gastrointestinal problems in patients who have type III osteogenesis imperfecta. *Journal of Bone and Joint Surgery* (American ed.), 77(9), 1352–1356.

McCullough, L. & Pellino, T. (1994). Congenital and developmental disorders. In Maher, A., Salmond, S., & Pellino, T. (Eds.) *Orthopaedic Nursing*. Philadelphia: W. B. Saunders, pp. 617–700.

Paterson, C., Burns, J., & McAllion, S. (1993). Osteogenesis imperfecta: The distinction from child abuse and the recognition of a variant form. *American Journal of Medical Genetics*, 45(2), 187–192.

Perrin, J., & Saturen, P. (1992). Skeletal disorders, musculoskeletal pain, and trauma in children. In Molnar, G (Ed.) *Pediatric Rehabilitation* (2nd ed.). Baltimore: Williams & Wilkins, pp. 455–480.

Raghunath, M., Mackay, K., Dalgleish, R., & Steinmann, B. (1995). Genetic counseling on brittle grounds: Recurring osteogenesis imperfecta due to parental mosaicism for a dominant mutation. *European Journal of Pediatrics*, 154(2), 123–129.

Sillence, D. (1981). Osteogenesis imperfecta: An expanding panorama of variants. *Clinical Orthopaedics and Related Research*, 159, 11–12.

Sillence, B., Butler, B., Latham, M., & Barlow, K. (1993). Natural history of blue sclerae in osteogenesis imperfecta. *American Journal of Medical Genetics*, 45(2), 183–186.

Tachdjian, M. (1990). *Pediatric Orthopedics* (2nd ed.) (Vol. 2). Philadelphia: W. B. Saunders.

Thompson, E. (1993). Non-invasive prenatal diagnosis of osteogenesis imperfecta. *American Journal of Medical Genetics*, 45(2), 201–206.

Verkh, Z., Russell, M., & Miller, C. (1995). Osteogenesis imperfecta type II: Microvascular changes in the CNS. *Clinical Neuropathology*, 14(3), 154–158.

Wang, T., Yang, G., & Alba, A. (1994). Chronic ventilator use in osteogenesis imperfecta congenita with basilar impression: A case report. *Archives of Physical Medicine and Rehabilitation*, 75(6), 699–702.

Wong, R., Follis, F., Shively, B., & Wernly, J. (1995). Osteogenesis imperfecta and cardiovascular diseases. *Annals of Thoracic Surgery*, 60(5), 1439–1443.

Resources

Osteogenesis Imperfecta Foundation, Inc., 804 W. Diamond Ave., Suite 210, Gaithersburg, MD 20878; (800)–981–BONE; fax (301) 947–0456; Internet http://members.aol.com/bonelink/main.htm.

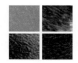

Chapter 17

Alterations in Cardio-respiratory Function

Nancy M. Youngblood

Adequate cardio-respiratory function is critical to survival. Advancements in medical technology during the past two decades have enabled children with congenital or acquired cardio-respiratory dysfunction, who, in the past, could not have survived, to live healthy and longer lives. These children are often faced with monumental physical limitations that require long-term, intense medical interventions to sustain life. Additionally, these children are often candidates for rehabilitation to maximize their cognitive and physical function, thereby giving themselves and their family control, to the degree possible, over their quality of life. It is likely that, regardless of whether the cardiac or respiratory system has the primary dysfunction, both systems are involved. Therefore, treatment is frequently focused on the management of both systems.

The pediatric rehabilitation nurse must be aware of the constant changes that are occurring in the fields of pediatric cardiology and pulmonology and understand cardio-respiratory dysfunctions and their impact on a child who is also experiencing other conditions (e.g., cerebral palsy, muscular dystrophy, myelodysplasia). The cardio-respiratory dysfunctions that are addressed in this chapter are bronchopulmonary dysplasia, asthma, and congenital heart disease.

BRONCHOPULMONARY DYSPLASIA

Bronchopulmonary dysplasia (BPD) is a chronic lung disease that may develop in the lungs of infants, primarily those who are born prematurely. It develops in infants secondary to treatment at birth for other conditions, such as respiratory distress syndrome, meconium aspiration, and persistent pulmonary hypertension. BPD is iatrogenic, caused by the therapies used to treat lung disease: exposure to high oxygen concentrations and use of these therapies, fluid overload, and patent ductus arteriosus. The more immature the infant is at the time of birth, the more susceptible the infant's lungs are to injury. As the survival of infants who are premature and of very low birth weight (i.e., less than 1500 g) continues to increase, the incidence of BPD will also continue to increase (Parker, Lindstrom, & Cotton, 1992).

Etiology and Incidence

The infant who is at greatest risk for BPD is the one born prematurely. The low-birth-weight infant may need mechanical ventilation with high concentrations of oxygen for extended periods of time. It is the combination of low birth weight and mechanical ventilation that results in injury to the immature lung. In neonates weighing less then 1500 g, 20% to 40% develop BPD, and up to 70% of premature infants weighing less than 1000 g develop BPD. Death from complications of BPD occurs in 23% to 40% of those infants with severe BPD (Moores & Abman, 1990). A majority of deaths occur during the first year of life. For infants who survive the initial disease process and recover, pulmonary function abnormalities, such as frequent respiratory exacerbations resulting in hypoxia and susceptibility to infection, are common for the first few years of life (Barnhart & Czervinskes, 1995).

Pathophysiology

The exact mechanism of injury is unclear, although there are several contributing factors, most of which are iatrogenic. BPD is the developing lung's response to acute injury. The injury to the lung is the result of treatments that may be necessary to maintain the life of a premature infant. When an infant is born prematurely, normal lung development is interrupted. The immature lung is then subjected to numerous insults that result in pulmonary changes. Initially, the alveoli do not inflate on inspiration because of low surfactant levels. The alveoli have difficulty expanding, and atelectasis develops. The atelectasis causes decreased lung compliance, which leads to increased airway resistance and air trapping. Decreased compliance requires increased peak pressure and tidal volume to ventilate the infant's lungs. The progressive stages of BPD are demonstrated in Table 17–1.

Diagnostic Criteria

The diagnosis of BPD is usually made based on history, clinical presentation, pulmonary function tests (PFTs), and chest radiographs. PFTs can be used to diagnose BPD but are difficult to obtain in an infant. If PFTs can be performed, the findings in an infant with BPD are increased airway resistance, decreased

Table 17–1 PATHOPHYSIOLOGY OF BRONCHOPULMONARY DYSPLASIA

Immature lungs
↓
Ventilatory support
↓
Inflammation of capillary bed (barotrauma)
↓
Decreased lung function
↓
Alveoli collapse or overinflate
↓
Interstitial emphysema
↓
Right-sided heart failure

Adapted from Betz, C., Hunsberger, M., & Wright, S. (1994). *Family-centered nursing care of children* (2nd ed.). Philadelphia: WB Saunders.

compliance (increased lung stiffness), and increased functional residual capacity.

The need for increased respiratory support is monitored by determining arterial blood gas values and peripheral oxygen saturation values. Treatment is also indicated if serum electrolyte studies reveal an increased bicarbonate level. This finding is associated with chronic respiratory failure.

The chest x-ray film of the infant with long-term or chronic BPD shows interstitial emphysema, which can be either unilateral or bilateral with coarse interstitial markings. The lung fields may be complete "whiteout," which reflects the decrease in lung compliance. The decrease in lung compliance increases pulmonary vascular resistance, thereby increasing the workload of the right side of the heart. This leads to right-sided heart failure or cor pulmonale.

Diagnostic testing for the infant includes the careful monitoring of blood gases or peripheral oxygen saturations to determine the adequacy of respiratory function. The regulation of the respiratory support depends on the evaluation of respiratory function through the measurement of oxygen and carbon dioxide in the blood. As the infant's condition stabilizes and the child is in the chronic phase of the disease, the tests can be performed on a less frequent basis as the infant's condition warrants. Chest radiography is a valuable aid in the management of BPD. A chest x-ray film should be ordered to monitor the progress that the infant is making as well as to identify a recurrence of lung infections. Chest radiography can also be used to monitor the size of the infant's heart and the changes in the right side of the heart related to the lung pathology. Cultures of tracheal secretions can provide information about the type of infection that is present if a respiratory tract infection is suspected. Chest films reveal the characteristic streakiness with areas of hyper-inflation and atelectasis. Electrocardiography and echocardiography may show evidence of right-sided heart hypertrophy secondary to increased pulmonary vascular resistance in severe cases. Echocardiography shows the condition of the valves.

Course

Northway, Rosan, and Porter (1967) first described the course of BPD in four stages. The stages are based on clinical and respiratory findings.

Stage I   occurs in the first 2 or 3 days after birth. The clinical presentation at this time is the same as it is for acute respiratory distress syndrome (RDS). The radiograph will have the "ground glass" appearance.

Stage II   lasts from 4 to 10 days after birth and is a period of regeneration, with repair of necrotic alveolar and bronchial epithelium.

Stage III   occurs at 10 to 20 days and is a period of transition to chronic lung disease. During this period there is increased proliferation, edema, and metaplasia of bronchial epithelium.

Stage IV   occurs after 1 month of age. It is the period of chronic disease in which there is hyperplasia of the smooth muscle in the small airways and pulmonary vessels. The lungs are emphysemic, and the emphysemic lung tissue is interspaced with areas of fibrosis and collapse.

The period of chronic illness may last for several years. The infant may require ventilation and increased oxygen therapy for the first few years after birth. These children have frequent respiratory tract infections requiring hospitalizations. Some infants have marked clinical improvement after 2 years of age, probably owing to intense alveolar multiplication occurring around this time (Wong, 1995). It is common for the infants who survive the first 2 years to have respiratory problems, such as recurrent hypoxic episodes and frequent respiratory tract infections, that persist into late childhood and early adolescence (Abman & Groothius, 1994).

Physical Impact and Evaluation

Because of the impact of the course of the disease on most body systems, these children may have delayed motor development, poor growth, and lethargy. Neurodevelopmental disabilities in infants with BPD are fairly common. Cerebral palsy is the major impairment seen.

These infants also have growth retardation and may be in the 5th to 25th percentile for age. The below-average growth percentiles may persist throughout childhood. Altered growth may adversely affect the long-term outcomes of infants with BPD. The lack of adequate nutrition impairs lung growth and development. The infants with poor growth rates commonly have persistent hypoxemia. Altered growth can also develop because of poor caloric intake resulting from adverse

oral stimulation from endotracheal or nasogastric tubes and frequent suctioning. Gastrostomy may be necessary to provide necessary nourishment. Therapists who specialize in oral motor feeding problems, such as speech therapists, occupational therapists, and nurses, intervene with infants who have the feeding problems. Registered dietitians are also a necessary part of the management team. These infants may have problems with gastroesophageal reflux, which often accompanies chronic lung disease (Abman & Groothius, 1994).

Functional Limitations

The infant or child with BPD has the limitations related to the neurodevelopmental problems that result from prematurity and the hypoxia that results from the BPD disease process. These infants may be globally developmentally delayed and need therapeutic intervention for some time after birth. Premature infants are at risk for severe developmental delays. These infants have twice the normal incidence of learning and behavior problems (McCormick, Gormaker, & Sobol, 1990). When assessed at 8 years, the overall incidence of severe disability in the low-birth-weight infant is about 18% compared with 3% in the normal population (Victorian Infant Collaborative Study Group, 1991). It is not unusual for these children to have more than one disability. More of these children have cerebral palsy, impaired vision, hearing impairment, and mental retardation.

The infants are often cared for in the home by their families, regardless of the level of advanced technology, care, and therapy that they need. The use of respiratory support such as oxygen therapy and ventilation can be provided in the home. The parents must be prepared to care for the child at home through an in-depth educational program. Management of home oxygen therapy is stress provoking, but most families become comfortable with the equipment and can manage the child at home. Home nursing for follow-up, coordination of care, and education is critical during the transition and acute illnesses.

Because of their functional limitations, these children benefit from individual therapy and early intervention programs. The infants should begin a program as soon as possible and maintain it even after discharge from the hospital. The early intervention programs can incorporate a number of different strategies. The infant can receive treatment at home, or, if possible, the infant can be transported to a child development center where the child receives multidisciplinary therapy with a 1:3 to 1:4 ratio of teachers to students (Batshaw & Perret, 1992).

Therapeutic Management

Infants with BPD have significant growth, nutritional, neurodevelopmental, and cardio-respiratory problems. Clinical management of the infant must focus on the simultaneous management of several problems. The major therapeutic modalities are mechanical ventilation, oxygenation, chest physiotherapy, medication therapy, nutritional management, support of growth and development, and home management.

Mechanical Ventilation

Most infants who develop BPD are born prematurely and require mechanical ventilation immediately after birth (Conte, 1992). After being placed on a ventilator the infant is at risk for BPD. As the infant develops BPD, positive-pressure ventilation is required for prolonged periods of time. Some infants with BPD require a tracheostomy. A tracheostomy will decrease the risk for airway scarring due to translaryngeal intubation and allow for greater patient comfort for the infant who must be ventilated for long periods of time (Abman & Groothius, 1994). Additionally, a tracheostomy reduces the amount of noxious oral stimulus that can result in feeding difficulties when the infant is ready to take food by mouth.

The goal is to remove an infant from the ventilator as soon as the child can tolerate weaning. However, the treatment team may decide to prolong the ventilator support with slow weaning, which will allow the infant an opportunity to grow and not use most of the caloric intake to support respiratory effort.

Oxygenation

The severity of lung disease determines the need for supplemental oxygen therapy. The lung damage that occurs with BPD prevents the exchange of gases resulting in marked hypoxemia. Supplemental oxygen is required to maintain the PaO_2 greater than 50 mm Hg. As the infant's condition improves, the amount of supplemental oxygen can be decreased. The level of supplemental oxygen should be such that the blood oxygen saturation is greater than 90% (Jackson & Saunders, 1993). The oxygen saturation can be monitored by pulse oximetry continuously or intermittently depending on the infant's level of activity. It is common practice to do intermittent monitoring during the time that the infant is awake and continuous monitoring when the infant is asleep.

Oxygen can be administered by mask, nasal cannula, oxygen tent, or oxygen hood.

Mask: The infant can breathe through the nose or mouth because the mask covers most of the face. Oxygen concentrations can be administered within a fairly accurate range. The problem with the mask is that it is very difficult to keep on the face of a small infant.

Nasal cannula: The infant can receive oxygen and continue activities such as playing and eating without significant interference. The problem with the nasal cannula is that it is difficult to control oxygen concentrations if the infant breathes through the mouth.

Oxygen tent: The infant can receive a constant flow of oxygen regardless of the infant's activity. The problems with the oxygen tent are the environment is cold and damp, the infant must stay in bed, and an active infant may crawl out of the plastic cover.

Oxygen hood: The infant can receive high concentrations of oxygen when in the hood. It is also easier to see the rest of the infant's body. The difficulty with the hood is the fact that it needs to be removed for care such as suctioning and the oxygen concentrations can drop dramatically.

Chest Physiotherapy

Infants with BPD produce large amounts of thick secretions. Chest physiotherapy (CPT) is a procedure that facilitates the drainage and clearance of these secretions. Chest percussion, vibration, and postural drainage are effective procedures that facilitate the removal of secretions. CPT may be most beneficial in the early morning, before meals, and before sleep. The procedures can be stressful to the infant and increase the need for oxygen. A careful assessment should be performed before chest physiotherapy is started so the infant's response can be monitored. Chest physiotherapy should be adjusted for the child's developmental age. Small children may be placed on a pillow or on the nurse's lap, and an older child can be placed in different positions on the bed (Fig. 17–1). Also, depending on the child's condition, the procedure may need to be modified. Therapy should be done to the child's tolerance level (Wong, 1995).

Medication Therapy

Long-term management of infants with BPD often includes treatment with multiple drugs. Medical management is aimed at the promotion of bronchodilation, control of the pulmonary inflammatory changes, and the control of cor pulmonale. Inhaled bronchodilators are used in ventilated and in spontaneously breathing infants. Several agents can lower airway resistance and improve lung function. Commonly used inhaled bronchodilators include albuterol, metaproterenol (Alupent), and isoetharine.

Systemic corticosteroids may be used to reverse the inflammatory process found in BPD. Corticosteroids are beneficial during acute respiratory illness and may facilitate the weaning process. Long-term treatment with corticosteroids has resulted in significant side effects; therefore, therapy should not exceed 5 days. Diuretics are commonly used in the long-term management of recurrent pulmonary edema in BPD and cor pulmonale in children with BPD. The diuretics include furosemide, chlorothiazide or hydrochlorothiazide, and spironolactone. Frequent or high doses of diuretic therapy have significant side effects, such as volume depletion, chloride deficiency, hypokalemia, and metabolic alkalosis. Fluid balance, electrolytes, and acid-base balance must be monitored. Potassium chloride replacement therapy is usually required. Spironolactone is often added to the treatment regimen because it is a potassium-sparing diuretic.

Table 17–2 is a summary of the medications used in the treatment of BPD.

Nutritional Management

Children with BPD are very sensitive to excessive amounts of fluid intake. The inability of these children to handle extra fluid results in pulmonary edema. These children are on severe fluid restrictions to reduce pulmonary edema. Because of the need to restrict fluids it is difficult to provide adequate nutritional intake. Caloric requirements in children with BPD are higher than their peers, up to 150 to 200 kcal/kg/day (Jackson & Saunders, 1993).

Total parenteral nutrition may be necessary to provide the necessary nutrition for these infants. High-calorie formulas are given to promote nutritional intake while maintaining fluid restrictions. These children may have an oral aversion and delayed oral motor skills. It is necessary for them to have intensive work with the therapist. The child who is difficult to feed by mouth may require gastrostomy feedings.

Support of Growth and Development

The infant with BPD is premature and requires hospitalization for long periods of time, which contributes to developmental delay. The delays often are motor and cognitive but can be global. Early intervention stimulation programs are critical to the management of these delays. The pediatric rehabilitation nurse is in a position to perform frequent assessments of the growth and development of the child. If the child does not grow and develop at an expected rate, interventions must be implemented that address these issues. See Chapter 10 for more specific information on growth and development.

Home Management

Caring for a child with BPD at home can provide a supportive environment that will facilitate the child's growth and development. The family and child can develop bonds that achieve positive relationships. Additionally, home care is considered to be a more cost-effective way to care for these children. In spite of the benefits of home care, home care can be very stressful for the family. The family routine is dramatically altered, and family members must make many adjustments to existing lifestyles. The child with BPD may need large areas of space for equipment and storage of supplies (see Teaching Topic: Oxygen Administration in the Home). Sleeping areas may be rearranged, and siblings may have to share space that was previously the dominion of one child. Living areas that were shared by family members may have to be converted into a space that is used for the child with BPD. When nursing care is provided, family members will have to adjust to having people who they do not know caring for their child and sharing their private moments. Additional information on family-centered nursing care can be found in Chapter 9.

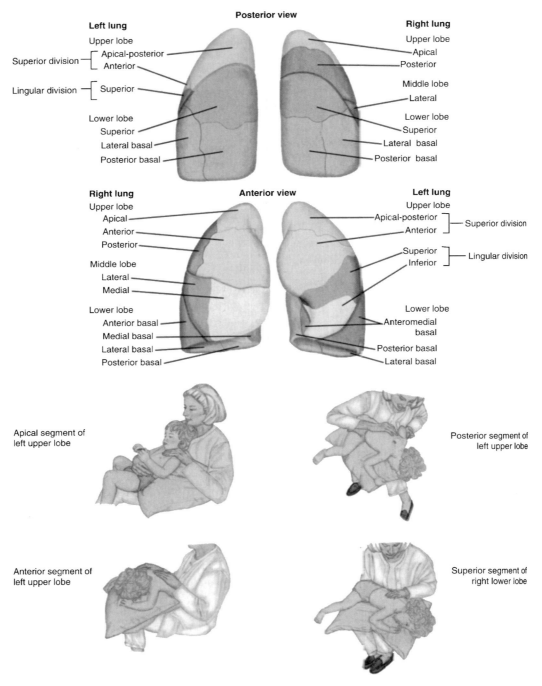

Figure 17-1 Chest physiotherapy for an infant or small child. (From Ashwill, J.W., Droske, S.C. (1997). *Nursing care of children*. Philadelphia: WB Saunders, pp. 474–475.)

Application of the Nursing Process

Assessment

Assessment of the child with BPD should begin with a thorough history to evaluate the pre-natal and post-natal course and the severity of the disease. Past treatments and responses to the treatment should be recorded, including any that were used to manage respiratory dysfunction, such as tracheostomy or

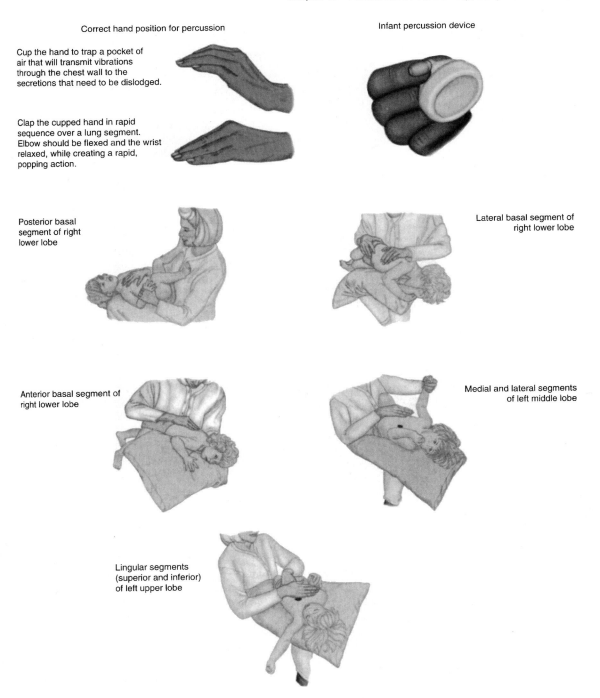

Correct hand position for percussion

Cup the hand to trap a pocket of air that will transmit vibrations through the chest wall to the secretions that need to be dislodged.

Clap the cupped hand in rapid sequence over a lung segment. Elbow should be flexed and the wrist relaxed, while creating a rapid, popping action.

Infant percussion device

Posterior basal segment of right lower lobe

Lateral basal segment of right lower lobe

Anterior basal segment of right lower lobe

Medial and lateral segments of left middle lobe

Lingular segments (superior and inferior) of left upper lobe

Figure 17–1   *Continued*

mechanical ventilation. The medications that have been prescribed for the infant in the past and current medical management should be indicated. The current physical status and medical management should be obtained from the infant's caregiver. The data that are necessary for the development of a plan of care for the infant include feeding problems, oxygen requirements, pharmacologic support, activity tolerance, growth and development issues, other medical conditions, and home equipment utilization.

Respiratory assessment of the infant with BPD should include examination of the respi-

Table 17–2 MEDICATIONS USED IN THE TREATMENT OF BRONCHOPULMONARY DYSPLASIA

Classification	Name	Side Effects
Diuretics	Furosemide (Lasix), 1–4 mg/kg/day in one to two divided doses	Photosensitivity, hearing loss, excessive diuresis, fluid or electrolyte imbalance, gastrointestinal upset, vertigo, orthostatic hypotension
	Chlorothiazide (Diuril), 15–30 mg/kg/day in two divided doses	Electrolyte disorders (esp. hypokalemia), hyperglycemia, orthostatic hypotension, photosensitivity
	Spironolactone (Aldactone), 2–4 mg/kg/day	Hyperkalemia, confusion, hyponatremia, gynecomastia, headache, rash, gastric ulcers
Bronchodilators	Beta-adrenergic agonists (Albuterol): inhalation 2 puffs every 4–6 hours	Tachycardia, hypertension, anaphylaxis, tremor, headache, insomnia, paradoxical bronchospasm, local irritation
	Anticholinergics: ipratropium (Atrovent), 0.02–0.1 mL/kg/dose every 4–6 hours	Exacerbation of symptoms, nervousness, dizziness, gastrointestinal upset, headache, palpitations
	Methylxanthines: theophylline, 4–6 mg/kg every 6 hours	Dysrhythmias, nausea, headache, irritability, restlessness, tachypnea, diuresis
Anti-inflammatory agents	Corticosteroids: prednisone, 1 to 2 mg/kg for 3 to 5 days of acute exacerbations	Hypothalamic-pituitary-adrenal axis suppression, masks infection, hypokalemia, hypocalcemia, peptic ulcer, dermal atrophy
	Cromolyn sodium (Intal) inhaled, nonsteroidal anti-inflammatory agent, 20 mg two to four times per day	Throat irritation, anaphylaxis, nasal congestion

Adapted from Bernbaum, J.E., Friedmon, S., Hoffman-Williamson, M., et al. (1989). Preterm infant care after hospital discharge. *Pediatrics in Review,* 10, 195–208. Reproduced by permission of *Pediatrics in Review.*

ratory rate, work of breathing, color, and breath sounds (Brown & Swannson, 1993).

Respiratory rate: The infant with BPD may normally have an increased rate because of restrictive lung disease. It is necessary to obtain a baseline rate so that changes can be identified. An increased respiratory rate is an indication of worsening respiratory status. Tachypnea may be an early sign of distress. Other factors, such as activity and elevated body temperature, can elevate the respiratory rate and should also be evaluated to determine the cause of the increased rate.

Work of breathing: As respiratory rate increases, the work of breathing is increased. The work of breathing is manifested by such signs as nasal flaring, retractions, or grunting.

Color: Cyanosis occurs when there is insuf-

ficient oxygen in the blood. Although cyanosis is usually a late sign of hypoxia, a baseline assessment should be made to determine if the presence of cyanosis is a significant finding, because many of these children are normally slightly cyanotic. If this is a new condition, it requires prompt attention on the part of the caregiver to ensure adequate respiratory function.

Breath sounds: The infant with significant reactive airways may present with wheezing. The onset of wheezing or an increase in baseline could indicate a worsening condition. Grunting is another sound that can be heard in the chest. It generally indicates an increase in respiratory distress. Fluid overload and pulmonary edema are manifested by the presence of rales, wheezing, and increased work of breathing.

Other signs of a worsening respiratory condition are activity intolerance and poor feeding, which are nonspecific signs of worsening hypoxia. Clubbing of the fingers is a sign that indicates chronic hypoxia. Cardiac function should be assessed because the heart rate during rest can indicate the effect of the BPD on cardiac function. Perfusion should be appraised by determining capillary refilling time, pulses, and skin temperature. Peripheral edema can indicate right-sided heart failure secondary to pulmonary vasoconstriction.

The infant's developmental level should be assessed. The assessment should include the infant's ability to interact with the environment and caregivers. Activity intolerance usually is noted in infants with BPD because of the inability of the lungs to meet the increased oxygen demands that result from increased activity.

The infant's feeding patterns should be assessed. The time that it takes for the infant to eat and the type and amount of food that the infant takes in should be recorded. The infant's behavior after feeding is significant in addition to any special positioning that may be required during or after feeding. The infant should be weighed and measured for height. These measurements should be compared with previous data to determine if the infant is growing at an appropriate rate. Assessment of nutritional status is important because adequate intake is critical for the growth and development of these fragile children. The balance between the caloric need for respiratory work must be maintained with the caloric need for growth. Table 17–3 is the plan of care for the nutritional needs of a child with BPD.

Nursing Diagnoses

Based on the assessment data, the following nursing diagnoses may apply to the family and infant with BPD.

- Ineffective Airway Clearance related to reactive airways and poor cough
- Activity Intolerance related to chronic hypoxia
- Impaired Gas Exchange related to reactive airways and airway inflammation
- Inability to Sustain Spontaneous Ventilation related to respiratory muscle fatigue
- Altered Growth and Development related to chronic hypoxia and decreased nutrition
- Anxiety related to knowledge deficit of home oxygen therapy, bronchodilator administration, and diuretics
- Altered Nutrition: Less than body requirements related to decreased oral intake
- Ineffective Family Coping related to chronic illness
- Social Isolation related to time spent in the infant's care
- Altered Home Management related to necessary care of a child with a chronic illness

Planning and Intervention

Based on the history and nursing assessment of a child with BPD and family, the following should be included in the nursing plan of care.

Table 17–3   NURSING PLAN OF CARE

Nursing Diagnosis: Nutrition, Altered: Less than body requirements

Related to: Intake of nutrients insufficient to meet metabolic needs

Goals	Nursing Interventions/Teaching
Increase caloric intake	Review factors that may prevent adequate intake. Note pattern of food tolerance. Assess weight. Provide diet modifications as indicated.
Promote a therapeutic environment to decrease stress	Provide primary caregivers to feed child. Maintain a calm environment. Develop a structured routine.

Expected Outcomes

Demonstrate progressive weight gain toward goal
Be free of signs of malnutrition
Tolerate increased amount of calories and food

Provide a balance between rest and activity.

Assess respiratory status for changes or distress.

Assess the child's response to respiratory treatments.

Monitor fluid intake and output.

Administer nutritional support and monitor the infant's response to feedings.

Weigh and monitor for rapid weight gain or loss.

Maintain growth records.

Administer chest physiotherapy and monitor infant's response to treatment.

Administer and monitor the effects of medications.

Provide developmentally appropriate visual, auditory, and tactile stimulation.

Promote infant-parent bonding.

Teach caregivers the procedures that are necessary to care for the child.

Evaluate the child's response to interventions.

Evaluation

Periodically, the nurse and family evaluate the outcomes of care given. The nurse needs to evaluate the infant's respiratory status and the effectiveness of respiratory therapies. The child needs to be evaluated to determine if developmental milestones have been facilitated. The interventions directed at nutritional support are evaluated. The child should be evaluated to determine if there is adequate weight gain and if the child is getting enough rest. Fluid intake and output should be evaluated to determine if the child is dehydrated or if the child is at risk for fluid overload. The parents' participation in infant care and their need for continuing education are evaluated.

As the evaluation of the effectiveness of interventions is carried out, the child's progress toward expected outcomes is established. If the outcomes have not been achieved, then the plan must be revised to reflect new interventions that will facilitate achievement of goals.

Conclusion

Many advances have occurred in the management of infants with BPD over the past 25 years (Abman & Groothius, 1994). However, BPD remains a significant complication for children who are born prematurely. More infants are surviving, but the complications that

---

> **Teaching Topic: Oxygen Administration in the Home**
>
> **Important Areas:**
> Maintaining adequate concentration
> Administer with humidity to prevent drying of the mucous membranes
> Schedule for changing and cleaning equipment
> Proper storage of clean equipment
> Safe storage of oxygen
> Phone number of equipment supplier

result from BPD can affect the child and family's quality of life for an extended period of time. Thus, as health care has improved the survival rate for the infant with BPD, the management of the chronic health problems remains a continuing challenge. The infants who are surviving are medically fragile and in need of high-technology care. The case study that follows is an example of a situation with a child with BPD.

The survival rate for infants with BPD has increased significantly. Survival means that infants are medically fragile and in need of sophisticated technologic equipment to sustain life. The care of these infants is moving rapidly into the home setting. The role of the nurse has expanded from the provision of care to the infant to the education and support of the caregivers who manage the infant in the home setting.

CASE STUDY

Richard is an 18-month-old boy with BPD. He was born at 28 weeks' gestation to a G2P1102, 20-year-old woman. After birth, Richard was placed on a ventilator with high oxygen concentrations. At 1 month of age he received a tracheostomy. Richard was weaned from the ventilator at 1 year of age and is currently on 25% oxygen with humidification through a trach collar. He does not take food by mouth but is fed through a gastrostomy tube. Richard is ready for discharge to his home, to be cared for by his mother who is 6 months pregnant with her third child. She has not visited Richard on a consistent basis and has not learned his care or how to manage his equipment.

You are coordinating Richard's care for the transition to home. Your priorities are to ensure a safe home environment and to teach Richard's mother how to care for him so he will grow and develop and eventually be able to attend school. You begin by focusing on a plan for preparing the mother for the pending discharge. Areas to stress are:

- Evaluating the mother's feelings about taking the child home and having a new baby to care for
- Developing a contract with the mother to ensure that she visits enough times to learn the necessary care of the child
- Having the mother do all of the procedures independently at least three times
- Having the mother identify a backup person who will learn all of the child's care in case the mother is unable to care for the child
- Requesting that the interdisciplinary team make decisions about the extent of the need for outpatient therapy so that a schedule can be developed that is convenient for the mother to ensure that she is compliant with it

Continued evaluation will be necessary to provide safe adequate care for Richard.

ASTHMA

Asthma is a common disease of childhood, and its incidence seems to be on the rise. Asthma is a lung disease that is characterized by reversible airway obstruction, inflammation of the airways, and increased airway responsiveness to a variety of stimuli.

Etiology and Incidence

Asthma is a common chronic disease. It is estimated that between 9 and 12 million persons in the United States have this disease. The incidence, severity, and mortality associated with asthma have risen steadily throughout the past 20 years. The prevalence rate for asthma has increased 38% from 6.8 million to 10.3 million from 1980 to 1990 (Bloomberg & Strunk, 1992). The increase in statistics may be the result of increasing air pollution and other contaminates in the environment. Asthma is the most common disease of childhood (Murphy & Kelly, 1993). Males predominate over females younger than the age of 10 years, but the incidence of the disease be-

comes approximately equal by the early teen years, and incidence in women becomes greater thereafter (Wong, 1995).

Airway hyper-responsiveness is almost always present in individuals with asthma. Viral upper respiratory tract infections are commonly associated with increased airway hyperactivity, but the relationship to this event in the induction of an asthmatic response is poorly understood. Air pollutants can precipitate an attack in an asthmatic person, but it is unknown if air pollution causes the disease. Both active and passive smoking may also predispose subjects to the development of asthma. Children with asthma improve by the time they reach adulthood; however, an early onset of disease is associated with a less favorable prognosis.

Pathophysiology

The primary characteristic of asthma is airway hyper-responsiveness. A number of stimuli—physical, chemical, and pharmacologic—can cause the hyperactivity. The primary immune mechanism of asthma involves the association of antigen IgE bound to the cell surfaces, which triggers the release of histamine and a variety of other factors that promote both bronchospasm and local inflammation. Histamine increases the leakage of protein and fluid from the venules, increasing airway secretions, and can stimulate irritant receptors in the airway walls. This, in turn, leads to reflex vagal release of acetylcholine near smooth muscles, promoting bronchospasm. Once the cycle is started, there is an accumulation of tenacious secretions, which may further decrease the diameter of airways. Bronchoconstriction increases airway resistance to air flow. Increased resistance in the airway causes forced expiration through narrowed lumens. The volume of trapped air in the lungs increases. As the severity of asthma increases, the airways close at higher residual volumes. This gas trapping forces the individual to breathe at a higher lung volume. The elastic work of breathing is increased, and the mechanical efficiency of the respiratory muscles is decreased. More energy is expended to overcome the tension of already stretched elastic lung tissues. The expenditure of effort causes fatigue, decreased respiratory effectiveness, and increased oxygen consumption and cardiac output at a time when respiratory functions are already compromised (Wong, 1995).

Bronchial changes related to asthma are shown in Figure 17–2.

Extrinsic asthma is the type of asthma that is the anaphylactic type 1 immune reaction to one or more allergens. Asthma that is unrelated to atopic predisposition or to specific environmental antigens is designated as intrinsic. Pollens, molds, house dust, and animal danger are common antigens. Antigens associated with skin mites are the principal factors in household dust that cause allergic reactions. Cockroaches are a common cause of asthma, particularly in economically disadvantaged urban areas. Exposure to specific foods and additives such as sulfites can induce serious attacks. Intrinsic asthma attacks can be triggered by a wide variety of nonspecific stimuli, including cold air, perfume, smoke, and sulfur dioxide. Vigorous exercise is not infrequently followed by asthmatic symptoms in asthmatics. Intrinsic and extrinsic factors that can trigger an asthmatic attack are listed in Table 17–4.

Clinical Manifestations

The classic manifestations are dyspnea, wheezing, and coughing. An asthmatic episode usually begins with feeling of irritability and restlessness. There may also be a feeling of tightness in the chest. The respiratory symptoms progress to a hacking, nonproduc-

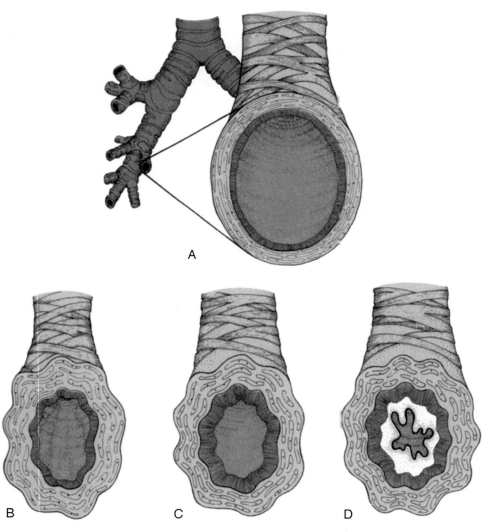

A

B   C   D

Figure 17–2 Bronchial changes related to asthma. (From Betz, C.L., Hunsberger, M.M., Wright, S. (1994). *Family-centered nursing care of Children*, 2nd edition. Philadelphia: WB Saunders, p. 1231.)

Table 17–4 TRIGGERS THAT PRECIPITATE AND/OR AGGRAVATE ASTHMATIC EXACERBATIONS

Allergens: grass, trees, molds, pollen, dust mites, cockroach antigen

Irritants: tobacco smoke, wood smoke, perfumes, atmospheric changes, respiratory tract infections, allergic rhinitis

Exercise: strenuous and associated with shortness of breath

Emotional factors

Gastroesophageal reflux

tive cough caused by the irritation from bronchial edema. Accumulating secretions, acting as a foreign body, stimulate the cough to become productive. As the secretions become more profuse, the cough becomes rattling and productive of frothy, gelatinous sputum. Coughing may be so severe that the child becomes exhausted.

Wheezing is the most common physical finding in asthma and is usually audible during both inspiration and expiration. The child is frequently short of breath. As the child tries to breathe more deeply, the expiratory phase becomes prolonged. The child may be pale, with progressive cyanosis of the mucous membranes and fingernails. Children may assume an upright sitting position to ease the work of breathing. The child speaks with panting phrases. The child may perspire, and the degree of the perspiration is indicative of the seriousness of the attack.

Status asthmaticus is a term used to identify children who continue to display respiratory distress despite vigorous treatment. It is a medical emergency that can result in respiratory failure and death.

Diagnostic Assessment

Laboratory studies include a complete blood cell count and sputum analysis for eosinophilia or elevated serum IgE. Eosinophilia is common regardless of whether allergic factors can be shown to have an etiologic role. In many asthmatics, the degree of eosinophilia may correlate with the asthma's severity. Multiantigen radioallergosorbent test (RAST) has been developed to screen children younger than age 7 years for atopic disease. Skin testing for specific antibodies to common allergens can also contribute to the diagnosis of asthma. Sputum in a child with uncomplicated asthma is highly distinctive. It is tenacious, rubbery, and whitish. If an infection is present, it is yellow. Microscopically, eosinophilia are numerous and arranged in sheets. Large numbers of histiocytes and polymorphonuclear leukocytes are present.

Pulmonary function test results will be abnormal. In assessing respiratory function, the parameters most often measured include lung volumes, flows, times, volumes, and airway reactivity. Spirometry can generally be performed reliably on children older than age 4 years. A key measurement is the peak expiratory flow rate, which is the greatest flow velocity that can be obtained during a forced expiration.

Determination of arterial blood gases and pH is essential to reveal hypoxemia and hypocapnia. Blood gases are particularly valuable in determining the need for hospitalization. Chest x-ray findings vary from normal to hyperinflated. Lung markings are increased in chronic disease. Atelectasis in the right middle lobe is common in children.

Course

Remissions and exacerbations are characteristic of asthma. During remission the children may be essentially asymptomatic, but in more severe forms of the disease some bronchospasm may persist even between attacks.

Physical Impact

Children with asthma are often excluded from exercise because of their general state of fatigue and the fear that exercise will induce an attack. This can seriously hamper normal physical and psychological development. The child with asthma may experience an attack related to physical exercise. The child is often discouraged from participation in physical activity by parents, teachers, and medical personnel. Because physical activity is a major form of activity for children, limitation of physical activity limits the child's ability to interact with the peer group. As the child becomes more isolated, the more difficult it will be for the child to become involved with peers in any activity. Functional limitations are usually attributed to the shortness of breath and muscle fatigue related to the work of breathing.

Therapeutic Management

The overall goal of asthma management is to prevent disability and to minimize physical and psychological morbidity. The child with asthma should have as happy and normal a life as possible. The child should be able to attend school and pursue recreational interests. Treatment is based on the following principles.

Treatment requires a continuous-care approach to prevent exacerbations.

Prevention of exacerbations is an important goal of therapy. This includes avoidance of factors that will bring on an attack and the use of medications as needed.

Therapy during an acute attack should be directed at reduction of inflammation and management of airway narrowing.

Asthma therapy includes pharmacologic therapy, environmental control, and patient education (National Heart, Lung, and Blood Institute, 1991).

Medication Therapy

The goal of pharmacologic treatment is to reduce inflammation and prevent bronchoconstriction. Treatment should be provided in accordance with the severity and chronicity of the disorder. The classifications of the medications include anti-inflammatory, bronchodilator, and anticholinergic.

Anti-inflammatory: Corticosteroids are the most effective anti-inflammatory drugs in reducing bronchial hyperactivity (National Heart, Lung, and Blood Institute, 1991). Corticosteroids may be administered parenterally, orally, or by aerosol. Intravenous administration is particularly valuable in patients with severe episodes of asthma. These drugs may not have an effect for 12 hours, so it is accepted practice to administer these drugs as soon as possible. High doses are recommended until peak flow returns to baseline and then taper over 1 to 2 weeks. Oral glucocorticoids can be used in home management with appropriate tapering schedules. Aerosolized corticosteroids are used to exert maximal local activity while minimizing absorption and systemic effects.

Cromolyn (disodium cromoglycate) is the best nonsteroidal anti-inflammatory drug for asthma (National Heart, Lung, and Blood Institute, 1991). The exact mechanism of how it works is not known, but it may inhibit mast cell degranulation. It is helpful in some children but does not work in others. It is not usually used in an acute attack because the response to this medication may take up to 2 months.

Bronchodilators: Beta-adrenergic agonists (primarily albuterol, metaproterenol, and terbutaline) are the medications of choice for treatment of acute exacerbations and exercised-induced asthma. They can be given by inhalation (see Teaching Topic: Use of Inhaled Medication) or as oral or parenteral preparations. The inhaled bronchodilators are the most commonly used medication in the treatment of a child with asthma. The inhaled drug can be administered by metered-dose inhaler or nebulizer.

Anticholinergic Drugs: Anticholinergic drugs (atropine or ipratropium [Atrovent]) work by reducing the intrinsic vagal tone to the airways and blocking bronchoconstriction. These drugs are not widely used because of the length of time for onset and the side effects such as drying of respiratory secretions, blurred vision, and central nervous system stimulation.

Other Medications: Methylxanthines (theophylline, aminophylline) are considered third-line agents and may not be very helpful in the management of asthma. It is a relatively weak bronchodilator. The drugs may be given intravenously, intramuscularly, orally, or rectally. The drug is also available in sustained-release form for oral ingestion. Theophylline is a central respiratory stimulant and increases respiratory muscle contractility.

Allergen Control

The goal of nonpharmacologic therapy is prevention and reduction of the child's exposure to allergens and irritants. The child's environment must be controlled so that the child has limited exposure to allergens. Once the child has been tested and the specific allergens identified, allergens must be removed or the child prevented from coming in contact with the allergen. This involves intense education of the child and family. The parents must understand the necessary modification that must be made to the home environment. If the child is allergic to dust mites, everything that can harbor mites must be removed from the home. That includes curtains, rugs, blinds, and possibly picture frames. The child may need to have bedding covered with protective covers to prevent contact with dust and dust mites. If the child has problems with cigarette smoke, smoking should not be allowed in the house. Perfumes, strongly scented soaps, and cleaning products should not be used in the home; and the child should not be taken to an environment that would result in exposure to these products. Family pets may need to be removed from the home. Nonspecific factors that may trigger an episode, such as extremes of temperature, are sometimes controlled by dehumidifiers or air conditioners.

Hyposensitization

The role of hyposensitization in childhood asthma has not been clarified. In cases in which the child has many allergies, this type of treatment would be impractical because of the large volume that would have to be injected. Immune therapy should only be considered in children whose asthma is difficult to control. Additionally, immune therapy should not be considered for allergens that can be removed from the environment. A small amount of the allergen is injected subcutaneously. The amount is increased on a weekly basis depending on the size of the reaction. When tolerance is achieved, injections are then given at 4-week intervals and successful treatment is continued for a minimum of 3 years and then stopped. If no symptoms appear, acquired immunity is said to be retained. If symptoms recur, treatment is reinstituted.

Physical Therapy

Physical therapy is directed at teaching the child breathing exercises and relaxation techniques. The latter can be helpful in the management of severe attack, because panic and anxiety may worsen the situation. The ability to relax will help the child control hyperventilation, which leads to a worsening of the condition.

The physical endurance of a child with asthma is generally affected, and excessive exercise may facilitate breathing difficulties. This child needs an exercise that begins with short exercise periods and slowly builds so that the child's physical endurance is strengthened. The child should also be taught how to manage exercise and problems that

result from exercise, possibly by taking a bronchodilator before exercise.

Application of the Nursing Process

Assessment

An adequate assessment of the asthmatic child is critical to determine the health status of the child and the appropriate interventions. A detailed history is an important first step in the assessment process. A history of atopic disease in the child or other family members is a common finding. A history of allergic reactions is often found in family members. Other data that are important in a health history are the onset of symptoms, progression of the attack, and treatment that relieves the attack. Often the child and family can identify the known triggers and the amount of exposure necessary to precipitate an attack.

The physical assessment should begin with an inspection by standing in front of the child and assessing the child's sitting position and any signs of respiratory distress. The degree of respiratory effort should be determined. Auscultation of the chest is performed to determine alterations in air flow. Wheezing is a common sound and signifies obstruction, and the phase of the respiratory cycle where it is most present should be noted. Decreased wheezing in the presence of increased work of breathing indicates a severe asthmatic condition and an almost complete airway obstruction.

Cardiovascular assessment includes evaluation of heart rate, blood pressure, systemic perfusion, and pulsus paradoxus. Pulsus paradoxus is present when the systolic blood pressure taken during inspiration is more than 15 mm Hg below the systolic pressure during expiration.

Level of consciousness should be evaluated. Children with respiratory distress are restless and agitated as the result of systemic hypoxia. Lethargy is a sign of hypercapnia.

Nursing Diagnoses

Based on assessment data the following nursing diagnoses may apply to the family and child with asthma.

- Activity Intolerance related to reactive airways
- Ineffective Airway Clearance related to reactive airways
- Decreased Cardiac Output related to changes in intrapleural pressure

- Impaired Gas Exchange related to reactive airways
- Inability to Sustain Spontaneous Ventilation related to respiratory muscle fatigue
- Fluid Volume Deficit related to poor oral intake
- Anxiety related to lack of information about the disease, treatment, and long-term outcomes
- Ineffective Family Coping related to chronic illness

Planning and Intervention

Self-management is the key to the successful control of the pathologic process. The nurse may care for the child with asthma in the rehabilitation setting or on an outpatient basis. There are many interventions that are directed at acute care management. In this section the focus is on the long-term interventions.

Regular exercise is recommended. Routine exercise improves pulmonary function if the disease is under control and also improves self-esteem. Activities that involve interaction with other children should be encouraged to promote socialization.

For children with exercise-induced asthma, a treatment with cromolyn before exercise may help prevent an attack. Minimizing airway moisture loss can prevent an exercise-induced attack. Adequate hydration with oral fluids is used to maintain airway moisture as well as nose breathing.

Additionally, adequate hydration is essential to decrease mucus viscosity and improve mucociliary airway clearance. Dehydration can occur from insensible water loss through increased breathing rate or the diuretic effect of theophylline. Hydration is critical to the management of the child with asthma.

Self-care is the cornerstone for effective asthma management. Education for the child and family is essential to the successful management of asthma. The goal of self-care is the control of asthma so that the child can have as many normal life experiences as possible. The role of the pediatric rehabilitation nurse is to help the family learn as much as possible about the factors that precipitate an asthma episode and the most effective means of bringing the disease under control.

Self-care does not mean that the family should try to manage the disease by themselves. Therefore, it is important that the treatment plan is developed by the interdisciplinary team, including the child and family.

The child and family should be knowledgeable enough to care for the child at home but should also have the confidence in the health care team to seek periodic re-evaluations and ask for help if the child does not respond to treatment. The family needs to realize that asthma is a common disease and that individuals with asthma can live full active lives. Support groups can help the child and family interact with other families who are managing similar issues.

The overriding principle for the management of asthma is that prevention of an attack is the goal of self-care. It is easier to prevent than it is to treat an asthmatic episode. Compliance must be stressed. Allergens must be removed from the child's environment. Taking medication as prescribed can prevent a recurrence of the attack. The family should be taught the maneuvers necessary to handle a child's asthmatic episode once it begins. Effective techniques for the administration of inhaled medications are essential.

Impact on Child and Family

The child and family are affected in a number of ways by the diagnosis of asthma. Family relationships can be altered by the stress of having a child with a chronic illness. The attention of the parents may be needed by the child who has the disease, and other children may feel left out or neglected. The child may control the family by threatening to have an asthma attack if the child does not get what is wanted, and, likewise, one parent

---

Teaching Topic: Use of Inhaled Medication

Important Areas:

The inhaler must be shaken before every activation.

A slow, deep inspiration is required, with the inhaler activated at the beginning of inspiration.

The inhaler is activated once for each inspiration.

Holding the breath for 5 to 10 seconds at the completion of inspiration improves drug deposition.

Remove inhaler and breathe out slowly through the nose.

Wait 1 minute between puffs.

may use the child to manipulate the other. The family should make every attempt to integrate the child's care into the normal routine. The family may need help setting priorities and learning how to manage the behavior of each family member.

School and Community

Children with asthma have the highest rate of absenteeism than any other chronic condition. To help the child make a successful transition into school life, the teacher and school nurse should be included in the team. The teacher and school nurse should know the child's routine and need for medication and provide opportunities for compliance with these treatments. The child's exercise tolerance should be shared with anyone working with the child, and the child's limits should not be exceeded. The peer group should be taught the signs of a beginning attack and the treatment that will manage the episode.

Long-Term Outlook

The outlook for children with asthma is unpredictable. Many children become symptom free as they enter puberty. There is no way to predict which child will become asymptomatic. Some children outgrow the asthma attacks but develop other forms of allergic responses in adulthood. In general, the children who have had severe episodes of asthma and have a family history of allergies have a poor prognosis. Deaths from asthma have been increasing, with the young adolescent being the most vulnerable. Self-management and compliance with therapy seem to play an important role in the outcome for the child with asthma.

Conclusion

The outlook for children with asthma varies widely. Many children outgrow the condition in puberty. However, as the total number of cases continues to grow, the morbidity for some children continues to increase. The pediatric rehabilitation nurse must be aware of the effect of exercise on the management of the child with asthma and have input into the interdisciplinary team plan for the management of symptoms. The greatest impact that the nurse can have is in the complete education of the child and family so that self-management is possible. Continued advances in the treatment of the disease means that it

is necessary for the nurse to keep abreast of the changes so that the care of these children can be effectively and safely managed.

CONGENITAL HEART DISEASE

Congenital heart disease (CHD) refers to structural or functional heart anomalies that are present at birth. The diagnosis of CHD is particularly difficult for families to accept. The heart represents the center of life, love, and feelings. Even a relatively simple heart condition provokes fear and concern for the family. In addition to the technical care, the pediatric rehabilitation nurse is challenged to provide sensitive and effective psychosocial care of the child and family.

Etiology and Incidence

The specific cause of CHD is not clearly understood. Many factors have been identified as possible causes of CHD.

Environmental factors: radiation, pollution, chemicals, viruses such as rubella, and certain drugs have been related to the incidence of CHD

Maternal factors: age older than 40 years, insulin-dependent diabetes, alcoholism, and drug use

Heredity seems to play a role in occurrence of CHD. The risk of recurrence in families with an affected parent is variable: 1% to 3% if the father is affected and 2% to 10% if the mother is affected (Nora & Nora, 1988). CHD is closely associated with a number of syndromes, including Down, Turner, and others.

The incidence of CHD has wide variation. CHD has been reported as between 4 to 10 in every 1000 live births (Hoffman, 1990). The lack of consistency probably results from the differences in reporting. Also, there are some conditions that can be diagnosed at birth and others that are not detected until the child has matured. There is a high incidence of CHD in stillborn and aborted infants. If these infants were included in the statistics, the number would be much higher.

Pathophysiology

Normally, blood moves through the different sections of the heart as a result of the pumping action of the heart and the pressure differentiation, following the path of least resistance from the areas of higher pressure to areas of lower pressure. Defects in the heart allow the blood to flow from areas of high pressure to areas of low pressure that is not the normal path for the blood. This results in excess blood in areas that are not designed to manage such large volumes. Additionally, there may be strictures that prevent a normal movement of blood from one area to another. The traditional classification of CHD is the presence or absence of cyanosis. This classification system is problematic because it implies that clinically the diagnosis can be made related to the amount of cyanosis that is present. In reality, the child with a cyanotic condition may be pink and the child with an acyanotic condition may become cyanotic as the symptoms become more acute.

Acyanotic CHD With Normal or Decreased Blood Flow

Acyanotic CHD lesions that result in normal or decreased pulmonary blood flow are caused by some degree of impairment to the flow of blood either within the heart or within the great vessels. In this type of lesion, blood follows the normal circulatory pathway. Because the pathway of blood flow is normal, even in the presence of decreased pulmonary blood flow, the blood in the systemic system is not desaturated unless the anomaly is severe. The hemodynamic effects depend on the severity of the lesion, and the degree of obstruction is described as mild, moderate, or severe. The most common obstructive lesions are pulmonary stenosis, aortic stenosis, and coarctation of the aorta.

Pulmonary stenosis is a narrowing of the right ventricular outflow tract. The most common lesion is valvular stenosis, in which the cusps of the pulmonary valve are thick and restrict the flow of blood into the pulmonary system.

Aortic stenosis is narrowing or obstruction in the path of systemic blood flow leaving the left ventricle. The defect can occur above the aortic valve (supravalvular), below the valve (subvalvular), or at the valve annulus (valvular). Valvular stenosis is the most common defect.

Coarctation of the aorta is a narrowing of the aorta that causes an obstruction to blood flow on the left side of the heart. This results in a decreased perfusion to the areas below the obstruction.

Acyanotic Congenital Heart Defects With Increased Pulmonary Blood Flow

Acyanotic congenital heart lesions with increased pulmonary blood flow are those that permit blood to pass between the systemic and pulmonary circulation through an abnormal opening. This results in a left-to-right shunt because the pressures in the left side of the heart are higher than those on the right side and blood flows through the abnormal openings in the septum, increasing flow to the pulmonic system. The acyanotic congenital heart defects with increased pulmonary blood flow are patent ductus arteriosus, ventricular septal defect, atrial septal defect, and atrioventricular septal defect.

Patent ductus arteriosus occurs when the normal muscular fetal structure connecting the pulmonary artery and aorta fails to close completely after birth. This occurs frequently in premature infants.

Atrial septal defect is an abnormal communication between the right and left atria that permits blood to be shunted from the left to right through the atrial septum.

Ventricular septal defect is an abnormal communication between the right and left ventricles that permits blood to shunt from the left ventricle into the right ventricle. This defect is the most common congenital cardiac lesion.

Atrioventricular septal defect is a lesion of incomplete fusion of endocardial cushions. It consists of a low atrial septal defect that is continuous with a high ventricular septal defect and clefts of the mitral and tricuspid valves, creating a large central atrioventricular valve that allows blood to flow between all four chambers of the heart.

Cyanotic Congenital Heart Defects With Normal or Decreased Pulmonary Blood Flow

Cyanotic congenital cardiac defects cause a decrease in blood flow to the pulmonary system. Systemic venous blood returns to the body without being oxygenated through a shunt that takes the blood from the right side of the heart to the left side of the heart. The child with cyanotic congenital heart defects has cyanosis of the mucous membranes and nailbeds, and skin become hypoxic. These cardiac anomalies include tetralogy of Fallot, tricuspid atresia, and pulmonary atresia.

Tetralogy of Fallot is an anomaly that has four specific abnormalities. They are (1) a large

VSD, (2) right ventricular outflow tract obstruction (sometimes called pulmonary stenosis), (3) displacement of the aorta toward the right side (overriding of the aorta), and (4) right ventricular hypertrophy.

Tricuspid atresia is the absence of the tricuspid valve or the presence of an imperforate tricuspid valve, which is located on the right side of the heart. An atrial septal defect or patent foramen ovale is usually present, which permits blood to flow to the left side of the heart. There is a mixing of deoxygenated blood and oxygenated blood in the left side of the heart.

Pulmonary atresia is the narrowing at the entrance to the pulmonary artery. Resistance to blood flow causes right ventricular hypertrophy and decreased pulmonary blood flow.

Clinical Manifestations

Clinical manifestations of the anomalies vary greatly depending on the hemodynamic effects of the lesions. The children may have heart murmurs at the site of the lesion. They may have altered growth patterns, dyspnea, and exercise intolerance. Peripheral pulses may be decreased, and peripheral circulation may be impaired or the peripheral pulses may be bounding. Some children may have such severe lesions that the signs are present at birth. On the other hand, the child may be asymptomatic and the lesion may not be discovered until a heart murmur is picked up at a routine examination.

Diagnostic Assessment

A major function of the cardiovascular system is to transport oxygen to the organs. When a chronic lack of oxygen exists, the body compensates by producing increasing amounts of hemoglobin, resulting in polycythemia. Blood gases may be drawn to determine Pao_2, $Paco_2$, pH, and oxygen. The child may be placed on pulse oximetry to monitor the oxygen saturation in the blood, especially during exercise.

Cardiographic studies include electrocardiography, echocardiography, and cardiac catheterization. An electrocardiogram is a measurement of the electrical activity of the heart. It records the conduction, magnitude, and duration of the electrical activities of the heart and provides information regarding the heart rate, abnormal rhythms, chamber size, and myocardial ischemia.

Echocardiography is a noninvasive test that provides data on cardiovascular structures and functions. They are the reflections from the tissues of ultra-high-frequency sound waves that are passed through the chest wall and heart. The ultrasonic impulses are sent to a recorder and visualized on a video screen; a permanent videotape may be made.

Cardiac catheterization refers to the insertion of a radiopaque catheter through an artery or vein to the heart. Fluoroscopy is used to monitor the location and movement of the catheter. Catheterization provides pressure measurements within the heart chambers and great vessels. Oxygen saturations indicate the presence and proportion of shunting within the heart.

Physical Impact and Functional Limitations

Exercise tolerance is an important indicator of cardiac function. Children with severe heart disease may have limited tolerance for exercise. Many children with heart disease do well to regulate their own exercise. These children are sensitive to internal cues that indicate the need to rest and need few external limitations on their activity.

Some children need to have activity limitations. In some types of heart disease, there are medical indications for restricted activity. Activity may cause myocardial ischemia, dysrhythmia, and death. The child may seem asymptomatic and therefore not understand the need for activity limitations. The activity limitation is a challenge for parents because they may overprotect the child, fearing a worsening of the child's condition. Therefore, the situation arises that the child is not even allowed to do the amount of exercise that has been prescribed.

Therapeutic Management

When an infant is diagnosed with cyanotic CHD shortly after birth, prostaglandin E_1 is given to keep the ductus arteriosus open so that pulmonary blood flow is maintained. The cyanotic infant and child should be well hydrated to keep the hematocrit and blood viscosity within acceptable limits. Older children may require serial phlebotomy to reduce blood viscosity and minimize the risk of a cerebrovascular accident. Palliative surgery may be necessary in severely hypoxic infants. A shunt is performed to create a communication between the right and left sides of the heart. A procedure that is frequently performed is the modified Blalock-Taussig shunt, which uses a Gore-Tex graft to act as the communication between the right and left sides of the heart. The child may develop congestive heart failure. If congestive heart failure develops, the child may need to be treated with digoxin and diuretic therapy.

The definitive treatment for most children with CHD is corrective surgery. The type and extent of surgery depends on the kind of defects that are present and the condition of the child. Palliative surgery may be performed early in the child's life; and when the child is stabilized and can tolerate surgery, the major surgical procedure is performed. Cardiac transplantation is becoming a more common procedure for the treatment of severe CHD.

Application of the Nursing Process

The child with CHD may require rehabilitation either before surgery to stabilize the child or after surgery to facilitate stabilization and normalize function of the child. The pediatric rehabilitation nurse is in the position to coordinate the care of the child so that interdisciplinary treatments are maximized. The nurse is also in the position to teach the family about the disease and the treatments necessary for the child's survival. Table 17–5 is a plan of care for fatigue related to the cardiac condition.

Table 17–5 NURSING PLAN OF CARE

Nursing Diagnosis: Fatigue related to cardiac condition.

Goal: Child will maintain adequate energy levels without additonal stress

Nursing Interventions/Teaching
Allow for frequent rest periods and uninterrupted periods of sleep.
Encourage quiet games and activities.
Provide multiple activities appropriate to age, condition, and capabilities.
Implement measures to reduce anxiety.
Respond to complaints of fatigue.

Expected Outcomes
Child receives appropriate amount of exercise
Child receives appropriate amounts of rest/ sleep (specify)
Child engages in developmentally appropriate activities

Nursing Diagnoses

Based on the needs of the child and family with a congenital cardiac condition the nursing diagnoses might include but not be limited to:

- Activity Intolerance related to imbalance between oxygen supply and demand
- High Risk for Altered Growth and Development related to growth failure, poor muscle tone, poor feeding, and decreased appetite
- High Risk for Decreased Cardiac Output related to structured defect
- High Risk for Infection related to reduced body defenses
- High Risk for Altered Parenting related to stress of chronic illness
- High Risk for Social Isolation related to complex care and other problems related to CHD

Planning and Intervention

Growth and Development: An infant or child with cardiac disease needs but may not receive the same type of developmental stimulation as a normal child. The nurse works with the parents to develop strategies to help the child experience normal activities without undue cardiac stress. These children may be physically small and passive rather than active, causing parents to think that they are younger and less capable then they may actually be. The nurse helps the parents provide appropriate activities that foster normal development.

Nutrition: Growth retardation is common in children with CHD, and these children often have special nutritional needs. Providing adequate intake of nutrients and calories is a major nursing goal. The children have to pause frequently to rest while eating, and the meal can take a long time with the child becoming exhausted. The child should be given small frequent feedings of high-calorie, nutritionally dense food. The food should be offered at times when the child is rested.

Oxygen: The body's demand for oxygen directly affects cardiac workload. Therefore a major nursing goal is to minimize the oxygen needs of the body. This can be accomplished by positioning the infant in a semi-Fowler position to prevent the abdominal organs from exerting pressure on the diaphragm and to allow greater expansion of the lungs.

Clothing should be loose to prevent chest constriction.

Supplemental oxygen may be necessary to improve tissue oxygenation. The oxygen is warmed to prevent chilling and humidified to prevent drying of the mucous membranes. Supplemental oxygen is not always beneficial for children with heart disease who have a right-to-left shunt and in whom the blood is not receiving proper oxygenation.

Self-Esteem: Several factors determine the effect of the heart problem on the child's sense of self. Children with CHD are frequently small for their age and cannot keep up with their same-age peers. They may lack confidence in their ability to perform activities. The lack of self-confidence may lead to overdependence on adults to provide care, and the child may have a sense of hopelessness. The child's sense of self is enhanced by the degree of confidence that others place in him or her. The child should be encouraged to take on appropriate responsibilities and independence.

Children may demonstrate strong reactions to having problems with their heart, depending on their perception of the disease. They may be afraid of death or have misconceptions about the meaning and cause of their illness. They may have inaccurate cause-and-effect reasoning, believing that their condition is the result of bad behavior. The nurse can determine the child's understanding of the disease and provide education so that the child understands that he or she is not responsible for the condition. The child may be angry because of the limitation of the disease and the discomfort that results from treatment. The nurse should acknowledge the child's feelings and make a referral to appropriate therapists.

Medication Therapy: Digoxin may be necessary if the child has congestive heart failure. Digoxin increases cardiac contractility and slows conduction through the atrioventricular node. Because toxic levels are easily possible, parents need careful instruction on administration of this medication (see Teaching Topic: Digoxin Administration). The child may also have diuretics prescribed. Excessive sodium intake should be avoided. Oral intake of fluid may or may not be restricted. Potassium supplements may be required.

Impact on Child and Family

The response of parents to the diagnosis of CHD is one of fear and anxiety. Parents may

> **Teaching Topic: Digoxin Administration**
>
> **Important Areas:**
> Medication should be given at the same time every day. If a dose is missed, do not make up for the missed dose. If two doses are missed, call the physician.
> If the child vomits the medication, give the next dose on time. If two doses are vomited, call the physician.
> For accidental overdose, take the child to the emergency department.
> Monitor the child for signs of anorexia, diarrhea, vomiting, lethargy, and difficult breathing. These are signs of digoxin toxicity and should be reported to the physician.

not be able to deal with their own feelings because of the intensity of the needs of the child. Every member of the family is affected by the diagnosis and treatment demands of the child with CHD. The parents may be afraid to discipline the child for fear of precipitating a cyanotic spell. The pediatric rehabilitation nurse can help the family members express their feelings and set consistent limitations for the family including the child with CHD.

The family may become exhausted by the continuing unrelenting financial and emotional stresses of care. Families should be encouraged to find respite care to get needed rest. The pediatric rehabilitation nurse can educate other family members or neighbors to care for the child to give the parents a break. Parents should also be encouraged to meet with other families with similarly affected children as a support to help them adjust to the daily stresses.

School and Community

The child needs opportunities for social development. Parents are often reluctant to expose these children to people who may have infections. The parents need to take reasonable precautions; however, if the child is not allowed to interact with other people, the child may develop overdependence on the family and become limited in independent growth and development. If possible, the child should attend school, although modifications may have to be made in the amount of activity the child should be allowed to do. The child may have to have several rest periods during the day. The interdisciplinary team and the parents need to work with teachers and other school personnel so that everyone who works with the child understands the need for a particular schedule.

Long-Term Outlook

The long-term outlook for children with CHD is variable and depends on the type of defect, severity of the defect, and child's response to treatment. Many children recover after surgery and do not require further treatment. New therapies, including cardiac transplant, have prolonged the life of children who would not have survived until recently. These children now survive but require intensive treatment for the rest of their lives. These children are usually cared for in the home by their families, who become very adept in the management of complicated medical conditions.

Conclusion

The child with CHD may be asymptomatic or have severe activity limitations. The symptoms that a child experiences are related to the type of lesion that the child has and the severity of the defect. Many new surgical procedures have resulted in the treatment of many children so that they can have a full and normal life. On the other hand, many children are surviving who would not have done so in the recent past. These children are surviving with disabilities that require long-term care. The pediatric rehabilitation nurse can help the family cope with the child before and after surgery. The nurse must keep up to date on the newest treatments and the nurse's role in the management of these therapies.

REFERENCES

Abman, S., & Groothius, J. (1994). Pathophysiology and treatment of bronchopulmonary dysplasia. *Pediatric Clinics of North America*, 41(2), 277–315.

Batshaw, M., & Perret, Y. (1992). *Children with disabilities: a medical primer.* Baltimore: Paul H. Brookes.

Barnhart, S., & Czervinskes, M. (1995). *Perinatal and pediatric respiratory care.* Philadelphia: WB Saunders.

Betz, C., Hunsberger, M., & Wright, S. (1994). *Family-centered nursing care of children* (2nd ed.). Philadelphia: WB Saunders.

Bloomberg, G., & Strunk, R. (1992). Crisis in asthma care. *Pediatric Clinics of North America*, 39(6), 1225–1241.

Brown, M., & Swannson, C. (1993). Understanding children with chronic lung disease. II. Respiratory supports and treatments. *Infants and Young Children*, 5(3), 57–66.

Conte, V. (1992). Bronchopulmonary dysplasia. In P. Jackson & J. Vessy (Eds.). *Primary care of the child with a chronic condition.* St. Louis: Mosby–Year Book.

Harvey, K. (1996). Bronchopulmonary dysplasia. In P. Jackson & J. Vessy (Eds.). *Primary care of the child with a chronic condition* (2nd ed.). Philadelphia: Mosby–Year Book.

Hoffman, J. (1990). Congenital heart disease: incidence and inheritance. *Pediatric Clinics of North America*, 37(1), 25–43.

Jackson, D., & Saunders, R. (1993). *Child health nursing: a comprehensive approach to the care of children and their families.* Philadelphia: JB Lippincott.

McCormick, M., Gormaker, S., & Sobol, A. (1990). Very low birth weight children: behavior problems and school difficulty in a national sample. *Journal of Pediatrics*, 117, 687–693.

Moores, R., & Abman, S. (1990). Bronchopulmonary dysplasia: persistent cardiopulmonary sequelae of neonatal respiratory distress and its treatment. *Seminars in Respiratory Medicine*, 11, 140–151.

Murphy, S., & Kelly, W. (1993). Asthma, inflammation and hyperresponsiveness in children. *Current Opinions in Pediatrics*, 5, 255–265.

National Heart, Lung, and Blood Institute (NHLBI), National Institutes of Health. (1991). *Guidelines for the diagnosis and management of asthma.* Publication No. 91-3042. Bethesda, MD: NHLBI.

Nora, J., & Nora, A. (1988). Update on counseling the family with a first degree relative with a congenital heart defect. *American Journal of Medical Genetics*, 29, 137–142.

Northway, W., Rosan, R., & Porter, D. (1967). Pulmonary disease following respiratory therapy of hyaline-membrane disease. *New England Journal of Medicine*, 276(7), 357–368.

Parker, R., Linstrom, D., & Cotton, R. (1992). Improved survival accounts for most, but not all, of the increase in bronchopulmonary dysplasia. *Pediatrics*, 90, 663–668.

Victorian Infant Collaborative Study Group. (1991). Eight-year outcome in infants with birth weight of 500 to 999 grams: continuing regional study of 1979 and 1980 births. *Journal of Pediatrics*, 118, 761–767.

Wong, D. (1995). *Whaley & Wong's nursing care of infants and children* (5th ed.). Baltimore: CV Mosby.

ADDITIONAL RESOURCE

Vohr, B., Bell, E., & Oh, W. (1982). Infants with bronchopulmonary dysplasia: growth pattern and neurologic and developmental outcome. *American Journal of Disease in Childhood, 136,* 443–447.

RESOURCES

American Lung Association
800-586-4872
"If Your Baby Has BPD: A Guide for Parents"

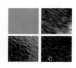

Chapter 18

Autoimmune and Endocrine Conditions

Nancy M. Youngblood and
Patricia A. Edwards

Autoimmune diseases occur when the body produces an inappropriate immunologic response against itself. Normally, the body develops immune defense mechanisms to substances that are foreign. The body is able to distinguish between the substances that are normal to the body and those that are not. In autoimmune disease, the immune system is no longer able to determine the normal parts of the body from those that are foreign. The immune system becomes defective and begins to produce antibodies against normal body systems. The antibodies attack the normal system and try to destroy it, causing tissue injury that may result in destruction that needs life-long management. The diseases that affect children and adolescents and that are encountered by the pediatric rehabilitation nurse are addressed in this chapter. These conditions are Guillain-Barré syndrome, juvenile arthritis, and diabetes mellitus. Also included is cystic fibrosis, which is an autoimmune disease that affects the body's exocrine glands, including the pancreas, sweat glands, and the lungs.

GUILLAIN-BARRÉ SYNDROME

Guillain-Barré syndrome (GBS) is an inflammation of a large number of nerves that results in progressive muscular weakness of the extremities, which may lead to paralysis. This syndrome usually follows an infectious disease. The signs of the infection usually have disappeared before the signs of GBS begin. The symptoms may last a few weeks or longer. Thirty percent of patients still have residual weakness after 3 years (Guillain-Barré, 1996). The child with GBS may have mild to severe physical disabilities. The child and the family may experience emotional distress because of the physical manifestations of the disease and the impact of the disabilities on activities of daily living.

The pediatric rehabilitation nurse may encounter the child in a variety of settings. The child will need hospitalization during the initial phase for diagnosis and the management of the respiratory system. The child will then enter a phase of intense rehabilitative therapy. This may take place in the child's home, ambulatory care, or inpatient setting. The nurse may have to assume the role of caregiver, educator, or case manager as the child progresses through the stages of recovery. It is especially important that the nurse provide the necessary emotional support for the child and family during this stressful time.

Etiology and Incidence

The exact cause of GBS is not known. It usually follows a minor infection, a respiratory tract infection, or gastrointestinal infection. GBS may also occur after a diagnosis of acquired immunodeficiency syndrome (AIDS) or AIDS-related complex. It may also be preceded by *Mycoplasma* infection; measles, herpes simplex virus infection, or other viral infections; major surgery within the past 6 weeks; systemic lupus erythematosus; Hodgkin's disease; other malignant diseases; and vaccination with vaccines such as the antirabies vaccine and the swine flu vaccine (Guillain-Barré, 1996). This disorder was first described in 1859 by Landry (McCance & Huether, 1994). It affects approximately 8 in 100,000 persons. It is worldwide in distribution and affects both sexes equally. GBS can occur at any age but is most frequent in individuals between the ages of 30 and 50 (Guillain-Barré, 1996).

Pathophysiology

In GBS the immune system functions abnormally and begins to destroy the myelin sheath that surrounds the axons and even the axons themselves. When the myelin sheaths are injured, the nerves cannot transmit signals efficiently. The loss of nervous stimulation results in the inability of the muscles to respond to the signals to and from the brain. The motor and sensory pathways are both affected, so, in addition to the loss of movement, the person with GBS may be unable to experience sensations. Sensory impulses may also be distorted, resulting in tingling, "crawling skin," or painful sensations (GBS: Fact Sheet, 1992). Because the nerves that enervate the arms and legs are some of the longest in the body, they are therefore the most vulnerable to interruption. The symptoms of GBS usually start first in the hands and feet. The changes in nervous function most generally occur in an ascending order. However, there are variations that begin in the brain stem and descend, often affecting respiratory function.

It is commonly believed that when GBS is preceded by a viral infection the virus damages the nerves in such a way that the immune system identifies them as foreign cells. A second theory is that the virus affects the immune system in such a way that the immune system is unable to determine the difference between cells in the body and foreign cells.

Clinical Aspects

In general, GBS is characterized by motor weakness and areflexia. The onset is usually rapid; symptoms develop quickly from days to about 1 month (GBS: Fact Sheet, 1992). The symptoms are manifested in a symmetric manner. The feet and hands are affected first, and then the symptoms spread upward through the body. The motor and sensory nerves are affected at the same time. GBS occurs in phases. The first phase is one of rapid symptom development. This phase lasts for up to 3 weeks (Hickey, 1996). The

next phase is a plateau phase during which there are no changes in the child or adolescent's condition. This phase may last for several days to 2 weeks (Hickey, 1996). The last phase is the recovery phase. During this phase, remyelination and axonal regeneration occur. This phase may take up to 2 years for maximal recovery. However, permanent deficits may result to a greater or lesser degree (Hickey, 1996).

Clinical manifestations may vary from paresis to complete quadriplegia. Systemic weakness or paralysis may include the extremities, the trunk, and perhaps the neck and face. The autonomic and respiratory systems may be affected. If the autonomic nervous system is involved, the child or adolescent may have tachycardia, hypertension, or hypotension. The ventilatory capacity is often decreased. Additionally, the child may have a respiratory arrest if the respiratory system is involved. The child may have hypotonia, and the deep tendon reflexes may be absent (McCance & Huether, 1994). Additional symptoms that may occur in GBS are blurred vision, dizziness, incontinence, and constipation. The symptoms indicating an emergency are difficulty swallowing, difficulty breathing, fainting, and apnea (Guillain-Barré, 1996).

Physical Impact and Functional Limitations

The physical limitations that occur depend on the extent of the nervous system involvement. Motor function may range from muscle weakness to complete paralysis. The paralysis is usually symmetric, with both sides of the body being equally affected. The paralysis results in the inability to move and perform activities of daily living. The child is unable to perform the usual activities that were functionally possible before having GBS. If the child does retain function, it may be limited, so that the child needs assistance with normal activity. Sensory abnormalities may follow a stocking-and-glove pattern, with position and vibratory sense predominantly affected (Noble, 1996). If the child has an extreme form of GBS, the respiratory system may need support to maintain life. The paralysis may be so severe that the child becomes "locked in" or unable to communicate (Steinberg, 1996).

Because the severity of GBS is variable, it is difficult to describe the usual functional limitations. There is no "typical" functional limitation. Each child needs to have an individual assessment because physical findings may vary significantly from case to case.

Diagnostic Assessment

A complete health history must be performed. Several disorders have symptoms similar to those found in GBS. In addition, the initial and subsequent abnormalities in GBS can be quite varied, making it difficult for the physician to identify the syndrome. The diagnosis is made by careful history and physical examination until collectively the signs and symptoms form a certain pattern that supports the differential diagnosis of GBS. The pattern generally appears on both sides of the body, and the symptoms appear in an orderly sequence. As compared with other neurologic disorders, GBS progresses more rapidly. Deep tendon reflexes are decreased or absent. A nerve conduction velocity test can aid in the diagnosis. In GBS, the cerebrospinal fluid contains an elevated protein with a normal cell count (Hickey, 1996). Electromyography identifies the response of the muscle to electrical stimulation.

Therapeutic Management

There is no cure for GBS. However, there are therapies that lessen the severity of the illness in most children and adolescents. The medical treatment of GBS includes the administration of corticosteroids, possible plasmapheresis, respiratory support, and supportive therapy. The goals of therapy depend on the phase of the syndrome.

Medication Therapy

The use of corticosteroids is controversial. In some reports, corticosteroid therapy has been of benefit in the early stages (Vallee et al., 1993). However, a controlled study using a short course of intravenous corticosteroids found no benefit (Guillain-Barré Syndrome Steroid Trial Group, 1993). Further research studies need to be done to determine if the use of these agents is beneficial or detrimental. The use of corticosteroids is a treatment decision made by the physician. If corticosteroids are given for their anti-inflammatory effect, they may be administered in high doses (Hickey, 1996).

Problems related to immobility must be managed. Immobility causes a decreased blood flow in the legs and pelvic veins. Edema can develop as well as the formation of deep vein thrombosis. The child or adolescent may be given heparin injections to prevent the formation of thrombosis.

Immobility and changes in the child's usual diet can result in the development of constipation. Stool softeners are used to treat the constipation. The child is started on a bowel program (see Chap. 12 for an explanation of a bowel program), and sodium sulfosuccinate (Colace) or psyllium (Metamucil) is given at scheduled times along with suppositories or enemas.

If the autonomic nervous system is involved, the child may need to be treated for hypertension, hypotension, tachycardia, or bradycardia. The medications may include beta blockers, calcium blockers, or digoxin, depending on the signs and symptoms of the autonomic nervous system dysfunction.

Pain, defined as severe muscle spasms, is a complaint of children and adolescents with GBS. The pain is worse at night and is not relieved by nonsteroidal agents or non-narcotics (Hickey, 1996). Narcotics may be given for pain that cannot be relieved by other methods.

Plasmapheresis

Plasmapheresis is a process in which some of the child's blood is removed and the plasma that contains the antibodies that are attacking the nervous tissue is removed. Then the blood cells are returned to the body. When plasmapheresis is used, timing of the initiation of this treatment is critical. To be effective it should be started 7 to 14 days after the onset of the disease. According to Steinberg (1996), on average, those treated early in their illness fare better than those who do not receive this treatment.

One course of plasmapheresis is done three or four times, 1 to 2 days apart. If the child does not improve or if the condition deteriorates after the first course of treatment is completed, a second course may be ordered.

Respiratory Support

Respiratory mechanical failure secondary to neuromuscular weakness is common in GBS. Vital capacity decreases and the cough becomes weaker. When the vital capacity decreases, the child or adolescent is at risk for atelectasis and hypoxemia. If the vital capacity falls below a predetermined amount for age and weight and respiratory failure is imminent, the child will need to be intubated and mechanical ventilation is usually indicated. The vital capacity should be monitored frequently. The optimal level for vital capacity is 12 to 15 mL/kg (Hickey, 1996). The length of time that a child remains on the ventilator depends on the severity of the disease, any pre-existing conditions, and the occurrence of respiratory complications during the recovery.

Even if the child does not need to be ventilated, airway protection may still be needed. The airway is particularly compromised if the ninth and tenth cranial nerves are affected. If this is the case, the gag and cough reflexes may be weakened or nonexistent. The child will have difficulty handling secretions. Because the gag and cough reflexes protect the airway, there is an increased risk of aspiration and the development of aspiration pneumonia. The child may need to be intubated to remove secretions and keep the airway clear. This may be necessary for an extended length of time.

Supportive Care

Supportive care is the cornerstone of treatment. Recovery from GBS is usual, but it may take an extended length of time for this to occur. During the first phase of the illness the child may need hospitalization in an acute care hospital. This hospitalization continues for a few days to a couple months until the child is stabilized, especially if there is autonomic nervous system involvement. Monitoring of the autonomic cardiac responses is required so that changes can be detected early. If a paralytic ileus occurs, a nasogastric tube is inserted for gastric decompression. Urinary retention is managed through an intermittent catheterization program. Finally, the problems related to immobility must be addressed through such treatments as frequent range-of-motion exercises and frequent position changes.

Interdisciplinary Therapy

During even the earliest part of the acute care hospitalization the rehabilitative process must be integrated into the child or adolescent's treatment plan. A rehabilitation program is optimally implemented with the physiatrist as part of the health care team. Depending on the residual effects of the disease process, the child will continue to need physical therapy during the recovery phase of the disease (Batshaw & Perret, 1992). The early focus of the

program is the prevention of muscle loss and the prevention of contractures. As the child begins to recover, the goal of treatment is to improve mobility and adapt to functional limitations. Special attention is usually given to the joints in the extremities to maintain complete range of motion. Limb movement may also help maintain proprioception (Steinberg, 1996). The return of function is usually in a descending pattern, so that the upper extremities become functional before the lower extremities.

The physical therapist emphasizes exercises to maintain muscle tone in the lower extremities and teaches the child to walk as independently as possible. Hydrotherapy may be used to support the child while learning partial weight bearing. As leg strength returns, parallel bars and a wheeled walker may be used for support during walking. Orthotic devices such as a molded ankle foot orthosis may be necessary for persisting muscle group weakness (see Chap. 14 for additional information about orthotic devices).

An occupational therapist develops interventions that focus on the upper extremities. The occupational therapist retrains the child on activities of daily living. Exercises are designed to strengthen the weaker muscles, such as the small muscles of the hand. Because of the severe fatigue experienced by these children, energy-conserving techniques are implemented. Splints may be used to support extremities during movement to maximize hand use and prevent fatigue.

Application of the Nursing Process

The pediatric rehabilitation nurse uses the nursing process to identify the nursing needs and coordinate care for the child or adolescent and family. The child that is affected with GBS may be cared for in a variety of settings and require the skilled care of a number of health care professionals.

Assessment

Nursing management of a child with GBS begins with a health history and physical and functional assessments. A comprehensive baseline respiratory and neurologic assessment is critical so that the nurse can identify changes when they occur.

An assessment of the respiratory focus should include vital capacity and signs of respiratory distress such as cyanosis, diaphoresis, dyspnea, confusion, and anxiety. The child should have frequent assessments of breath sounds to identify changes that might indicate the development of pneumonia or atelectasis.

A neurologic assessment should focus on motor and sensory function. Cranial nerves should be assessed, especially the ones that are most frequently affected (i.e., III, V, VI, VII, IX, X, XI, and XII) (Hickey, 1996). Because the autonomic nervous system may be involved, the child should be assessed for cardiac arrhythmias and changes in blood pressure indicating hypertension or hypotension.

Nursing Diagnosis

Based on the assessment data, the following nursing diagnoses may apply to the child or adolescent with GBS and the family:

- High Risk for Ineffective Breathing Pattern related to neuromuscular weakness of the respiratory muscles
- Ineffective Airway Clearance related to weakness of the cough and gag reflexes
- High Risk for Disuse Syndrome related to immobility
- Impaired Physical Mobility related to paralysis
- Impaired Verbal Communication related to muscle weakness, intubation, or both
- Urinary Retention related to autonomic dysfunction
- Fear related to illness, treatment protocols, and loss of control
- Knowledge Deficit related to illness and changes in body function
- High Risk for Aspiration related to muscle weakness and decreased reflexes
- Impaired Social Interaction related to hospitalization and disease process
- Powerlessness

Planning and Interventions

Nursing interventions should include but are not limited to the following:

Monitor respiratory status.
Monitor breath sounds throughout lung fields.
Monitor vital capacity.
Use an oximeter to monitor adequate oxygenation.
If the child receives respiratory support, monitor setting and proper use of equipment.
Monitor the child's ability to manage secretions and keep the airway clear.

Administer assisted coughing every 4 hours.
Administer chest physical therapy every 4 hours.
Suction the airway PRN.
Maintain usual bowel elimination patterns by establishing a bowel program.
Prevent pressure ulcers by changing position every 2 hours; use pressure relief devices; and monitor skin for redness.
Promote venous return by applying thigh-high elastic stockings.
Provide a method of communication that is appropriate for the child's developmental level.
Establish a bladder retraining program.
Reduce environmental distractions and sleep interruptions.
Identify factors that interfere with sleep.
Assess factors that contribute to fear.
Make appropriate referrals as needed.
Develop a teaching plan for the child and parents so that they understand the disease process, treatment goals, and procedures and can become competent in the child's care.
Provide developmentally appropriate diversional activities.
Provide for educational opportunities to maintain academic level.
Provide an opportunity for the child and family to make some decisions about care.

Additionally, the pediatric rehabilitation nurse should assess the child with GBS for pain and implement the nursing plan of care in Table 18–1.

Education of the child and family is essential to help them understand the disease and specific treatments required for the management of the physical limitations that arise from GBS. The development of a teaching plan should be done shortly after admission to the health care system. The teaching plan should be developed to help the child and family understand the disease, health care routines, and procedures. Because it is likely that the family will need to care for the child at home and manage complex aspects of care, the family caregivers should begin to learn the procedures and be able to perform them before the child is discharged to home. The family may need to learn how to manage a ventilator, perform exercises, administer medication, and use adaptive equipment and orthoses (see Teaching Topic: Application of Molded Ankle Foot Orthosis). The family

Table 18–1   NURSING PLAN OF CARE—PAIN

Nursing Diagnosis: Pain

Related to: Sensory nerve dysfunction

Goals	Nursing Interventions
Identify the type and severity of pain	Monitor for pain with a pediatric pain scale. Assess predisposing factors. Identify ways of minimizing pain.
Relief of pain	Enhance comfort with positioning and turning techniques. Use distraction and/or relaxation techniques if appropriate. Use application of heat if it relieves or lessens pain. Administer prescribed analgesic (usually a narcotic). Monitor for side effects of medication. Assess for effect of medication.

Expected Outcomes
The child will indicate relief from pain verbally or by a change in behavior.
A decrease in pain will be documented by a decrease on the pediatric pain scale.

---

caregivers will need to learn how to assess the child for changes in health status and how to handle an emergency situation if the child's condition should deteriorate.

Impact on Child and Family

The diagnosis of GBS is devastating to the child and family. The syndrome is frightening because of the speed in which symptoms develop. The symptoms increase over a short period of time compared with those of other neurologic diseases. The respiratory dysfunction and muscle weakness causes extreme anxiety and feelings of helplessness. Once the

acute phase is over, the possible long-term disability can be discouraging to the child or adolescent and family. The parents may feel guilty because they believe that they are responsible for the child's condition. The family's resources can quickly be depleted because of the intensity of the health care needs of the child with GBS. Depending on the support systems and coping abilities of the family, the child's illness may have devastating effects on them.

School and Community

School attendance will be disrupted, possibly for an extended period of time. The child may receive tutoring until able to return to school. When the child does return, provisions should be made for any special equipment. The child's classmates should have a chance to talk about the changes in the child and the experiences that have occurred. Adjustments may need to be made to the child's schedule so that the child can have rest periods. Opportunities for play and recreation need to be included in the schedule.

The child and family should make use of accessible community activities. The child and family need to participate in activities that encourage normal growth and development as long as the activities are adapted to the child's limitations. The family may need guidance in selecting the types of activities that are safe for the child with GBS.

Teaching Topic: Application of Molded Ankle Foot Orthosis

Important Areas:
Make sure application maintains functional position.
Inspect skin for breakdown under pressure points.
Schedule wearing time and time off—frequently the schedule is 2 hours on and 2 hours off or on at night and off during daytime activity.
Provide skin care.
Wash every other day with warm, soapy water; rinse and dry.
Assess circulation when orthosis is applied.

Evaluation

Evaluation of nursing interventions gives the pediatric rehabilitation nurse an opportunity to determine the adequacy of the care that the child and family are receiving. The nurse needs to evaluate the child's respiratory status and the effectiveness of respiratory therapies. The interventions for airway maintenance are evaluated to ensure a patent airway and decreased risk of aspiration pneumonia. Evaluation of the interventions to decrease the risk of disuse syndrome would be outcomes that show a normal bowel pattern, maximal peripheral blood flow without the development of deep vein thrombosis, and intact skin.

Interventions for communication, powerlessness, and impaired social interaction are adequate if the child and family are coping with the situation and are not exhibiting signs or symptoms of extreme emotional distress. If interventions have not resulted in the expected outcomes, then the pediatric rehabilitation nurse needs to reassess the situation and try to identify the necessary adjustments to the intervention plan that would lead to positive outcomes.

Long-Term Outlook

The overall outlook for the child with GBS is relatively optimistic. Fifty to 90 percent of the people with GBS have a nearly complete recovery (Steinberg, 1996). The better outcomes are found in children with the following characteristics (Wong, 1995; Steinberg, 1996):

- younger age
- minimal respiratory involvement
- relatively normal electromyographic studies
- receipt of early plasmapheresis
- mild muscle weakness

Severe cases have the poorest prognoses. Recovery may take up to 2 years or longer (Steinberg, 1996) with exacerbation of the muscle weakness.

CASE STUDY—Guillain-Barré Syndrome

Margie is a perky, vivacious, 16-year-old girl who is recovering from GBS. She had a "cold" 6 months ago that was followed by weakness in her legs that progressed to complete paralysis within a 24-hour period. Margie was hospitalized in an intensive care unit for 2 weeks for pulmonary muscle weakness. She received a tracheostomy tube for pulmonary care and oxygen administration. After she was discharged from the intensive care unit she was carefully monitored for changes in her breathing status. She began to recover function and is now ambulating independently.

Margie is ready for discharge to home to be cared for by her parents, who have been very involved in her care. Margie has expressed the feeling of being very frightened to go home because she is afraid that she will stop breathing again. She constantly talks about her paralysis and refuses to spend time with her friends when they visit, preferring the company of the nurses. The pediatric rehabilitation nurse should include the following points in the discharge plan:

- Stress the importance of keeping appointments with the psychologist.
- Assure Margie that it is not likely that she will have an exacerbation of the disease.
- Give her numbers of the physicians and emergency units that can be contacted if any symptoms arise.
- Contact the social worker for information on support groups for GBS, particularly those that have an adolescent membership.
- Involve Margie's friends in the interactions that Margie has with the nurses by playing card games and so on, and have the nurses slowly move out of the picture as Margie becomes more comfortable with her friends.
- Share Margie's concerns with her parents and develop a plan so that Margie can contact them at any time if she becomes fearful.
- Set up a weekend visit before discharge.

Conclusion

GBS is a devastating disorder; however, most of the children recover with minimal functional disabilities. Recovery may require long-term rehabilitation to either regain function or learn new functional activities to compensate for permanent disabilities. Pediatric rehabilitation nurses need to be aware of the possible disease trajectories and support the child and family through long-term treatment.

JUVENILE ARTHRITIS

Juvenile arthritis is a chronic inflammatory condition that begins before 16 years of age and is the primary cause of disability in children. It is a systemic disorder of connective tissue, joints, and viscera that includes arthritis-like manifestations. There are three onset types: systemic, pauciarticular, and polyarticular. Symptoms include joint swelling or restriction of movement with pain, tenderness, or heat.

The pediatric rehabilitation nurse may encounter the child in a variety of settings: hospital, home, school, and ambulatory care. The child may be hospitalized during the initial diagnosis, when the condition "flares up," when medications need to be re-evaluated, or when surgical procedures such as contracture releases or joint replacement need to be performed. The nurses' roles are very broad and include caregiver, teacher, advocate, and, in many instances, coordinator of therapeutic management for the child and family.

Etiology and Incidence

The cause is unknown, but it is thought to be due to a hypersensitivity response in which normal immune mechanisms are exaggerated or a reaction to unknown infectious agents. The disorder is probably multifactorial; and often an environmental trigger, infection, or trauma precedes the event. Age at onset is between 2 and 16 years and varies with each onset type. Prevalence in the United States is approximately 1 child in every 1000 in a given year, with slightly more females than males involved. Fortunately, many of the cases are a mild form of the condition (Lehman, 1996; Hartley & Fuller, 1997). Further insight into etiology and pathogenesis from recent immunogenetic studies suggests that bacterial heat-shock proteins may be significant in the chronic inflammatory response (Lindsley, 1995) and research investigating the relationship of the disease with viruses, stress, and immunodeficiency is being conducted.

Pathophysiology

Onset type is based on manifestations in the first 6 months of the illness, and the diagnosis is made by exclusion of other diseases, trauma, malignancies, joint or systemic infections, "growing pains," or congenital anomalies. Classification includes the concept of onset types as shown in Table 18–2, which are distinguished by the joint involvement in the first months after onset.

Inflammatory Process

The term *arthritis* indicates an inflammatory process occurring specifically in the synovium of a joint. This usually results in increased synovial fluid, which leads to swelling. When the joint is stretched during activity, the child experiences pain and tends to flex the joint to find a position of comfort. This can lead to flexion contractures. Heat, swelling, stiffness, and pain in the lining of the joint can lead to deformity and erode joint surfaces. Inflammation may alter the bones' growth centers and result in longer, shorter, or bigger than normal bones. Inflammation may also be found in the iris and ciliary body of the eye. This condition, called uveitis, is usually painless but can be a serious complication resulting in visual impairment.

Clinical Aspects

The signs and symptoms of juvenile arthritis may vary depending on the onset type and the responses of the individual child. Those symptoms most commonly seen are fever, morning stiffness, irritability, pain, limping, and heat and swelling of a joint. The child may be admitted to the hospital to assess spiking temperatures of undetermined origin before the onset of other arthritis symptoms. The onset types (see Table 18–2) are differentiated based on how they begin.

Systemic-onset type usually starts with a rash and a high temperature, which may go away for part of the day. Arthritis may be present in one or more joints, and the child is irritable and tires easily. The characteristic feature is the pink rash that is most noticeable during the temperature elevations.

In the *polyarticular* type, a greater number of joints are involved and the symptomatology may be more severe because the condition tends to worsen over time. Additional differentiation can be made in this group by testing for rheumatoid factor. Those with a positive rheumatoid factor will have clinical features more like the adult form.

The young child who is observed "walking funny" or is seen to have a swollen knee, without complaints of pain, has the *pauciarticular* type. Usually four or fewer joints are involved, most commonly the knees, ankles, and hips. A chronic eye inflammation, uveitis, may occur.

Course

Remissions and exacerbations characterize the course of the disease and vary among children. Late joint changes include adhesions and osteophytes, and surrounding tissues

Table 18–2 JUVENILE ARTHRITIS—ONSET TYPES AND CLINICAL ASPECTS

Systemic Onset	Any age; female = male; about 20% of cases Recurrent, intermittent fever greater than 103°F, usually high once or twice each day Rheumatoid rash—pale red, nonpruritic, macular on trunk and extremities Joint manifestations vary and lag behind systemic symptoms Internal organ involvement—liver, spleen, heart
Polyarticular Onset RF Negative	Females 4:1, any age but peaks 1–3 years and 8–10 years Involves four joints or more—wrists, knees, ankles, elbows, feet Insidious or precipitated by infection—progression early, tends to get worse over time Morning stiffness—systemic distribution
Polyarticular Onset RF Positive	Female, younger than 10 years of age Family history Clinical features as adult form—more likely to develop severe chronic arthritis Fever usually less than 103°F, rash, anemia, fatigue, anorexia, failure to gain weight
Pauciarticular Arthritis	Most common type, females younger than 4 years of age Four or less joints; knee most common, also ankles and hips Painless swelling, child is walking "funny" Few systemic signs—irritable, tired, poor weight gain, chronic eye inflammation

may undergo fibrosis, leading to contracture. Underlying bone may be scarred, and joint shape may become irregular, leading to subluxation.

Physical Impact and Functional Limitations

Overgrowth of bone may result in enlargement of the joint or a longer limb unless the epiphyseal plate is involved, in which case growth can be retarded and general stature reduced. Gait disturbance and altered posture might also result from the pain and swelling in the joints. Involvement of the mandibular rami may result in shortening and cause facial appearance and dental problems. Other physical abnormalities may be related to the effect of drugs. Two problems may develop with the pauciarticular type: eye inflammation leading to scarring of the lens, and differing leg lengths as the bones grow at different rates.

Functional limitations are usually attributed to stiffness, loss of range of motion, and deformity. Evaluation should be done in the home, school, and outdoors in the community. This can be done by interview, observation, and questionnaires. Tools that might be used for assessment include the Pediatric Evaluation of Disability Inventory (PEDI) and the Functional Independence Measure for Children (WeeFIM), discussed in Chapter 14, and the Juvenile Arthritis Functional Assessment Scale (JAFAS) and the Childhood Health Assessment Questionnaire (CHAQ). The JAFAS includes ten activities that must be completed within a specified time frame: elements of dressing, eating, standing, walking, and so on. The CHAQ is a checklist completed by the parent that covers similar activities plus hygiene and community mobility. Evaluation for accomplishing age-specific tasks is also important.

Diagnostic Assessment

A complete health history, including symptom progression, other infectious processes, and family history of arthritis, must be performed. The physical assessment should focus on joint inflammation, presence of rashes or nodules, and slit-lamp examination of the eyes for inflammation. Laboratory tests or procedures are performed to rule out other diseases, and the diagnosis is usually based on clinical findings. The most common serologic abnormality is the presence of antinuclear antibodies, but other laboratory tests might include identification of the rheumatoid factor, the erythrocyte sedimentation rate (which would be elevated), a hemoglobin test for the presence of anemia, and a urinalysis. Synovial fluid analysis to check for infections might find the predominant cells are neutrophils. X-ray films may be taken to document the stage and amount of joint involvement.

Therapeutic Management

There is no cure. Management focuses on suppressing the inflammatory process. A balanced program of medication, rest, and regular exercise, including physical therapy, is developed and is individualized to the child's needs, depending on the onset type and symptoms. Goals of treatment include controlling inflammation, relieving pain, preventing or controlling joint damage, and attaining the highest level of functional independence. Treatment includes medications, exercise and rest, eye and dental care, and healthy eating practices. Surgery may sometimes be recommended. Pain may be decreased by combining treatment with other techniques such as muscle relaxation, meditative breathing, and guided imagery.

Medication Therapy

Various medications may be prescribed to control pain, stiffness, and inflammation and treat chronic uveitis. Nonsteroidal, anti-inflammatory medications such as aspirin and indomethacin (Indocin) have analgesic, antipyretic, and anti-inflammatory effects. They act to decrease swelling, pain on movement, and tenderness and increase the range of motion in the involved joints. The aspirin dosage is based on the child's weight, 60 to 100 mg/kg/day in four divided doses, to maintain a consistent salicylate level. Knowing the side effects and signs of salicylate toxicity is very important. The most common side effect with aspirin is gastrointestinal upset; therefore, the drug should be taken with food (see Teaching Topic: Aspirin Therapy). In a study to determine the frequency of significant gastrointestinal side effects to nonsteroidal anti-inflammatory agents, it was found that, although mild gastrointestinal disturbance is a frequent side effect, clinically significant gastropathy is low (Keenan, Giannini, & Athreya, 1995).

Slow-acting antirheumatic medications affect the immune system but do not affect inflammation. One commonly used is gold salt (0.75 to 1 mg/kg/week for 20 weeks). Antimalarials, such as penicillamine and hydroxychloroquine, are oral agents that are slow acting and are also used in conjunction with aspirin.

Corticosteroids are infrequently used and definitely not used long term because of the side effects related to growth impairment. There may be reasons for short-term intra-articular injection to control inflammation in a particular joint.

Immunosuppressive drugs such as methotrexate are still experimental and have serious potential side effects. In a study to assess the response to and safety of long-term, high-dose drug therapy, it was found that although the high dose may be well tolerated the role in treatment may be limited. Outcome was assessed based on changes in therapy, laboratory parameters, physician assessment, and radiologic evaluation (Reiff et al., 1995).

Investigations have also begun on the use of oral type II collagen in the treatment of juvenile arthritis. Barnett, Combitchi, and Trentham (1996) found that it may be a safe and effective therapy and recommended that its use warrants further investigation.

Physical Therapy

Children with juvenile arthritis need a balanced program including rest and a regular schedule of exercise. The focus of this program is improving motion and strength, preventing musculoskeletal abnormalities, and promoting independence and controlling pain. The physical therapist develops a program with the child and family that allows for the greatest amount of independence while still ensuring that exercises are performed once or twice a day. Participating in regular daily activities is also important, but the joints must also move through their entire motion range on a regular basis. Rest periods and sleep time are also important parts of the program. A firm mattress is more supportive along with the use of a flatter pillow. The physical therapist may also incorporate hydrotherapy and the use of splints or casts.

Surgical Procedures and Post-surgical Rehabilitation

Surgery may be indicated for contracture release, but joint replacement is still controversial. If it is indicated, it should be postponed until bone growth has ceased and may pose other problems if the child is not prepared to be an active participant in rehabilitation.

Interdisciplinary Management

The management of the child with juvenile arthritis requires a team approach for both diagnosis and treatment. Pediatric rheumatology centers found in urban medical centers usually offer this type of approach. The team usually consists of a pediatric rheumatologist, nurse, physical therapist, occupational therapist, social worker, ophthalmologist, and orthopedist. Once the program is established, it can be coordinated by the pediatric rehabilitation nurse, who acts as a liaison between the child and family, the team, the school system, and other health care professionals. Periodic team meetings are helpful to reassess the needs of the child and family and make adjustments to the management program.

Application of the Nursing Process

The pediatric rehabilitation nurse as the coordinator of the care for the child and family interacts in a variety of settings with other nurses and health care professionals. The critical thinking skills inherent in the nursing process are essential in the provision of quality care that meets the needs of the child and family and obtains the desired outcomes.

Assessment

A health history and physical and functional assessment, focusing on neuromuscular and skeletal assessment, is an important initial element in determining the needs and problems of the child and family.

Nursing Diagnoses and Plan

After a thorough, individualized assessment of the child and family, a list of problems should be developed and nursing diagnoses and a plan of care identified. Two main problems that might be identified relate to physical mobility and pain, which can be closely related. If the nursing diagnosis of impaired physical mobility is identified, the plan as outlined in Table 18–3 can be initiated after it is specifically tailored to the age and abilities of the child and family.

Because pain is often reported by children and adolescents as a major symptom that affects their activities of daily living it is important to have information about the psychological, social, and environmental factors that influence their pain, which have been found to be different from those in adults.

One study (Hagglund et al., 1995) sought to determine which factors (demographics, disease status, social-psychological) contribute to a child's pain. Using a pain visual analogue scale as the measure and the Hopelessness Scale for Children, the Sadness Scale, and the Social Support Questionnaire, they found that reported pain was modestly correlated with age and duration of the disease. It is also very important to assess the pain and determine the best methods to relieve it. An observation method for assessing the pain behavior is useful in treatment outcome studies. In one study in which children were observed (Jaworski et al., 1995), total pain behaviors were significantly related to disability levels as well as subjective reports of pain.

Children have more pain than was previously appreciated. Limited data suggest that pain management interventions in children with active arthritis decrease pain-related behavior despite persistence of active disease. The recognition of pain-related behaviors and access to team members with skill in pain management fosters coping skills and increased compliance.

Self-esteem and body image concerns may also pose a problem for the child and family. The limitations that result because of the disease process may alter the child's perception of self-worth. It is important to assess the accuracy of these perceptions and assist the child and family with realistic expectations. An accurate understanding of the disease process can help the child and family see where interventions can have a positive impact. Support groups can be helpful for an older child because they provide opportunities to exchange concerns and ideas and verbalize feelings and frustrations.

Other problem areas that might be identified include deficits in self-care activities, such as dressing and grooming, alterations in nutrition and growth and development, ineffective coping, and alterations in family processes. Specific plans of care, based on information found in Chapters 12 and 13, can be developed to solve these problems as well.

Good nutrition is important to both normal growth and development and preventing complications from the condition. The pediatric rehabilitation nurse must recognize if caloric intake is meeting the child's nutritional needs and incorporate nutritional aspects into the educational program. For some children, decreased mobility may predispose the child to gaining weight, which will further stress inflamed joints. In other children, metabolic

Table 18–3   NURSING PLAN OF CARE—IMPAIRED PHYSICAL MOBILITY

Nursing Diagnosis: Impaired Physical Mobility

Related to: Intolerance to activity   Limited strength
                  Pain and discomfort   Musculoskeletal impairment

Goals	Nursing Interventions/Teaching
Increase or maintain strength and range of motion	Assist with active range of motion or perform passive range-of-motion exercises. Provide reinforcement of formal exercise program and encourage compliance. Encourage early morning shower or soak in warm water. Consult with physical therapist for indications for hydrotherapy, splints. Plan activities with adequate rest periods.
Promote independence in ambulation	Teach use of assistive devices and encourage appropriate use (splints, orthoses, etc.). Provide positive reinforcement during activity. Facilitate ambulation: provide diversional activities as needed.
Promote independence in activities of daily living	Encourage participation in self-care and recreational activities. Emphasize abilities and assist in understanding limitations.
Control or relieve pain	Determine pain characteristics and child's perceptions. Provide physical care such as application of heat and positioning. Provide comfort measures. Identify ways of minimizing pain.
Demonstrate use of activities for diversion and relaxation	Teach the use of distraction and relaxation techniques and exercises. Encourage use of relaxation exercises. Provide diversional activities.

Expected Outcomes

Willingness to participate in activities
Maintain or increase strength, joint mobility, and range of motion
Understand disease condition and treatment regimen
Report pain is relieved or controlled

needs may increase, resulting in inadequate weight gain, which interferes with normal growth.

Other nursing interventions that might be considered in the plan of care relate to

- monitoring medication effects—response and untoward effects
- collaborating with therapists in continuation of treatment program
- assessing psychological needs of the child and family and providing emotional support, especially during hospitalization
- encouraging compliance with the plan of care and evaluating it through follow-up at home and at school
- managing and coordinating long-term follow-up
- promoting activities that enhance the strengths of the child and family
- providing interaction with peers who share similar concerns and experiences
- informing the school nurse about the medication and exercise regimens and the need for movement frequently during the school day
- encouraging intervention by ancillary supports and outside resources

- educating the child and family about proper medication administration and precautions for medical therapy

Education is an ongoing process beginning at the time of diagnosis and involves all team members in providing appropriate information about the treatment program. The content and teaching sessions should be individualized to the needs and level of the child and family. Teaching needs include medications, dose, side effects, signs of toxicity, need for blood levels (see Teaching Topic: Aspirin Therapy), assessment of the child's physical condition, appropriate activities, nutrition, availability of community resources, and use of splints and casts. A common concern when teaching and establishing the management program is compliance with treatment recommendations. A higher level of compliance has been shown with medications than with the exercise regimen. Hartley and Fuller (1997) identified resources that serve to empower people and enhance the quality of life as they cope with chronic illness. These include

- knowledge about the disease and its management
- emotional and social support
- maintenance of mobility and function
- balancing energy use and rest to decrease fatigue
- increasing independence, motivation, and self-esteem

Impact on Child and Family

The diagnosis of juvenile arthritis affects both child and family. It impacts on family function and raises issues of dependence and independence. It has been determined that families benefit from a disciplined routine including time for therapies, rest, school, pleasure, and normal family activities. In a study of relationship between the child's cognitive development and conceptions of illness, it was shown that the child's understanding is at a concrete operational level even though the child has achieved higher cognitive levels (Pachman & Poznanski, 1993).

School attendance should be encouraged because it is an important part of normal development. Children with juvenile arthritis have more than double the school absences as other children (2.7 days over 2 months as compared with 1.1 days for others). They may need intermittent, variable-length home tutorial services available on short notice to "keep up" with class when attendance is difficult owing to surgery or disease exacerbations. They may also experience difficulty because schoolmates and teachers have no idea about the nature of the illness and may believe children do not get arthritis. Some adjustment may need to be made in the daily schedule to adapt activities to the child's limitations and to schedule regular exercises balanced with rest. Opportunities for play and directed school activities are essential and might include bike riding, rolling clay, daily living skills, and swimming. Those children participating in physical education at school should have an optimal exercise prescription. Information should be provided to the school staff, as outlined in the case study.

Community mobility is also important to the child and family. The team should be involved in evaluating for architectural barriers, recommending modifications, and assisting with the development of a planned program of recreation that is enjoyable for the child and family.

Long-Term Outlook

The outlook for most children is good, although there are no criteria for individual accurate prediction. The vast majority of children grow up to lead normal lives without significant difficulties. This includes successful attainment of developmental milestones, independence, and self-esteem. Long periods of spontaneous remission are typical, and the condition often remits or improves after puberty. Approximately 1 child in every 10,000 will have a severe case that does not go away;

Teaching Topic: Aspirin Therapy

Important Areas:
Therapeutic dosage (individualized to the child)
Administer with food to minimize gastric irritation. Discourage antacid use.
Therapeutic and side effects
Difference between salicylates and acetaminophen
Risks during flu season. Discuss with nurse or physician.
Safety issues for storage of medications.
Needed assessments to monitor benefit: changes in mobility and function and visual changes

and some, even with remission, may have long-term musculoskeletal complications. In outcome studies, Lindsley (1995) found risk factors for disability that included the presence of the rheumatoid factor and eye involvement.

CASE STUDY

Chandra is a 6-year-old girl with polyarticular juvenile arthritis. She has involvement of the elbows and wrists as well as the knees, ankles, and feet. She is taking aspirin to control inflammation and pain, and her most recent blood test showed a therapeutic salicylate level. You have been coordinating her care for the past few years and are now involved in preparation for the transition into school. She has been assessed by the team, and recommendations have been made for activities to improve gait, increase strength, decrease stiffness, and improve lower extremity range of motion. You are meeting with the school staff, including teachers, school nurse, and classroom aides, to assist them in integrating Chandra into the school setting and provide them with information about the condition and its effects. Areas to stress will be:

- frequent ambulation in the classroom
- equipment and activities that might be adapted for use during recess
- need for assistance with dressing skills
- education of peers regarding juvenile arthritis using an age-appropriate method
- medication effects
- assistance with activities of daily living at school with privacy for toileting
- use of computer for school work—may need to be voice activated.

   Continued assessment and education will be necessary during the school year to prevent social isolation and promote full inclusion in school activities.

Conclusion

New drugs are not needed for a large percentage of the children today with juvenile arthritis, but the multiple resources that are now available must be properly applied. Three important considerations for pediatric rehabilitation nurses working with children are proper diagnosis and recognition of the con-

dition, correct treatment with professional coordination and multidisciplinary support, and proper education of the child and family. Continued advances in knowledge of genetic and immunologic mechanisms operative in disease susceptibility and severity could lead to new therapeutic interventions, so it is also imperative that the nurse maintain current knowledge about the condition and its management.

DIABETES MELLITUS

Diabetes mellitus (DM) is a chronic disorder of carbohydrate metabolism characterized by a deficiency of the hormone insulin. The lack of insulin can be the result of an absence of beta cells in the pancreas or a relative lack of insulin related to insulin resistance. Type 1, or insulin-dependent diabetes mellitus (IDDM), is the most common type found in people younger than age 30 years.

   For carbohydrates to be metabolized correctly, insulin must be produced in adequate amounts in the pancreas in response to the amount of glucose in the blood. Without insulin, the serum glucose level rises until a condition of hyperglycemia exists. If hyperglycemia is not controlled, complications result, including blindness, end-stage renal disease, and premature cardiovascular death (American Diabetes Association, 1988).

   Successful management of diabetes is largely dependent on the child and family's commitment and involvement in a treatment plan that involves glucose monitoring, diet management, insulin management, and exercise. There are, however, many developmental and family issues that can prevent the optimal management of diabetes.

Incidence and Etiology

The cause of IDDM is unknown, but it is thought to be multifactorial. Genetics, autoimmunity, and environmental factors are linked to the destruction of the beta cells in the pancreatic islets of Langerhans. It is estimated that 16 million people in the United States have DM, although half are not aware they have the disease; and children and adolescents make up about 10% of all cases (American Diabetes Association, 1988). In chronic illnesses among school-aged children, diabetes ranks third. It usually develops between the ages of 6 and 13, with a peak incidence of age 10 to 12 years in girls and age 12 to 14 in boys. IDDM is more prominent in whites, with an incidence of 20 per 100,000. The incidence for blacks is 11.8 per 100,000, and the incidence in Hispanics is 9.7 per 100,000. Native Americans tend to have non–insulin-dependent diabetes mellitus (NIDDM) rather than IDDM, even if diagnosed during childhood (Kahn & Weir, 1994).

Genetic Factors: Genetic factors are known to play a role in the development of IDDM; however, the exact mechanism is not clearly understood. Genes within the human leukocyte antigen (HLA) region known as the major histocompatibility complex, located on chromosome 6, are related to the development of IDDM. There are several classes of genes that direct self-recognition and host defense mechanisms located on this complex. The frequency of certain HLA alleles (antigen DR3, DR4, or both) is five times greater in people who develop IDDM (Drash, 1986). Family studies also support a linkage of the HLA region with disease susceptibility and a genetic predisposition to the disease. However, someone who is genetically predisposed may never develop the disease unless exposed to another trigger, possibly environmental or viral (Cerrato, 1993).

Autoimmune Mechanisms: Anti–islet cell antibodies (ICAs) and insulin autoantibodies (IAA) have been found at the time of diagnosis of IDDM. ICAs are found in 70% to 85% of individuals newly diagnosed with IDDM (Drash, 1989). The ICAs may interact with the islet cell surface to inhibit insulin secretion. This is not believed to be the primary factor in the destruction of the beta cells but a secondary response to progressive beta-cell damage. Typically, nearly 90% of beta cells are destroyed by the time of diagnosis. There is a strong association between IDDM and other autoimmune endocrine disorders. Thyroiditis and Addison's disease are found in families and children with IDDM in which HLA-DR3 has been identified.

Environmental Factors: Evidence exists that implicates environmental factors in the development of IDDM. A number of viruses are implicated as the primary environmental factor in the etiology of IDDM. The virus may directly attack the beta cell or produce chemicals that damage the beta cell. The body reacts to this damage by an autoimmune response. Further evidence to support a viral trigger for diabetes relates to a seasonal variation in the onset of IDDM. There is an increase in IDDM during winter months that suggests an infectious disease relationship in the etiology of diabetes in children. Recent studies also suggest involvement of certain foods in the cause of IDDM, specifically the immune system's attack on pancreatic cells, making them unable to synthesize insulin (Cerrato, 1993). Several reports suggest that the trigger may be cow's milk.

Pathophysiology

In IDDM, destruction of the pancreatic beta cells results in a severe and eventual total depletion of insulin. With a deficiency of insulin, glucose is unable to enter the cell and it becomes concentrated in the blood. The increased concentration in the blood is called hyperglycemia. The increase of glucose in the blood produces a hyperosmolar osmotic gradient that pulls fluid from the intracellular space to the interstitial space and then to the extracellular space to be excreted by the kidneys. Normally the renal tubules reabsorb all of the glucose in the glomerular filtrate. When the glucose concentration in the glomerular filtrate exceeds the threshold of 160 mg/dL of glucose, it spills into the urine. The inability of the body to utilize glucose because of lack of insulin results in an ongoing catabolic state. The body begins to use alternative fuels. Therefore, glycogen, protein, and fat are mobilized from stores to meet the body's energy needs. However, in the absence of insulin, these substances cannot be used. The stores are depleted and cannot be replenished. The end result is a state of starvation.

Diabetic ketoacidosis (DKA) begins to develop when the body chooses alternate sources of energy, principally fat. The fat cannot be used by the body for energy and breaks down to fatty acids. The glycerol in the fat cells is converted by the liver to ketone bodies. Any excess is excreted by the kidneys in the urine (ketonuria) or lungs (acetone breath). The ketone bodies are strong acids that lower serum pH, producing ketosis. The state of acidosis is life threatening, and unless it is treated promptly, coma and death can result.

Clinical Aspects

The signs of IDDM occur in relationship to the amount of islet cell destruction. Eighty to 90 percent of the cells must be destroyed before there are symptoms of IDDM. Frequently, the first symptoms in children with IDDM are enuresis, irritability, and unusual fatigue. The child may also complain of abdominal discomfort as well as weight loss. The symptoms can be similar to those of the flu in children. The classic signs of DM are excessive thirst (polydipsia), increased food intake (polyphagia), and excessive urination (polyuria). Other symptoms include dry skin, increased infections, sores that are slow to heal, and blurred vision.

IDDM may not be diagnosed until the child has the symptoms of DKA. The increase in ketone bodies, resulting in DKA, are organic acids that produce excessive quantities of free hydrogen ions. The chemical buffers in the blood, particularly bicarbonate, combine with hydrogen ions to form carbonic acid, which breaks down into water and carbon dioxide. The body attempts to eliminate the excess carbon dioxide by increasing the rate and depth of respirations. This is called Kussmaul respirations. The breath will also have a fruity odor as the body attempts to blow off excess acetone. Table 18–4 lists the clinical manifestations with their appropriate therapeutic management and nursing care for children and adolescents who are newly diagnosed diabetics.

Course

Insulin-dependent DM is a disease that requires life-long treatment. Good control of the disease can result in normal activity for the children. With good control the long-term complications (retinopathy, nephropathy, and neuropathy) can be postponed for 20 or more years. Intensive insulin therapy may delay the onset and slow the progression of the long-term complications. One study, the Diabetes Control and Complications Trial (1995), enrolled children and young adults to evaluate the onset and progression of complications with both intensive therapy and conventional treatment. The result was a significant reduction in microvascular complications for those receiving intensive therapy that was related to the ability to control glucose levels (Beaser, 1995).

Physical Impact and Functional Limitations

The impact of IDDM on physical function is related to the long-term complications. These complications involve both the microvasculature and macrovasculature. Microvascular complications are retinopathy and nephropathy. Microvascular disease involves the thickening of the capillary basement membranes, tissue hypoxia, venous dilatation, and red blood cell aggregation. Cardiovascular disease and peripheral vascular events are macrovascular complications.

The kidneys may be involved. When the filtering system of the kidney is affected, the result is decreased renal function, followed by hypertension and end-stage renal disease. Visual problems occur when the capillaries in the retina break and bleed into the vitreous. The blood causes scarring to occur. New capillaries develop, but they are weak and poorly supported. This is called neovascularization. The scarring puts traction on the retina, causing retinal detachment. Cataracts can develop even in young children if glucose control is poor.

When the blood supply to the peripheral nerves is decreased, nerve dysfunction becomes a major problem. With decreased nerve function there is a loss of sensation, problems with proprioception, and a decrease in deep tendon reflexes. There may be injuries to the hands and feet of which the person is unaware because of decreased function of sensory nerves.

Diagnostic Assessment

Children of all ages can develop DM. It is not uncommon for the diagnosis to be made when the child becomes critically ill with ketoacidosis. DKA is defined by a glucose level over 300 mg/dL, a venous pH less than 7.3, a bicarbonate level less than 15 mEq/dL, glucosuria, and ketonuria.

Children can also be diagnosed after displaying the classic symptoms of DM and glucosuria. DM is diagnosed after a fasting blood sugar level of more than 200 mg/dL accompanied by classic signs of DM. Post-prandial blood glucose determinations and the traditional oral glucose tolerance tests are not necessary in children to establish a diagnosis.

A test that is helpful in the diagnosis is an index of long-term serum glucose levels, which is the determination of the glucose concentration in the erythrocytes. Hemoglobin A, or glycosylated hemoglobin, is hemoglobin to which glucose has been nonenzymatically coupled. This test reflects the average blood glucose concentration over the 120-day life span of the red blood cell.

Therapeutic Management

The management of the child with DM consists of an interdisciplinary approach involv-

Table 18–4 SYMPTOMS, MEDICAL MANAGEMENT, AND NURSING MANAGEMENT OF NEWLY DIAGNOSED DIABETIC PATIENTS

Clinical Manifestations	Therapeutic Management	Nursing Care
Diabetic Ketoacidosis (Acute Stage)		
Hyperglycemia, glycosuria, ketones Dehydration (polyuria, vomiting) Electrolyte imbalance (serum potassium ↑ or ↓, total body potassium ↓, serum sodium ↓, blood urea nitrogen ↑, plasma bicarbonate ↓, serum pH ↓)	Treatment with frequent doses of regular insulin (IV, SC, or IM) (common dosage: 0.1 unit/kg stat; 0.1 unit/kg/hr) Fluid and electrolyte therapy	Careful observation of patient receiving IV insulin and child's reaction to insulin Accurate intake and output
	Careful monitoring of glucose levels in blood and urine, electrolyte and abnormal laboratory values; monitor for cardiac irritability	
Kussmaul respirations Abnormal laboratory values (↑ WBC, RBC, and WBC ↑ in urine)		Constant observation of child's neurologic and vital signs
Cerebral edema-agitation, changes in level of consciousness	Informing both the family and the child of what is happening	
		Basic comfort measures for the child and family
Diabetic Ketosis		
Hyperglycemia Glycosuria	Treatment with regular insulin	Assessment of child's response to insulin, vital signs
Ketones (in both blood and urine)	Careful assessment of serum glucose levels, glycosuria, and ketones	
Possible dehydration	Careful monitoring of electrolytes and fluids	Careful monitoring of intake/output
	Information/education of the child and parents	
		Begin to encourage self-care when appropriate
Hyperglycemia		
Polyuria, polydipsia, polyphagia, fatigue Glycosuria No ketones	Careful assessment of insulin requirements (may require the addition of or ↑ regular insulin)	
	Careful assessment of serum glucose levels and glycosuria Encourage usual diet and activities (no exercise if blood sugar >300 mg/dL or if ketones +) Assess and plan education of the child and family	

From Betz, C., Hunsberger, M., & Wright, S. (1994). *Family-centered nursing care of children* (2nd ed.). Philadelphia: WB Saunders Co.

ing the family, the child, and health care professionals, including an endocrinologist, diabetic nurse educator, nutritionist, and a physical therapist or exercise physiologist to monitor the exercise program. The treatment plan is based on a balance between medica- tion therapy, nutrition, and exercise. The success of the treatment plan depends to a great degree on how well the family and child have been taught to manage the disease as well as their compliance with the treatment plan.

Medication Therapy

Insulin replacement is the critical element in the management of DM. Insulin dosage depends on the child's blood glucose level, diet, and amount of regular exercise. Insulin is available in highly purified beef, pork, and beef-pork preparations and in human insulin biosynthesized by and extracted from bacterial cultures. Human insulin is less likely to produce an allergic reaction and is therefore most often used to treat children. However, animal insulin is less expensive than the human insulin and may be used if cost may inhibit compliance with treatment. Insulin is available in rapid, intermediate, and long-acting preparations. All are supplied in the strength of 100 U/mL. Other concentrations can be obtained if small dosages are required.

The treatment of children with DM is fairly standard. A short-acting insulin is combined with an intermediate-acting insulin and administered before breakfast and the evening meals. This routine is preferred to one injection per day because it provides greater control over the coverage throughout the day. The short-acting insulin in the morning injection provides insulin for breakfast coverage, and the intermediate provides coverage for lunch. The short-acting insulin in the second injections provides coverage for the evening meal, and the intermediate-acting insulin meets the body's needs throughout the night. The disadvantage of the routine is the fact that the insulin injections and meals must be closely timed and given on schedule so that coverage is adequate for the meals and the child does not experience hypoglycemia if meals are not taken after the insulin injection has been given. The rigid routine may require significant lifestyle changes for the family.

There are other regimens that are designed to achieve tighter metabolic control. Multidose insulin regimens of three, four, or more injections per day provide control that is similar to the normal insulin secretion. When combined with frequent blood glucose monitoring and adjustment of insulin dosage based on test results, it can optimize control and limit complications.

Continuous subcutaneous insulin infusion, or insulin pump therapy, can be used. The pump is an electromechanical device designed to deliver fixed amounts of regular insulin continuously in a dilute solution that resembles normal insulin secretion. It is worn on a belt and injects insulin through a needle that is inserted into subcutaneous tissue such as the abdomen or thigh.

Nutrition

Dietary management is essential to the adequate metabolic control of DM. The goal is to assist children and adolescents in making changes in eating and exercise habits to minimize fluctuations in the blood glucose level to avoid hypoglycemia. Diet is the most difficult component of treatment to manage day to day. A major consideration is compliance, and sensitivity to ethnic, cultural, and financial factors is of utmost consideration. Most diets avoid refined and simple sugars, limit certain fats, and include adequate milk and calories for the child's desired weight and growth requirements. The dietary prescription should be based on nutrition assessment and treatment goals and individualized based on lifestyle, eating habits, and desired outcomes.

A balanced diet should include the basic food groups: vegetables, fruit, protein, fat milk, and starch. The meals can be planned using the exchange system approved by the American Diabetes Association. The exchange system is based on a prescribed amount of each food group and the number of each exchanges that can be eaten at the three meals and for snacks. If the diet is followed correctly, it allows for flexibility and the incorporation of preferred foods.

Exercise

Exercise should be incorporated into the treatment plan. Exercise helps to control DM because it helps to lower blood glucose levels. This decreases the need for insulin. The type and amount of exercise should be planned around the child's interests and developmental needs. The child's exercise activities, planned or unplanned, should be monitored by checking blood glucose levels because of the risk of hypoglycemia. If hypoglycemia does occur, the child should be given extra glucose before exercise. Exercise also increases circulation to muscle tissue, which increases the absorption of insulin. This can result in the development of hypoglycemia. If vigorous exercise is planned, insulin should be injected into a site that will not be exercised.

Application of the Nursing Process

The role of the pediatric rehabilitation nurse is focused on the coordination of care for the child and family as they interact with other health care professionals. Additionally, the nurse has the major responsibility of ensuring that the child and family receive the education necessary to manage the child's disease at home. Nursing interventions are developed so that optimal outcomes can be achieved; therefore, nursing actions are based on the nursing process.

Assessment

One of the most important functions is the assessment of the child or adolescent's and the family's knowledge about the disease and its management. This occurs in all settings and in each interaction between family and nurse. A health history will provide a background for the diagnosis and management of DM and should include eating habits, activity, medications, and glucose monitoring techniques.

Nursing Diagnoses

Based on the assessment data the following nursing diagnoses may apply:

- Alteration in Nutrition—depending on nutritional intake related to metabolic needs
- Potential for Infection/Impaired Skin Integrity
- Grieving, Disturbed Self-Concept/Body Image, Altered Growth and Development
- Powerlessness, Ineffective Individual/Family Coping
- Knowledge Deficit in the areas of dietary planning, medication management, glucose monitoring, appropriate exercise and activity regimen, complications, and community resources

The long-term goals for the child or adolescent with IDDM include:

Maintain optimum level of performance.
Prevent complications and pathologic changes.
Live within limitations of condition and integrate treatment regimen into lifestyle.
Resume normal role in home, school, and community.
Cope with and adapt to stressful events.

The health care emphasis has shifted from direct care to self-management and the acceptance by the child or adolescent and family of the responsibility for the day-to-day activities and care. Table 18–5 identifies the skills needed for survival as well as for health promotion and maintenance. Pediatric rehabilita-

tion nurses are key to successful management through the identification of knowledge and skill deficits and the provision of appropriate education to motivate and empower the child and family to develop confidence and set and achieve health care goals.

Psychosocial and Developmental Factors

Areas to consider are developmental level, school grade, stressors and coping mechanisms, family and other supports, habits, and interests. Table 18–6 lists specific concerns and suggested nursing interventions for each developmental level from infancy through adolescence. Davidson, Boland, and Grey (1997) concluded from their research that teaching coping skills to teens with IDDM helps with both the daily issues and long-term management. They noted that these teens "contend with the ever-present fear of hypoglycemia, fears of future medical complications and feelings of guilt for possible wrongdoing when faced with hyperglycemia" (p. 65). Teaching them skills to cope with stressful events can aid in their long-term adaptation and increase their ability to handle multiple demands. The areas suggested for training of teens are:

- coping skills especially social problem solving
- communication including assertiveness training
- cognitive-behavior modification
- conflict resolution

This can be accomplished in individual work sessions or with small groups of adolescents, allowing for sharing of ideas and the practice of behaviors.

School

The teacher and school nurse should be integral members of the diabetes management team and can assist in maintaining normal growth and development, keeping blood glucose levels within a normal target range, and promoting the child's well-being and emotional health. They should be knowledgeable about insulin needs and timing of injections, testing of blood glucose levels, schedule for meals and snacks, sports activities and regular exercise, and participation in school parties and other events. Efforts should be made to balance food intake and exercise with insulin levels and maintain a target range of blood

Table 18–5   LEVELS OF DIABETIC SKILLS

Survival Skills	Health Maintenance Skills	Health Promotion Skills
Need for insulin	Test blood and urine for glucose and ketones	Use of test results and records to make changes in insulin dose
Differentiate between types of insulin	Keep records	Insulin alteration
Relationship between meals and insulin	Rotate injection sites	Initiate illness regimen
Prepare and administer own insulin	Understand diabetic diet and how to modify during exercise or illness	Ability to modify regimen to maintain good metabolic control
Storage of insulin	How to prevent hypoglycemia	
Foods to avoid	Effect of stress, illness, and exercise	
How to recognize and treat hypoglycemic reaction	Meaning of metabolic control	

From Betz, C., Hunsberger, M., & Wright, S. (1994). *Family-centered nursing care of children* (2nd ed.). Philadelphia: WB Saunders.

glucose. A good plan (American Diabetes Association 1997) includes:

- eating on schedule, reasonable amounts
- regularly testing blood glucose levels
- regular exercise
- adjusting insulin to individual needs and as activities indicate

Long-Term Outlook

The future is promising with exciting prospects for slowing development or preventing the development of IDDM, and attention is given to the genetic basis of pathogenesis and prevention of complications. Also, work is being done in the areas of islet transplant and implantable insulin pumps.

CYSTIC FIBROSIS

Cystic fibrosis (CF) is a disease caused by an inherited genetic defect through an autosomal recessive trait that affects multiple systems, primarily the respiratory and digestive. It was first described in the late 1930s, and at that time nearly all children died in the first year of life. Characteristics of the condition include chronic pulmonary disease and digestive problems.

The pediatric rehabilitation nurse may encounter the child in a variety of settings: hospital, ambulatory care, home, school, and community. The child may be hospitalized during the initial diagnosis, during infections when vigorous pulmonary and antibiotic treatments are necessary, or for a lung transplant, which is now a treatment option. The nurses' roles are very broad and include caregiver, teacher, advocate, and, in many instances, coordinator of the plan of care and link to the comprehensive care program at a specialized center.

Etiology and Incidence

Although CF was first described in the 1930s, it was not until the late 1980s that the cause, a defective gene, located on the long arm of chromosome 7, was discovered. To inherit the condition a child must have a defective copy of the CF gene from each parent. This is the most common fatal genetic disease in the United States today, affecting nearly every race but mostly white Americans and northern European populations. It is rare in Native Americans and almost unheard of in Asian populations. In approximately 1 of every 3300 live births (approximately 1000 new cases/year) the child has CF, and more than 5% of the white population is believed to be heterozygous for CF. There are about 40,000 people in the United States with CF, and the incidence is equal initially for both sexes; but by age 20 years, males outlive females 6:1. Today 95% live to 16 years, 50% to 28 years, and some into their 30s and 40s, with a median survival age of 30.1 years; and the life span

Table 18–6   GROWTH AND DEVELOPMENT OF THE DIABETIC CHILD

Developmental Characteristics/ Developmental Tasks	Specific Concerns Posed by Diabetes	Suggested Nursing Interventions
Infancy		
Small physical size; rapid physical growth; physically active	Small insulin doses Frequent adjustments of insulin and diet Greater risks of hyperglycemia or hypoglycemia	Teach parents appropriate techniques for accurate measurement: use of 30-unit low-dose syringe, dilution of insulin Frequent visits to primary health care provider
Learning about environment; primitive language	Difficulty in detecting signs of changes on blood glucose	Instruct parents in age-appropriate signs of hypoglycemia: rapid heart beat, dilated pupils, irritability
Developing sense of self and physical capabilities; limited control of body functions	Increased susceptibility to vaginal and perineal infections because of moist glucose-laden environment of diapered infant	Educate parents about increased risks; encourage good hygiene practices and frequent diaper changes
Learning to trust	Pain of frequent injections and blood glucose monitoring can inhibit development of trust	
Dependent, requiring uninterrupted parental supervision	Difficult for parents to locate appropriate baby sitters	Encourage parents to bring other possible caregivers to diabetic teaching sessions; investigate baby-sitting programs with diabetic teens
Toddler		
Developing autonomy	Diabetes increases dependence on parents; parents may overprotect	Encourage use of alternative caregivers
Controlling body Making own choices	Frequent urination associated with hyperglycemic periods may make toilet training more difficult Hypoglycemic episodes may initiate temper tantrum behaviors Food selection may begin to be an issue	Suggest limited choices that parent can allow child to make in diabetic regimen: choice of allowed foods, site of injection
Preoperational thinking; cannot understand consequences of own actions		Encourage parents to set realistic limits and feel confident with them

Table 18–6   GROWTH AND DEVELOPMENT OF THE DIABETIC CHILD *Continued*

Developmental Characteristics/ Developmental Tasks	Specific Concerns Posed by Diabetes	Suggested Nursing Interventions
Preschooler		
Developing initiative	Realizes that diabetes makes him or her different from other family members	Acknowledge differences and focus on strengths Involve child in simple tasks of diabetic management
Developing social independence; may begin preschool	Relinquishing child to other caregivers may be anxiety provoking for parents Finding an appropriate preschool may be difficult	
Beginning moral judgments ("good" vs. "bad")	May see disease as "punishment"; may interpret "good" or "bad" blood or urine tests as a reflection on himself or herself	Avoid use of judgmental terms in describing test results or alterations from diet Encourage child to express feelings through play and art
Magical thinking; immature use of logic	Child may believe she or he "caught" diabetes from germs	Encourage parents to begin diabetes education using simple concepts and language; role play with dolls, stuffed animals
School-Age Child		
Developing industry; child wants to be successful in all tasks		Encourage child's independence and acknowledge small successes because children of this age need adult approval.
Development of concrete operational thinking and beginnings of formal operational thinking in older school-aged children	Ready for causal information; can understand the immediate consequences of his or her actions Child interested in the scientific nature of the illness (causes of hypoglycemia or hyperglycemia)	Educate child about the nature of diabetes with use of appropriate visual aids, toys. Reinforce or teach the child about ways to control symptoms (altering food intake, insulin, exercise).
Developing sense of personal responsibility	Parents are attempting to foster the child's independence but may have difficulty letting go of the diabetic management tasks they have been so accustomed to doing.	Encourage child to assume responsibility for larger portions of his or her own management of diabetes as he or she is ready.
Child makes social comparisons and is developing self-image through these comparisons	Being different from peers may be interpreted as a deficiency by the child. Diabetic management tasks that need to be performed in school may be a problem.	Encourage child to view diabetes as another example of differences between people and use appropriate comparisons with differences that are widely accepted (e.g., wearing glasses).

Table continued on following page

Table 18–6 GROWTH AND DEVELOPMENT OF THE DIABETIC CHILD *Continued*

Developmental Characteristics/ Developmental Tasks	Specific Concerns Posed by Diabetes	Suggested Nursing Interventions
		Encourage parents and child to establish a good working relationship with the school nurse.
		Be sure privacy is available for the child for management tasks.
		Encourage child to wear MedicAlert bracelet.
		Encourage interaction with other diabetic peers through support groups or diabetic camp.
Fine-tuning of small motor muscles		Gradually encourage child to assume responsibility for insulin administration and blood glucose testing.
Adolescent		
Developing a sense of identity; becoming more independent	May rebel against diabetic management regimen, which is seen as hampering independence; inappropriate food choices May isolate self from family or health care providers	Encourage adolescent to assume full responsibility for diabetic management; advise parents that adolescents still need to have their parents available for consultation and guidance. Encourage open discussion of issues; encourage participation in adolescent support group for diabetic teenagers. Teach the individual about food choices that may be appealing to adolescents.
Period of rapid physical growth, change, and sexual maturation	May make diabetic control difficult; menstrual periods may lead to reactions related to hormonal changes and effect on glucose metabolism	Reinforce signs and symptoms of hypoglycemia or hyperglycemia; maintain frequent contact with primary health care provider. Encourage adolescents to enlist the help of friends and educate them about appropriate actions in case of a reaction. Educate girls about possible effects of menstrual cycle.
Developing sexual interest; preferences	Rebellion can take the form of sexual experimentation	Provide information on the consequences of sexual activity; stress importance of planned preconception counseling for diabetic women.

Table 18–6 GROWTH AND DEVELOPMENT OF THE DIABETIC CHILD *Continued*

Developmental Characteristics/ Developmental Tasks	Specific Concerns Posed by Diabetes	Suggested Nursing Interventions
Selecting future lifestyle; career choices		Encourage parents to provide career counseling that acknowledges the demands of a diabetic regimen.
Self-image changes with dramatic physical changes; makes many physical comparisons with peers	Self-esteem may suffer because of differences from peers; may be anxious about possible reactions creating embarrassment	Use diabetic adolescent support group.
Developing own value system; comparing values of family and peers	May reject parental advice and counseling	Encourage relationships with other supportive adults or peers.
Formal operational thinking developing	Long-term consequences of disease will become real to the individual; may lead to depression	Encourage parents to keep discussions about the future open; observe for withdrawal or change in affect.

From Betz, C., Hunsberger, M., & Wright, S. (1994). *Family-centered nursing care of children* (2nd ed.). Philadelphia: WB Saunders.

continues to increase (Cystic Fibrosis Foundation, 1996a).

Pathophysiology

The disease is characterized by exocrine dysfunction involving the respiratory and digestive systems. Basically, the transport of sodium and chloride within epithelial cells is faulty. Specifically, the glands produce sticky, thick secretions that obstruct the small ducts of the bronchi of the lungs, the small intestine, and the pancreas, as well as the sweat glands. This makes digestion and breathing difficult. In the pancreas, enzyme secretion is inhibited so the digestion and absorption of fats and protein is impaired. This affects the small intestine and liver, resulting in malabsorption and steatorrhea (excessive amount of fat in the stool). In the lungs, the disorder interferes with normal ciliary action and the mucus, rather than acting as a lubricant, forms thick secretions that plug the airways, altering the exchange of oxygen and carbon dioxide. This provides a medium for microorganisms to grow, impairing the body's defenses and leading to infection. Additionally, the sweat glands are unable to conserve salt and skeletal maturation is retarded, leading to short stature and delayed bone aging.

Clinical Aspects

The most common presenting signs and symptoms are:

- recurrent respiratory infections or pneumonia
- poor weight gain despite good appetite
- persistent dry, nonproductive coughing with excessive thick, sticky mucus and wheezing
- salty taste of the skin and excessively salty sweat
- bulky, foul-smelling, numerous stools that float
- generalized hyperinflation and atelectasis of the lungs

The child may also have nasal polyps and varying degrees of hypoxia, cyanosis, hypercapnia, and acidosis. The anteroposterior diameter of the chest is increased, forming a barrel chest. Fibrotic lung changes may occur, and in severe cases pulmonary hypertension and cor pulmonale may be found. Additionally, there is poor weight gain or failure to thrive, clubbing of the fingers and toes, and thin extremities. Bowel obstruction (meconium ileus at birth), distended abdomen, malabsorption, and rectal prolapse are some of the other problems. Common complications that may occur are found in Table 18–7.

Table 18–7 COMMON COMPLICATIONS OF CYSTIC FIBROSIS

Gastrointestinal	Endocrine	Pulmonary
Cirrhosis	Diabetes mellitus	Emphysema
Pancreatitis	Heat prostration	Pneumothorax
Esophageal varices		Pulmonary pneumonia
Fecal impaction		Bronchiectasis
Hypertension		
Intussusception		
Cholelithiasis		
Pancreatitis		
Hemoptysis		
Rectal prolapse		

Physical Impact and Functional Limitations

Repeated infections and permanent damage to the lungs are common, and lower respiratory tract involvement causes over 90% of the morbidity and mortality. The obstructive disease begins in the small airways with a pattern of decreased vital capacity, forced expiratory volume in 1 second, peak expiratory flow, and increased residual volume indicative of air trapping. Pulmonary function and exercise testing typically show reduced lung capacity, exercise tolerance, and fitness; these are good techniques to use for following the progression of the disease in the older, cooperative child.

Clinical scoring systems can be used in assessment. In the Shwachman score, the four categories are (Ashwell et al., 1994, p. 693):

- chest radiography
- growth and nutrition
- pulmonary (physical findings and cough)
- case history, which includes subjective reports of exercise tolerance

If there is no impairment, the category is awarded 25 points, so a perfect score is 100. The child with a lower score has greater impairment.

Psychosocial concerns and developmental factors include participation in activities, self-image, fostering independence, acceptance of disease, and use of coping and problem-solving skills.

Diagnostic Assessment

A complete health history, including symptom progression, infectious processes, and family history of the disease must be performed, with a diagnosis made based on the clinical features. The current diagnostic criteria are:

- a positive sweat test—elevated concentrations of sodium and chloride in pharmacologically stimulated sweat
- chronic obstructive pulmonary disease
- exocrine pancreatic insufficiency
- family history of the disease

At least two criteria are required to establish the diagnosis; and almost always one of them is a positive sweat test, which is the most reliable. Prenatal determinations may be made by the presence of the mutated gene. Ten to 15 percent of infants have symptoms at birth, and many are diagnosed in the first 6 months, after an initial presentation for failure to thrive or gain weight; but the diagnosis may be made later in infancy or for up to 3 years.

Blood tests used in the diagnosis include albumin, blood urea nitrogen, creatinine, and aspartate aminotransferase and alanine aminotransferase to assess liver function. A urinalysis is performed to assess function of the kidneys; pulmonary function testing is done to diagnose and assess severity of the condition; a chest x-ray film confirms chronic obstructive lung disease; and stool samples are evaluated for fat content and trypsin. Research continues for an appropriate screening test. The child and parents need thorough explanation of the tests, procedures, and equipment to decrease their anxiety.

Therapeutic Management

There is no cure. Treatment is individualized and depends on the stage of the disease and which organs are involved but is aimed at promoting an independent life. Comprehensive, therapeutic management focuses on pulmonary and inhalation therapy with breathing exercises; gastrointestinal, digestive, and nutritional therapy; and psychosocial adjustment and genetic counseling, usually coordinated through a specialized center. The treatment team is composed of a physician, nurse, social worker, nutritionist, and physical therapist.

Pulmonary and Inhalation Therapy

Pulmonary and inhalation therapy is designed to prevent and treat pulmonary infection, clear secretions from airways, increase aeration, and reduce intensity of pulmonary infection. It involves techniques such as chest physiotherapy with percussion and postural drainage before and after therapy, two to four times daily in various positions, to stimulate coughing, loosen secretions, and maintain good pulmonary hygiene. Figure 18–1 shows chest physiotherapy with bronchial drainage positions and percussion points for major lung segments for older children. The same diagrams of positions and percussion points for the infant and small child are found in Figure 17–1. Mechanical percussion is shown in Figure 18–2. Daily breathing exercises aerate the lungs to maximum capacity, and inhalation therapy prevents and treats infection. Intermittent aerosol may be given 5 to 10 minutes before chest physiotherapy. Bronchodilators, decongestants, expectorants, and antibiotics are other treatments as well as double-lung transplantation, now a treatment option. A regular exercise program to increase breathing mechanics, posture, chest mobility, muscle strength, and aerobic fitness is also essential. Rehabilitation management focuses on maintaining or improving the efficiency of lung function so the child or adolescent can grow, play, and work as normally as possible.

Digestive and Nutritional Therapy

Digestive and nutritional therapy includes pancreatic enzyme replacement, dietary adjustment, and fat-soluble vitamin supplementation to promote growth, adequate nutrition, and normal bowel movements. Pancreatic enzymes (tablet or powdered form) are taken orally when food is consumed, and the amount varies with the child's diet, activity level, number of bowel movements each day, and type of stool. Salt is allowed in generous amounts.

Rehabilitation management focuses on

maintaining or improving the efficiency of lung function so the child or adolescent can grow, play, and work as normally as possible.

Application of the Nursing Process

The pediatric rehabilitation nurse obtains a health history and description of the current treatment regimen to establish a comprehensive nursing care plan. Respiratory assessment skills are essential to determine the child or adolescent's current status and response to treatment. Baseline information about nutrition, dietary habits, and bowel function provides additional information for determining goals and outcomes. Ongoing assessment of the child's status must be a part of the nurse's role because the disease progression is variable and the individualized needs of the child and family must be identified and met. The long-term goal is to have few or no complications and to maximize the coping skills required to live with chronic disease (see Teaching Topic: Prevention of Complications and Need for Compliance With Treatment Regimen).

After a thorough assessment, a list of problems and nursing diagnoses can be formulated and a plan of care identified. The primary nursing diagnosis areas to consider include:

- Ineffective Airway Clearance, Breathing Pattern and Impaired Gas Exchange related to increased pulmonary secretions, air trapping in the alveoli, and airways narrowed by mucus
- Alterations in Nutrition: Less than body requirements related to impaired metabolism of nutrients and vitamins, insufficient pancreatic enzymes and malabsorption
- Risk of Infection due to chronic tenacious secretions and lack of compliance with physiotherapy regimen
- Disturbance in Coping, Self-Concept, Self-Esteem and Role Performance
- Anticipatory Grieving related to perceptions regarding the diagnosis of an eventually fatal disease

During adolescence the issue of noncompliance may also become a factor. If the nursing diagnosis of ineffective airway clearance is identified, the plan in Table 18–8 can be initiated after it is specifically tailored to the age and abilities of the child and family.

The child with CF is unable to adequately digest and absorb fats and proteins, and the work of breathing also interferes with inges-

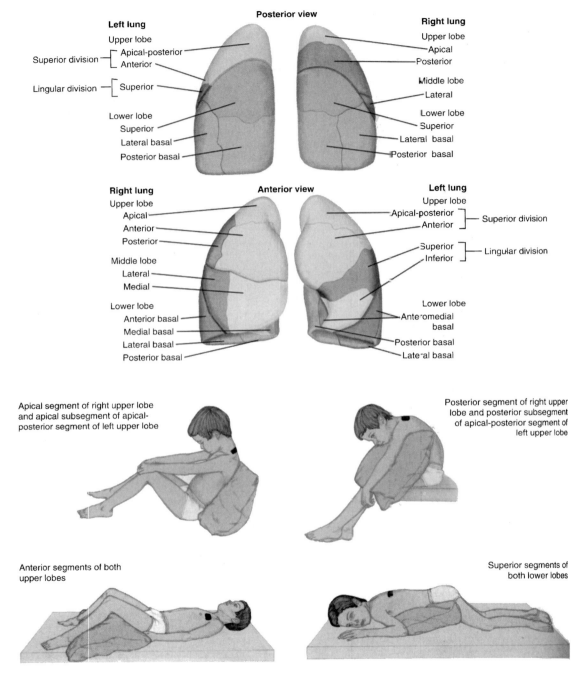

Figure 18–1 Chest physiotherapy for older children. Bronchial drainage positions and percussion points for major lung segments are shown. (From Ashwill, J.W., Droste, S.C. (1997). *Nursing Care of Children*. Philadelphia: WB Saunders, pp. 474–475.)

Correct hand position for percussion

Cup the hand to trap a pocket of
air that will transmit vibrations
through the chest wall to the
secretions that need to be dislodged.

Clap the cupped hand in rapid
sequence over a lung segment.
Elbow should be flexed and the wrist
relaxed, while creating a rapid
popping action.

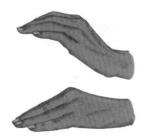

Lateral basal segments of right
lower lobe. Left lateral segment would be
drained by mirror image of
this position (right side down).

Posterior basal segments
of both lower lobes.

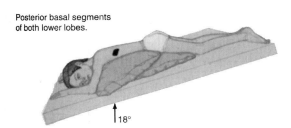

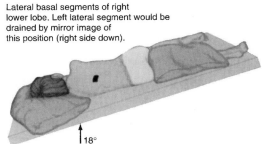

18°

18°

Anterior basal segment of left lower lobe;
right anterior basal segment would be
drained by mirror image of
this position (left side down).

Medial and lateral segments
of right middle lobe.

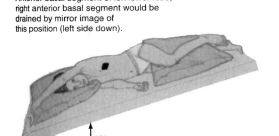

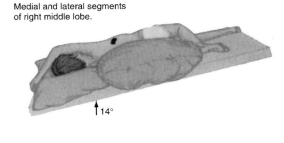

18°

14°

Lingular segments (superior and inferior)
of the left upper lobe (homologue of
right middle lobe).

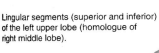
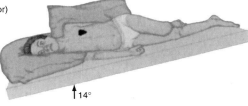

14°

Figure 18–1   *Continued*

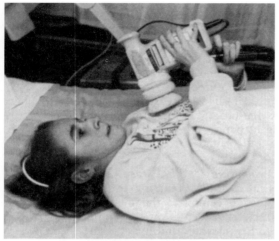

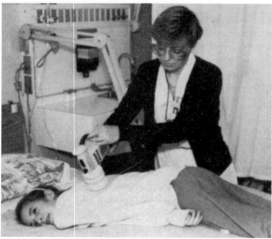

Figure 18–2 Hospitalized for cystic fibrosis, this 11-year-old girl performs parts of her own percussion. The nurse percusses the areas that the patient cannot reach. Mechanical percussion is now widely used and replaces manual percussion. (From Betz, C.L., Hensberger, M.M., Wright, S. (1994). *Family-Centered Nursing Care of Children, 2nd edition.* Philadelphia: WB Saunders, p. 1249.)

tion of nutrients and requires additional energy. Therefore, nutritional requirements are not met and weight gain does not progress according to a normal growth curve. The pediatric rehabilitation nurse must provide guidance and teaching for the child and family to plan well-balanced meals that incorporate food preferences, so that adequate nutrients are ingested for normal growth and development. Additionally, pancreatic enzymes are included, as well as vitamins and iron supplements and sodium chloride tablets in hot weather. The goals are for the child

to consume sufficient calories and nutrients needed for age and activity level, to progress normally along the growth curve, and to have stools of normal consistency, frequency, and color. Enzymes should be mixed with carbohydrate foods (e.g., applesauce) and administered at the beginning of the meal.

The child or adolescent may have an altered self-concept because of physical appearance, inability to participate in activities with peers, and other symptoms and treatments associated with the condition. It is important for the nurse to assess the child's or adolescent's feelings about CF, recognizing strengths and suggesting ways to excel, provide information about the disease progression, answer questions about peer relationships, and assist in making realistic plans for the future. The child should be encouraged to take an active role in the plan of care and treatment, and families should allow as much independence as possible in activities and choices.

In preparation for care at home, the pediatric rehabilitation nurse should instruct the parents and child about techniques of home management: dietary needs, postural drainage and percussion, intermittent positive-pressure breathing treatments, breathing exercises, and administration of medications. The nurse should also assist the family in contacting support systems for financial, psychological, and medical assistance. In as-

---

Teaching Topic: Prevention of Complications and Need for Compliance with Treatment Regimen

Important Areas:

Provide information on the disease and its impact on body systems.

Review postural drainage, percussion, use of equipment, diet, and administration of medications.

Review signs of pulmonary infection; encourage to seek health care immediately; avoid contact with persons with respiratory tract infections.

Provide opportunities for questions and voicing concerns.

Provide telephone numbers for contacts for questions, problems with equipment, or information about medications.

Table 18-8 NURSING PLAN OF CARE—INEFFECTIVE AIRWAY CLEARANCE

Nursing Diagnosis: Ineffective Airway Clearance

Related to: Increased pulmonary secretions
Difficulty in expelling mucus

Goals	Nursing Interventions/Teaching
Effectively clear the airways of mucus Free from dyspnea and respiratory tract infection	Percussion and postural drainage as indicated Teach/review breathing exercises and coughing Observe and monitor respiratory status Monitor effects of respiratory treatments Encourage physical activity Observe sputum color and quality

Expected Outcomes

Participate in normal activities
Experience minimal or no pulmonary complications

sessing home management, the nurse should focus on the specific activities found in Table 18–9.

Impact on Child and Family

Cystic fibrosis disrupts the life of the entire family and impacts on the ways in which the family members are coping. Family members should be encouraged to verbalize feelings about the child's illness and its impact on their lives and focus on their roles within the family as well as relating to the child with CF. It is important for the nurse to identify resources—community, information, supportive, and financial—for the family and assist them to use these appropriately. Parents and families should seek relevant support groups where they can share common knowledge and experience. They need help to promote optimal development and create a balance between protection/nurturance and autonomy/independence. Hymovich and Hagopian (1992) identified situational tasks that children and families face in relation to a chronic condition. These are found in Tables

Table 18-9 NURSING FOCUS IN ASSESSING HOME MANAGEMENT FOR THE CHILD WITH CYSTIC FIBROSIS

Plot height and weight on the growth curve and assess for steady progress.

Assess vital signs, breath sounds, and energy available to perform usual activities of daily living.

Determine effectiveness of expectoration with home chest physical therapy and inhalation therapy; have caregivers demonstrate techniques.

Ask the child and parent about gastrointestinal symptoms that would indicate malabsorption and inadequate enzyme replacement: bloating, abdominal cramping and distention, and diarrhea.

Have the child and parent record the dietary intake for the previous 24 to 48 hours to assess nutrient and caloric adequacy.

When appropriate, determine adherence to prescribed antibiotic therapy.

Encourage the child and parent to discuss psychosocial and developmental concerns and to ask questions about the technical aspects of home management.
    Yearly chest radiographs; unless chest condition changes between visits, then more often
    Pulmonary function tests done on all children older than 5 years every 3 to 6 months
    Blood and urine testing as necessary
    Exercise testing every 6 months
    Sputum culture every 6 months

From Betz, C., Hunsberger, M., & Wright, S. (1994). *Family-centered nursing care of children* (2nd ed.). Philadelphia: WB Saunders.

18–10 and 18–11. They also developed a Contingency Model of Long-Term Care that can be used by nurses to assess families and provide interventions unique to their needs. The nursing care component of the model is found in Figure 18–3. Broken lines indicate areas of overlap of nursing process and content. Examples are in lower-case type. The model should be used as a guide for organizing information and assessment areas and formulating the interdisciplinary plans of care.

Long-Term Outlook

There is no cure, but research and medical advances have improved life expectancy and quality of life. This is dependent on severity of the disease, the aggressiveness of the treat-

Table 18–10 SITUATIONAL TASKS OF CHILDREN AND ADULTS WITH CHRONIC CONDITIONS

Master, within limits of the condition, age-appropriate developmental tasks

Develop an age-appropriate understanding of the condition and its management

Develop and preserve a sense of control over the situation

Adjust to potential role changes

Maintain control of symptoms (e.g., pain, incapacitation, decreased control of bodily functions)

Deal with the uncertainty of the condition and prepare for an uncertain future

Develop or refine one's value system

Develop or preserve relationships with family and friends

Understand and cope with emotional impact of the condition

Master the ability to provide care for self, within the limits of the condition and one's developmental level

Make age-appropriate decisions regarding one's care

Develop trust in oneself and one's caregivers

Develop and maintain a positive self-concept and sense of self-esteem

From Hymovich, D., & Hagopian, G. (1992). *Chronic illness in children and adults: a psychosocial approach.* Philadelphia: WB Saunders.

Table 18–11 SITUATIONAL TASKS OF PARENTS OF CHRONICALLY ILL CHILDREN

Obtain adequate health care

Meet financial burden of the condition

Maintain health of all family members

Understand and manage the condition

Meet the developmental needs of each family member

Learn areas in which child's life and function are not affected by the condition and develop plan to ensure as much normalcy as possible

Maintain their own health

Maintain the individual integrity of each family member

Establish and maintain support system

Establish a philosophy of life to cope with the condition

Help child(ren) understand and cope with the condition

Assign condition management tasks to child appropriate for age and developmental status

Understand and cope with the emotional impact of the condition on family

Adjust family organization to accommodate person with the chronic condition

Adjust to changes in lifestyle

Become an advocate for self and family

Seek and use appropriate health and community resources

From Hymovich, D., & Hagopian, G. (1992). *Chronic illness in children and adults: a psychosocial approach.* Philadelphia: WB Saunders.

ment, and the element of contact with bacterial infections. The timing of diagnosis and treatment impacts the long-term prognosis. For example, children who are diagnosed and have treatment initiated before irreversible pulmonary damage have better function and survival (Orenstein, 1991). As medical advances have increased life expectancy, adolescents and young adults face new challenges: getting advanced education, getting a job and health insurance, and building relationships while maintaining a treatment regimen.

A new mucus-thinning drug (dornase alfa [Pulmozyme]) is improving lung function

NURSING CARE

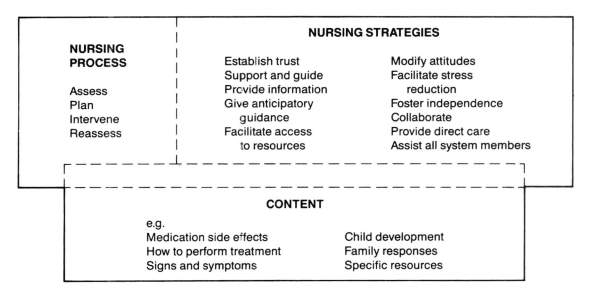

Figure 18–3   Nursing care component of the contingency model of long-term care. The broken lines depict the overlapping nature of nursing process and content. (From Hymovich DP, Hagopian GA. *Chronic Illness in Children and Adults: A Psychosocial Approach.* Philadelphia: WB Saunders, 1992, p. 32.)

and reducing the number of respiratory tract infections. Results of one study showed that ibuprofen reduced lung inflammation particularly in children (Cystic Fibrosis Foundation, 1996a). Another study showed a correlation between aerobic fitness and exercise and an increase in lung efficiency and utilization capacity (Zaborowski-Dunn, 1995).

Since the CF gene was found in 1989, research has taken major steps toward successful gene therapy treatment, and gene-transfer techniques and studies are continuing. Ultimately, enough normal genes will be added to airways to correct defective cells. This will be done by innovative delivery systems such as modified viruses and synthetic vectors (e.g., via nose drops or through a bronchoscope). Three areas of research that are underway are gene, protein, and drug therapies; eventually the technology used to treat the airways will be adapted to treat the other organs (Cystic Fibrosis Foundation, 1996b).

SUMMARY

Each of these conditions, Guillain-Barré syndrome, juvenile arthritis, diabetes mellitus, and cystic fibrosis, poses challenges for the pediatric rehabilitation nurse because of the long-term rehabilitation needs and chronic ef-

fects and the physical and psychosocial impact on the child or adolescent and family. It is very important for the nurse to maintain current knowledge and the requisite skills to provide the most appropriate nursing care and treatment regardless of the setting in which the nurse encounters the child and family. Research, as an integral part of the nurse's role, is expected to provide new therapeutic interventions and dramatic breakthroughs in the genetic basis of disease and the prevention of complications. It is an exciting and challenging time, and the pediatric rehabilitation nurse, with all the requisite knowledge and skills, will be a valuable, integral member of the interdisciplinary team.

REFERENCES

American Diabetes Association (ADA). (1988). *Physician's guide to insulin-dependent (type 1) diabetes: diagnosis and treatment.* Alexandria, VA: ADA.

American Diabetes Association. (1997a). *Diabetes facts and figures* [On-line]. Available: www.diabetes.com

American Diabetes Association. (1997b). *Children with diabetes: information for teachers and childcare providers* [On-line]. Available: www.diabetes.com

Ashwell, J., Agnew-Coughlin, J., Boyd, S., &

Brooks, D. (1994). Cystic fibrosis. In Campbell, S. (Ed.) *Physical therapy for children*, pp. 687–715. Philadelphia: WB Saunders.

Barnett, M., Combitchi, D., & Trentham, D. (1996). A pilot trial of oral type II collagen in the treatment of juvenile rheumatoid arthritis. *Arthritis and Rheumatism*, 39(4), 623–628.

Batshaw, M., & Perret, Y. (1992). *Children with disabilities: a medical primer* (3rd ed.). Baltimore: Paul H. Brookes.

Beaser, R. (1995). Putting DCCT into practice. *Patient Care*, Feb. 15, 15–30.

Cerrato, P. (1993). Does milk cause juvenile diabetes? *Rehabilitation Nursing*, (1), 56, 69–71.

Cystic Fibrosis Foundation. (1996a). *Facts about cystic fibrosis* [On-line]. Available: www.cff.org/factsabo

Cystic Fibrosis Foundation. (1996b). *Gene therapy* [On-line]. Available: www.cff.org/genether

Davidson, M., Boland, E., & Grey, M. (1997). Teaching teens to cope: coping skills training for adolescents with insulin-dependent diabetes mellitus. *Journal of the Society of Pediatrics Nursing*, 2(2), 65–71.

Drash, A. (1986). Diabetes mellitus in the child and adolescent: part 1. In J. Lockhart (Ed.). *Current problems in pediatrics.* Chicago: Year Book Medical.

Drash, A. (1989). Insulin-dependent diabetes mellitus in children and adolescents: genetics and etiology. *Current Opinions in Pediatrics*, 1, 61–73.

Guillain-Barré. (1996). *Health information* [On-line]. Available: www.Housecall.com/databases/ami/convert/000684.html

Guillain-Barré syndrome: fact sheet. (1992). NIH Publication No. 92-2902. Washington, DC: U.S. Department of Health & Human Services, National Institutes of Health.

Guillain-Barré Syndrome Steroid Trial Group. (1993). Double-blind trial of intravenous methylprednisolone in Guillain-Barré syndromes. *Lancet*, 341(8845), 580–590.

Hagglund, K., Schopp, L., Alberts, K., Cassidy, J., & Frank, R. (1995). Predicting pain among children with juvenile rheumatoid arthritis. *Arthritis Care and Research*, 8(1), 36–42.

Hartley, B., & Fuller, C. (1997). Juvenile arthritis: a nursing perspective. *Journal of Pediatric Nursing*, 12(2), 100–109.

Hickey, J. (1996). *The clinical practice of neurological and neurosurgical nursing* (4th ed.). Philadelphia: JB Lippincott.

Hunsberger, M., & Feenan, L. (1994). Altered respiratory function. In C. Betz, M. Hunsberger, & S. Wright (Eds.). *Family-centered nursing care of children* (2nd ed.) pp. 1167–1275. Philadelphia: WB Saunders.

Hymovich, D., & Hagopian, G. (1992). *Chronic illness in children and adults: a psychosocial approach.* Philadelphia: WB Saunders.

Jaworski, T., Bradley, L., Heck, L., Roca, A., & Alarcon, G. (1995). Development of an observation method for assessing pain behaviors in children with juvenile rheumatoid arthritis. *Arthritis and Rheumatism*, 38(8), 1142–1151.

Kahn, C., & Weir, G. (1994). *Joslin's diabetic mellitus* (13th ed.). Philadelphia: Lea & Febiger.

Keenan, G., Gannini, E., & Athreya, B. (1995). Clinically significant gastropathy associated with nonsteroidal antiinflammatory drug use in children with juvenile rheumatoid arthritis. *Journal of Rheumatology*, 22(6), 1149–1151.

Lehman, T. (1996). *Arthritis in childhood and adolescence* [On-line]. Available: www.wp.com/pedsrheum

Lindsley, C. (1995). Juvenile rheumatoid arthritis and spondyloarthropathies. *Current Opinions in Rheumatology*, 7(5), 425–429.

McCance, K., & Huether, S. (1994). *Pathophysiology: the biologic basis for disease in adults and children* (2nd ed.). Philadelphia: CV Mosby.

Noble, J. (Ed.). 1996). *Textbook of primary care medicine* (2nd ed.). Philadelphia: CV Mosby.

Orenstein, D. (1991). Cystic fibrosis. *Respiratory Care*, 36(7), 746–754.

Pachman, L., & Poznanski, A. (1993). Juvenile rheumatoid arthritis. In D. McCarthy & W. Koopman (Eds.). *Arthritis and allied conditions: a textbook of rheumatology* (12th ed.). Philadelphia: Lea & Febiger.

Reiff, A., Shahan, B., Wood, B., Bernstein, B., Stanley, P., & Sze, I. (1995). High dose methotrexate in the treatment of refractory juvenile rheumatoid arthritis. *Clinical and Experimental Rheumatology*, 13(1), 113–118.

Steinberg, J. (1996). *Guillain-Barré syndrome: an overview for the layperson.* Philadelphia: Guillain-Barré Syndrome Foundation International.

Vallee, L., Dulac, O., Nuyts, J., Leclerc, F., & Vamecq, J. (1993). Intravenous immune globulin is also an efficient therapy of acute Guillain-Barré syndrome in affected children. *Neuropediatrics*, 24(4), 235–235.

Wong, D. (1995). *Whaley & Wong's nursing care of infants and children* (5th ed.). Philadelphia: CV Mosby.

Zaborowski-Dunn, L. (1995). *Rewards after exercise linked to improved health of children with cystic fibrosis* [On-line]. Available: http://tns.sdsu.edu/infocom/news/cys-fib.html

Nutrition recommendations and principles for people with diabetes mellitus. (1994). *Diabetes Care*, 17(5), 519–522.

ADDITIONAL REFERENCES

Betz, C., Hunsberger, M., & Wright, S. (Eds.). (1994). *Family-centered nursing care of children* (2nd ed.). Philadelphia: WB Saunders.

Campbell, S. (Ed.). (1994). *Physical therapy for children.* Philadelphia: WB Saunders.

Logigian, M., & Ward, J. (Eds.). (1989). *Pediatric rehabilitation: a team approach for therapists.* Boston: Little, Brown & Co.

Orenstein, D. (1989). *Cystic fibrosis: a guide for patient and family.* New York: Raven Press.

Stullenbarger, B., Norris, J., Edgel, A., & Prosser, M. (1987). Family adaptation to cystic fibrosis. *Pediatric Nursing*, 13(1), 29–31.

Scipien, G., Chard, M., Howe, J., & Barnard, M. (1990). *Pediatric nursing care.* Philadelphia: CV Mosby.

RESOURCES

American Diabetes Association
1660 Duke Street
Alexandria, VA 22314
www.diabetes.org

Arthritis Foundation
800-542-0295

Cystic Fibrosis Foundation
6931 Arlington Boulevard
Bethesda, MD 20814
800-FIGHT-CF 301-951-4422
www.cff.org info@cff.org

Guillain-Barré Syndrome Foundation International
P.O. Box 262
Wynnewood, PA 19096
610-667-0131
www.webmast.com/gbs
gbint@ix.netcom.com

Joslin Diabetes Center
Boston, MA
800-344-4501

National Institute of Neurological Disorders and Stroke
P.O. Box 5801
Bethesda, MD 20824
301-496-5751
800-352-9424
www.ninds.nih.gov/healinfo/disorder/guillain

National Jewish Medical and Research Center
1400 Jackson Street
Denver, CO 80206
800-222-LUNG (5864) 303-388-4461
www.njc.org

Chapter 19

The Child With HIV

Lynn Czarniecki and *Mary G. Boland*

Human immunodeficiency virus (HIV) infection in children is not one disease but rather is a multi-organ systemic illness producing a combination of acute and chronic processes mediated both by the virus itself and the resulting suppression of the immune system. The diverse clinical presentation of HIV infection and acquired immunodeficiency syndrome (AIDS) demands evaluation of the rehabilitative needs of infected children to ensure a multi-disciplinary, comprehensive approach that treats the child with multiple disabilities while supporting the family's efforts to help their child lead as normal a life as possible (Oleske, 1995).

Children with HIV infection develop a range of problems that are both similar to and different from those of adults with HIV. HIV differs from other conditions encountered by rehabilitation nurses. This disease will continue to progress, with new symptoms emerging and aggressive chemotherapy treatment ongoing, while the child is receiving rehabilitation. While a child is receiving care in a residential setting, an understanding of the progression of the disease is critical to ensure that the immune system is monitored and new symptoms treated.

This chapter presents an overview of HIV disease and describes the common symptoms, diseases, and developmental and functional effects, as well as their implications for pediatric nurses working in a variety of settings. The emphasis is placed on those manifestations that produce chronic effects requiring habilitation and rehabilitation. Family and social concerns are emphasized, with

suggestions provided for nursing interventions. Understanding of HIV and AIDS continues to evolve, and new treatments emerge based on laboratory findings and experience with clinical trials of investigational drugs. It is critical that nurses recognize the need to obtain or maintain knowledge regarding the understanding and treatment of this disease.

BACKGROUND

The first reports of pediatric AIDS were published in 1983. Since that time, 6948 U.S. children have been reported with AIDS and an additional 1350 children have been reported with HIV infection (Centers for Disease Control and Prevention [CDC], 1996). Worldwide, it is estimated that 3 million children are infected with HIV (Joint United Nations Programme on HIV/AIDS, 1996). Perinatal transmission accounts for the majority of cases of infection in children. The risk of HIV transmission from a woman to her infant is about 25%. Zidovudine administered to the mother during pregnancy and at delivery and to the infant for the first 6 weeks of life has been shown to decrease this transmission rate to about 8%, with no deleterious effects on the infant. Studies assessing the role of additional agents in interrupting perinatal transmission are ongoing. Throughout the United States there is an aggressive effort to counsel all pregnant women regarding HIV infection and to encourage HIV testing during pregnancy. The goal of such efforts is to improve the health care provided to infected women and offer the woman the opportunity to interrupt transmission to her infant. Such initiatives are showing signs of success, with some communities already reporting decreases in the number of infected babies born to women who are taking the zidovudine regimen.

It is believed that transmission can happen in utero, at the time of delivery, and through breastfeeding. Infection in a child can be diagnosed as early as 1 month of age through the use of HIV culture and polymerase chain reaction (PCR). These diagnostic methods are not currently commercially available and are typically performed at research centers. For the child older than 18 months, a positive HIV antibody test using enzyme-linked immunosorbent assay (ELISA) and Western blot is acceptable. Once diagnosis is documented, the child is evaluated to identify the stage of infection and placed into a diagnostic category using the CDC classification scheme. This scheme, pertaining to children through the age of 12 years, defines the spectrum of the disease based on both immunologic status and clinical symptoms (Table 19-1).

NATURAL HISTORY

As a result of early diagnosis, supportive care, and specific HIV treatment, perinatally infected infants are frequently living to school-age and occasionally early adolescence. HIV-infected children fall into two groups: rapid progressors and slow progressors. Both groups of children will be seen in rehabilitation settings. Rapid progressors have, as a rule, severe HIV encephalopathy with associated disabilities, and some older children develop neurologic disease associated with HIV and consequent disabilities (see Problems Related to Neurologic System Dysfunction).

About 10% to 15% of children with HIV are thought to be rapid progressors and develop severe and life-threatening symptoms in infancy, some as early as 6 months of age. *Pneumocystis carinii* pneumonia (PCP), an opportunistic infection (OI), can be life-threatening; however, it can be prevented if the infant is identified as the child of an HIV-infected woman and prophylaxis is begun. More difficult to treat are encephalopathy and failure to thrive, which are the two other hallmarks of the rapidly progressing infant (discussed later). Even with aggressive and complex treatments, such children rarely survive longer than 5 years (Blanche et al., 1990).

Children with late onset of symptoms, sometimes referred to as "long-term survivors," have a better prognosis. For these slow progressors, immunodeficiency and clinical symptoms develop gradually over a period of several years, sometimes as late as 10 years. These children usually have milder symptoms and may be clinically asymptomatic for long periods. It is this group that is most likely to benefit from combination anti-retroviral drug therapy.

The use of plasma HIV RNA concentration, which measures viral load, in conjunction with CD4 T-lymphocyte counts has become a standard tool to evaluate the progression of HIV disease. Palumbo and colleagues (1998) reported that the presence of a high HIV RNA concentration with a low CD4 T-lymphocyte count can be prognostic of more rapid disease progression.

TREATMENT

Human immunodeficiency virus causes illness in two different but equally severe ways. Direct infection of cells by the virus itself can occur in organ systems throughout the body, and the virus has a particular affinity for the nervous system. Second, as HIV infects and

Table 19-1   CLASSIFICATION SYSTEM FOR HUMAN IMMUNODEFICIENCY VIRUS INFECTION IN CHILDREN YOUNGER THAN 13 YEARS OF AGE

	Clinical Categories			
Immunologic Categories	No Signs/ Symptoms	Mild Signs/ Symptoms	Moderate Signs/ Symptoms	Severe Signs/ Symptoms
No evidence of suppression	N1	A1	B1	C1
Evidence of moderate suppression	N2	A2	B2	C2
Severe suppression	N3	A3	B3	C3

Both category C and lymphoid interstitial pneumonitis in category B are reportable as acquired immunodeficiency syndrome to state and local health departments.
From Centers for Disease Control and Prevention. (1994). 1994 Revised classification system for human immunodeficiency virus infection in children less than 13 years of age. *Morbidity and Mortality Weekly Report* 43, RR-12.

destroys the T-helper or CD4 cells, the immune system is weakened, increasing susceptibility to infections. Because of this pathogenesis, the course of disease cannot be predicted for any one individual. It is the interaction of both these processes that produces clinical illness. Thus, the manifestations and progression of HIV in each child is unique.

Management of HIV infection and the resulting manifestations is complex. Anti-retroviral treatment that can "cure" the illness is a long way off for children. Although dramatic results have been reported for adults receiving combination therapy, studies have yet to begin in children. Anti-retroviral drugs currently available for use in infants, children, and adolescents include the following:

> Nucleoside analogue reverse-transcriptase inhibitors (NRTIs): zidovudine, didanosine, lamivudine, stavudine, and zalcitabine
>
> Non-nucleoside reverse-transcriptase inhibitors (NNRTI): nevirapine
>
> Protease inhibitors: indinavir, nelfinavir, ritonavir, saquinavir

These agents should be used in combination. Zidovudine has been found to decrease neurologic manifestations. The decision to initiate anti-retroviral treatment is a complex one, made even more complicated by the emergence of viral load as a recognized surro-gate marker for disease progression. Treatment guidelines for children were published in 1998 (CDC, 1998). These guidelines outline the recommended anti-retroviral treatment for infants and children with HIV. Goals of symptomatic care include eradicating or slowing down the virus, maintaining or strengthening the immune system, treating OIs, and providing symptomatic treatment of organ system disease.

CLINICAL MANIFESTATIONS OF HIV IN CHILDREN AND NURSING INTERVENTIONS

The clinical manifestations of HIV infection in children reflect the action of the virus on the immune system and other organ systems throughout the body. The nursing care of children with HIV is therefore organized around these problems.

Problems Related to Immunosuppression

Opportunistic Infections

Opportunistic infections are those caused by organisms that normally do not produce illness in immunocompetent individuals. The depletion of the immune system by HIV allows these organisms to take the opportunity to cause symptoms. Table 19–2 lists com-

Table 19–2 CLINICAL MANIFESTATIONS OF HUMAN IMMUNODEFICIENCY VIRUS INFECTION IN CHILDREN

Opportunistic Infections	Clinical Manifestations	Treatments
Pneumocystis carinii pneumonia (PCP)	Acute tachypnea, dyspnea, fever, dry cough, hypoxemia, bilateral pulmonary infiltrates; occurs in 25% of pediatric AIDS cases	Trimethoprim sulfa Pentamidine Steroids Oxygen, ventilatory support
Mycobacterium avium complex (MAC) (*M. avium-intracellulare*)	Recurrent fevers, chills, abdominal pain, failure to gain or maintain weight, diarrhea, anemia, hepatosplenomegaly, anorexia; occurs in 6%–11% of children with AIDS	Clarithromycin Ethambutol Rifabutin Amikacin Nutritional support
Cryptosporidosis (*Cryptosporidium*)	Fever, frequent large watery diarrhea, cramps, abdominal pain, weight loss, dehydration, lactose intolerance, anorexia	Azithromycin Bovine colostrum Nutritional support/total parenteral nutrition
Candidiasis (*Candida*)	Oral thrush, esophagitis, dermatitis, sepsis	Nystatin Terconazole vaginal cream Fluconazole Amphotericin
Cytomegalovirus (CMV)	Interstitial pneumonia, encephalitis, chorioretinitis, colitis	Ganciclovir Foscarnet

Table 19–2   CLINICAL MANIFESTATIONS OF HUMAN IMMUNODEFICIENCY VIRUS INFECTION IN CHILDREN *Continued*

Opportunistic Infections System	Clinical Manifestations	Treatments
Gastrointestinal	Failure to thrive Weight loss Anorexia Abdominal pain Abdominal distention Gastroenteritis Hepatitis, pancreatitis	Nutritional support: nasogastric or gastrostomy feeds, total parenteral nutrition Appetite stimulants Pain management Antimicrobials as indicated Supportive care
Central nervous	Progressive encephalopathy Infections Seizures Developmental delay or loss of milestones and functional activities of daily living Behavioral changes: memory loss, confusion, agitation, psychosis	Steroids Antimicrobials Anticonvulsants Habilitation and rehabilitation therapies Psychiatric interventions: anti-psychotic and anti-depressant therapy
Pulmonary	Lymphoid interstitial pneumonitis (chronic progressive interstitial lung disease resulting in disruption in O_2-CO_2 exchange) Recurrent respiratory infections Reactive airways disease	Steroids Oxygen Antimicrobials Bronchodilators
Cardiac	Cardiomyopathy Decreased left ventricular contractility and dilatation resulting in congestive heart failure	Cardiotropic drugs Diuretics
Renal	Nephropathy B- and T-cell lymphoma Electrolyte abnormalities Hypertension	Electrolyte replacement Anti-hypertensives
Hematologic	Anemia Neutropenia Thrombocytopenia	Iron, blood transfusions Erythropoietin G-CSF (Neupogen) Platelet transfusions Steroids, gammaglobulin Change in medications as needed
Dermatologic	*Candida* skin rashes Tinea Molluscum contagiosum	Antifungal topical and systemic therapy Removal of lesions or liquid nitrogen or tretinoin cream
Oral	Thrush Aphthous ulcers Herpes Dental caries and periodontal disease	Antifungals Steroids Acyclovir Dental care

mon OIs in children and the appropriate medical treatments.

Nursing care of children with HIV is first aimed at preventing these infections whenever possible, either primarily or secondarily (after a primary infection has occurred). Pharmacologic primary prophylaxis for most OIs (except PCP, discussed later) is currently being investigated Secondary prophylaxis is achieved by prescribing medications used for treatment, usually on a daily basis. Families and children can be taught basic infection-control measures such as hand washing, careful food preparation, and avoidance of certain organisms in an attempt to prevent infection, although by their nature, OIs are usually present in the patient or environment and difficult to avoid. Once a patient has developed a specific OI, available treatments are usually lifelong.

Pneumocystis carinii pneumonia is the most common OI in children and is potentially life-threatening (Connor et al., 1991). Guidelines for the primary prevention of PCP have been developed (CDC, 1995). The administration of prophylaxis for PCP is based on age and immune status as measured by CD4 count. All HIV-exposed infants between 4 to 6 weeks and 1 year of age should receive PCP prophylaxis until HIV infection has been ruled out. From 1 to 5 years of age, prophylaxis is given to patients who have CD4 counts below 500 cells/μL or 15%. From 6 to 12 years of age, prophylaxis is given for patients who have CD4 counts below 200 cells/μL or 15%. Trimethoprim-sulfamethoxazole (TMP-SMX) is the drug of choice for prophylaxis, and if TMP-SMX is not tolerated, the second-line drug is dapsone. Children who have had PCP should receive lifelong prophylaxis. Children and parents sometimes have difficulty understanding the need for taking medication when they are not sick. Adherence to a prophylactic regimen can best be accomplished when the nurse takes the time to educate the family about the life-threatening nature of PCP, the side effects of the medication, and how the child is monitored for these side effects. Children taking multiple medications for treatment or prophylaxis need assistance in devising dosing schedules that work for them, and parents must be taught how to prepare and measure medications safely.

Acute PCP requires the continued assessment of respiratory status, the administration of TMP-SMX intravenously, and the concurrent administration of steroids and oxygen for hypoxemia (Hughes, 1994). Some children

---

Teaching Topic: PCP Prophylaxis

Important Areas:
What is PCP?
Symptoms of PCP
Mortality connected to PCP
Medication
  Names
  Doses
  Amount to give
  When to give
  Side effects and monitoring
   required

---

develop respiratory failure requiring mechanical ventilation.

Candida infections of the oral mucosa (thrush), skin, esophagus, and trachea are treated with systemic and topical anti-fungal agents, Children with recurrent candidal infections are treated continuously. Nursing interventions such as good mouth care (including dental hygiene) and good skin care (keeping the skin clean and moistened) can help decrease the incidence of *Candida* infections. Careful assessment of the patient for the earliest signs of candidiasis and early treatment can prevent more serious candidal infections such as esophagitis and sepsis.

Tinea corporis and *Tinea capitis* are two other fungal infections that can become chronic and difficult to eradicate in the immunosuppressed person. *T corporis* should be treated early and consistently with topical clotrimazole 1% cream, whereas *T capitis* may require systemic treatment with an anti-fungal agent such as griseofulvin as well as topical treatment. Caregivers must be taught to continue treatment even as lesions resolve to prevent recurrence and drug resistance.

Opportunistic infections of the gastrointestinal tract with organisms such as *Mycobacterium avium-intracellulare, Cryptosporidium,* and cytomegalovirus (CMV) are more difficult to prevent. Available treatments slow the progress of these diseases but do not cure them. Nursing interventions must be focused on supportive care: monitoring weight, fluids, and electrolytes; controlling fever; managing pain, providing nutritional support, preventing dehydration, and providing skin care. Again, teaching families about the various medications and their side effects, dosing schedules, and preparation is necessary.

Viral infections such as CMV and herpes can effect numerous organ systems. CMV is seen in children most frequently as retinitis, pneumonitis, hepatitis, and enteritis (Van Dyke, 1995). Thus far, anti-viral therapies for CMV, such as ganciclovir and foscarnet, are not curative. Children with retinitis and vision loss should be referred for assistance from organizations serving the visually impaired which can provide assistive devices and teaching about negotiating activities of daily living with such an impairment. If intravenous medications are to be administered in the home, appropriate teaching of the family must take place and referrals should be made to home care agencies that provide infusion therapy. Families must be taught to observe for signs of the side effects associated with these potent drugs, including renal impairment, disturbances in fluids and electrolytes (foscarnet), and neutropenia and thrombocytopenia (ganciclovir), and given instructions how to manage these conditions.

Recurrent herpes (zoster or simplex) can cause painful and uncomfortable lesions. Acyclovir is the drug of choice for treating herpes, and it can be given orally or intravenously for acute exacerbations or chronically for recurrent infections. Attention must be paid to the symptoms of herpes: pain and itching. The pain of herpes is neuropathic in nature and can sometimes be helped by tricyclic anti-depressants. Itching can be somewhat alleviated by cool baths, lotions, and anti-histamines.

Bacterial Infections

Children with HIV/AIDS have more frequent bacterial infections that are less amenable to standard treatment (Dankner, 1995). Frequently, these children must receive intravenous antibiotics and long courses of oral antibiotics. Bacterial infections often seen include pneumonia (*Streptococcus pneumoniae*, the most common), *Haemophilus influenzae* type b, group A streptococci, *Staphylococcus aureus*, and *Mycoplasma pneumoniae*. Otitis media, sinusitis, gastroenteritis, meningitis, and skin infections may also occur as a result of bacterial infections in the immunosuppressed child.

The best prevention of bacterial infections is scrupulous hand washing by caregivers and staff, strict attention to sterile technique when doing invasive procedures, appropriate immunization if available, and prophylaxis with oral antibiotics. Children who have had two or more serious bacterial infections may receive monthly infusions of immune globulin. Children with HIV can attend school and are at no greater risk for developing or transmitting bacterial infections.

Problems Related to Neurologic System Dysfunction

Many children with HIV/AIDS have neurologic involvement as a result of direct damage to brain tissue caused by the virus itself (Brouwers, Belman, & Epstein, 1994). The most common computed tomographic (CT) finding was cerebral atrophy. Children with neurologic involvement present with either static or progressive encephalopathy. Common signs and symptoms include inability to achieve developmental milestones or loss of milestones, impaired brain growth, weakness with bilateral pyramidal tract signs, ataxia, and less commonly, seizures and coma. Many of these children also have hypertonicity, spasticity, rigidity, and hyper-reflexia. Static encephalopathy is characterized by non-progressive cognitive or motor deficits, hyperactivity, or attention deficits.

Treatment of neurologic involvement includes zidovudine (AZT, Retrovir) and rehabilitation services such as Early Intervention Programs for infants and toddlers and pre-school handicapped programs for pre-schoolers. Physical therapy is provided for children with major motor deficits. Adaptive seating, wheelchairs, and other equipment are ordered by the therapist as needed. Speech therapy is helpful for children with language delays, and dysphagia therapy can assist children with oral motor skills. School-aged children must undergo a child study team assessment (i.e., a multi-disciplinary evaluation of the child's motor, speech, cognitive, psychological, and social functioning) to be placed in the correct learning environment. Although many children with HIV can function in a normal classroom, those with special needs require special education.

Central nervous system involvement can occur at any time in the course of the disease and may begin quite subtly, with families reporting subtle to obvious changes in functioning. Children with HIV must be monitored frequently for such changes. Every physical examination should include a basic neurologic evaluation, and it is advisable for children to undergo neuro-psychological testing at frequent intervals.

HIV also makes children more susceptible to central nervous system infections such as meningitis, encephalitis, and tumors. Opportunistic infections of the central nervous system such as CMV, cryptococcal meningitis, and toxoplasmosis, although less common in young children, are seen in school-aged and adolescent patients. Occasionally, the older child may develop altered cognitive functioning and changes in personality similar to the dementia seen in adults with AIDS. The cause of these changes is not usually understood while the child is alive. Post-mortem examinations may show CMV or massive atrophy.

Nursing care of the child with encephalopathy is mostly directed at assessing the child for changes in functioning or personality and then ensuring that the child is referred for all possible services. These include a visiting nurse to monitor the child's progress and reinforce treatment plans, physical therapy, speech and dysphagia therapy, and special education. The nurse must anticipate the complications associated with immobility and develop plans of care to prevent them. Caregiver education is also critical.

Problems Related to Gastro-intestinal Dysfunction

Gastrointestinal dysfunction can have severe effects on nutrition, immune status, and growth. Many complications of HIV lead to malnutrition (Winter & Chang, 1993), including *decreased intake* due to oral disease, esophagitis, nausea, anorexia, encephalopathy, depression, or lack of appropriate food in the home; *increased losses* due to vomiting, diarrhea, pancreatic insufficiency, lactose intolerance, and OIs; and *increased nutrient requirements* caused by fever and altered metabolic requirements. Nutritional deficits in infants and toddlers can contribute to developmental delays due to poor brain growth.

Treatment of failure to thrive or wasting must be multi-focused and multi-disciplinary; the team should include a gastroenterologist, nutritionist, speech therapist, nurse, and social worker. Treating underlying diseases is imperative, and a diet high in calories and protein should be offered. Counseling by a nutritionist knowledgeable regarding HIV is important. Children and families must be offered a diet that is high in nutrients, palatable to the child, and affordable. Teaching families to offer foods that are cold or warm or to avoid acidic or spicy foods can alleviate problems with taste and discomfort. Attention must be paid to mouth care. Oral lesions, poor dentition, and gum disease can be painful and contribute to anorexia, and these can best be prevented by scrupulous mouth care.

Commercially available nutritional supplements may be helpful. When necessary and appropriate, artificial nutrition interventions such as enteral and parenteral nutrition can be given. The decision to institute enteral or parenteral nutrition depends on the child's overall medical condition and prognosis, caregiver willingness and ability, and the child's willingness. Not all children with HIV/AIDS will benefit from these interventions because of the advanced stage of the disease and multiple organ problems.

Problems Related to Multi-Organ Failure

In addition to the many infections of the respiratory system that children with HIV can get, many HIV-positive children develop a chronic lung disease known as *lymphoid interstitial pneumonitis (LIP)*. LIP is characterized by infiltration of the interstitium by lymphocytes causing a disruption in oxygen–carbon dioxide exchange (Pitt, 1991). Signs and symptoms of LIP include chronic pulmonary infiltrate, tachypnea, cough, wheezing, and hypoxemia. LIP is a progressive disease that eventually mimics cystic fibrosis. Treatment includes bronchodilators, oral antibiotics, and steroids.

Children with advanced LIP frequently develop bronchiectasis. This condition is treated with chest physiotherapy, prophylactic intravenous antibiotics every 2 to 3 months, and oxygen, in addition to bronchodilators and steroids. Children and caregivers need to be taught to use nebulizers and oxygen in the home safely, to perform chest physical therapy, to position the child to maximize ventilation (especially at night), and to use a fan or air conditioner when available.

Children with HIV can develop cardiac problems, the most common of which is progressive left ventricular dysfunction (Lane-McAuliffe & Lipshultz, 1995). This condition is seen most frequently in children with advanced HIV or HIV encephalopathy. Treatment of cardiomyopathy in children with HIV includes cardiotropic drugs and diuretics. The nurse must monitor the child for signs of congestive heart failure, which include increased fatigue, shortness of breath, rapid heart rate, pulmonary congestion, and edema. Teaching caregivers the signs and symptoms of congestive heart failure and the proper administration of cardiac medications are also critical nursing responsibilities.

Renal problems arise in some children with HIV/AIDS. Children with renal problems present with abnormal electrolytes, protein-uria, edema, intermittent hematuria, azotemia, and hypertension (Strauss et al., 1990). Treatment is supportive and includes replacement of electrolytes and anti-hypertensive agents. Once again, nursing care involves much caregiver education regarding medication administration, monitoring of blood pressure in the home, and watching for signs of renal failure. Due to the silent nature of hypertension, it is extremely important that families fully understand the child's problem to encourage adherence to the treatment regimen.

Abnormalities of the hematologic system are frequently seen in children with HIV. These abnormalities include anemia, thrombocytopenia, and neutropenia (Mueller, 1994). Causes of hematologic abnormalities can include OIs such as *Mycobacterium avium* complex (MAC), viral infections such as parvovirus, or drugs such as TMP-SMX or zidovudine. If possible, the underlying cause is treated; other treatments include transfusions of packed red blood cells or platelets, supplemental iron, granulocyte colony-stimulating factor (G-CSF, Neupogen), gamma-globulin (intravenous immune globulin [IVIG]), high-dose steroids, and changes in medications as indicated. Nurses caring for children with HIV must monitor the patient's complete blood count (CBC) and differential regularly, particularly those patients receiving drugs like TMP-SMX and zidovudine. When patients are receiving G-CSF at home, the caregiver must be taught how to administer a subcutaneous injection in a manner that is safe for both the patient and the caregiver, or a referral for a visiting nurse must be made. Caregivers must also be taught to recognize the side effects of high-dose steroids and the importance of regular gamma-globulin infusions.

The multiple complications of HIV and their associated treatments can be overwhelming for the child and family. Children often feel abnormal compared with their peers and have difficulty adhering to the complex treatment plan. School-aged children and adolescents often rebel and refuse treatments. Parents and caregivers feel anxious and frustrated by the heavy burden of their child's care. Some parents may be sick themselves and must balance their own medical needs with those of their child. Most parents of HIV-infected children put their child's needs for help ahead of their own, making sure that the child receives medicines, keeps appointments, and undergoes necessary tests.

CARING FOR THE CHILD WITH HIV IN THE HOME AND COMMUNITY

As HIV disease progresses and the child's condition worsens, it is still in the child's best interest to remain at home and to engage in as many normal activities as possible. Certain conditions, such as encephalopathy, may plateau, and some function may be restored. However, a great deal of support is necessary for the child to remain at home. Coordination and planning by health providers, including nurses, social workers, physicians, psychologists, nutritionists, habilitation and rehabilitation specialists, and community outreach workers, is necessary. Services from health care agencies and educational providers may be needed. Case management can ensure good planning and implementation of services and help avoid duplication of services. When done in collaboration with the family, necessary services are provided to the child while striving for minimal disruption to daily family life. Community-based home care services, including visiting nurses, home health aides, pharmacies, infusion therapy services, and respiratory therapy services, can assist the family in caring for the child at home for a long period of time. Good communication with these agencies is essential.

Children can be enrolled in day care, preschool, and school. Disclosure of the diagnosis to the day care or school is a difficult issue. For example, in New Jersey, families are not required to disclose their child's condition; however, it is sometimes advantageous for at least the principal or school nurse to be aware of a child's HIV status to ensure appropriate treatment of illnesses and injuries and administration of medications during school. It is also helpful when there is an outbreak of a contagious disease in school such as measles or varicella. Schools are required to adhere to the same confidentiality laws regarding HIV as health care professionals. School teachers and administrators who demand disclosure need to be informed about the law in their state. All schools must adhere to universal precautions. Children with HIV should remain out of school for the same conditions other non-infected children must: contagious conditions such as varicella, skin infections, and lice. The child with HIV infection and advanced disease may not be able to tolerate an entire day of school and may require a modified schedule. When the child is too weak or sick to attend school, a home tutor should be used.

For HIV-infected children to remain in their homes, their families must be able to care for them safely and comfortably. Providing this care can present a big challenge to the family and health providers. Although children with HIV live in many types of family situations, the majority of young children live with their biologic mother and siblings. As the child ages, the probability that he or she lives with relatives as a result of illness or death of a parent increases. At the Children's Hospital AIDS Program in Newark, New Jersey, 44% of children older than 9 years lived with their biologic parents (Grubman et al., 1995). Possible change in the structure of the family situation due to parental illness, hospitalization, and death should be anticipated and planned for. Although some families are able to plan for the care of their children with assistance from social workers, other family, and AIDS service organizations, some are not.

Caregiver education about the child's problems, treatments, and medications is essential. Information must be provided repeatedly, with opportunity for the caregiver to provide feedback on his or her understanding of the material. Tools such as medication schedules, calendars, and diaries are helpful. Assessing the home before implementing oxygen or parenteral therapy is mandatory because changes may need to be made in the physical organization of the apartment or home to effectively manage the care. The nurse must assess whether there is enough space for equipment; appropriate electricity, plumbing, heat, or air conditioning; and whether there is a telephone. Cleanliness of the house or apartment is important; frequently, at least one area of a home can be made suitably clean for the sick child. Infestation of insects and rodents must be resolved if at all possible. For an immobile child, there must be a safe and rapid means of exiting the home in the event of fire. Some environments may be deemed unsafe, and alternate living arrangements may be required. Infrequently, the child's family, even with home care services, may not be able to carry out the treatment plan.

The care of the HIV-infected child may be so complex and demanding that it is exhausting and threatens the health of the parent. In this situation, discussion with the family of options such as foregoing some treatments or placement of the child in a group setting such as a residential facility or nursing home must be considered. Often, residential placement means that child is in a community at some distance from the family, making visits difficult even with assistance. Such separation is painful for both child and family. In our experience in an urban setting with few services, the majority of children have been able to remain in their homes; however, it takes a committed family member and the persistence of dedicated staff willing to weave and re-weave fragmented services into a quilt that covers the child and family.

Family Responses to the Disease

Many models exist to explain the challenges faced by children with chronic illness and their families. Most models presume that these families consist of an ill child and well parents; whereas with HIV, both child and parent may suffer the same illness. Regardless of the model applied, families are required to develop and adapt as they cope with the illness and its treatments. Family members often are in different phases of the disease simultaneously, putting further stresses on the family and extended family (Boyd-Franklin et al., 1995).

The manner in which a biologic, extended, or foster family copes with the HIV diagnosis is related to its previously established ways of dealing with crises and stresses. Parents of children with HIV experience many of the same stresses and concerns as any parent whose child has a chronic condition; however, biologic parents may face these stresses as well as a potential for their own impaired health status or while managing their own HIV infection. Ongoing assessment of the family response is an important component of nursing care.

Caring for the Child With End-Stage HIV/AIDS

It is apparent that HIV/AIDS causes many progressive and irreversible complications. When a child has experienced multiple OIs and other multi-organ complications, it is often recognized that the patient is in the terminal phase of the disease. The thrust of care then moves to palliation of symptoms and preparation of the child and family for death. Many of the treatments already discussed are continued in an effort to decrease uncomfortable symptoms while other treatments are discontinued. These decisions are made collaboratively between the health care team, the child (depending on his or her ability to participate in decision making), and the caregivers. A primary goal at this time, as throughout the course of HIV, is to relieve pain and decrease uncomfortable symptoms as much as possible. Children with HIV/AIDS experience many different untoward symptoms, and pain is a common problem (Czarniecki, Dollfus, & Strafford, 1994; Czarniecki, Boland, & Oleske, 1993). Failure to treat these uncomfortable symptoms and pain can lead to further complications and negatively impact on the child's quality of life; therefore, the nurse must continually assess the child for pain and other symptoms and report these to physicians for appropriate treatment. There are many pain assessment tools available for children. Two that are very helpful are a faces scale, in which the child chooses a face that matches his or her degree of pain, and a body outline tool, in which the child colors in the location of his or her pain on an outline of the human body. Pain is managed, as in other children, with good pharmacologic analgesia (e.g., acetaminophen, non-steroidal anti-inflammatory agents, weak opioids, strong opioids, muscle relaxants, anxiolytics, antidepressants, anticonvulsants) and non-pharmacologic interventions (e.g., relaxation, distraction, visualization, hypnosis, heat, cold, massage). A preventive approach with around-the-clock dosing is better than as-needed doses. During end-stage HIV/AIDS, doses of opioids necessary to control pain may be very high. Fears of respiratory depression and drug addiction are unfounded and should not influence pain management decisions in terminal patients.

Other symptoms experienced during end-stage disease should be treated as aggressively as pain; these include cough, nausea, itching, insomnia, and depression. Rehabilitation approaches can help a child maintain as much independence as possible, even during physical decline. Again, a multi-disciplinary approach is vital in providing the best symptom relief possible.

In addition to treating physical symptoms, end-of-life care also includes attention to the psychological, social, and spiritual needs of the child and family (Czarniecki, 1996). Meeting the needs of families at this time requires a multi-disciplinary approach using the services of nurses, social workers, psychologists, child life workers, teachers, and clergy. Decisions regarding where a child should die, do-not-resuscitate orders, and autopsy must be faced by the child and family. Health care professionals must respect the wishes of the child and family as much as possible. Com-munity services such as hospice care can be involved to maintain children at home if they wish. Hospice care includes implementing comfort measures, reducing the amount of painful or invasive tests and treatments, providing psychosocial support to the child and family, maintaining the child's dignity, and offering spiritual care. Children in hospitals and nursing homes can still be helped to die with dignity and with the least amount of suffering if a hospice-type approach is implemented. Support for hospice staff may become as important as support for families.

CASE STUDY

Mindy, a 4-year-old girl, has been cared for in the hospital for the past 6 weeks. Her problems have included disseminated *Mycobacterium avium* complex (MAC), wasting, anorexia, vomiting, abdominal pain and distension, thrush, recurrent zoster, transfusion-dependent anemia, neutropenia, and chronic cough. The MAC has become resistant to treatment. While she was in the hospital, nasogastric feedings were attempted but not tolerated, and total parenteral nutrition (TPN) via a Broviac catheter was begun. Mindy has been pleading to go home, and her family (a mother who is also infected, a grandmother, and a 14-year-old sister) have decided they wish to take her home on TPN. They have also agreed to not have her resuscitated (DNR) or placed on a ventilator. They wish to continue only those treatments that will increase her comfort. In preparing this child to go home, the nurse must work with the family and community-based agencies to develop a plan of care. This plan must include:

- Teach family the administration of TPN: Broviac care, use of pump, trouble-shooting, signs and symptoms of complications (e.g., hypoglycemia, sepsis, tunnel infection).
- Teach family management of untoward symptoms such as pain (e.g., administration of pain medication, non-pharmacologic interventions, side effects of medications, prevention of side effects).
- Prepare family for complications that may occur at home and help them think about a plan for each possibility (e.g., fever, bleeding, seizures).
- Assist family in contacting local emergency services to alert them to a child in the community and the desire for DNR orders.

- Make referrals to an infusion company, infusion nursing agency, and hospice program, discuss the case with each agency in detail, and provide a written plan of care.
- Make sure family has 24-hour-a-day access to health care professionals for symptom management, trouble-shooting, and support.
- Make referrals to community-based social service programs as needed.
- If desired, connect family with a spiritual caregiver.

Ultimately, the child, the family, and the staff caring for them can experience the last days of the child's life as quality time to be treasured and remembered rather than as a time of unbearable suffering.

SUMMARY

HIV/AIDS is a relatively new chronic and ultimately fatal disease that affects children from infancy through adolescence. Daily breakthroughs in research change the course and prognosis of this disease. As treatment advances extend the lives of children with HIV/AIDS, the need for skilled nursing care at varying points, including rehabilitation nursing, will grow. Children with chronic illnesses do best when they can be maintained in the home with competent caregivers. Nurses play a crucial role in ensuring that families can care for their child safely and with a high level of comfort. By bringing together knowledge of pediatrics, rehabilitation, and home care, the nurse can make a valuable contribution to the life of a child with HIV/AIDS.

REFERENCES

Blanche, S., Tardieu, M., Duliege, A., et al. (1990). Longitudinal study of 94 symptomatic infants with perinatally acquired human immunodeficiency virus infection: evidence for a bimodal expression of clinical and biological symptoms. *American Journal of the Diseases of Children*, 144, 1210–1215.

Boyd-Franklin, N., Aleman, J., Steiner, G., Drelich, E., & Norford, B. (1995). Family systems interventions and family therapy. In N. Boyd-Franklin, G.L. Steiner, & M.G. Boland (Eds.). *Children, families and HIV/AIDS: psychosocial and therapeutic issues*, p. 117. New York, Guilford Press.

Brouwers, P., Belman, A., & Epstein, L. (1994). Central nervous system involvement: manifestations, evaluation and pathogenesis. In P. Pizzo & C. Wilfert (Eds.). *Pediatric AIDS: the challenge of HIV infection in infants, children and adolescents*, pp. 433–455. Baltimore: Williams & Wilkins.

Centers for Disease Control and Prevention. (1998). Guidelines for the use of antiretroviral agents in pediatric HIV infection. *Morbidity and Mortality Weekly Report*, 47(RR-4).

Centers for Disease Control and Prevention. (1997). *HIV/AIDS surveillance report 1997: year-end edition*, 9:2. Atlanta: U.S. Department of Health and Human Services Public Health Service of the Centers for Disease Control and Prevention.

Connor, E., Bagarzzi, M., McSherry, G., et al. (1991). Clinical and laboratory correlates of *Pneumocystis carinii* pneumonia in children infected with HIV. *Journal of the American Medical Association*, 265, 1693–1697.

Czarniecki, L. (1996). Advanced HIV disease in children. *Nursing Clinics of North America*, 31(1), 207–219.

Czarniecki, L., Boland, M.G., & Oleske, J. (1993). Pain in children with HIV disease. *PAAC Notes*, 5, 492–495.

Czarniecki, L., Dollfus, C., & Strafford, M. (1994). Children with pain and HIV/AIDS. In D. Carr (Ed.). *Pain in HIV/AIDS*, pp. 48–52. Washington, DC: France-USA Pain Association.

Dankner, W.M. (1995). Bacterial infections in HIV infected children. *Seminars in Pediatric Infectious Diseases*, 6(1), 10–16.

Grubman, S., Gross. E., Lerner-Weiss, N., et al. (1995). Older children and adolescents living with perinatally acquired human immunodeficiency acquired infection. *Pediatrics*, 95, 657.

Hughes, W. (1994). *Pneumocystis carinii* pneumonia. In P. Pizzo & C. Wilfert (Eds.). *Pediatric AIDS: the challenge of HIV infection in infants, children, and adolescents*, pp. 405–418. Baltimore: Williams & Wilkins.

Joint United Nations Programme on HIV/AIDS. (1996). *Fact sheet*. July 1. Geneva, Switzerland: Joint United Nations Programme on HIV/AIDS.

Lane-McAuliffe, E., & Lipshultz, S.E. (1995). Cardiovascular manifestations of pediatric HIV infection. *Nursing Clinics of North America*, 30 (2), 291–316.

Mueller. B. (1994). Hematological problems and their management in children with HIV infection. In P. Pizzo & C. Wilfert (Eds.). *Pediatric AIDS: the challenge of HIV infection in infants, children, and adolescents*, pp. 591–601. Baltimore: Williams & Wilkins.

Oleske, J. (1995). In P. McCardle & L.A. Quatrano (Eds.). *Pediatric AIDS Rehabilitation Research: Report of a Research Planning Workshop*, March 17, 1994, NIH Publication No. 95-3850. Washington DC: USDHHS

Pitt, J. (1991). Lymphocytic interstitial pneumonia. *Pediatric Clinics of North America*, 38(1), 89–96.

Strauss, J., Abitol, C., Zilleruelo, G.L., et al. (1990). Renal disease in children with the acquired immunodeficiency syndrome. *New England Journal of Medicine*, 321(10), 625–630.

Van Dyke, R.B. (1995). Opportunistic infections in HIV-infected children. *Seminars in Pediatric Infectious Diseases*, 6(1), 10–16.

Winter, H., & Chang, T. (1993). Nutrition in children with HIV. *Pediatric HIV Forum: Focus on Nutrition*, 1(2), 1–5.

4

Chapter 20

Perspectives on Pediatric Rehabilitation Cancer

Michael Comeau and *Janet Duncan*

A diagnosis of cancer will produce fear and anxiety in every child, parent, or caregiver. However, recent technology and treatment options have made some cancers serious but potentially curable illnesses. The American Cancer Society (ACS) estimated that in 1996 over 10 million Americans were alive who had a history of cancer, 7 million of whom were diagnosed for 5 years or more. In 1996, over 8300 new cases of pediatric cancer were diagnosed in the United States and an estimated 1700 children died of the disease. Cancer, although rare in the pediatric population, is the chief cause of death by disease in children younger than 15 years of age (ACS Cancer Facts and Figures, 1996). It is predicted that "by the year 2000 an estimated one out of every 900 young adults will be a survivor of childhood cancer" (DeLaat & Lampkin, 1992, p. 263). Many children and adult survivors of cancer therapy have health problems resulting from their particular cancer. These survivors will be living with chronic conditions and have specialized rehabilitation needs.

Nursing rehabilitation of the child with cancer incorporates many aspects of nursing care. The challenge of oncology rehabilitation involves the oncology nurse incorporating rehabilitation strategies into the plan of care as well as the rehabilitation nurse incorporating oncology practices into the rehabilitation and home care setting. For example, the neutropenic child in the induction phase of treatment who is transferred to the intensive care unit for sepsis must be approached with rehabilitation concepts so that complications such

as footdrop are prevented and range of motion is incorporated into the plan of care. Likewise, the home care nurse working with the child with a brain tumor on chemotherapy must have an understanding of neutropenia as it relates to children with cancer. Rehabilitation is a continuous process and involves many members of the nursing team working collaboratively in various settings. Table 20–1 presents an example of the phases of illness, the nurse who would utilize rehabilitation concepts in practice, and the nursing goals.

Caring for the child with cancer can be a challenging and rewarding experience for the nurse as he or she develops an individualized plan of care that addresses all phases of the illness and the complications that arise throughout the stages of cancer treatment. By its very nature, cancer treatment requires a health care team, including, but not limited to, the child and family, primary oncologist, nurse, social worker, psychologist, radiation therapist, surgeon, and physical therapist. Additional information about the interdisciplinary care team can be found in Chapter 8. The expanded team may also include a dietitian or nutritionist, chaplain, child life therapist, assistive personnel, volunteers, and those professionals offering complementary therapies such as acupuncture, Reiki therapy, herbal medicine, and spiritual healing.

It is the nurse, as the member of the health care team who has the most contact with the child and family, who coordinates care among the disciplines and serves as a liaison between members of the team. It is the nursing team

Table 20-1 NURSING REHABILITATION PROCESS FOR THE CHILD WITH CANCER

Phase	Nurse	Goals
Acute phase	Acute care oncology nurse Outpatient nurse Home care nurse Rehabilitation nurse	Obtaining remission status Preventing/controlling side effects of treatment Patient and family education Psychological adjustment
Intensification/chronic phase	Outpatient nurse Home care nurse School nurse Rehabilitation nurse	Rehabilitation from side effects of treatment and complications Habilitation Reintegration to school and community
Palliative phase	Hospice nurse Home care nurse Outpatient nurse Acute care oncology nurse Rehabilitation nurse	Comfort Quality of life issues Facilitating wishes of child and family Emotional support Preparation/transition work Symptom management

members who follow the plan of care, including goals directly related to the rehabilitation process, throughout the illness continuum (Hydzik, 1990). The Association of Rehabilitation Nurses in its 1994 *Standards and Scope of Rehabilitation Nursing Practice* (p. 3) defines rehabilitation nursing as:

> . . . a specialty practice area of professional nursing. Rehabilitation nursing is the diagnosis and treatment of human responses of individuals and groups to actual or potential health problems relative to altered functional ability and lifestyle. The goal of rehabilitation nursing is to assist the individual who has a disability and/or chronic illness in restoring, maintaining, and promoting his or her maximal health. This includes preventing chronic illness and disability. The rehabilitation nurse is skilled at treating alterations in functional ability and lifestyle that result from physical disability and chronic illness.

It is the nurse who assists the child and family through the process of rehabilitation, through education, support, and empowerment, to achieve a maximum level of functioning (Potter & Perry, 1995). Through implementation of the nursing process the nurse identifies the needs of the child and family, performs an assessment, develops a plan of care, and evaluates its effectiveness. Rehabilitation strategies must begin at diagnosis and continue throughout the cancer experience as the child and family attempt to adjust to the diagnosis, illness, and treatment. The goals of rehabilitation begin in the induction phase and continue throughout the cancer treatment process whether the child completes therapy and goes on to become a long-term survivor or the cancer returns and the goal of care becomes palliation and comfort.

EPIDEMIOLOGY

Cancer is a significant public health problem not only in the United States but all over the world. It affects all age groups and races and both genders It is important to understand the statistical values to place emphasis on the fact that as people live longer more people will be affected by the diagnosis of cancer. Pediatric cancers remain the second leading cause of death in children, second only to accidents. As cancer treatments improve, the number of people surviving cancer and adapting to the long-term side effects of cancer will increase. This fact is important to the nurse who will be assisting with the rehabilitation process for cancer survivors and others in various stages of treatment for cancer as a chronic illness.

In 1997, the ACS published its report on cancer statistics. Several important reported observations were:

The present lifetime risk of cancer for males is 1 in 2, and for females it is 1 in 3.

African Americans continue to be diagnosed at less favorable stages of the disease than white Americans.

The rate of survival for common pediatric cancers has improved dramatically over the past 30 years.

In 1997, it was estimated that there would

be about 1,382,400 new cases of cancer diagnosed in the United States.

The three most common cancers for children younger than age 15 years were leukemia, brain and nervous system cancers, and lymphoma.

Each year more than 1600 children die of cancer in the United States.

Approximately 8200 children annually will be diagnosed with cancer in the United States (Wong, 1995).

In general, there have been many advances in the treatment of childhood cancers. This is in part because children have otherwise healthy vital organ systems. The health of children is usually better than that of many adults who have other pre-existing medical and physical problems. To understand the nature of the difference between childhood and adult cancers it is important to recognize factors that result in the development of pediatric cancer. Childhood cancers develop differently from those that affect adults. Many cancers of childhood arise from the embryonal germ layer of the mesoderm. In fetal development, these tissues give rise to organs such as connective tissue, bone, muscle, cartilage, blood vessels, sex organs, kidney, lymph, and lymphoid organs. This results in the more common cancers of childhood leukemia, lymphoma, and sarcomas (Mooney, 1993). Adult cancers tend to arise from tissues of epithelial cell nature. These cancers are called carcinomas, which are less frequent in the pediatric population. According to Mooney (1993), the difference between adult and childhood cancers remains until age 15 years, and from ages 15 to 19 years the types of cancers tend to become more similar to the adult population. Table 20–2 outlines the differences between childhood and adult cancers.

PATHOPHYSIOLOGY

To understand cancer and its treatment it is necessary to have a basic understanding of cellular function and reproduction. During embryogenesis, cells divide and multiply at a rapid rate. After birth, the rate decreases and for some cells (heart, nervous system) replication ceases completely. The cells of the liver, bone marrow, and lining of the gastrointestinal tract continue to divide and multiply throughout a person's life. Cell growth normally occurs in response to a physiologic need for the organism to grow, repair, and

differentiate, thus ensuring the survival of the organism (Mooney, 1993). The initiation of growth and the process of division are influenced by hormone-like chemicals in the body called growth factors. Growth factors are proteins produced by cells, and they may influence the growth of cells other than those that produced them. Growth factors stimulate cells to increase or decrease the rate of reproduction. Examples of growth factors are erythropoietin, which effects red blood cells, and granulocyte colony-stimulating factor, which increases the number of granulocytes (a type of white blood cell). The cell cycle is the process by which cells reproduce their DNA and split into two identical daughter cells. Both normal cells and cancer cells go through the same steps or phases of the cell cycle. There are five phases of the cell cycle: G_0, G_1, S, G_2, and M. Each phase of the cell cycle is composed of a sequence of events that lead to the duplication of the genetic material and the division into two identical daughter cells. The G phases represent periods of time when preparation occurs between the S phase and mitosis (Groenwald et al., 1993).

The *G_0 phase* is also called the resting phase. In this phase, normal cellular function occurs and the cells are not actively involved in the process of division. A stimulus such as the death or destruction of a like cell causes the cell to enter the G_1, or growth, phase.

The *G_1 phase* is a period of decreased metabolic activity. This phase can last from 12 to 14 hours and begins at the completion of the previous cell division and lasts until the cell prepares to enter the S phase.

The *S phase* involves the synthesis of RNA, which is necessary for the synthesis of DNA. It lasts from 7 to 20 hours. DNA is synthesized during this phase, and cells are most vulnerable during this phase (Otto, 1994).

The *G_2 phase* occurs after the completion of the replication of DNA and lasts until the start of the mitotic phase (1 to 4 hours). It is a period of decreased activity but consists of protein synthesis and additional RNA synthesis.

The *M phase* is the process of mitosis and cell division. It lasts from 40 minutes to 2 hours. This phase consists of four stages: prophase, metaphase, anaphase, and telophase. During this four-stage process

Table 20–2 DIFFERENCES BETWEEN CHILDHOOD AND ADULT CANCERS

Factor	Childhood Cancer	Adult Cancer
Incidence	Rare; <1% of all cancers	Common; >99% of all cancers
Sites	Involves tissue (e.g., reticuloendothelial system, central nervous system, muscle, bone)	Involves organs (e.g., lung, breast, colon, prostate)
Histology	Most common type: nonepithelial—sarcomas, embryonal, leukemia, lymphoma	Most common type: epithelial carcinomas
Latency (from initiation to diagnosis)	Relatively short period	Long period: can be well over 20 years
Influence of environmental factors in causation	Some environmental factors; few lifestyle factors; overall not strong influence shown; more likely interaction of genetic alterations and environmental factors (i.e., ecogenetics)	Strong relationship to environmental exposures and lifestyle factors
Prevention	Minimal strategies known to date	80% estimated as preventable
Early detection	Generally accidental; small percentage known as genetically at high risk can be followed more closely	Possible with adherence to early detection screening tests and examination recommendations
State at diagnosis	Metastatic disease present in 80%	Local or regional disease
Response to treatment	Very responsive to chemotherapy; tolerate higher doses	Less responsive to chemotherapy
Treatment side effects	Less difficulty with acute toxicity but more significant long-term consequences	More difficulty with acute toxicity but fewer long-term consequences
Prognosis	>60% cure	<60% cure

From Mooney, K. (1993). Biologic basis of childhood cancer. In G. Foley, D. Fochtman, & K. Mooney (Eds.). *Nursing care of the child with cancer* (2nd ed.). Philadelphia: WB Saunders.

the nuclear membrane breaks down and chromosomes first clump, then move to the middle of the cell, and then to each side. At this time, the cycle moves to the last stage and cell division occurs and two identical daughter cells are produced.

The phases, events, and time frames for the cell cycle are shown in Figure 20–1.

ETIOLOGY

Mechanisms of Carcinogenesis

Cancer is a highly complex group of diseases involving many factors, and thus there is no single preventable cause. The process through which cancer develops is called *carcinogenesis*.

Normally, cells divide and multiply to replace cells that have either died or been damaged. Cells divide in a highly ordered process, through a number of specific steps. Yabro (1993, p. 29) provided an explanation of cell division in normal and cancer states:

Animals have evolved an elaborate set of controls regulating cellular growth and repair. There are signals to turn growth on and off as needed. There are complex fail-safe mechanisms to prevent the overgrowth of a mutant clone. However, cancer escapes this regulation. Step by step—that is, mutation by mutation—cancer overcomes this protection against uncontrolled growth. This happens because the mutations that lead to cancer are mutations of the very same genes that regulate normal growth. Indeed, many of the genes that regulate normal growth were discovered, almost by accident,

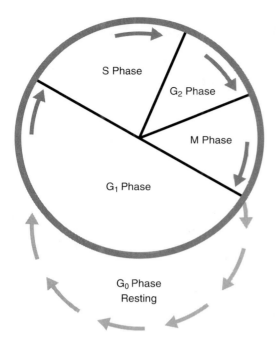

Figure 20–1   The cell cycle.

during the search for cancer genes in oncogenic viruses.

There are two types of genes that control growth. One gene stimulates cells to grow (oncogenes), and the other suppresses cell growth (anti-oncogenes). It is believed that there are two distinct types of mutations that occur that influence the development of cancer. The first mutation is one the individual inherits, and it can then be passed along in families, for example, colon and breast cancer in adults and Wilms' tumor and retinoblastoma in children. The other type results from the mutation of normal cells, which, when exposed to a carcinogen, mutate and by mutating can go on to form cancer (e.g., smoking leading to lung cancer) (Mooney, 1993; Yabro, 1993). Other factors believed to be related to human carcinogenesis, such as viruses, dietary fat, and physical carcinogens, are listed in Table 20–3.

CHARACTERISTICS OF CANCERS

The human body responds to the need for repair and replacement of cells that have been injured or destroyed by means of cell division. Normal cells respond to growth factors by speeding up cell proliferation. Cancer cells no longer respond to the regulators that control growth and cell division. Cancer cells have characteristics that differentiate them

from normal cells. These are the ability to invade; produce factors that influence the ability to produce new and continuous blood vessels (angiogenesis), which provide the tumor with oxygen and essential nutrients; and spread (metastasize). Normally, when one cell is damaged or destroyed it is replaced with one cell. Cells have a property called contact inhibition. This maintains organization and the ability of the tissue to function normally. Cancer cells lack contact inhibition, and the orderly arrangement becomes clumped and disorganized. Cells impinge on and invade surrounding structures. Cell-to-cell communication is lost, and the normal adhesive properties that attach two aligned cells are disrupted. This eases the ability of the cancer cells to move about, invading local tissue and blood vessels.

Cancer cells have the ability to spread and to invade the surrounding tissue by a process known as metastasis. The cells clump and begin to build their own supply of blood vessels. The cancer cells invade these vessels and are transported to distant sites in the body. They are also able to invade neighboring lymph vessels and are also carried in the lymph fluid to lymph nodes, usually in the immediate area of the tumor. It is believed that there are properties at the site of metastasis that influence the cancer's ability to grow at that site. They include hormones, growth factors, genetics, age, tumor angiogenesis factors, immune status, and blood flow (Mooney, 1993).

SIGNS AND SYMPTOMS ASSOCIATED WITH PEDIATRIC CANCERS

Cancers affecting children are different from those that affect adults. Adult tumors tend to originate from the epithelial lining of organs and are called carcinomas. Carcinomas are believed to be related to long-term exposure to chemicals such as smoke, alcohol, and sunlight. Pediatric tumors more commonly originate from the mesodermal germ layer, which in the embryo becomes connective tissue, bone, cartilage, muscle, blood, blood vessels, kidneys, sex organs, lymphatics, and lymphoid organs (Mooney, 1993). Because of the type and location of the tumors, pediatric cancers tend to be diagnosed late, usually after the tumor has already metastasized. Symptoms that may develop are usually specific to the tumor and its site. Some general symptoms that may occur include pain, cachexia, bruising, swelling, fever, anemia, fa-

Table 20–3 FACTORS RELATED TO CARCINOGENESIS

Carcinogen	Specific Carcinogen	Type of Cancer
Viruses	Human T-cell lymphotropic virus type I	Lymphoma, leukemia
	Human papillomavirus	Cervical
	Hepatitis B	Hepatocellular carcinoma
Physical carcinogens	Ultraviolet radiation	Melanoma
	Radon	Lung cancer
	Asbestos	Mesothelioma
Diet	Fat	Colon, breast

tigue, cough, and bleeding. Table 20–4 outlines common symptoms and complications and their underlying causes.

STRUCTURE AND FUNCTION: SPECIFIC CONDITIONS

Leukemia and Lymphomas

Leukemia is the most common pediatric malignancy in children younger than 15 years old. In 1993, it resulted in almost 600 deaths of children younger than 15 years of age (Parker et al., 1997). Approximately 2000 cases are diagnosed in the United States annually (Margolin & Poplack, 1997). There are two major types: acute leukemia and chronic leukemia. Of the acute leukemias there are acute lymphocytic leukemia (ALL) and acute nonlymphocytic leukemia (ANLL). ALL accounts for nearly 75% of all cases of childhood leukemia. Children diagnosed with ALL since 1990 have a projected long-term survival rate of 80% (Cohen, 1993). ALL occurs most commonly around the age of 4 years, is more common in whites than blacks, and is higher among boys than girls. It is more common in developed countries, related to industrialization (Margolin & Poplack, 1997).

The cause of leukemia is unknown, but there are several factors that have been implicated as potential sources. They include viral infections (human T-cell lymphotropic virus type I [HTLV-I], Epstein-Barr), radiation, genetics (increased incidence among twins, Down syndrome), and immunodeficiency (Margolin & Poplack, 1997).

ALL is the most common and treatable form of childhood leukemia, and more than 80% of children with ALL will be long-term survivors. Presenting symptoms of leukemia include pallor, dyspnea, bleeding, fever, and pain. These occur because the bone marrow is no longer functioning properly and the production of normal cells, such as red cells and

platelets, has been obstructed by the leukemic cells. The typical treatment regimen for ALL occurs over 2 years and is composed of three stages: induction, consolidation, and maintenance. Combination therapy, with chemotherapy, radiation, and, in some cases, bone marrow transplantation, may be included in the treatment regimen.

Tumors of the Central Nervous System

Brain tumors are the most common solid tumor of childhood, affecting about 1500 children in the United States each year. They occur almost as frequently as ALL. Figure 20–2 illustrates the anatomic structure of the brain and the most common sites.

The cause of brain tumors is unknown. Brain tumors in children may have a better outcome than in adults because of the type and location. Children rarely develop two of the more highly malignant types of brain tumors commonly found in adults, and they are less likely to have types of cancer that tend to metastasize to the brain. Table 20–5 outlines the types of brain tumors and their symptoms.

Pediatric brain tumors are treated with combination therapy, including chemotherapy, radiation, and surgery. Currently, the use of chemotherapy is more widespread than in recent history with the development of new drug regimens. There are three main problems associated with pediatric brain tumors: they are often misdiagnosed; the effects of treatment may have long-term consequences because of the effects of therapy on the developing brain; and because there are several types and the occurrence rate is low, it is difficult to enroll large numbers of children in research protocols (Petriccione, 1993). The long-term consequences have implications for the nursing plan of care in many areas, as discussed later in this chapter.

Table 20–4   DISEASE MANIFESTATIONS AND COMPLICATIONS OF CHILDHOOD CANCER

Manifestations/Complications	Cancer-Related Cause
Anemia	Replacement of bone marrow with tumor cells or leukemic cells
Bruising, bleeding, hemorrhage	Thrombocytopenia due to replacement of bone marrow with tumor cells or leukemic cells
Cachexia	Hypothesized as a combination of factors: increased energy expenditure, decreased food intake, altered metabolism, by-products of tumor metabolism
Cardiac tamponade	Tumor involving cardiac muscle or pericardium, resulting in accumulation of fluid in pericardial space
Disseminated intravascular coagulation	In children with acute leukemia release of enzymes from leukemic cells that activate coagulation system (rare) or consequences of sepsis, particularly with gram-negative organisms
Effusions (pleural, pericardial, abdominal)	Local invasion or metastatic spread to chest or abdomen
Fatigue	Hypothesized as a combination of factors: altered metabolism, increased energy expenditure, decreased food intake, anemia, by-products of tumor metabolism
Fever	Infection from cancer-related neutropenia and immunosuppression or non–infection-related fever from tumor stimulation of cells that produce interleukin-1, a pyrogen (hypothesized)
Hyperleukocytosis or hyperviscosity of blood	Leukemia with peripheral white blood cell count $>100,000/mm^3$
Immunosuppression	Release of immunosuppressive factors by cancer cells
Increased intracranial pressure	Pressure from primary or metastatic brain tumors, resulting in headache, visual disturbances, nausea and vomiting, and/or behavioral changes
Infection or sepsis	Cancer-related neutropenia and immunosuppression and local tumor growth that disrupts normal pathogen barriers
Pain	Tumor infiltration and stretching or compression of pain-sensitive structures
Respiratory distress	Mediastinal tumors
Spinal cord compression	Tumor-related compression of the spinal cord, resulting in edema and ischemia of the cord and possible destruction from direct tumor infiltration
Superior vena cava syndrome	Mediastinal tumor compression of the superior vena cava resulting in airway obstruction, respiratory distress, and edema
Tumor lysis syndrome	Cancers with high-growth fractions and rapid cell lysis, resulting in hyperuricemia, hyperkalemia, hyperphosphatemia, hypocalcemia, and possible renal failure

From Mooney, K. (1993). Biologic basis of childhood cancer. In G. Foley, D. Fochtman, & K. Mooney (Eds.). *Nursing care of the child with cancer* (2nd ed.). Philadelphia: WB Saunders.

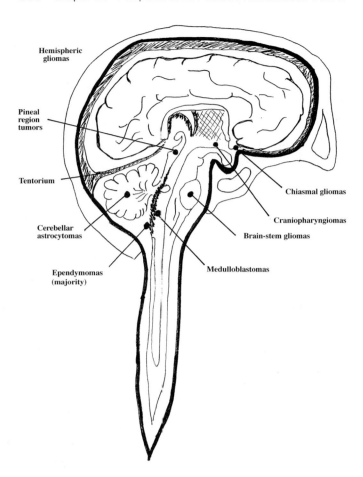

Hemispheric gliomas

Pineal region tumors

Tentorium

Cerebellar astrocytomas

Ependymomas (majority)

Chiasmal gliomas

Craniopharyngiomas

Brain-stem gliomas

Medulloblastomas

Figure 20–2 Lateral view of the brain and spinal cord showing the location of common pediatric brain tumors. (Adapted from Albright, A. L. (1993). Pediatric Brain Tumors. *Cancer Journal for Clinicians*, 43(5), 272–288.)

DIAGNOSTIC ASSESSMENT

The diagnosis of cancer involves all members of the health care team. Treatment options are based on the type of disease, location, extent, and age of the child. The diagnostic process for cancer is similar to many illnesses, and it involves three stages. The first stage is the history and physical examination. The past medical history includes past illnesses, surgeries, current medications, allergies, childhood illnesses, family illnesses, and presenting signs and symptoms. It is also important to ask about the use of complementary therapies. A nursing assessment includes the history and physical examination as well as particular attention to learning styles, barriers to learning, how the child and family deal with stress, religious and cultural implications, and family support structure. It is important to remember to include the older child and adolescent when taking the initial history because this will set the tone for their involvement and participation in their treatment.

The second stage includes all tests and diagnostic procedures used to determine the cause of the child's symptoms. There are many different diagnostic procedures that may be employed to make a diagnosis of cancer. Many of them are disease specific and used to confirm or rule out the suspected cause of the symptoms. Such procedures may be invasive or noninvasive. Noninvasive procedures include radiologic studies such as chest radiography, barium studies, computed tomography (CT), magnetic resonance imaging (MRI), ultrasonography, nuclear medicine studies (bone scans), laboratory studies (complete cell blood count or liver function tests), and tumor markers. Tumor markers are substances measurable in the blood that are either not produced in healthy individuals or are produced in lesser amounts. They can be used to measure the presence of tumors as well as the response to therapy. Invasive pro-

Table 20–5   BRAIN TUMOR LOCATION, TYPE, AND SYMPTOMS

Location	Type	Symptoms
Supratentorial hemispheric tumors	Low-grade astrocytomas High-grade astrocytomas Ependymomas	Generalized: headache, dull and steady, can occur at any time of day although usually in the morning; nausea Localized: seizures, changes in behavior. Symptoms correlate with the function of the area involved by the tumor Frontal lobe: personality and movement Parietal tumors: affect ability to read, awareness of contralateral extremities Temporal lobe: seizures, fluent aphasia Occipital lobe: visual field deficits
Supratentorial tumors (midline)	Optic chiasm tumors Craniopharyngiomas Pineal region tumors (germ cell tumors)	Chiasmal tumors may cause visual field and acuity deficits; if large can cause hydrocephalus Craniopharyngiomas: may cause short stature, visual field deficits, hormonal insufficiency, and hydrocephalus, and endocrinopathies Pineal region tumors: impair upward gaze and affect accommodation; may cause hydrocephalus and headache
Infratentorial tumors (posterior fossa)	Astrocytomas (brain-stem gliomas) Medulloblastomas Ependymomas	Hydrocephalus Progressively worsening morning headache Vomiting, unsteadiness, double vision, papilledema Morning vomiting Brain stem tumors may cause: cranial nerve palsies, crossed eyes, hemiparesis, and increased intracranial pressure

cedures include surgery to excise a specimen of the tumor, bone marrow biopsy, lymph node biopsy, needle biopsy, and any procedure that requires entering the body or a cavity to procure specimens for diagnosis.

THERAPEUTIC MANAGEMENT

Cancer treatment is mainly composed of three modalities: surgery, radiation, and chemotherapy. Advances in each area have changed the survival rates dramatically over the past 30 years. Cancers that were relatively incurable 20 to 30 years ago now have significantly improved survival rates. For example, the three most common cancers of childhood, acute lymphocytic leukemia, brain tumors, and lymphomas, have increased survival rates. Table 20–6 outlines current survival rates.

Surgery

Indications for Surgery

About 80% of patients with a suspected neoplasm will be referred to a surgeon (Barr,

Cowan, & Nicolson, 1997). The surgical oncologist is knowledgeable about the therapeutic benefits and risks associated with surgery. The surgeon, as part of the health care team, collaborates in the development of a surgical plan of care that best meets the child's needs

Table 20–6   TRENDS IN CANCER SURVIVAL FOR CHILDREN YOUNGER THAN AGE 15 IN THE UNITED STATES

Cancer	1960–1963	1986–1992
Acute lymphocytic leukemia	4	71
Brain and nervous system	35	61
Hodgkin's disease	52	92
Non-Hodgkin's lymphoma	18	71

Adapted from Parker, S., Tang, T., Bolden, S., & Wingo, P. (1997). Cancer statistics, 1997. *CA—A Cancer Journal for Clinicians, 47*(5), 5–27.

for diagnosis and treatment. Often in children, a central line or venous access device is inserted to make the future intravenous chemotherapy treatments, antibiotic administration, and transfusions safer and more tolerable for the child or adolescent and family.

Surgery has four functions in the treatment of childhood cancer: biopsy, staging, resection, and palliative surgical procedures. Surgical procedures may take place at any stage of the illness and throughout the illness experience. Often the child with cancer has multiple experiences with surgical interventions during the course of the illness. The biopsy is usually the first surgical experience for the child with cancer.

Biopsy

Biopsy allows the surgeon to obtain a specimen of suspected tissue to make or confirm the diagnosis. The biopsy may be done in several ways, depending on the location and depth of the tumor. Biopsy procedures may range from a less invasive procedure such as a needle biopsy to highly invasive surgical procedures requiring a longer recovery time.

Staging

Staging allows for confirmation of the extent of the disease by means of pathologic analysis and determines the level and extent of treatment. For example, a child with stage I neuroblastoma has a good prognosis and is monitored closely, whereas a child with a stage IV tumor has a poorer prognosis and requires surgery and intensive chemotherapy. In some tumors, the lymph nodes are examined for microscopic evidence of the spread of tumor cells. Recent advances in scanning allow for noninvasive means to stage the disease. There are disease-specific staging criteria for some childhood cancers, and further information may be found in an oncology textbook.

Curative Resection

Curative resections are performed when the cancer is non-metastatic, the lesion is resectable, and the benefit of survival outweighs the risks and possibility of functional disability.

Palliation

The role of surgery in palliation includes procedures that are believed to make the child more comfortable, relieve distressing symptoms, and prolong an acceptable quality of life. Surgical procedures associated with palliation include stents to bypass blockages, ostomies to relieve blockage or compression, and resection for removal of large fungating tumors.

Chemotherapy

Chemotherapy is used in combination with surgery and radiation therapy. Similarly, chemotherapy can be used to cure, control, or provide palliation. Chemotherapy is usually given in the oral, intravenous, or injectable forms and may also be given intra-arterially, intrathecally, intra-cavitarily, or intraperitoneally. Chemotherapeutic agents may be given in the hospital over a period of days, in an ambulatory clinic over the course of hours, or in the home by parents or the home care nurse.

Chemotherapy interferes with the stages of the cell cycle or the particular cellular process in the metabolism of the dividing cell. Chemotherapeutic agents work by several methods. Some drugs require that the cancer cell be in a certain stage of the cell cycle. These chemotherapeutic agents are called cell cycle phase specific. These agents are most effective against growing tumors that have large numbers of cells entering the cell cycle. Examples of cell cycle phase-specific drugs include antimetabolites and *Vinca* alkaloids.

Agents that do not require the cell to be in a certain phase are called cell cycle phase nonspecific. These are active throughout the phases of the cell cycle against tumors with cells that are in less active phases of cell division. Examples of cell cycle phase-nonspecific drugs include alkylating agents, anti-tumor antibiotics, nitrosoureas, hormones, and steroids. Table 20–7 describes several types of chemotherapeutic agents.

In the United States, all drugs must undergo careful pre-clinical testing. Animal testing allows for the discovery of toxicities, side effects, and initial dosage before the drug is used in human trials. There are four phases of human cancer drug trials, each requiring informed consent. Each phase allows for a specific focus that contributes to the scientific knowledge of the particular drug being tested. Phase I studies of anti-cancer drugs are done in cancer patients whose cancer has not responded to standard treatment or who have a cancer for which no current effective standard therapy exists. The objective of

Table 20-7   COMMON CHEMOTHERAPEUTIC AGENTS AND THEIR GENERAL MECHANISM

Family	Examples	Common Name	General Mechanism of Action
Antimetabolites	Methotrexate	MTX	Blocks enzymes necessary for DNA synthesis.
	6-Mercaptopurine	6MP	May be incorporated into new nuclear material or combined with vital cell components to inhibit division or metabolism of the cell.
	6-Thioguianine	6TG	
	5-Fluorouracil	5-FU	
	Cytarabine	Ara-c	
Vinca alkaloids	Vincristine	VCR	Arrests metaphase by binding to microtubules preventing microtubule and spindle formation.
	Vinblastine	Velban	This process is necessary for cell division; cell loses the ability to divide and dies.
	Etoposide	VP-16	
	Tenoposide	VM-26	
Cell Cycle Phase-Nonspecific Agents			
Alkylating agents	Mechlorethamine	Mustard	Form covalent bonds with molecules.
	Cyclophosphamide	Cytoxan	Affects DNA helix preventing the separation of the two strands
	Ifosfamide	Ifos	Also affects the separated DNA strands preventing them from acting as templates for formation of new DNA
	Mephalen		
	Cisplatin		
	Carboplatin		
	Dacarbazine	DTIC	
Anti-tumor antibiotics	Doxorubicin	Adriamycin	Inhibit DNA and RNA synthesis
	Anthracycline		
	Daunomycin		Increases cell membrane permeability.
	Anthracycline		
	Bleomycin		Blocks DNA replication.
	Dactinomycin	Actinomycin D	
Antitumor enzyme	Asparaginase		Inhibits DNA and RNA synthesis; inhibits protein synthesis in tumor cells that are dependent on asparaginase.

Phase I clinical trials is to discover and evaluate toxicities and to determine the maximum tolerated dose. Phase I trials are experimental and usually require special schedules of laboratory testing, such as multiple-timed blood studies, around the time of administration of the drug.

Phase II trials are used to determine the anti-cancer effectiveness of a drug. These are commonly used as first-line agents in cancers that have shown little response to conventional therapies. These trials provide researchers with knowledge regarding tumor biology, administration of the drug, dosage, toxicities, and necessary supportive care (e.g., transfusion requirements, growth factors) (Knobf & Durivage, 1993).

Phase III studies are used to compare a study drug to a standard drug in terms of effectiveness, whether administered alone or in combination with other drug regimens. These studies allow for the evaluation and comparison of factors such as response, toxicities, and quality of life issues.

Phase IV studies are used to compare standard therapies for new uses, compare different administration and dosing schedules, and determine the associated toxicities, risks, and possible benefits. Most children are treated according to pre-established protocols that outline the plan of care. Protocols are composed of dosing schedules, dosages, side effects, and consents for treatment and supportive care. A single protocol may be carried out over a period of a few months or up to 2 years.

Management of the Toxicity of Therapy

The management of treatment-related symptoms is one of the greatest challenges of oncology nursing. Symptom management is an area where the oncology nurse plays a crucial role. It is the nurse who administers much of the chemotherapy in both inpatient and outpatient settings. Attention to the individual needs of the child can have direct effect on how the therapy is tolerated. In symptom management the nurse has a significant level of autonomy in teaching children and families how to manage the side effects of treatment. Teaching includes both pharmacologic and non-pharmacologic interventions that influence compliance with symptom management that may improve the quality of life and decrease side effects of therapy.

Side effects of therapy are related to several factors, such as dose, drug, drug combinations, and concurrent therapies. There are drugs that are known to cause myelosuppression and mouth sores and are highly emetogenic. The nurse assesses prior experience with therapies and ensures the appropriateness of the antiemetic regimen for a particular therapy. The nurse reinforces patient education for the child and family, empowering them to do what they can to alleviate symptoms, maintain a schedule, and control the unpleasant side effects of nausea and vomiting. Side effects of treatment can be classified in short- and long-term categories. Nausea and emesis may be predicted to occur in minutes to hours and alopecia in days to weeks, and neurotoxicity and cardiac myopathy may occur early in treatment or many months later. Table 20–8 outlines the short- and long-term effects of several chemotherapeutic agents.

Radiation

Ionizing radiation is used with surgery and chemotherapy to increase tumor cell kill. Radiation is a highly effective cytotoxic agent. It affects both healthy cells and cancer cells in a way similar to chemotherapy. Radiation produces free radicals that cause damage to the DNA by disrupting the bonds within the double helix. Radiation may cause irreversible or reversible damage, with cancer cells having less ability to repair the damage caused by radiation. Cells may continue to perform normal activities but may be unable to divide, causing decreased growth of the tumor. Radiation therapy can be used alone to treat certain cancers or used in combination with chemotherapy and surgery. The goal of therapy is to cure, control, or palliate cancer, depending on the type, location, and extent of disease. Radiation therapy can be used to immediately treat tumors that are life threatening, such as tumors causing acute respiratory distress, intracranial pressure, or spinal cord compression.

There are several types of machines and beams used in radiation therapy. The main classifications of radiotherapy are teletherapy (radiation from a source outside the body) and brachytherapy (radiation from a source placed within a cavity inside the body).

Teletherapy involves the use of x-ray beams, gamma beams, and particle beams. In brachytherapy (interstitial and intra-cavitary) cesium or cobalt is used. The side effects of radiation therapy depend on site, volume of body area treated, dose administered, and individual differences. Symptoms usually develop 10 to 14 days into treatment and last for 2 or more weeks after treatment stops. Potential side effects of radiation include but are not limited to:

- mucositis
- anorexia
- xerostomia
- dental caries
- esophagitis
- nausea
- vomiting
- diarrhea
- alopecia
- skin reactions
- bone marrow depression
- anemia
- thrombocytopenia
- leukopenia
- dysphagia

The late effects of the radiation treatments for brain tumor can have a profound effect on the child's ability to function. Side effects of treatment include significant intellectual impairment, cognitive dysfunction, endocrine deficiencies, neurologic impairment, second malignancies, and nerve damage (Lew & Lavally, 1995; Shiminski-Maher & Shields, 1995). This may be due to the type of tumor, location, or treatments (surgery, chemotherapy, and radiation). One way of attempting to reduce long-term effects of radiation is the use of stereotactic radiation. Stereotactic radiation uses radiation beams in a precise and focal delivery to the targeted area. It is believed that the use of this form of highly defined radiation delivered to a smaller volume of the brain will decrease the long-term sequelae of treatment (Lew & Lavally, 1995).

Hematopoietic Stem Cell Transplant

Hematopoietic stem cell transplant (HSCT) is a relatively new modality of cancer therapy and involves the use of surgery, chemotherapy, and radiation therapy. Bone marrow transplantation (BMT) was first used in the late 1960s and involves the use of transplanted bone marrow from one of several sources: self (autologous), identical twin (syngeneic), and genotypically human leukocyte antigen–matched donor (allogeneic). Peripheral blood stem cells are also being used with success in BMT. Peripheral blood stem cells are harvested from the child by means of apheresis through a pheresis catheter.

During the process of BMT, the bone marrow stem cells are harvested by means of multiple bone marrow aspirates. In a peripheral blood stem cell transplant the stem cells are harvested by means of apheresis. Depending on the protocol a child undergoing transplantation would then receive ablative chemotherapy, radiation therapy, or both to eradicate residual disease. After ablative therapies, the harvested bone marrow, peripheral blood stem cells, or both are infused intravenously, and engraftment begins.

HSCT is often considered in the treatment of the following illnesses:

- immunodeficiencies such as severe combined immunodeficiency syndrome (SCIDS)
- genetic abnormalities: osteopetrosis, Hurler's disease
- hematologic problems: aplastic anemia, Fanconi's anemia

- malignancies: acute lymphoblastic and acute monocytic leukemias, chronic leukemias
- certain solid tumors: rhabdomyosarcoma, neuroblastoma
- lymphomas: relapsed Hodgkin's disease, relapsed non-Hodgkin's lymphoma

Toxicity and Complications

HSCT is a highly complex process that has many potential side effects, some of which are life threatening. Possible side effects include infection and sepsis, graft failure, relapse of the initial disease, graft-versus-host disease, and pulmonary, cardiac, neuromuscular, and renal toxicities. In general, the more intensive the therapy the child has before and during the transplant, the greater is the chance of having long-term complications (Abramovitz, 1991). In terms of the rehabilitation of the child who has undergone BMT and is experiencing side effects, the rehabilitative processes would be specific to the organ system affected. The child with decreased renal function has similar rehabilitation needs to the child in renal failure, and care of the child with cardiac sequelae would follow cardiac rehabilitation principles. A condition called graft-versus-host disease (GVHD) is a specific BMT complication when the marrow came from a donor other than the self. It is a reaction in which the donated bone marrow has T lymphocytes that reject the tissue of the bone marrow of the recipient (Caudell, 1991). There are two types: acute and chronic. Acute GVHD can affect several organ systems, mainly the "epithelium of the skin, the gastrointestinal tract, the small intrahepatic biliary ducts and the lymphoid system. It is unknown why these specific epithelial cells are recognized (as foreign) and targeted in the process of GVHD" (Caudell, 1991). Chronic GVHD may be manifested similar to a collagen-vascular disease such as lupus or rheumatoid arthritis and usually occurs 3 to 6 months after the transplant (Wagner et al., 1990; Caudell, 1991). Chronic GVHD may affect the skin, causing atrophy, erythema, and sclerosis. It may affect the liver, causing elevations of liver transaminases, and the gastrointestinal tract, causing dysphagia, pain, mucosal fibrosis, and diarrhea. GVHD may also affect the lungs, causing frequent infections, cough, and bronchospastic airway disease (Wagner et al., 1990). Treatment of GVHD involves the use of corticosteroids and immunosuppressive agents such as cyclosporine.

Table 20–8   SHORT- AND LONG-TERM SIDE EFFECTS OF CHEMOTHERAPY

Family	Drug	Short Term	Long Term
Cell Cycle Phase-Specific Agents			
Antimetabolites	Methotrexate	Myelosuppression, stomatitis, alopecia, anorexia, diarrhea, rash, photosensitivity	Neurotoxicity, renal toxicity, hepatotoxicity
	6-Mercaptopurine	Myelosuppression, anorexia, stomatitis, rash	Hepatotoxicity
	6-Thioguianine	Myelosuppression, nausea, vomiting, diarrhea, stomatitis	Hepatotoxicity
	5-Fluorouracil	Diarrhea, myelosuppression, stomatitis, rash, alopecia, esophagitis	Acute cerebellar syndrome, photosensitivity
	Cytarabine	Myelosuppression, anorexia, alopecia, conjunctivitis, erythema, diarrhea, rash	Neurotoxicity, hepatotoxicity
Vinca alkaloids	Vincristine	Constipation, stomatitis, fatigue, fever, jaw/bone pain, paralytic ileus	Neurotoxicity, syndrome of inappropriate antidiuretic hormone (SIADH), neuropathies
	Vinblastine	Alopecia, constipation, myelosuppression, jaw/bone pain, malaise	Neurotoxicity, neuropathies, paresthesias
	Etoposide	Hypersensitivity, myelosuppression, hypotension, stomatitis, alopecia, anorexia, bronchospasm	Fatigue, somnolence
	Tenoposide	Hypersensitivity, myelosuppression, hypotension, hypertension	Hemolytic anemia

Cell Cycle Phase Nonspecific Agents

		Reproductive toxicity
Alkylating agents	Mechlorethamine	Myelosuppression, severe nausea and vomiting, fever, rash	
	Cyclophosphamide	Alopecia, cystitis, hepatic toxicity, nausea and vomiting	Neurotoxicity, cardiac toxicity, renal toxicity, reproductive toxicity
	Ifosfamide	Cystitis, myelosuppression, nausea and vomiting, alopecia, ataxia	Neurotoxicity, renal toxicity, seizures, weakness
	Cisplatin	Nausea and vomiting, electrolyte imbalance, myelosuppression	Neurotoxicity, renal toxicity, ototoxicity, cardiotoxicity
	Carboplatin	Myelosuppression, nausea and vomiting, diarrhea, hematuria, SIADH	Neurotoxicity, nephrotoxicity, hepatotoxicity
	Dacarbazine	Alopecia, myelosuppression, hepatotoxicity, facial flushing, nausea and vomiting, flu-like syndrome	Hepatotoxicity
Anti-tumor antibiotics	Doxorubicin Anthracycline	Alopecia, red-pink urine for first few postadministration voids, nausea and vomiting, stomatitis, myelosuppression, mucositis, hyperpigmentation	Cardiac toxicity, hepatic toxicity, radiation recall
	Daunomycin	Alopecia, myelosuppression, nausea and vomiting, stomatitis, dermatitis, fever and chills, urticaria	Cardiac toxicity, hepatoxicity, nephrotoxicity
	Bleomycin	Hypersensitivity, fever, chills, stomatitis, hypotension, alopecia, hyperpigmentation, myelosuppression	Pulmonary toxicity, renal toxicity
	Dactinomycin	Potentiates the effects of radiation, myelosuppression, alopecia, acne, hyperpigmentation	Hepatotoxicity
Antitumor enzyme	Asparaginase	Anaphylaxis, anemia, anorexia, depression, hypersensitivity	Hepatotoxicity, pancreatitis

Rehabilitative nursing care includes the identification of GVHD, which may present as symptoms of rash, diarrhea, or elevated results of liver function tests. Symptom management to prevent complications includes skin care, measurement of intake and output, monitoring signs and symptoms of infection and electrolyte imbalance and bleeding, and monitoring serum levels of immunosuppressive agents (e.g., cyclosporine levels).

GVHD may affect multiple organ systems. The rehabilitation of the child with acute GVHD includes strategies that promote effective management of the changes in skin condition and elimination and interventions that maintain mobility and function. BMT and GVHD require a collaborative, multidisciplinary team approach in the management and support of the associated side effects experienced by the child. Whedon (1991) provides an outline showing the BMT rehabilitation team members and their functions. The functions of the oncology-rehabilitation nurse include evaluation (compliance, activities of daily living, range of motion, and serial assessments), assisting the primary caregiver in management, and providing the patient and family support and education about disease and medication effects and appropriate interventions.

Complementary Therapies

Research is increasingly documenting the threads between the body and the mind and the consumer's interest in connecting them. Wells (1990) stated that as many as 50% of cancer patients were seeking complementary therapies in addition to orthodox medical treatment and noted that nurses have the opportunity to learn such skills and treatments and then incorporate them into their care rather than have families seek these services elsewhere. Eisenberg and colleagues (1993), in studying adult use of unconventional therapies for all kinds of medical problems, found that one in three respondents used at least one unconventional treatment in the previous year. Currently, many families enter tertiary care centers asking not only about chemotherapy but also about complementary therapies, such as dietary supplements, alternate therapies for pain control, healing, acupuncture, and relaxation exercises. For example, one mother, after her 3-year-old son was diagnosed with a rare solid tumor, researched complementary therapies and found ways to supplement the child's diet with processed seaweed and, after every chemotherapy treatment, would take him for Reiki therapy (energy healing through light touch) on the way home from the hospital. There is much interest in diet and its effects on cancer. Many articles focus on prevention and what foods or supplements are beneficial (ACS, 1996), but little has been proven in humans. Communication between families and the health care team is essential to facilitate mutual learning and prevent adverse reactions with chemotherapy.

In her article "Imagine the Possibilities!" Ott (1996) clearly shows how guided imagery can work for toddlers and pre-schoolers to increase coping and self-esteem. Moreover, nurses can easily incorporate this technique into their practice in the hospital or home. For example, a 4-year-old girl who requires bone marrow aspirates and biopsies for diagnostic purposes uses guided imagery for distraction throughout the procedures. She receives moderate doses of conscious sedation (fentanyl and midazolam [Versed]) and uses imagery to maintain a focus and distraction. She blows out imaginary birthday candles on the tips of the fingers of her coach while talking about the candles, cake, and party activities of the imaginary birthday host. Imagery is very successful but must be introduced before the painful experience.

Many children and their families benefit from a health care team that includes nurses specializing in the physical and emotional cancer care as well as in relaxation and stress management techniques, therapeutic touch, and guided imagery. A holistic team might also include those specializing in acupuncture, homeopathy, naturopathic medicine, herbalism, and meditation. Nurses would be able to teach about the chemotherapy as well as dietary supplements, benefits of massage, and ways to naturally increase the body's endorphins. In this way it is acknowledged that each child, although treated with the same medicines, will heal differently. Employing complementary therapies with conventional treatments allows for the best holistic care of each unique child. Chapter 26 provides additional information on alternative treatment modalities.

GROWTH AND DEVELOPMENTAL ASPECTS OF CANCER THERAPY

Cancer does not discriminate. It affects people of all ages throughout the life span from newborn through childhood and into adulthood.

To provide specialized care for children with cancer it is necessary to have an understanding of the intrinsic growth and developmental needs of each age group that influence behavior. Knowledge of growth and development allows the nurse to formulate a plan of care at an appropriate developmental level. Developmental concepts influence the care, treatment, and rehabilitation of the child as well as provide a framework from which to base strategies for rehabilitation. These concepts are a thread woven throughout all aspects of nursing care for the child with cancer.

Much research has gone into the area of growth, development, and behavior. Theorists such as Freud, Piaget, and Erikson have specific theories on the science of growth and development, and these are explained in more detail in Chapter 10. One example of a growth and developmental theory is the work of Erik Erikson. His research has been used extensively to put child behavior and development in context. The nurse caring for a child undergoing cancer treatment must utilize knowledge of growth and development and incorporate techniques into practice to create understanding and a framework in which the child can understand what is happening. In doing so the nurse enlists the cooperation of the child and, depending on the age level, adapts nursing care and medical interventions accordingly. For example, with a school-aged child who must take oral medication, the nurse may create a game by using stickers or another reward system to accomplish the task. When an adolescent must be separated from peers to be admitted for chemotherapy treatments, the nurse may respond by encouraging friends to visit during the periods the adolescent is feeling well. Having an understanding of the developmental issues provides the nurse with a framework from which to understand the ill child's behavior. Table 20–9 provides an overview of the normal developmental characteristics of each age group.

DISCHARGE PLANNING ISSUES

From the moment of diagnosis there are questions from the family of prognosis, number of treatment days, and hospital stays, but the health care team is also thinking about discharge and home care issues. For instance this may mean helping the family determine what kind of intravenous access device the child most likely will need to facilitate treatment and which one will maximize ease of treatment but also allow for maximum quality of life. Even those children with an excellent prognosis, as in ALL, may have a myriad of complications and need extensive care and rehabilitation.

Before discharge from the hospital, teaching is of paramount importance. The obstacles to learning, however, may be overwhelming for some families. There is the shock of the diagnosis, the foreign language of medical terminology, and the fear and anxiety of painful procedures, and grief surrounding the loss of "life before cancer." For some, coping means a hunger to read, talk, and learn as much as possible right away. For others, it means supporting the child, gathering family and friends, letting the impact sink in, and letting the health care team take care of the other issues. The child and family may have a 1-month stay or less than a week, and so teaching begins informally from the first meeting or the "Day One" diagnosis talk. Thereafter, the parents' and child's learning style is assessed and a plan of teaching through modeling, videos, written material, and return-demonstration is developed. The health care team must include the child as a member in planning and teaching, emphasizing his or her expert knowledge about his or her own body to encourage their reporting of symptoms, fears, and fantasies.

The transition from the hospital to home is often facilitated by nurses who are able to determine which home care agency is best suited to the family's needs by making initial inquiries. For the school-aged child, a visit to the classroom is offered to facilitate the return to that environment. The continuation of treatment is a combination of outpatient visits, home visits, and hospital admissions. The continuing follow-up is usually with the outpatient nurse who is in close contact with the home care nurse to facilitate smooth transitions and continuity of care.

HOME MANAGEMENT

Acute Phase

Home management for children with cancer is essential. As more children with cancer are being discharged earlier or treated on an outpatient basis, the home care nurse is becoming an increasingly important part of the health care treatment team. Assessing, intervening, and evaluating, from diagnosis through treatment to cure or death, are essential components of the role. It is the home care

Table 20-9 DEVELOPMENTAL MILESTONES AND PHYSICAL ATTRIBUTES BY AGE GROUP

Critical Period	Description	Developmental Milestones	Physical Attributes
Neonate (birth to 1 mo) Erikson: Trust versus mistrust. The quality and consistency of care provided can influence the child's feelings and attitudes toward him/herself and the world.	Negotiates the transition from intrauterine to extrauterine life. Role of the rehabilitation nurse in the oncology setting is to maintain consistency of care. Establish a schedule for feeding, sleeping, nursing care. Monitor appropriate laboratory values and vital signs. Encourage parents to participate in newborn's care and utilize time for teaching.	Central nervous system is the fastest growing system; brain cells continue to develop in size and numbers. Holds head up when prone, hands fisted, startle reflex, attracted to moving bright objects; lusty cry, movements uncoordinated. The team may consider outside agencies such as early intervention to assist with developmental issues of this period.	Temperature: 97.9-98.0°F; 36.5-37.0°C axillary. Cardiovascular: color good, warm extremities, color increases with stress. Heart rate 100-180 awake/resting. B/P 75-85/ systolic. Respiratory: Respiratory rate rapid and irregular (avg. 35 breaths/min). Immune system: Antigen-antibody response is present 6-8 weeks (immunizations may be started if applicable). *Note:* In the oncology population it is imperative that the ill child not be given live vaccines. Check with the primary oncologist first. Maternal antibodies present.
Infancy (1-12 mo) Erikson: Major emotional task of infancy is the development of a sense of trust. The hospitalized infant will require consistent caregivers. Encourage the parents to assist with aspects of care. Continue routine as much as possible.	Goals include meeting the infant's needs for nutrition, warmth, sucking, comfort, sensory stimulation, safety, and love. Environment that is consistent and loving creates the sense that the world is a safe place. Stranger anxiety: 8 months. Object permanence is present. Becomes more mobile: creeping > crawling > standing (6-8 mos).	Central nervous system: head not held at midline, random movements of arms, hands fisted thumbs inside, startle reflex less intense. Gastrointestinal: strong sucking reflex, stomach is larger, holds more food. Solid food is initiated at 6 months. First teeth 5-10 months. Immune system: susceptible to infections because own immune system is weak and maternal protection lessens.	Cardiovascular: heart rate: 1 week to 3 months—100-220 beats/ min resting; 3 months to 2 years—80-150 beats/min resting. Blood pressure: 6 weeks 95-112 mm Hg systolic; 6 months 92-115 mm Hg systolic; 1 year 92-112 mm Hg systolic. Respiratory: Normal rate, 30 breaths/min. Monitor for signs of infection. Fever in the oncology population in presence of low white blood count can quickly lead to sepsis.

Toddler (12–36 mo)	Toddlers develop physical control of both body and activities. Language acquisition continues, and they begin to use words to control the environment.	Mobility: refine fine and gross motor skills. Walking alone is usually accomplished by age 15 months, and a more steady gait is evident by 24 months. The need for independence is strong, as is separation anxiety and fear of strangers. Elimination: Begins to be aware of soiling. Toilet training process begins; girls train earlier than boys, and small children earlier than larger children. Sleeps better at night, naps shorter in morning, longer in afternoon. Speech: jargon conversations develop into words that gain attention/express feelings.	Temperature: 99.7°F; 37.7°C. Cardiovascular: heart rate 80–150 beats/min resting 3 months to 2 years; 70–110 beats/min 2–10 years Blood pressure: 96–115/60–79 mm Hg. Respiratory: 25–30 breaths/min. Safety: decreased ability to control behavior or depth perception; therefore it is important to monitor activity which may be dangerous. Institute added safety measures when platelet count less than 50/mm³. Continue to monitor for signs and symptoms of infection.
Negotiating the passage from trust to autonomy. Balance set between independence and need to become member of society. Incorporate the use of age-approach interventions in daily care. Encourage parents to maintain normal pattern of limit setting and structure to provide sense of safety for child.			
Pre-school child (3–5 yr)	Period of exploration and discovery. Imagination is active and initiative is strongly developed. Explain all procedure to pre-schooler. Encourage child to ask questions to assess level of understanding and direct answers to alleviate fears.	Motor: coordination improves. Immune system: ability to produce antibodies improves; immunoglobulin production unstable.	Temperature: 98.6–99.0°F; 37.0–37.2°C Cardiovascular: heart rate 70–110 beats/min. Blood pressure: 96–115/60–79 mm Hg Respiration: 21–23 breaths/min.
Erikson: Initiative versus guilt. Actions become purposeful. Begins to determine right from wrong. Increasing confidence and independence. Participates in activities away from home/primary caregiver.			
School-aged child (6–12 yr)	Dynamic and complex time of transition. The school-aged child is challenged to learn new skills and to adapt to new environments. Develops independence and the ability to problem solve. Is able to plan strategies. The world outside the home becomes increasingly important. Encourage participation in teaching sessions. Encourage questions and continue to explore fears and clarify information.	Sleep: 10 hours, realizes when needs to rest. Elimination: independent, develops routine. Speech: articulates all sounds, vocabulary increases.	Temperature: 97.9–98.3°F; 36.6–36.8°C Cardiovascular: heart rate 55–90 beats/min. Blood pressure: 98–115/64–80 mm Hg (boys); 115–134/74–88 mm Hg (girls). Respiratory: normal average respiratory rate 19 breaths/min.
Erikson: Industry versus inferiority. The child feels able to manage the routine. These children are enthusiastic, enjoy companionship, seek approval and affection from caretaker, begin to turn to teachers and peer group for this support.			

Table continued on following page

Table 20-9 DEVELOPMENTAL MILESTONES AND PHYSICAL ATTRIBUTES BY AGE GROUP *Continued*

Critical Period	Description	Developmental Milestones	Physical Attributes
Adolescence (13–20 yr). Erikson: The adolescent continues the development begun in preadolescence, continues to establish identity, independence, self-sufficiency, and caring.	Adolescents attempt to sort out the roles they have played and the roles they hope to achieve. This period is exemplified by peer pressure and preoccupation with how they appear. Development of a sex-role identity. Explore high-risk behaviors. Incorporate teaching into periods when adolescent willing to listen. Encourage participation in treatment plan to increase cooperation. Adjust schedule when appropriate to allow for control of the environment.	Individual growth patterns, rapid physical body changes, secondary sexual physical characteristics appear. Sexual identity emerges and body image plays important role. The adolescent with acute lymphocytic leukemia undergoing chemotherapy and possibly radiation therapy will have the psychological and physiologic adjustment to changes that will have dramatic effects on body image (e.g., weight loss/gain, hair loss). The adolescent's ability to socialize with his/her peer group will be affected. Rehabilitation will include participation of the whole team.	Temperature: 98.6°F; 37.0°C. Cardiovascular: heart rate 55–90 beats/min. Blood pressure 128–150/75–95 mm Hg (boys); 122–145/75–95 mm Hg (girls). Respiratory: 16–18 breaths/min.

Data from Wong, D. (1995). *Whaley & Wong's nursing care of infants and children* (5th ed). St. Louis: C. V. Mosby.

nurse who communicates with the hospital-based treatment team and collaborates to deliver a care plan and facilitate care across the continuum. The primary goals of the home care nurse might include the following (Frierdich, 1990):

- reinforcement of discharge teaching
- prevention and early identification of complications
- rehabilitation to optimum physical ability
- provision of access to community resources
- promotion of family cohesion, communication, and positive adaptation to the chronic illness

However, as Selekman (1991) points out, rehabilitation is not just related to physical activity but may also encompass emotional, psychological, social, and vocational aspects. For the child, this must also include issues relevant to growth and development, chronicity of the disease, and family involvement. This means that the home care nurse must have readily available resources and the ability to assess, teach, and evaluate the care needs of a child with cancer. Just as the acute care oncology nurse has incorporated rehabilitation concepts, so the home care nurse incorporates oncology principles.

APPLICATION OF THE NURSING PROCESS

The rehabilitation needs of the child with cancer are related to the diagnosis, treatment, and side effects of therapy. These rehabilitation needs can be classified into three general groups (Gerber & Binder, 1993):

1. Those associated with the early phase of treatment as with a newly diagnosed cancer. For example, the nurse can encourage the child who is bald, gaining weight from steroids, and walking abnormally due to neuropathy from a chemotherapeutic agent to continue involvement in normal activities as able.
2. Those associated with the intermittent or chronic phase of treatment—children with long term effects from chemotherapy, radiation, or surgery. For example, the nurse can recognize symptoms of congestive heart failure in children who receive anthracyclines.
3. Those associated with the palliative phase of treatment—the needs of children with multiple relapse with little hope of cure. For example, the nurse can encourage the

parents and child to determine what is most meaningful in their lives. This will enable them to make choices about treatments, being in school, going on special trips, and having quality time together at the end of life.

The unique needs of the child and family must also be considered. Although the diagnosis and even treatment may be the same, the individuals involved are different. The nurse needs to build on the strengths and provide help where family needs are identified. For example, if a parent shudders at the thought of doing a central venous line dressing change, the older child may be willing to do his or her own dressing.

Nursing assessment and management of the child with newly diagnosed cancer will aid in the detection and prevention of many problems (Panzarella & Duncan, 1993). The early nursing interventions include identification and assessment of the problems as well as the rehabilitation needs of the child. Table 20–10 outlines four early potential problems of the newly diagnosed child and their etiology and management.

Of the problems listed—impaired skin integrity, alteration in comfort, impaired physical mobility, and alteration in nutrition—it is the last one that parents often focus on because this seems within their realm. Adequate nutrition is essential because this helps children better resist infection and tolerate treatment. This becomes quite a challenge because often children experience an altered sense of taste and nausea and vomiting secondary to chemotherapy, radiation, or both. Favorite foods often do not taste the same, and hospital food almost never compares favorably with home-cooked food.

Children must be assessed for height, weight, muscle tone, skin turgor, and energy and activity level. Parents and children should work with the nurse and dietitian for reasonable ways to supplement the child's diet by adding more protein, fat, or carbohydrate. For instance, suggesting adding instant breakfast drinks to milk is a simple, easy way to enhance nutrition. Whenever possible, enteral feeding is encouraged, with nasogastric tube feedings for short times or via a gastrostomy tube. If this is not feasible, children with cancer often may have parenteral nutrition.

Often a primary concern of the health care team working with children with cancer and their families is teaching about the risk of injury due to immunosuppression. It is also

Table 20-10 NURSING ASSESSMENT AND MANAGEMENT OF PHYSICAL CARE NEEDS

Problem	Etiology	Rehabilitation Nursing Management
Impaired skin integrity	Tumor/disease Surgery Invasive procedures Infiltration of vesicants Radiation therapy	Wound management Infection control Maximize comfort

Alteration in comfort	Tumor/disease progression
	Radiation
	Chemotherapy
	Surgery
		Maximize comfort
		Pharmacologic and non-
		  pharmacologic interventions
		  (imagery, relaxation techniques)
		Long-term coping

Impaired physical mobility	Fatigue as a result of
	  treatment
	Surgery
	Pain
	Chemotherapy
	Depression
		Physical therapy to decrease muscle
		  wasting
		Plan activities to increase activities
		  of daily living
		Pain management to facilitate
		  movement
		Minimize side effects of
		  chemotherapy
		Emotional support

Alteration in nutrition	Decreased appetite
	Nausea and vomiting related
	  to chemotherapy/radiation
	Mouth sores
	Esophagitis
	Dysphagia
	Increased appetite related to
	  corticosteroids, boredom
		Small frequent meals with a variety
		  of foods
		Medicate before meals for nausea
		  or pain
		Minimize offensive sights or smells
		Encourage weight gain with
		  appropriate exercise
		Facilitate alternate feeding methods

essential that the home care nurse understands this concept and can reinforce teaching begun in the initial stages of treatment. A plan of care using the nursing diagnosis of High Risk for Injury is found in Table 20-11. This includes the necessary interventions and teaching for the child or adolescent and family. Another useful method is to give parents teaching material, which reinforces the verbal instruction they have received. *Neutropenia: A Parents Guide* (see Appendix), is one example of helpful teaching material.

In addition to the physical aspects of care, there are important emotional aspects that affect children and their families. Specific nursing diagnoses and their related assessed areas might include:

- Knowledge Deficit related to new diagnosis, physical care needs, and emotional care needs
- Anxiety/Fear related to diagnostic tests, waiting for results, medical personnel, the unknown, and death

- Self-Esteem Disturbance related to physical changes, isolation from peers, loss of control, and loss of mastery
- Altered Role Performance/Coping related to sick vs. healthy role, disrupted family patterns, loss of control, new expectations, and fatigue
- Body Image Disturbance related to alopecia, weight gain or loss, and surgical interventions
- Anticipatory Grieving related to loss of life as anticipated, loss of limb, and loss of friends
- Spiritual Distress related to questions like "Why me?", questioning God's intentions, and questioning the meaning of life

LATE EFFECTS AND LONG-TERM CONSEQUENCES

Chronic Phase

As children with cancer recover from acute side effects and intensive treatment, the home

Table 20–11   NURSING PLAN OF CARE

Nursing Diagnosis: High Risk for Injury

Related to: Immunosuppression secondary to chemotherapy

Goals	Nursing Interventions/Teaching
Verbalize signs and symptoms of infection	Demonstrate use of thermometer by mouth and under axilla only and what is a temperature (38.5°C). Check skin for breakdown, redness/swelling especially of mouth, central venous access sites, perirectal area, previous areas of surgery or invasive procedures. Assess for pain. Note if white blood cell count is low, response to infection may not be present. Note signs and symptoms of respiratory compromise.
Know when and how to call the health care provider	For fever, signs and symptoms of infection Complaints of pain Difficulty breathing Prolonged diarrhea, constipation Emesis or poor fluid intake (greater than 24 hr) Know telephone numbers of providers and how to page the physician
Reduce risk of infection in the home	Reinforce frequent handwashing. Restrict visitors with illness. Teach importance of proper food handling and storage.
Reduce risk of infection outside the home	Minimize exposure to large groups of people. Instruct school personnel to inform family of contagious diseases. Immunize only as advised by health care provider. Discuss with siblings and peers the importance of "infection control."

Expected Outcomes

The child/family demonstrate behaviors that reduce the risk of injury.
The child/family seek appropriate medical attention in a timely manner so that interventions keep child free from injury.

---

care nurse needs to continue assessment for long-term and late effects of treatment. The nurse plays a crucial role in following the growth and development and progress of the child at home and in the school and community. The nurse must be aware of potential long-term consequences of therapy and be able to detect abnormalities based on history and physical assessment. There are many potential late effects of childhood cancer and treatment that involve major systems such as cardiovascular, neurologic, pulmonary, immune, renal, endocrine, and reproductive. Orthopedic, dental, and visual problems may be identified as well. The development of second tumors is unfortunately also a possibility. Of particular concern with children are psychosocial and developmental issues, especially relating to education (Robinson, 1992).

Physical Late Effects

Second Malignancies

For children previously treated for a malignancy, there is an increased risk of developing a different second malignancy. This risk is reported to be between 3% and 12% within 20 years of initial diagnosis (Meadows & D'Angio, 1982). This may be due to genetic predisposition, radiation therapy, or certain chemotherapeutic agents and varies in frequency and type based on the original childhood cancer. Childhood cancers with the highest risk of developing second malignancies are retinoblastoma, Ewing's sarcoma,

Wilms' tumor, and Hodgkin's disease. It is essential that, as the health care team members continue to work with the child throughout life, they are aware of the previous disease, treatment, and side effects. Children also need to be educated about how to have a healthy lifestyle. This education might include information about the following:

- alcohol
- smoking
- healthy diet
- regular exercise
- use of seat belts in cars
- use of helmets when bike riding
- safe sex practices
- drug use
- routine checkups
- identifying and practicing stress reduction activities
- breast self-examination
- testicular self-examination

Cardiac Sequelae

Most commonly cited causes for cardiac problems are the anthracyclines, cyclophosphamide, and radiation. Anthracyclines damage the myocytes and cause a shift in intracellular calcium. This increases the risk of myocardial dysfunction and arrhythmia (Hobbie et al., 1993). This risk is thought to be dose and age dependent, but there is no prescribed "safe dose" (Carter, Thompson, & Simone, 1991). Children are followed for years with diagnostic tests such as echocardiography and electrocardiography. Cardiac decompensation may happen suddenly or during particularly high-stress events such as pregnancy, weight lifting, or anesthesia. It may evolve similar to a cardiac failure condition and require long-term management with cardiac medications. Cyclophosphamide in high doses such as those used in BMT has been associated with cardiotoxicity in acute events. These side effects usually diminish after therapy, but the long-term side effects are not yet known (Hobbie et al., 1993). Radiation therapy also has an effect on the heart. This may be seen as acute or delayed pericarditis, myopathy, coronary artery disease, damage to the valves, and conduction defects. Preventative strategies include combining chemotherapy with lower doses of radiation when possible, using protective blocks to shield the heart and lungs, and more precise delivery of the radiation (Halperin et al., 1994).

Pulmonary Changes

Pulmonary changes may be due to radiation, surgery, or chemotherapy. Radiation may cause both acute pneumonitis and chronic fibrosis, particularly when total body irradiation is used before a BMT (Hobbie et al., 1993). Even though chemotherapy or the dose of radiation may be adjusted to decrease side effects and children may not exhibit any symptoms, the pulmonary function tests and chest x-rays will show the changes. Surgery, such as a thoracotomy, may also affect pulmonary function because the lungs are often a site of metastases. Chemotherapy agents, particularly the nitrosoureas, have been shown to cause pulmonary fibrosis. Survivors undergoing operative procedures, previously treated with bleomycin, should tell their physicians of their increased risk for pulmonary complications if given high concentrations of oxygen intraoperatively or postoperatively. Careful fluid management in these situations is also essential.

Neurologic Deficits

Although radiation therapy is more readily attributed to neurologic deficits in the child with cancer, there is also evidence of damage from intrathecal chemotherapy and particularly the synergistic effect of the therapies (Butler et al., 1994). Higher doses of radiation often cause more significant side effects; and the younger the child is at the time of treatment, the more harm. Children younger than age 3 years with brain tumors may be given chemotherapy initially instead of extended-field radiation to allow further brain maturation. There are also some data to suggest that girls are at greater risk and are more severely affected than boys (Waber et al., 1990). The cognitive deficits that have been identified show a significant decrease in IQ scores by 10 to 20 points. These side effects may not become apparent for 2 to 5 years; therefore, it is essential for families, nurses, pediatricians, and school personnel to be aware of the problems that may become apparent in school work and interactions. These include deficits in memory, attention, perceptual abilities, verbal skills, and arithmetic. Surgery to remove a tumor or the tumor itself may also cause neurologic deficits. Careful assessment and a thorough health history of the child with cancer is essential. Periodic testing is recommended, particularly for those known to be at risk for these deficits. Early intervention can often help normalize a child's education.

Endocrine System

The effects of cancer therapy on the endocrine system may occur through direct damage to the gonads and thyroid gland or damage to the "controlling hypothalamic-pituitary axis" (Hobbie et al., 1993). Beside the initial worry of hair loss, many parents focus on whether their child with cancer will be able to bear children. The gonads are sensitive to both radiotherapy and certain chemotherapy agents. The insult may depend on the dose delivered, the nutritional status of the child at diagnosis, the stage of puberty at diagnosis, and the duration of therapy. For males, therapy may result in a lack of secondary sex characteristics, lack of change in libido, and low sperm counts (Hobbie et al., 1993). Some male adolescents do attempt sperm banking before beginning therapy. Radiation to the hypothalamic-pituitary axis can also cause testicular dysfunction. Therefore, it is essential that males at risk continue to have physical examinations and blood work to be alert to the need for hormonal therapy. They may also need psychological counseling to support them through the issues of sexual dysfunction.

The ovaries may be affected by radiation and chemotherapy; however, it may be possible to shield or surgically move them to accommodate radiation therapy. The effect of chemotherapy may be dependent on several factors, such as dose of drug, length of treatment, and sexual development at the time of treatment. The symptoms of ovarian failure might include amenorrhea, decreased libido, and failure to develop secondary sex characteristics. Radiation to the hypothalamic-pituitary axis can affect ovarian function and also result in the development of precocious puberty, which is "any secondary sex characteristics in a female before the age of eight years" (Hobbie et al., 1993, p. 471). Premature menopause may be a treatment-related side effect as well as an increased risk of breast or uterine cancer if estrogen replacement therapy is used (Robinson, 1993). There is the need for continued assessment of sexual development and menses, with appropriate referrals, including psychological counseling if identified as a need.

Another long-term effect on the neuroendocrine system is growth hormone deficiency and short statures (Moore, 1995). Many cancer survivors struggle with body image as they are often small and appear much younger than their chronological age. Irradia-

tion of the brain or nasopharynx can cause hypothalamic-pituitary dysfunction and put these children at risk for severe growth retardation. Additionally, children receiving total-body irradiation in preparation for receiving a transplant show a growth hormone deficiency, which contributes to decreased rate of growth. Growth problems also may be related to the age and nutritional status of the patient at the time of receiving radiation therapy, as well as the dosing, methods, and length of the treatments (Hobbie et al., 1993). Table 20–12 outlines in greater detail the long-term effects on these systems and others.

As survivors move into and through the chronic phase of their disease, it may be overwhelming to think of the potential long-term or late effects. It is a balancing act between being aware and not living life as a "sick" individual. The nurse in every setting involved with the child or adolescent and family must remain astute in assessing for physical and psychological late effects, referring to appropriate resources and encouraging and promoting health and return to normalcy. The following case study illustrates some of the acute and chronic needs of an adolescent diagnosed with cancer and the plan of care.

CASE STUDY

Louise is an 18-year-old who was diagnosed at age 14 years with ALL. She was entered on a 2-year protocol involving chemotherapy: intravenous doxorubicin (Adriamycin), methotrexate, and vincristine; intramuscular asparaginase; oral prednisone and 6-mercaptopurine; intrathecal cytarabine and methotrexate; and 2 weeks of cranial radiation. She experienced many complications during her induction chemotherapy the first several months of treatment. For instance, her implanted central venous access device became unusable, presumably due to a precipitate, and had to be removed and replaced by an external central line. She had one episode of bacteremia and one of fungemia, most likely from endogenous bacteria and *Candida*, which flourished due to treatment-induced neutropenia. She also had hepatitis of unknown etiology and pancreatitis, most likely from the chemotherapeutic agent asparaginase. She had a significant weight loss due to loss of appetite and taste alteration and had to receive parenteral nutrition. She was depressed because of an altered body image from weight loss and

Text continued on page 485

Table 20-12 EVALUATION OF LONG-TERM EFFECTS

Body System	Health Problem	Associated Treatment Modality	Method of Assessment	Management and Nursing Considerations
Endocrine				
Ovaries	Ovarian dysfunction	Procarbazine, cyclophosphamide, nitrogen mustard, busulfan	Careful health history and physical examination	Oophoropexy before treatment
	Primary	400–800 cGy	Tanner staging	Refer to endocrinologist
	Secondary	High risk	Serum determinations of LH, FSH, estradiol at age 12 yr if no secondary sex characteristics	Replacement hormone
		Older patients		Refer for counseling
		Poor nutrition		Anticipatory teaching:
		Longer length of treatment		Lack of secondary sex characteristics
		Combination therapy		Loss of menses, irregularities
				Decreased libido, vaginal dryness
Testes	Testicular dysfunction	Procarbazine, cyclophosphamide, nitrogen mustard, busulfan	Careful health history and physical examination	Sperm banking at treatment
	Primary	400–600 cGy; azoospermia	Tanner staging	Refer to endocrinologist
	Secondary	≥2400 cGy; Leydig cell damage	Testicular volumes	Replacement testosterone
			Semen analysis	
		High risk	Serum determination of LH, FSH if no secondary sex characteristics after 14 yr of age	Refer for counseling
		Poor nutrition		Anticipatory teaching:
		Combination therapy		Small testicles
		Longer length of treatment		Possible impotence
				Decreased libido
				Lack of secondary sex characteristics
Thyroid	Hypothyroidism Overt and compensatory	No known chemotherapy	Careful health history and physical examination	Refer to endocrinologist
		>2000 cGy; overt or compensatory hypothyroidism; Graves' disease	Free T$_4$, TSH, T$_3$	Replacement hormone
				Anticipatory teaching:
				Hypothyroidism or hyperthyroidism—signs and symptoms
	Graves' disease	≥750 cGy total body irradiation; hypothyroidism		
		High risk		
		Younger patients		

System	Effect	Risk Factors	Evaluation	Management
Hypothalamic-pituitary axis	Hypothalamic dysfunction Panhypothalamic dysfunction Panhypopituitary dysfunction	No known chemotherapy ≥2400 cGy; hypothalamic dysfunction ≥4000 cGy; pituitary dysfunction	Careful health history and physical examination Growth charts Tanner staging GH: stimulation tests, pulsatile tests Somatomedin-C LH, FSH, estradiol, testosterone, prolactin, free T_4, TSH, T_3	Refer to endocrinologist Replacement hormone Bromocriptine (for hyperprolactinemia) Anticipatory teaching: As above Poor growth Short stature
Cardiovascular	Cardiomyopathy	Anthracycline chemotherapy Risk increased with Lifetime cumulative dose ≥550 mg/m² Mediastinal radiation	ECG, echocardiogram, or MUGA History of symptoms of congestive heart failure (CHF) Stress testing	Careful monitoring of anthracycline dosage to limit lifetime dose If CHF develops, supportive care with Referral to cardiologist Digoxin, diuretics Sodium restriction
	Pericardial damage	Mediastinal radiation	Physical examination, echocardiogram History of chest pain, dyspnea, fever, pulsus paradoxus, venous distension	May be subclinical If pericardial effusion develops, treatment may include Referral to cardiologist Anti-inflammatory drugs Pericardial tap If restrictive pericarditis occurs, treatment may include pericardiectomy

Table continued on following page

Table 20–12 EVALUATION OF LONG-TERM EFFECTS *Continued*

Body System	Health Problem	Associated Treatment Modality	Method of Assessment	Management and Nursing Considerations
	Early coronary artery atherosclerosis	Mediastinal radiation	ECG, echocardiogram History of chest pain with exertion, decreased exercise tolerance	Referral to cardiologist Dietary restriction of fat and salt intake Program of moderate exercise If significant obstruction to coronary artery flow develops, treatment may include Thrombolytic drugs Calcium channel blocking agents Balloon dilation angioplasty Coronary artery bypass surgery
	Atrioventricular (AV) valve tissue damage	Mediastinal radiation	Physical examination, ECG, echocardiogram	Referral to cardiologist If significant AV valve insufficiency develops, treatment may include Diuretics Afterload reducing agents Surgical implication of replacement of valve
	Ventricular arrhythmias	Anthracycline chemotherapy	ECG, Holter monitor, exercise test	Referral to cardiologist If significant arrhythmias develop, treatment may include antiarrhythmic drugs
Musculoskeletal	Scoliosis, kyphosis	Radiation therapy for intra-abdominal tumor in which vertebrae absorb radiation unevenly	Regular physical examination May not become apparent until adolescent growth spurt	Referral to orthopedist for rehabilitative measures Instruction about normal weight maintenance to make problem less noticeable

Late Effect	Cause	Detection	Management
Spinal shortening (sitting height)	Spinal irradiation (e.g., for medulloblastoma); direct effect of radiation on growth centers of vertebral bodies	Serial measurements of sitting height (crown to rump)	Referral to orthopedic surgeon Anticipatory teaching about disproportion between shorter-than-usual trunk and normal leg length as full growth is attained; reassurance that disproportion probably will not be obvious to others but may be a problem in fitting clothing
Increased susceptibility to fracture, poor healing, deformities of shortening of extremities	Irradiation to lesions in long bones (e.g., with Ewing's sarcoma)	Regular physical examination	Referral to orthopedic surgeon Teaching about protective measures such as avoiding rough contact sports
Facial asymmetry	Surgery plus irradiation to head and neck area (e.g., for rhabdomyosarcoma), causing altered growth of facial bones	Physical examination Early evaluation by reconstructive surgeon	Anticipatory guidance about possible adjustment problems with visible deformity Referral to family counseling to manage or prevent adjustment and behavioral problems
Dental problems Gingival irritation and bleeding, tooth loosening, migration (can lead to periodontal disease) Delayed or arrested tooth development	Radiation therapy to maxilla and mandible Chemotherapy	Clinical observation with dental examination	Many dental problems can be minimized or prevented with Good oral hygiene with flossing and brushing, gingival massage, use of plaque-disclosing tablets or solutions Preradiation therapy fluoride prophylaxis Frequent dental evaluation Extraction of damaged, nonfunctional teeth

Table continued on following page

Table 20-12 EVALUATION OF LONG-TERM EFFECTS *Continued*

Body System	Health Problem	Associated Treatment Modality	Method of Assessment	Management and Nursing Considerations

Vision	Cataracts	Cranial radiation
		Corticosteroids (long term)
			Eye examination
			  Visual inspection
			  Slit-lamp examination
				Ophthalmology consult
				Surgical removal
				Corrective lense fitting

Hearing	Hearing loss (high-tone range)	Cisplatin
		Increased risk
		  Recurrent ear infections
		  Ototoxic antibiotic therapy
		  Radiation to auditory area
			Monitor with hearing tests	Hearing aid
				Speech therapist consult

Respiratory	Pulmonary fibrosis	Lung irradiation
		Some chemotherapeutic agents
		Risk increased with
		  Larger lung volume in
		  radiation field
		  Dose, 4000 cGy
		  Radiation-sensitizing
		  chemotherapeutic agents
			Clinical observation for dyspnea, rales, cough, decreased exercise tolerance, pulmonary insufficiency
			Monitor with
			  Physical examination
			  Chest x-ray studies
			  Pulmonary function tests
				Health education for smoking prevention or cessation
				Supportive care with provision of adequate rest periods
				Vigilance for development of pulmonary infection
				Pneumococcal vaccine
				Yearly influenza vaccination
				Careful oxygen administration (busulfan)

Gastrointestinal	Chronic enteritis	Radiation therapy
		Risk Increased with
		  Dose, 5000 cGy
		  Previous abdominal surgery
		  Radiation-sensitizing
		  chemotherapeutic agents
			Clinical observation for pain, dysphagia, recurrent vomiting, obstipation or constipation, blood- or mucus-containing diarrhea, or malabsorption syndrome	Nutritional consultation for diet plan to diminish symptoms while providing adequate nutrition for growth and development and to fit family routine, ethnic, or cultural customs
				Dietary modifications may include low-fat, low-residue, gluten-free diet free of milk and milk products
				If enterostomy is performed, coordination with enterostomal therapist for patient and family teaching about stoma care

Body System	Late Effect	Causes	Screening/Monitoring	Management
	Hepatic fibrosis, cirrhosis	Radiation therapy Some chemotherapeutic agents	Clinical observation for pain, hepatomegaly, jaundice Monitoring with liver function tests and liver scans may be inconclusive so periodic liver biopsy may be necessary	Supportive care with nutritional consultation
Kidney and Urinary Tract	Chronic nephritis (may lead to renal failure, cardiovascular damage)	Radiation to renal structures Risk increased with concomitant chemotherapy	Clinical observation and monitoring with Blood pressure readings Urinalysis Creatinine levels Complete blood count (CBC)	If progressive renal failure develops, supportive care (possibly dialysis and/or transplantation)
	Chronic hemorrhagic cystitis	Chemotherapy (cyclophosphamide) Risk increased with Pelvic irradiation Inadequate hydration before, during, and after chemotherapy	Clinical observation for dysuria, urinary frequency, hematuria Monitoring with urinalysis, blood pressure	Ensure adequate hydration before, during, and after chemotherapy (3000 mL/m²/24 hr) Bladder hemorrhage may be treated with formalin instillation and/or fulguration of bleeding sites

Table continued on following page

Table 20-12 **EVALUATION OF LONG-TERM EFFECTS** *Continued*

Body System	Health Problem	Associated Treatment Modality	Method of Assessment	Management and Nursing Considerations
	Unilateral kidney	Nephrectomy for Wilms' tumor	Clinical observation for dysuria, urinary frequency, hematuria Monitoring with urinalysis, blood pressure	Health education to avoid injury to remaining kidney (e.g., avoid contact sports) Wear kidney guard during sports If urinary tract infection develops: Identification of causative organism Antibiotic treatment Urinalysis Medic-Alert identification bracelet
Hematopoietic	Prolonged immunosuppression	Chemotherapy (high dose, extended periods) Radiation to marrow-containing bones Splenectomy (e.g., for Hodgkin's disease)	Monitoring with: CBC, platelet count Tests of immune function Bone marrow examinations as indicated	Health education about infection Pneumococcal vaccine and prophylactic antibiotics for asplenic individuals Prompt treatment if infection occurs

From Hobbie, W., Ruccione, K., Moore, I., Truesdall, S. (1993). Late effects in long-term survivors. In G. Foley, D. Fochtman, & K. Mooney (Eds.) *Nursing care of the child with cancer* (2nd ed.), pp. 466–496. Philadelphia: W.B. Saunders.

alopecia; immobile because of inertia, fatigue, and neuropathy secondary to vincristine; and minimally interactive with family and staff.

Interventions were attempted to motivate Louise and involve her in her care. The nurse formulated the following plan of care:

Problem	Intervention	Outcome
Potential for injury due to pancytopenia	Monitor counts. Assess for signs and symptoms of infection. Assess for signs and symptoms of bleeding, low hematocrit. Transfuse as needed. Administer antibiotics as ordered. Encourage excellent hygiene.	Louise will be free of injury.
Alteration in nutritional status	Daily weights. Encourage small frequent meals chosen by Louise. Have dietitian visit twice a week. Supplement with high-calorie, high-protein nourishment. Reduce distractions at meal times.	Nutritional requirement will be met.
Alteration in coping secondary to change in body image and hospitalization	Encourage Louise to ask questions. Introduce Louise to other teens. Schedule meetings with psychologist two to three times a week. Schedule physical therapy two to three times a week. Set daily schedule with Louise. Encourage Louise to go to teen room. Allow time for visitors, phone calls. Allow private time. Introduce literature/tapes. Explore wig options. Show ways to "hide" central venous line. Introduce relaxation techniques, guided imagery.	Louise will cope with hospitalization.

While in the hospital Louise was mostly supported by her mother. She lived at home with her disabled father, mother, and older sister, who had a 3-year-old daughter. She had a few school friends, who mostly called but did not visit, and extended family, who occasionally visited or sent presents to the hospital.

Louise was discharged from the hospital 6 weeks after diagnosis needing psychological support, parenteral nutrition for 12 hours at night, and physical therapy to walk and regain strength. She required frequent assessment of, and intervention for, the above nursing diagnoses. These now had to be translated into the home setting. Louise was referred to a home care agency for daily nursing visits. While the home care nurse assessed Louise for potential complications, the teaching begun in the hospital was reinforced. The nurse worked with the mother and Louise to develop a food plan for the day and taught them parenteral nutrition therapy for overnight administration. Finally, the home care nurse continued to assess the family's coping strategies and facilitated a manageable daily routine with support from the community and school.

Louise also continued weekly visits to the outpatient clinic to see her oncologist, nurse, and psychologist. After 2 months on parenteral nutrition, Louise was found to have a clot impeding the use of her central venous line, and the line was removed. At 3 months post diagnosis she was still considered malnourished and had continuous feeds via a nasogastric tube at night with bolus feeds during the day for the next month. She began to maintain and gradually gain weight without supplement. Louise continued with a physical therapist at home and in-water therapy to increase her mobility, which gradually improved. By 6 months post diagnosis she was able to return to school, going to the clinic 1 day every 3 weeks for chemotherapy, while receiving chemotherapy at home during the other weeks. Over the next year she experienced intermittent symptoms of sinusitis, pneumonia, and mucositis, all of which were treated on an outpatient basis.

Now 2 years off therapy she has thin hair on her head, striae on her trunk and legs due to previous corticosteroid therapy, borderline ventricular function due to her anthracycline therapy, which does not limit her physical activity at this point, and a small cataract in one eye. She is in high school, sexually active with her boyfriend, still living at home, and cancer free. She returns to the clinic once every year for a physical examination, tests, laboratory work, and monitoring.

LONG-TERM OUTLOOK

As we move into the twenty-first century it is clear that there will be increasing numbers of pediatric cancer survivors. With an overall 5-year survival rate around 70% for ages 1 through 15 years (Parker et al., 1997) there will be an estimated 180,000 to 220,000 childhood cancer survivors in the year 2000 (Bleyer, 1990). Because pediatric cancer affects children from birth through adulthood, there will be many services needed along the continuum. For some it is truly rehabilitation—restoring, retraining, relearning that which they knew or did in a different way. For others it is habilitation, learning something new, or growing to reach their fullest potential (Selekman, 1991). For a 13-year old with osteogenic sarcoma and a new allograft, it will be rehabilitation first, learning to walk with a prosthesis, then habilitation learning to accommodate the prosthetic device in a new sport.

As more children survive cancer, it is important to look at what the current studies report about the needs of these children and adolescents. Despite rigorous cancer treatment, it appears that most cancer survivors do not suffer from severe psychopathology. Furthermore, whereas studies report increased risk taking in adolescents during treatment, this is not carried into adulthood (Zeltzer, 1993). Also, despite remembering many of the treatments and their unpleasant side effects, long-term survivors are able to report positive outcomes of having had cancer. They developed a maturity earlier than their peers and an appreciation for life and what is important. They also express concerns about their future. Late effects of the cancer, fertility issues, employment, and health insurance are some of the concerns they mention (Lozowski, 1993). The health care team needs to be vigilant in raising society's awareness of the obstacles facing survivors and what kind of support is needed. Currently, Candlelighters Childhood Cancer Foundation publishes *The Phoenix*, a newsletter for adult survivors, and there are also camps and retreats or programs that may be offered solely for survivors and their significant others. Some needs may be met by late effects follow-up clinics, which can provide support, education, and medical follow-up as necessary.

IMPACT ON CHILD AND FAMILY

Although it is the child who has cancer, it is recognized immediately that cancer affects the entire family and it is a life-changing event. Peers, parents, siblings, and grandparents may feel their lives have been forever altered. As the working group for psychosocial issues reported at the ACS workshop in 1991 "Psychosocial care is, and should be seen as essential to improving the chances for disease-free life-enhancing futures for everyone affected by childhood cancer. It is fundamental to the promotion of physical and mental health and social productivity" (Chesler et al., 1993, p. 3210). This is a strong mandate to the health care team to begin at diagnosis the assessment and interventions to promote psychosocial well-being. Some of the factors that must be considered are:

- age at diagnosis
- prior coping mechanisms
- community supports available
- communication pattern of child
- cultural background, including primary language, religious or spiritual customs
- anticipated length of treatment
- family constellation
- previous life stresses and experiences
- parents' coping abilities

The interventions must begin in the hospital or clinic setting at diagnosis and be evaluated and modified as the child progresses through treatment, meeting new stressors along the continuum. The outpatient and home care nurse will continue to assess the coping and survival skills of the family members as they live with cancer as a chronic condition.

Many questions arise, but one of the first to be considered is who will be the primary caregiver. Will there be a rearrangement of roles? If there is only one parent, then who will be the "back up"? Most often one parent will take a leave of absence or quit a job while the other must continue to maintain income and benefits such as health insurance. Other questions and concerns include:

Who will care for the other children at home?

How can a husband and wife support each other and keep communication clear when they are trading the increased responsibilities between hospital and home?

What services does the family need at home?

Does the family speak English? Who is available to translate both language and culture for the health care team?

What are the existing supports for the family? Will extended family members be helpful in caring for the child, parents, or siblings?

How will the family manage transportation, out of pocket expenses for food, travel, and complementary therapies?

Will the school be ready and willing to educate and support the classmates and the returning student?

How can the siblings be included and their stress minimized?

Interventions for the child or adolescent need to be developmentally appropriate. Once diagnosed with cancer, they enter another world, one of different rules, with pain, few choices, and little control. It is helpful for nurses to see the similarities in working with these children. Tasks to be accomplished at each age are:

1. Allow for physical and personal self-identity formation. The first goal in the hospital is to reduce fear. This means developing trust, forming bonds, and making a connection. For example, with a toddler that could mean the nurse playing ball before taking vital signs while the child sits on mom's lap; for the school-aged child it may mean helping the child gather information and enjoy fantasy play in the playroom; for the adolescent it could mean interpreting medical jargon, watching the nonverbal cues, encouraging questions, and not interrupting phone calls from friends. For all it means being honest, allowing expression of feelings, encouraging positive thinking, and being mindful of comfort objects such as blankets, stuffed animals, quilts, and pictures of loved ones.

2. Help the child continue to become autonomous and increase control over the environment. For example, with a toddler this might be having the choice of taking medicine from a cup or an oral syringe and then choosing the sticker to go on the chart; school-aged children might be allowed to "do a dressing" on a doll before they have their central line dressing changed; and adolescents might be allowed to sleep late and later enlisted to participate in their care and advocate for personal needs and concerns.

3. Help make future plans, to develop "normalization strategies." This is one way children and families know the team is working toward a cure (O'Connor & Blesch, 1992). For example, the parents of a toddler should be reassured that regression is a temporary coping mechanism and that the child will get "back to normal." School-aged children should be reassured that they will get home, and birthdays and holidays are celebrated in the hospital. Adolescents should be told that keeping up with schoolwork is possible and that they should make weekend plans and continue peer relationships.

Katz and Varni (1993) introduce an interesting model of social skills training for newly diagnosed children aged 5 to 13 years. They note that as chronic illnesses are known to cause increased stress over a lifetime, teaching children new skills early may help their coping. They propose individual sessions in which children learn how to deal with being teased (due to their altered body image or cognitive skills), how to be assertive, and how to problem solve. As these authors say, "Empirical methods for improving social support, such as social skills training, are now emerging as critical interventions in cancer control and rehabilitation" (p. 3318). This sentiment is echoed by Hockenberry-Eaton, Dilorio, and Kemp (1995), who report that children are able to learn coping techniques early in treatment and at a young age, which then serve them well later in dealing with "chronic cancer stressors."

Psychosocial Support

Each child is at a different developmental stage, and each child and family is confronting different psychosocial concerns. The goal should be to have the child and family either maintain or gain a higher level of psychological functioning. The strengths and weaknesses of each family member should be assessed to individualize psychosocial interventions effectively (Walker et al., 1993). Topics to be considered by the health care team include:

- impact of cancer on the family
- stressors throughout the illness
- physiologic problems
- special needs of adolescent
- changes in family relationships
- impact on siblings

The health care team in conjunction with the family needs to plan optimum interventions to facilitate coping, adaptation, and growth. This way the team will promote mental health and normal development.

Just as children and adolescents need special treatment, so do siblings and parents of children with cancer. Many siblings feel left out, guilty, and jealous. There is an increasing awareness that the health care team must also involve siblings by offering counseling, special workshops, and opportunities for them to be involved. Many parents feel angry, exhausted, confused, guilty, and devastated. Some are able to seek support from friends, family, and spouses, whereas others may need individual counseling or encouragement to attend a parent support group.

SCHOOL AND COMMUNITY

Because school and play are the work of the child and being with peers becomes increasingly important, a school re-entry program is offered by most cancer treatment centers. This is offered for pre-school through high school classes. It usually involves members from the health care team making a visit and doing a presentation with slides, videos, or a puppet show (Baysinger et al., 1993). The child with cancer may be present, depending on his or her preference, but is always consulted as to the content of the program. Class members, teachers, guidance counselors, nurses, and family members are encouraged to be present. One teacher wrote after such a visit that she could feel the anxiety level decrease in the classmates as they anticipated the return of their friend.

Adolescence

Adolescence has always been recognized as a particularly challenging, difficult, growth-filled, and unique time. The main tasks of children in this age group are identity formation of the physical and personal self, becom-

ing autonomous from parents, and making career and future plans (Walker et al., 1993). These tasks are severely compromised when teens are diagnosed and undergo treatment for cancer. Their physical self is challenged by hair loss, altered body image, possible long-lasting side effects of disfiguring but lifesaving surgery, or even the possibility of death. Most teens do not see cancer as a chronic illness. Their attitude tends to be "let's do this and get it over with." They still see themselves as invincible even when faced with a life-threatening illness. Their personal self is assaulted because they now deal with a new role—that of patient. They feel their space and body are invaded. They worry about peer relationships and issues related to sexual identity. Most are struggling to gain some control over their lives and become autonomous from their parents and yet cancer puts them back in the dependent role.

Whether it is providing transportation, caring for teens when they feel sick, or watching for side effects, parents are forced into a protective, "caring for" mode rather than the "letting go" that should be happening. And instead of making future plans, it often seems that everything must be put on hold. Seniors in high school may delay college or pick one closer to home so that follow-up visits will be possible. They quickly must focus on the here and now and save dreams for the future. Particularly for teens, transitions between the hospital and home are extremely difficult. Although some children are able to make "cancer friends," they may not be in the hospital on the same days and they might feel too sick to support one another. Many centers instead offer support groups or social activities for teens when not hospitalized. There are also camps that offer not only family sessions but sessions specifically for teens as well.

TERMINALLY ILL CHILD

Palliative Phase

Although many children will survive, for others the treatment will not be successful. There are some whose treatment course is short and not effective, and the care quickly focuses on palliation. For others, long remissions occur with good quality of life even into the palliative phase. The home care nurse, like the acute care nurse in the hospital, may have the experience of intense time spent with the child and family, a hiatus of months or years perhaps not in contact, and then again being in an intense relationship. At the time of diagnosis there is usually anticipatory grieving by parents and perhaps the child, and this recurs with each relapse. Families will often say that the relapse is much harder than the initial diagnosis. They know the chances for survival are diminished: they know "what they are in for" in relation to more treatment, hospital or outpatient visits, and home care; and, there is often much anger that "I did everything right the first time—this isn't fair—how could it come back?"

There is a point at which there is a change in the intent of treatment from cure to palliation. At this point the health care team tells the family that further therapy is not likely to be curative and the focus should move to support and the relief of symptoms. Most families will choose to continue treatment until close to the time of the child's death. The home care nurse may sense mixed messages coming from families at this point when they are still pursuing treatment but seemingly coming closer to the time of death. There is a strong theme that is universal at this point with parents who fervently wish for the health care team to "not take away my child's hope." It is at this point that it is helpful to talk about hope, not for cure, but for healing and wholeness, a time for making memories and having closure. For many families this is a concept only realized after the physical death. For the death of a child is recognized as "the worst loss," and it is usually after death that families can talk about the specialness, the healing, and the lives touched and changed.

And how do these children understand death? They understand it from a developmental, emotional, cognitive, and spiritual viewpoint. Age is often how the understanding is delineated, but this only serves as a guideline. For infants, death means separation. They cannot tell time, but they can sense and feel the difference in caregivers and pick up cues from them. For toddlers and preschoolers, death may be seen as temporary and reversible. Magical thinking is paramount, and death is not permanent for them. They may also have fears about death, such as dying in their sleep or that they may have caused another person's death. They begin to learn about death from their parents, church, and the media. School-aged children begin to have a sense of time and permanence. They are curious about aspects of death and believe it to happen mostly to old people. Somewhere between the ages of 7 and 10 years there is

concrete understanding of death. This is the point at which the child can understand the concepts that everyone dies (universality), that it is permanent (irreversibility), that the body does not work (non-functionality), and that there are many ways and reasons that people die (causality) (Faulkner, 1993). It is known that children who have been sick for a long time and know other children who die may come to understand death for others and themselves in a different timeline. Bluebond-Langner (1978) proposed the model in which children move from being diagnosed with cancer but considering themselves to be well to having a disease with remissions and relapses and therefore dying.

Many children tell us by their actions that they know they are dying even if they, or their parents, have not been able to talk about it. For example, a 9-year-old boy who was thrilled to have his own art show for community and hospital friends several months later insisted on giving presents to his family on Christmas Eve and then died on Christmas Day. Some families seek guidance about how to talk with their child about death, and many others choose to never speak directly about death. It is important for the health care team to honor a family's style of communication and coping and yet bring realistic possibilities to them. Knowing that after the death, most families are comforted by having had direct communication with the child, the nurse might suggest ways to talk to the child. One child was able to pick songs she wanted at her funeral mass, while another was able to give away special belongings to special friends. Above all it is important to be honest with the child in answering questions, remembering that what is most important is the sincerity and caring that is conveyed, not the words.

Foley and Whitam (1990) have several helpful suggestions for the health care team when facing this situation:

Know yourself: your own beliefs, opinions, and loss history.
Validate personal opinions with research and literature.
Strengthen the role of family members so that they can speak openly with the child.
Remember the importance of nonverbal communication and symbolic language.
Use a variety of means to communicate. Children may prefer imaginary play or to express themselves by drawing.

Think about words. Use simple words like "dying" and "death" rather than euphemisms.

Be aware of the needs of all of the children involved with the dying child, particularly siblings.

When the child is in the palliative phase there comes a time when death seems to be more imminent. The health care team in the hospital, clinic, and home can work smoothly like a revolving door so that the child and family move from one to another to gain resources and strengths. The physical and emotional needs may be met in any one of these places at different times. With the ever-increasing benefits realized in children dying at home, the home care nurse can be the provider, advocate, organizer, and facilitator.

Hospice Services

An increasingly accepted concept is that of hospice care for children. While fairly well established for adults, it has been slow to gain popularity for children. Some families have equated accepting hospice care as "giving up" rather than as holistic care aimed at improving the quality of life for the child and family in the palliative phase. Furthermore, the child with cancer and the family often have an extended care team with whom they have developed a close relationship and may dread meeting "more new caregivers." The home care nurse may be the bridge or the linkage between the family, hospice, and the hospital or clinic team. The key is for the family to feel prepared for what might occur (Martinson & Moldow, 1991; Pazola & Pugsley, 1992); to feel that there is excellent communication between the team members; to have 24-hour availability and support; and to have the choice to die at home or in the hospital. James and Johnson (1997) summarized the needs of parents: to have the child recognized as special while still preserving normality, to feel cared for and connected to the health care professionals, and to retain responsibility of parenting their dying child.

The hospice staff can also help families think about and plan for the funeral. They can reinforce that planning ahead does not hasten the death; and if the child is included, the family members may be comforted in knowing that they are doing what the child wished. They may also think about the siblings and how to best meet their individual needs.

The physical needs of the dying child encompass many aspects, but for most children adequate pain control is the most important. This may range from a pharmacologic approach including simple narcotic elixirs to megadoses of medications delivered intravenously. It also includes non-pharmacologic interventions, including distraction, massage, relaxation techniques, positioning, and being present. Even with all the "best" therapies available there is the realization that a painless death may not be possible, whether at home or in the hospital. The home care nurse must know the resources available to help the child or adolescent and family manage pain effectively. Pain management often brings side effects such as constipation, pruritus, nausea, and vomiting; and these should be dealt with prophylactically. Other physical signs may include fever, dehydration, dyspnea, seizures, bleeding, anorexia, and restlessness. These may be cared for by controlling versus treating, and again the nurse must take cues from the family and child as to "how much" to do. For some, giving acetaminophen (Tylenol) for the fever is sufficient; others will argue for instituting antibiotics. Hopefully during discussions with the family, preliminary decisions have been made that make this easier. With many families it is possible to institute Do Not Resuscitate (DNR) orders that can delineate interventions, whether in the hospital or home. This painful but necessary discussion can allow families, and sometimes the child, to choose which medical interventions they want or do not want. Most importantly, the family and child must know that a DNR order does not mean "caring" and involvement will cease. The focus becomes caring, comfort, and healing, which will continue.

During this time it is also important to address the emotional needs of the child. Most children want very much to go on living until they die, and many children want to attend school even if it is only a few hours a day. This is their work, it is distraction, it lets them be "normal." Most want their friends and family around. Adolescents particularly need their peer group to be present. They need the opportunity to experience control over what they want to still accomplish, what wishes they want to fulfill, and how they might die (Pazola & Gerberg, 1990). Younger children may be helped to express their feelings and wishes through art or play. Stories, such as *Lifetimes* by B. Mellonie & R. Ingpen or *Badger's Parting Gifts* by S. Varley, which speak about life and death as something that happens to everyone, may help bring the opportunity for questions and answers.

After the child's death, another transition occurs for the family that the home care nurse can facilitate. Much of their time has been focused on the child with cancer, treatments, and physical care. Now the family must integrate back into the community. Letting family members know what to expect of themselves, where to find the resources, and that the health care team continues to care about them is important. Many hospital oncology units, hospices, and churches have bereavement programs and outreach such as sending printed materials and support groups. The home care nurse may be able to direct parents and siblings to supportive activities, groups, and professionals. Each family member is forever changed and may need individualized support for years to come. The nurse can help the family move toward growth and healing from the beginning.

SUMMARY

Rehabilitative oncology nursing offers a wide range of experience and opportunities for the inpatient, clinic, school, and home care nurse. At any given point the child with cancer may have several nurses on the health care team, each with a special focus and background. The treatments and management of a cancer diagnosis offer a wide range of technologic opportunities as well as intense psychosocial interactions with the child and family. Changes and advances in treatment have made cancer a chronic illness with each stage requiring a special focus and skills. Throughout the illness continuum the focus is on rehabilitation promoting strategies, which will allow the individual to reach his or her maximum potential and level of functioning despite the stage, phase, or age of the child. Throughout the experience, nurses become the united thread that assists the child and family in negotiating the health care environment as well as the rehabilitative course of the disease and treatment process.

REFERENCES

Abramovitz, L. (1991). Perspectives on pediatric bone marrow transplantation. In M. Whedon (Ed.). *Bone marrow transplantation principles, practice, and nursing insights*, pp. 70–104. Boston: Jones & Bartlett.

American Cancer Society 1996 Advisory Committee on Diet, Nutrition and Cancer Prevention. (1996). Guidelines on diet, nutrition and cancer prevention: Reducing the risk of cancer with healthy food choices and physical activity. *CA—A Cancer Journal for Clinicians*, 40(16), 325–341.

Association of Rehabilitation Nurses. (1994). *Standards and scope of rehabilitation nursing practice*. Skokie, IL: Association of Rehabilitation Nurses.

Barr, L., Cowan, R., & Nicolson, M. (1997). *Churchill's pocketbook of oncology*. New York: Churchill Livingstone.

Baysinger, M., Heiney, S., Creed, J., & Ettinger, R. (1993). A trajectory approach for education of the child/adolescent with cancer. *Journal of Pediatric Oncology Nursing*, 10(4), 133–138.

Bleyer, W. (1990). The impact of childhood cancer on the United States and the world. *CA—A Cancer Journal for Clinicians*, 40(6), 355–357.

Bluebond-Langer, M. (1978). *The private worlds of dying children*. Princeton, NJ: Princeton University Press.

Butler, R., Hill, J., Steinherz, P., Meyers, P., & Finlay, J. (1994). Neuropsychologic effects of cranial irradiation, intrathecal methotrexate, and systemic methotrexate in childhood cancer. *Journal of Clinical Oncology*, 12(12), 2621–2628.

Carter, M., Thompson, E., & Simone, J. (1991). The survivors of childhood solid tumors. *Pediatric Clinics of North America*, 38(2), 505–526.

Caudell, K. (1991). Graft-versus-host disease. In M. Whedon (Ed.). *Bone marrow transplantation principles, practice and nursing insights*, pp. 160–181. Boston: Jones & Bartlett.

Chesler, M., Heiney, S., Perrin, R., Monaco, G., Kupst, M., Cincotta, N., et al. (1993). Principles of psychosocial programming for children and cancer. *Cancer Supplement*, 71(10), 3210–3212.

Cohen, D. (1993). Acute lymphocytic leukemia. In G. Foley, D. Fochtman, & K. Mooney (Eds.). *Nursing care of the child with cancer* (2nd ed.), pp. 208–225. Philadelphia: WB Saunders.

DeLatt, C., & Lampkin, B. (1992). Long-term survivors of childhood cancer: evaluation and identification of sequelae of treatment. *CA—A Cancer Journal for Clinicians*, 42(5), 263–282

Eisenberg, D., Kessler, R., Foster, C., Norlock, F., Calkins, D., & Delbanco, Y. (1993). Unconventional medicine in the United States. *New England Journal of Medicine*, 328(4), 246–282.

Faulkner, K. (1993). Children's understanding of death. In A. Armstrong-Dailey & S. Goltzer (Eds.). *Hospice care for children*, pp. 9–21. New York: Oxford University Press.

Foley, G., & Whitam, E. (1990). Care of the child dying of cancer: I. *CA—A Cancer Journal for Clinicians*, 40(6), 327–354.

Frierdich, S. (1990). Impairment of the hematopoietic system. In P. McCoy & W. Votroubek (Eds.). *Pediatric home care*, pp. 190–254. Gaithersburg, MD: Aspen Publishers.

Gerber. L., & Binder, H. (1993). Rehabilitation of

the child with cancer. In P. Pizzo & D. Poplack (Eds.). *Principles and practice of pediatric oncology* (2nd ed.), pp. 1079–1090. Philadelphia: JB Lippincott.

Groenwald, S., Frogge, M., Goodman, M., & Yarbro, C. (1993). *Cancer nursing: principles and practice* (3rd ed.). Boston: Jones & Bartlett.

Halperin, E., Constine, L., Tarbell, N., & Kun, L. (1994). *Pediatric radiation oncology*. New York: Raven Press.

Hobbie, W., Ruccione, K., Moore, I., & Truesdell, S. (1993). Late effects in long-term survivors. In G. Foley, D. Fochtman, & K. Mooney (Eds.). *Nursing care of the child with cancer* (2nd ed.), pp. 466–496. Philadelphia: WB Saunders.

Hockenberry-Eaton, M., Dilorio, C., & Kemp, V. (1995). The relationship of illness longevity and relapse with self-perception, cancer stressors, anxiety and coping strategies in children with cancer. *Journal of Pediatric Oncology Nursing*, 12(2), 71–79.

Hydzik, C. (1990). Late effects of chemotherapy, implications for patient management and rehabilitation. *Oncology Clinics of North America*, 25(2), 423–444.

James, L., & Johnson, B. (1997). The needs of parents of pediatric oncology patients during the palliative care phase. *Journal of Pediatric Oncology Nursing*, 14(2), 83–95.

Katz, E., & Varni, J. (1993). Social support and social cognitive problem-solving in children with newly diagnosed cancer. *Cancer Supplement*, 71(10), 3314–3319.

Knobf, T., & Durivage, H. (1993). Chemotherapy: principles of therapy. In S. Groenwald, M. Frogge, M. Goodman, & C. Yarbro (Eds.). *Cancer nursing principles and practice* (3rd ed.), pp. 270–292. Boston: Jones & Bartlett.

Lew, C., & Lavally, B. (1995). The role of stereotactic radiation therapy in the management of children with brain tumors. *Journal of Pediatric Oncology Nursing*, 12(4), 212–222.

Lozowski, S. (1993). Views of childhood cancer survivors. *Cancer Supplement*, 71(10), 3354–3358.

Margolin, J., & Poplack, D. (1997). Acute lymphoblastic leukemia. In P. Pizzo, & D. Poplack (Eds.). *Principles and practice of pediatric oncology* (3rd ed.), pp. 409–462. Philadelphia: JB Lippincott.

Martinson, I., & Moldon, D. (1991). *Home care for seriously ill children: a manual for parents*. Alexandria, VA: Children's Hospice International.

Meadows, A., & D'Angio, G. (1982). Incidence of second malignant neoplasms in children: results of an international study. *Lancet*, 2(8311), 1326–1330.

Mooney, K. (1993). Biologic basis of childhood cancer. In G. Foley, D. Fochtman, & K. Mooney (Eds.). *Nursing care of the child with cancer* (2nd ed.), pp. 25–55. Philadelphia: WB Saunders.

Moore, I. (1995). Central nervous system toxicity of cancer therapy in children. *Journal of Pediatric Oncology Nursing*, 12(4), 203–210.

O'Connor, L., & Blesch, K. (1992). Life cycle issues affecting cancer rehabilitation. *Seminars in Oncology Nursing*, 8(3), 174–185.

Ott, M. (1996). Imagine the possibilities! Guided imagery with toddlers and pre-schoolers. *Pediatric Nursing*, 22(1), 34–38.

Otto, S. (1994). *Oncology nursing* (2nd ed.). St. Louis: CV Mosby.

Panzarella, C., & Duncan, J. (1993). Nursing management of physical care needs. In G. Foley, D. Fochtman, & K. Mooney (Eds.). *Nursing care of the child with cancer* (2nd ed.), pp. 335–352. Philadelphia: WB Saunders.

Parker, S., Tang, T., Bolden, S., & Wingo, P. (1997). Cancer statistics, 1997. *CA—A Cancer Journal for Clinicians*, 47(5), 5–27.

Pazola, K., & Gerberg, A. (1990). Privileged communication—talking with a dying adolescent. *MCN: American Journal of Maternal Child Nursing*, 15(1), 16–21.

Pazola, K., & Pugsley, S. (1992). *The journey homeward*. Boston: Pediatric Nursing Service, Massachusetts General Hospital, Friends of the MGH Cancer Center.

Petriccione, M. (1993). Central nervous system tumors. In G. Foley, D. Fochtman, & K. Mooney (Eds.). *Nursing care of the child with cancer* (2nd ed.), pp. 239–253. Philadelphia: WB Saunders.

Potter, P., & Perry, A. (1995). *Basic nursing theory and practice* (3rd ed.). St. Louis: CV Mosby.

Robinson, L. (1993). Issues in the consideration of intervention strategies in long-term survivors of childhood cancer. *Cancer Supplement*, 71(10), 3406–3410.

Selekman, J. (1991). Pediatric rehabilitation from concepts to practice. *Pediatric Nursing*, 17(1), 11–13.

Shiminski-Maher, T., & Shields, M. (1995). Pediatric brain tumors: diagnosis and management. *Journal of Pediatric Oncology Nursing*, 12(4), 188–198.

Waber, D., Uron, D., Tarbell, N., Niemeyer, C., Gelber, R., & Sallan, S. (1990). Late effects of central nervous system treatment of acute lymphoblastic leukemia in childhood are sex-dependent. *Developmental Medicine and Child Neurology*, 32(3), 238–248.

Wagner, J., Yeager, A., & Beschorner, W. (1990). Pathology of bone marrow transplantation. In F.L. Johnson & C. Pochedly (Eds.). *Bone marrow transplantation in children*. New York: Raven Press

Walker, C., Wells, L., Heiney, S., Hymovich, D., & Weekes, D. (1993). Nursing management of psychosocial care needs. In G. Foley, D. Fochtman, & K. Mooney (Eds.). *Nursing care of the child with cancer* (2nd ed.), pp. 397–434. Philadelphia: WB Saunders.

Wells, R. (1990). Rehabilitation: making the most of time. *Oncology Nursing Forum*, 17(4), 503–507.

Whedon, M. (1991). *Bone marrow transplantation principles, practice and nursing insights*. Boston: Jones & Bartlett.

Wong, D. (1995). *Whaley & Wong's nursing care of infants and children* (5th ed.). St. Louis: CV Mosby.

Yabro, J. (1993). Milestones in our understanding of the causes of cancer. In S. Groenwald, M. Frogge, M. Goodman, & C. Yarbro (Eds.). *Cancer nursing principles and practice* (3rd ed.), pp. 28–46. Boston: Jones & Bartlett.

Zeltzer, L. (1993). Cancer in adolescents and young adults: psychosocial aspects. *Cancer Supplement,* 71(10), 3463–3468.

ADDITIONAL RESOURCES

Cunningham, M. (1997). Giving life to numbers. *CA—A Cancer Journal for Clinicians,* 47(1), 3–4.

Fochtman, D. (1993). The terminally ill child or adolescent. In G. Foley, D. Fochtman, & K. Mooney (Eds.). *Nursing care of the child with cancer* (2nd ed.), pp. 450–465. Philadelphia: WB Saunders.

Gibbons, M. (1993). Psychosocial aspects of serious illness in childhood and adolescence. In A. Armstrong-Dailey & S. Goltzer (Eds.). *Hospice care for children,* pp. 60–74. New York: Oxford University Press.

Hoeman, S. (1996). *Rehabilitation nursing process and application* (2nd ed.). St. Louis: CV Mosby.

McCoy, P., & Votroubek, W. (Eds.). (1990). *Pediatric home care: a comprehensive approach.* Rockville, MD: Aspen Publishers.

Thompson, J. (Ed.). (1990). *The child with cancer—nursing care.* London: Scotari Press.

RESOURCES

American Cancer Society
1599 Clifton Road, N.E.
Atlanta, GA 30329
404-320-3333

Association for Brain Tumor Research
2910 West Montrose Avenue
Chicago, IL 60618
312-286-5571

Association of Pediatric Oncology Nurses (APON)
11512 Allecingie Parkway
Richmond, VA 23235
804-379-9150

Cancer Information Service
454 Brookline Avenue
Boston, MA 02115
800-422-6239

The Candlelighters Childhood Cancer Foundation
1313 18th Street, N.W., Suite 200
Washington, DC 20036
202-659-5136
800-366-2223

Children's Hospice International
330 North Washington Street, Suite 3
Alexandria, Va. 22314
703-684-0330

Compassionate Friends
P. O. Box 3696
Oak Brook, IL 60522
312-990-0010

Leukemia Society of America
800 Second Avenue
New York, NY 10017
212-573-8484

National Cancer Institute
Cancer Information Clearinghouse
Office of Cancer Communications
Building 31, Room 10A18
9000 Rockville Pike
Bethesda, MD 20892
800-638-6694

National Rehabilitation Information Center
8455 Colesville Road, Suite 935
Silver Springs, MD 20917
800-346-2742 or 301-588-9284

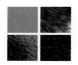

Chapter 21

Pediatric Burn Rehabilitation

Cynthia H. Himes and *Kathleen Ryan Kuntz*

■

Rehabilitation of the child with burns requires physical, emotional, and psycho-social interventions to achieve reintegration into a normal environment. The goal of nursing care is to assist the child with things he or she cannot do independently, enabling the child to regain skills and return to optimal functional ability. This goal can be reached only through close collaboration of the interdisciplinary team to provide consistency in an approach to care. Nurses must understand the importance of all aspects of the child's physical care and therapeutic regimen. An important goal in planning nursing care is to be able to perform interventions within the child's daily activities; this potentiates the therapeutic effect of the occupational and physical therapeutic services received. The nurse must also be aware of the emotional component of care with regard to both the child and the caregiver. It is important for the nurse to identify his or her ability to deal with the need to perform procedures that are painful to the child.

INCIDENCE

Injury by burn is a frequent occurrence in the pediatric population. Most children sustaining a burn injury are younger than 5 years of age. Eighty-five percent of burn injuries in this population are the result of scalds from hot tap water or liquid spilled from cooking pots (Schweich, 1994). Burns occurring in adolescents are more commonly the result of gasoline or other flammable liquids. Adolescents are also at risk for burns, as well as mutilation and loss of eyesight, from igniting

fireworks. In the United States, the number of childhood deaths from burn injuries is estimated to be approximately 1400 each year (Tarnowski, 1994). Most burn-related deaths are the result of house fires, and the usual cause is smoke inhalation. As many as 25% of burns in children are the result of some type of abuse; in some cases, the infliction of burns may be used as a method of discipline.

CAUSES AND PREVENTION

There are four primary causes of burns: thermal, electrical, chemical, and irradiation. Thermal burns refer to those caused by agents such as steam, boiling water, flame, hot water bottles, heated metals, or hot grease. Chemical burns are the result of exposure to acids, caustic soda, strong alkalies, phosphorus, or similar chemical agents. Electrical burns are related to exposure to electrical voltage entering the body and resulting in disturbances in respiratory, circulatory, and central nervous system function. Irradiation refers to burns caused by ultraviolet rays, x-rays, and radium. Burns from exposure to x-rays and radium may take a prolonged period of time to develop.

In burn injuries, as with other accidents, the best way to decrease morbidity and mortality is through preventative efforts. Death and injury resulting from house fires can be greatly reduced by educating children and adults, increasing adult supervision of children, and increasing the use of smoke detectors and sprinkler systems.

Parents, teachers, and other caregivers

should regularly develop and review scenarios depicting the plan of action in the event of a house fire. Children should know how to evacuate the home or other building and have alternate escape routes to follow. Fire-fighting decals should be placed on each child's bedroom window to alert the fire department that children may be trapped inside. Safety programs are carried out in pre-school settings through stories, fire drills, and instruction regarding what to do if clothes catch fire (i.e., "Stop, Drop, Roll"). In elementary schools, the fire department provides presentations, literature, and teaching materials to support education of students in the classroom and children in the community.

Burns can easily be caused by exposure to hot water. Table 21–1 illustrates the effects according to the time exposed as well as the temperature of the water.

The maximum temperature setting of the hot water heater should be no higher than 49°C (120°F), when small children are in the home. This helps to reduce the number of accidental scald burns, a leading cause of injuries in young children. When cooking, pots and utensils should have the handles turned inward so that the child cannot see or reach them. Handles extending over the edge of the stovetop may invite the child to reach up and pull on them.

Flammable and caustic substances should be locked safely away from the reach of children. A child who has demonstrated fire-setting tendencies should receive counseling and intervention from someone trained in this area who can help both the child and the family.

Table 21–1 SCALD BURNS IN CHILDREN: TIME OF EXPOSURE VERSUS TEMPERATURE TO CAUSE SERIOUS BURNS

Water Temperature	Time (seconds)
49°C (120°F)	>300
52°C (125°F)	>120
54.5°C (130°F)	30
57°C (135°F)	10
60°C (140°F)	5
63°C (145°F)	3
66°C (150°F)	1.5
68.5°C (155°F)	1.0

Adapted from Fratianne, R.B., & Brandt, C.P. (1994). Medical management. In K.J. Tarnowski (Ed.). *Behavioral aspects of pediatric burns,* p. 33. Plenum Press. New York: Reprinted with permission.

Electrical injuries in the home can be prevented by covering outlets with plastic protectors and not using appliances with worn or frayed cords. Electrical appliances with detachable cords can also pose a risk if the cord is left in the outlet. A curious toddler may pick up the unattached end and put it in their mouth, causing a serious electrical burn.

The ultraviolet rays of the sun can be dangerous to children, especially those who are very young. Precautions should be taken to avoid long periods of exposure to the sun. Light-colored clothing covering exposed skin surfaces, hats, and sunscreen with a minimum sun protection factor (SPF) of 15 are essentials to protect skin from the sun's damaging rays.

SEVERITY

The skin is the largest organ of the body. Its primary purposes are to protect and contain the internal organs and to regulate the body's temperature. There are three layers of skin. The epidermis is the outermost layer, and through exposure to environmental elements it can become rough and dry. Dead tissue cells are shed at this level. The dermis is the second layer, and it contains sebaceous and sweat glands as well as the hair follicle. The third layer is the subcutaneous tissue. This layer holds fat stores and has an increased blood supply.

The extent of a burn is identified by the layers of skin that are affected. Burns can be identified by degree (i.e., first, second, or third), indicating the depth of the skin affected, or by the thickness of the burn affecting the area (i.e., superficial, partial-thickness, or full-thickness). Table 21–2 illustrates the severity of the burn by its depth and thickness, as well as by its appearance and sensation.

In addition to the depth of the burn, it is important to consider the amount of the body's surface that is affected. Figure 21–1 illustrates the "Rule of 9s," which is used to identify areas of the body that constitute a higher severity of injury. The extent of the burn is expressed in the percentage of total body surface area (TBSA). Burns covering greater than 30% TBSA are considered life threatening in children.

A comprehensive history is necessary to facilitate the correct course of treatment, including the identification of the causative agent and possible complications. For example, it is important to determine whether

Table 21–2   SEVERITY OF BURNS

Depth of Burn	Thickness	Appearance of Burn	Sensation	Example of Cause
First degree	Superficial epithelium	Erythema	Painful	Sunburn
Second degree	Partial thickness Destruction into, but not through, epidermis	Blisters Peeling epidermis Swelling White or red mottling Weeping, wet	Painful Hypersensitive to air, touch	Very deep sunburn Scalds
Third degree	Full-thickness destruction of skin into hypodermis Death to all skin appendages and subcutaneous tissue	Translucent Mottled white or tan Waxy Leathery Basically dry	Painless (initially)	Fire Prolonged exposure to hot liquid Electricity

there was inhalation if the child was in a closed area, whether the child had a fall, whether there was exposure to an explosive or caustic substance, and whether there is any evidence of child abuse.

Initial treatment for burns includes the removal of clothing in the burned area and assessment of the child's airway, breathing, and circulation. Smoke inhalation contributes to upper airway edema or swelling of the face and neck due to soft tissue edema; therefore, the child may need oxygen and other interventions to ensure a patent airway is maintained. Intravenous access is necessary for all inhalation injuries and when more than 10% to 15% of the TBSA is burned. Chemical burns require immediate irrigation with copious amounts of water.

PHYSIOLOGY OF A MAJOR BURN INJURIES AND INITIAL TREATMENT

Cardiovascular

The loss of extracellular fluid through the stratum corneum of the epidermis occurs when large areas of skin are burned. Additionally, the physiologic response to the burn injury results in an alteration of capillary endothelium and a shift of fluid from the vascular space into the extracellular space. This is called "capillary leak syndrome," and it permits loss of water, electrolytes, and albumin, which results in edema and hypoalbuminemia. Any child with burns greater than 15% TBSA requires fluid resuscitation via intravenous fluid replacement (Graves et al.,

1988). The goals of resuscitation are to maintain vital signs within the normal range for the child and urine output of 1 to 2 mL/kg/hour. Intravenous fluid replacement varies in composition and volume based on the weight of child and the TBSA burned. Crystalloid solutions such as lactated Ringer's or normal saline solution are the primary fluids administered. If more than 20% of the TBSA is burned, a colloid may be added to the rehydrating solution to reverse intravascular protein loss. This occurs most significantly 6 to 8 hours after the injury.

The intravascular fluid is the first to be depleted, followed next by interstitial fluid, and then by intracellular fluid. The intravascular loss, or fluid volume reduction, is accompanied by an increased hematocrit (volume of red blood cells compared with whole blood), blood cell agglutination, and stasis of circulation in smaller vessels. Without fluid substitution, hypovolemic shock can result.

Edema develops when the rate at which fluid is filtered from the microvessels is greater than the rate in which the lymphatic vessels can drain the fluid away (Dutcher & Johnson, 1994). Edema is one of the first sequelae considered by the pediatric burn rehabilitation team. After positioning and/or splinting the involved areas, caregivers must closely monitor for adequate blood flow. External pressure from positioning or splinting devices, as well as internal pressure from the increase in interstitial fluid, can cause occlusion of small vessels. Activity must be encouraged to maintain joint mobility and to promote circulation to the injured area or areas.

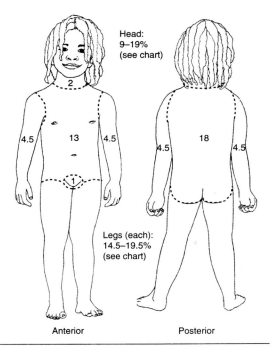

Head:
9–19%
(see chart)

4.5   13   4.5   4.5   18   4.5

Legs (each):
14.5–19.5%
(see chart)

Anterior   Posterior

Child Burn Size Estimation Table
(percent total body surface area)

Burn area	Age (years)				
	1	1–4	5–9	10–14	15
Head	19	17	13	11	9
Neck	2	2	2	2	2
Anterior trunk	13	13	13	13	13
Posterior trunk	18	18	18	18	18
Genitalia	1	1	1	1	1
Upper extremity (each)	9	9	9	9	9
Lower extremity (each)	14.5	15.5	17.5	18.5	19.5

Figure 21–1 Calculating total body surface area burned in children. The standard "rule of nines" and standard body surface charts must be adapted because of the difference in body proportions between adults and children. (From Ashwill, J. W., & Droske, S. C. [1997]. *Nursing Care of Children: Principles and Practice.* Philadelphia: WB Saunders, p. 1066.)

Pulmonary

Two types of airway obstruction can occur in the child with burns. When burns are in the area of the neck, chest, and upper abdomen, an extrinsic obstruction can occur from constriction as the damaged tissue becomes tight and forms a crust. Obstruction may also be caused by foreign material entering the nose, mouth, or throat. Another type of obstruction can occur when the child inhales superheated air, steam, gases, flames, or smoke while in an enclosed space, causing upper airway edema and an intrinsic airway obstruction. The severity of this type of obstruction can range from requiring humidified air and stim-

ulation of a productive cough to the need to establish an airway, administer oxygen, provide mechanical ventilation, and suction to remove secretions.

Good pulmonary hygiene is essential for patients with burns. Pneumonia is a frequent type of infection in these individuals. Adequate oxygenation is impaired by an increase in mucus in the lungs. Coughing, deep breathing exercises, and incentive spirometry should be used for the patient who is not intubated. If intubation is necessary, chest percussion and postural drainage and suctioning are indicated to avoid these complications.

Thermal Regulation

With large surface burns, thermal regulation of the body is compromised due to rapid heat loss. The thalamus automatically resets the internal temperature thermostat, causing a dramatic increase in metabolism—as much as 2.5 times normal. This metabolic increase results in increased cardiac output and oxygen usage, and additional stress is placed on the hepatic, renal, and pulmonary systems. This status continues until the burned areas are closed over. Once covered, the body seeks a level of homeostasis. The metabolic rate remains elevated for a period of time as the body uses protein and other nutrients to rebuild the damaged tissue.

Infection

As the damaged tissue begins to separate from viable tissue under the surface, further complications can occur. The open, moist areas resulting from burns are an excellent culture medium for bacteria that reside on the surface of the skin, hair follicles, and sebaceous glands. Prompt debridement and early grafting must be instituted so the wounds will close quickly and decrease the opportunity for infection.

When grafting is necessary, it is preferred to use an autograft, which is the patient's own skin from another site. When this is not possible, temporary grafts obtained from cadaver skin through a graft bank can be used (i.e., homograft or allograft). It is also possible to use pig skin (i.e., heterograft or xenograft). These temporary grafts are used until an autograft can be performed.

The burn site is initially covered by damaged, necrotic tissue (i.e., eschar), which forms a crust across the wound. This crust has no blood supply and does not help the body fight infection. Methods used to combat the severe complication of infection include exposure, occlusive dressings, leaving the wounds open and using a topical agent, and excision.

The exposure method controls bacteria by exposing the area to light and maintaining a cool environment. This is most commonly used with burns to the face, neck, perineum, and trunk. Over 2 to 3 days, the wound dries and forms a hard crust that can protect the underlying skin.

The occlusive dressing method is typically used with burns to the feet and hands. A fine gauze impregnated with an antimicrobial agent is applied to the wound and maintained with a tubular mesh over-dressing. This over-dressing applies light pressure to the area, and circulation to the extremity should be frequently monitored. Debridement is achieved with the dressing changes, thereby promoting healing.

The most frequently used method of treatment is the open method with a topical agent. An antimicrobial agent is applied to the area while leaving the skin open to air or with only a light covering. This method provides two advantages: caregivers can more easily monitor the progress of the wound, and physical therapy can be initiated earlier in the recovery phase.

In the excisional method of treatment, all damaged tissue is surgically removed to the level of viable tissue. This method reduces the risk of infection and promotes quicker healing of the underlying tissue.

Nutrition

The increased metabolic needs of the child with burns in conjunction with associated immunosuppression increases the risk for complications in wound healing. Increased losses of intracellular nutrients such as nitrogen, potassium, and phosphorus indicate a state of catabolism, or breakdown of compounds in the body. The breakdown of muscle compounds, particularly protein, leads to atrophy and loss of body weight. The nitrogen metabolized from these amino acids brings the body into a negative nitrogen balance.

The increased rate of glucose production and utilization and the decreased rate of lipid metabolism can affect the immune system. Up to 2 to 3 times the normal caloric requirement, particularly in the form of protein, is necessary to achieve a positive nitrogen bal-

ance. The larger the area of the burn, the greater the body's caloric need. Other factors that influence the individual needs of the patient include pre-injury nutritional status, age, gender, weight, and height. Methods for achieving nutritional requirements may include oral supplements, tube feedings, intravenous supplements, or total parenteral nutrition (TPN).

It has been noted in cases of trauma, including burns, that gastric dilatation and paralytic ileus occurs in response to shock, pain, or fear. In the past, these patients were not given oral nutrition for the first 72 hours, or until bowel sounds were detected, at which point it was felt safe to progress the diet. Waymack and Herndon (1992) have more recently identified that the ileus is limited to the stomach and colon, and the small intestine continues to function normally. Therefore, a continuous enteral feeding delivered to the small bowel assists in maintaining the patient's nutritional needs. Enteral feedings are preferred to TPN, which has been shown to result in atrophy of intestinal mucosa, increases in serum insulin, and decreases in fat metabolism. Elevations in insulin contribute to the increased use of protein for energy and therefore further the risk of protein catabolism.

SECONDARY PROCESSES AND THEIR IMPACT ON FUNCTIONAL OUTCOME

Escharotomy

An escharotomy, or surgical incision into the dermal fascia, is performed on the chest or the limbs if there is a restriction causing a decrease in chest movement or arterial circulation resulting from edema beneath the burn tissue. The escharotomy allows the skin to separate freely and restores normal pulmonary and circulatory dynamics.

Contractures

The immobility experienced as a result of the child's discomfort contributes to the development of contractures. The result is a significant reduction in normal range of motion in a joint. This occurs if the joint is maintained in an immobile position for a prolonged period of time, resulting in a tightening and shortening of the tendons, muscles, and associated structures.

Loss of motion in any joint results in a

decrease in functional ability. Impairment to the joints in the toes, feet, ankles, knees, and hips imposes significant limitations in mobility and a decrease in independence. However, loss of motion in the fingers, hands, wrists, elbows, or shoulders, particularly on the dominant side, may have the greatest impact in terms of the individual's self-care and social and vocational abilities.

The most effective treatment for contractures is prevention. It is essential to initiate the rehabilitation process as early as possible. Aggressive therapy can facilitate increased motion and ability. Once fixed, they can be treated with specific surgical procedures determined by the severity and location of the contracture.

Hypertrophic Scars

Another threat to mobility and function is the development of hypertrophic scars. This type of scarring in burn patients results from an increased production of collagen fibers on the skin surface. The process begins with healing and reaches a peak in 2 to 4 months post-injury. In addition to their effect on motion, hypertrophic scars have a significant effect on cosmetic appearance. The location and degree of the scar can adversely affect the child's self-concept, sense of self-worth, and ability to develop interpersonal relationships.

A primary treatment of hypertrophic scarring is the use of compression garments. These garments are carefully measured and individually constructed. They are tight-fitting and apply an even pressure against the healing skin to reduce scar formation. Because these garments are worn over a long period of time, however, these too may result in problems with body image. When scar formation continues to develop to a significant degree, reconstructive plastic surgery should be considered.

Alteration in Sensation

Individuals with burns frequently lose sensation as a result of their injuries. Diminished or absent responses to sharp/dull, hot/cold, and light touch sensations appear to be related to the depth of the burn injury. Caution must be exercised to avoid further injury to these areas, where protective responses are decreased as a result of loss of sensation.

Another frequent complaint of individuals sustaining burns is an increased sensitivity to ambient or environmental temperatures. A cold environment, as opposed to a warm environment, is particularly uncomfortable for these persons

An additional complication that occurs with burns is pruritus, or itching, as the healing process continues. Although this may seem to be a minor concern, it should be considered a risk, because scratching could result in damage to the new, healing skin and an opportunity to introduce infection. Pruritus can be easily treated with oral systemic or topical agents.

Hypersensitivity of the skin may become a concern in the plan for scar management. The patient may not adhere to the wearing of pressure garments as a result of uncomfortable or even painful stimuli. Incorporating strategies to desensitize these areas early in the treatment regimen may be helpful.

Heterotopic Ossification

Heterotopic ossification (HO) is a condition in which new bone is formed in tissue that does not normally ossify (i.e., soft tissue surrounding a joint). HO is a complication associated with burns and other injuries such as spinal cord injury, head injury, cerebral vascular accident, and musculoskeletal trauma. In some instances, this abnormal deposition of bone resolves spontaneously. In many cases, however, the development of this bony matter limits the functional ability of the individual and requires surgical intervention.

The precise cause of HO remains unknown, although it is believed to be related to calcium metabolism and may be influenced by prolonged periods of immobility. The incidence of HO does not appear to be related to age, gender, race, cause of burn injury, or location of burn. It is, however, found more commonly in patients with more than 20% full-thickness burns and in those with wounds that remained ungrafted for an extended period (Dutcher & Johnson, 1994).

NURSING ASSESSMENT

History and Physical Assessment

The nursing assessment begins with a comprehensive health history, including information regarding the mechanism of the burn and any other contributing factors (i.e., suspected child abuse, history of risk-taking behavior). A complete physical assessment serves as the foundation for evaluating the child's response to the care provided. A body diagram should be used to document the location and appearance of the burns, grafted areas, and donor sites; marking measurements; and indicating the areas being dressed and splinted. An associated table can be used to provide a description of the site and precise measurements (Fig. 21–2). This documentation assists in evaluating the healing process.

A functional assessment can be performed to determine the degree of loss of function sustained and to provide an objective measure of the child's progress. Periodic evalua-

tion using this measure provides valuable information that can assist in directing the course of treatment. Although there are many functional measurement tools available for use with adults, fewer tools address the special needs of pediatric patients and their families. Rehabilitation teams may find it useful to adopt two or more tools, tailoring aspects of them to capture the needs of a specific patient population.

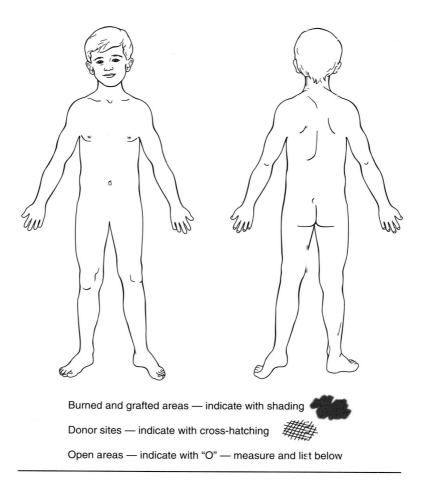

Burned and grafted areas — indicate with shading

Donor sites — indicate with cross-hatching

Open areas — indicate with "O" — measure and list below

Date	Description/Site	Measurement

Figure 21–2 Sample chart and table for recording burned, grafted, and open areas.

The Battelle Developmental Inventory (BDI, DLM Teaching Resources) is a test that can be administered to children from birth to 8 years of age. Although many of the motor and adaptive items are developmental in nature, there is a subset of items related to the functional assessment of a child with a disability.

The Vineland Adaptive Behavior Scale (VABS, American Guidance Service) assesses children and adolescents between birth and 19 years of age in their ability to perform necessary activities of daily living, covering areas including communication, daily living skills, and motor ability.

The Functional Independence Measure for Children (WeeFIM, Research Foundation, State University of New York) was developed for use with children aged 6 months to 7 years and older and modeled after the FIM used for adults. The WeeFIM captures measurements of levels of dependence or independence in the following areas: eating, grooming, bathing, dressing the upper body, dressing the lower body, toileting, bladder management, bowel management, transfers to chair or wheelchair, transfers to toilet, transfers to tub or shower, locomotion, stairs, comprehension, expression, social interaction, problem solving, and memory.

The Pediatric Evaluation of Disability Inventory (PEDI, Department of Rehabilitation Medicine, New England Medical Center Hospitals) provides a comprehensive clinical assessment of key functional capabilities and performance in children between the ages of 6 months and 7 years, but it can also be used for the evaluation of older children if their functional abilities fall below that expected of 7-year-old children without disabilities. The PEDI measures both capability and performance of functional activities in three content domains: self-care, mobility, and social function.

The Scale of Independent Behavior (SIB, DLM Teaching Resources) is part of the Woodcock-Johnson Psychoeducational Battery, which identifies functional skills needed at home and in social and community settings. The test is applicable for infant to adult levels but is best used for the child older than 6 years of age through adolescence. Content addresses four adaptive skill clusters: motor, social interaction and communication, personal living, and community living.

Family Assessment

A comprehensive assessment of the family structure, dynamics, and support systems is a critical aspect of caring for the child with burns. It is important to objectively consider the role of family members in the incident and the expectations that are held regarding the child's treatment and recovery. Planning should be done in collaboration with the parents or primary caregivers to ensure that the treatment regimen can be continued and that the child will have maximal independence in the home environment.

Knowledge and Skill Assessment

The child with burns and his or her family must develop knowledge and skill related to their own health status as well as the child's treatments, personal care, nutritional needs, the process of recovery and rehabilitation, and new ways to perform activities. Traumatic injuries frequently leave children and their families unable to accommodate and assimilate a great deal of information at one time. It is important to recognize the learning ability and capacity of each individual.

Nursing Diagnosis in the Rehabilitation Phase

Key nursing diagnoses can be identified in the care of the child with burns as related to the location and severity of burns, the developmental level of the child, and the support and environment of care provided by the family.

Alteration in Skin Integrity: A burn injury interrupts the integrity of the skin, and frequently structures beneath the skin as well. A primary focus of care is related to the care of wounds, the prevention of infection via the wound, the protection of developing and healing tissue, and the prevention of scars. The location of the burns, scars, or both may also impact on the functional ability of the child (i.e., should contractures develop).

Potential for Infection: The open area of the skin where the burn was sustained is a prime route of entry for infectious organisms. Meticulous precautions must be maintained when performing dressing changes, providing hydrotherapy, and applying topical agents. In addition, other sources of infection should not be overlooked. Respiratory infections are common in burn patients, primarily as a result of the insult to the mucosa from the inhalation of smoke, steam, or chemicals. Pulmonary hygiene is critical and entails assistive measures to facilitate the mobilization of secretions such as chest percussion and postural drainage, coughing and deep breathing exercises, incentive spirometry, and suctioning (if indicated). Immobility and alterations in metabolism may also contribute to the formation of urinary tract infections. It is important to maintain a positive nitrogen balance and maintain adequate hydration of cells. Urine output should be monitored closely.

Alteration in Comfort: Pain management is a primary concern when caring for the child with burns. Fear and anxiety may intensify the pain that the child experiences related to caretaking and dressing change activities. Every effort should be taken to promote pain relief and facilitate these procedures. Analgesics can be administered orally or intravenously. Topically, precautions can be implemented to protect healthy granulation tissue (e.g., soaking dressings before removal).

Alteration in Mobility: Positioning and splinting are essential components of care for the child with burns to promote healing, protect function, and prevent the complications of contractures. It is important to monitor skin integrity while implementing these techniques. Pressure garments may be used to prevent scar formation. Mobility is important to maintain adequate circulation to the affected areas for healing to take place.

Potential Alteration in Nutrition: Adequate nutrition is paramount to the healing of injured tissue and the maintenance of energy to preserve functional ability. Dietary management should provide up to 2 to 3 times the normal caloric requirement, particularly in the form of protein, to facilitate a positive nitrogen balance and prevent a catabolic effect.

Alteration in Body Image, Disturbance in Self-Concept, Alteration in Self-Esteem, and Alteration in Coping: The developmental level of the child strongly affects their perception of themselves. The location and severity of the burn also influences the child's body image. Peer and family relationships may change or be interrupted as a result of the injury and the extensive care required. It is important to address these areas with the child and the family, incorporating support services such as counseling whenever possible.

Alteration in Urinary Elimination, Alteration in Bowel Elimination, and Ineffective Airway Clearance: Physiologic functions may be interrupted as a result of the severity of burn injuries. Children may become incontinent of urine; constipation may result from immobility or pain medications; alternate means for elimination may be necessary related to the wounds (i.e., a colostomy or urinary catheterization); and the child may require intubation or aggressive respiratory treatment.

Knowledge Deficit: The burned child and his or her family members have a great deal to learn regarding health status, treatments, nutritional needs, and the process of recovery and rehabilitation. Traumatic injuries frequently leave children and families unable to accommodate and assimilate a great deal of information at one time. It is important to recognize the learning ability and capacity of each individual. Including the child and the family in the care as early as possible will enhance their ability to learn.

KEY AREAS OF PLANNING AND IMPLEMENTATION

Skin, Garments, and Dressings

A major risk of occlusive and semi-occlusive dressings is infection, which can develop insidiously beneath the dressing. For this reason, regular replacement is required if these dressings are used. Some antibiotic topical creams and ointments are effective for only 8 to 12 hours after application. The wound should be cleansed and antibiotic cream reapplied 2 to 3 times per day, depending on the stage of healing, to decrease the risk of infection. Topical agents are applied using a sterile glove, tongue blade, or cotton swab and are administered as thickly as the manufacturer recommends (generally just until you cannot see through the cream).

Open areas are usually covered with a generous amount of topical antibiotic cream and dressed with dry gauze followed by a conforming wrap gauze, elastic tubular dressing, or both. Non-adherent or petroleum gauze dressings may also be used to prevent the dressing from adhering to the wound.

Treatments with topical agents vary. Antibiotic ointments are used until the wounds are completely closed over. Moisturizers are used on a long-term basis to assist in maintaining flexibility of the tissue. Custom-made compression garments can be initiated after most open areas are healed. If a few small areas remain open, they can be covered by a dressing prior to donning the garments.

Daily bathing can be accomplished by soaking in a tub or whirlpool bath with a gentle cleansing agent in the water. Careful inspection of the skin after bathing is critical. A moisturizing cream is applied over all donor sites and scar tissue. Small open areas are dressed and garments worn with the seams on the outside. Much care must be given to ensuring that garments are wrinkle-free, especially in joint areas, because skin breakdown can occur rapidly due to the increased pressure and friction from fabric overlap.

The nursing plan of care must be extremely thorough and specific regarding dressings and garments to achieve 100% compliance of all caretakers. The body diagram should reflect the burned areas, grafts, and donor sites. Healing of open areas and any new open areas must be indicated and dated on this diagram.

A body diagram in the nursing plan of care ensures the correct application of elastic tubular dressings, compression garments, and splints. Elastic tubular dressings may be used in layers to add to the degree of pressure provided. The number of layers to be worn should be clearly indicated in the plan. It is also helpful to use a laundry marker to label the elastic tubular dressings (e.g., thigh, calf, wrist) to avoid excessive stretching as a result of incorrect application. The occupational therapist should also monitor these dressings and make recommendations regarding replacement when excessive stretching occurs. At least one extra set of elastic tubular dressing should be available; two or more sets should be available for infants and toddlers. These dressings should be washed daily in mild soap, rinsed, and hung to air dry. Compression garments are also cared for in this way. These dressings and garments should never be machine dried due to the deleterious effect of heat on elasticity. The duration of treatment with elastic tubular dressings or compression garments varies according to the severity of scar development. Generally, these items are worn continually throughout the day except during bathing, and are continued on a long-term basis as part of the treatment regimen until optimal healing is noted.

Mobility, Positioning, and Splints

Proper positioning of the child with burns is a challenge. Children do not routinely cooperate when they are instructed to maintain a position. A child's normal positioning may encourage the formation of contractures. The use of traction, restraints, and splints may be necessary to achieve optimal positioning in this population.

Gentle active or active-assistive range of motion should be initiated within the first 24 to 48 hours post-injury. Passive stretching and massage of healed burn tissue helps the tissue to lengthen and prevents contractures. If scar tissue can be kept flexible, normal growth will not be adversely affected, especially in the hands and feet. Developmentally and age-appropriate recreation and play activities can enhance the child's participation in active and active-assistive exercises. These activities can encourage active stretching and reaching (e.g., basketball and balloon play), increase strength and endurance (e.g., Simon says, riding a tricycle), and enhance fine motor coordination (e.g., puzzles, crafts).

Age-appropriate self-care activities such as feeding, bathing, dressing, toileting, and assisting with dressing changes should be encouraged as soon as the child is able to participate in them. Self-care activities can be used as a way to increase physical activity and assist the child in exerting control and independence over the situation.

Splints are used to maintain the essential functional position of an extremity. In an acute care setting, the medical status is the first priority. Splints may be fabricated for positioning, but modification may be necessary until the patient is medically stable and active rehabilitation can begin.

The splinting regimen is established by the occupational therapist for the upper extremity and the physical therapist for the lower extremity. With the exception of severe hand and foot burns, prophylactic positioning splints are not always necessary. When a patient is alert and cooperative, splinting may not be necessary except to preserve the integrity of the joint. Splinting is sometimes reserved for use while sleeping.

The most common types of splints used with burn patients are neck, axilla, elbow, wrist, hand, hip, knee, and ankle (Fig. 21–3). Correct application is important to maximize joint function and to ensure that the skin integrity beneath the splint is not compromised. Any change in the appearance of the skin or problems with splint application should be brought to the attention of the therapist. Resolution of the problem should be a collaborative effort.

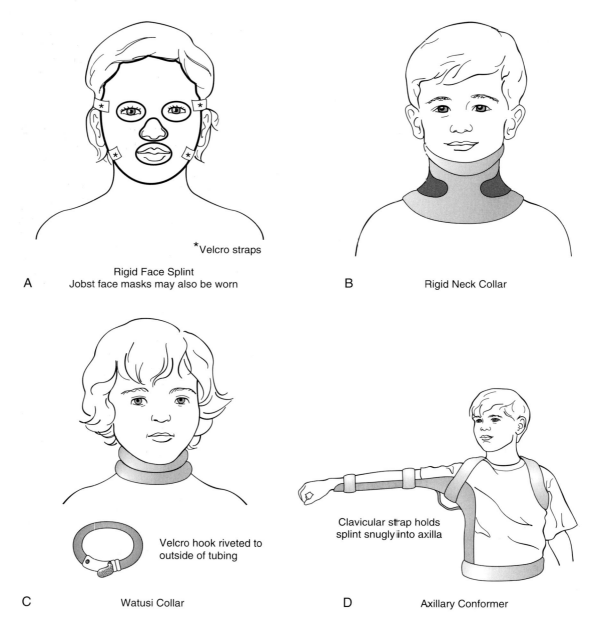

Figure 21–3 Rehabilitation devices for pediatric burn patients. *A*, Rigid face splint. *B*, Rigid neck collar. *C*, Watusi collar. *D*, Axillary conformer.

The nursing plan of care must contain clear, step-by-step instructions and diagrams regarding splint applications. All caregivers should be familiar with the child's splint and positioning regimen to maintain continuity of care. The child's level of tolerance of splints should be conveyed to the therapy team.

Splints can be washed with a mild soap and cool water. They should be kept with the dressings and garments in one place, preferably in a designated area in the child's room.

A large, covered, transparent storage box is ideal for holding dressings and splints. It is easy for small items to be lost, and retracing an active child's steps to recover a face mask or a thumb splint can prove frustrating and time consuming.

Cognitive and Sensory Management

If the child did not sustain brain injury related to a fall or hypoxia, his or her level of cognitive and sensory ability should remain the same as prior to the burn. The lengthy hospital stay may necessitate providing educational services while the child is an inpatient. School records and assignments can be obtained with the parents' permission.

Development

Developmental considerations should be integrated into every aspect of care provided by the rehabilitation team. The child's pre-existing cognitive and socio-emotional level serves as a guide in determining the approach to care. The child's separation from home, family, and familiar activities intensifies his or her feelings of fear and anxiety. Consideration of the child's perception of events and ability to cope should be integrated into each activity (i.e., dressing change, medication administration, therapy).

Behavior Management

Many pediatric rehabilitation nurses caring for children with burns consistently identify one behavior in the young child and adolescent alike: procrastination or avoidance is frequently exhibited when it is time for burn care to be performed. Certainly, no one is enthusiastic about having a painful procedure done, just as the caregiver is not eager to inflict pain on the child. Interventions to decrease anxiety and pain are very important. The nurse may have great difficulty enlisting the child's cooperation, turning a 30-minute dressing change into a 3-hour ordeal that distresses both the child and the nurse.

Before beginning any painful treatment, the child should receive analgesics. This may be in the form of a narcotic or over-the-counter pain medication, depending on the child's degree of healing and stage of rehabilitation. In addition, offering the child a drink and an opportunity to use the toilet eliminates these options as possible diversions for the child to use once the procedure has begun. Enlisting the child's assistance in removing garments and dressings is a way to provide the child with some degree of control over the situation while accomplishing the task at hand.

If dressings adhere to the skin, soaking them in warm, sterile saline solution will help loosen them as well as providing a comforting sensation to the skin. Having all supplies prepared and ready prior to beginning the procedure eliminates the need for unnecessary interruptions. Talking with the child about his or her interests or singing along with music playing are two diversions that may be helpful. Sometimes, the toddler or pre-school aged child may prefer to watch a favorite television show or videotape while the nurse provides burn care. Scheduling a brief, pleasurable activity after the dressing change and application of garments may provide some incentive to complete the treatment in a shorter period of time.

Psycho-social Support

The emotional and behavioral responses of a child become intensified following a traumatic injury. Separation from family and friends and a sense of loss of control over their own actions and the environment compound these responses. The child's sense of body image and self-concept are directly related to the location and severity of the injury as well as possible feelings of guilt and responsibility. Ever present is the problem of pain and the child's fear of pain. These concerns may be directly evident or may manifest themselves as aggressive behavior, depression, regression, withdrawal, or eating disturbances.

If the event in which the burn was sustained is in conjunction with other injuries or the death of a friend, parent, or other family member, psycho-social problems become intensified. It is important to access professional support for the child in dealing with these complex issues. The psycho-social care of the burned child is closely associated with the physical treatment, compounding the complexity of the total rehabilitation.

Family Support

The family and home environment is a critical component of the child's long-term psycho-social adjustment following a burn injury. Positive adjustment is evident when the child sees his or her family acting as a unit, with a commitment to the child and to each other. When families understand the steps to recovery and rehabilitation, they more readily encourage their children to resume their previous roles and activities. A supportive social network (i.e., family and friends) leads to better self-esteem following a burn injury, and the child is able to achieve a more positive adjustment and outcome. Unfortunately, many children who sustain burns live in unsupportive environments. Visits by family or friends may be infrequent or absent. This situation causes the child to feel helpless and hopeless and to have low self-esteem. When this occurs, there is a risk that the child will pursue a relationship with staff members to "substitute" for family members. Staff members should recognize this and be prepared to provide the necessary caring and support while supporting the familial relationships that exist, even though they may be tenuous. Efforts should also be put forth to try to involve family members in the care and support of the child as much as possible. This is necessary to ensure a successful transition back to the home environment.

Regardless of actual culpability, parents and other family members often express feelings of guilt about the burn incident. It is natural to want to have been able to prevent such a traumatic injury. This guilt is compounded by feelings of powerlessness and helplessness when the parents cannot eliminate their child's suffering and "make it better." The family may be further burdened by issues related to the financial aspects of care or possible personal loss. In addition, when a child is hospitalized, parents frequently lose time at work and the related income. Separation from other family members such as a spouse or other children places an additional stress on the parent.

The rehabilitation of a burn injury may progress slowly, and the outcome may be uncertain. Support is needed to assist the child and family to see the progress achieved and look forward to ongoing progress with patience. The nurse and other members of the interdisciplinary team, together with the child and the family, must support each other through this period.

The goals of the interdisciplinary team are to collaborate with the child's family in all aspects of the plan of care while promoting the child's independence and ability. This level of collaboration is the key to helping the child make a positive transition to home and return to school. At times the family may require interventions to promote appropriate interactions so that they can adequately support the burned child and manage his or her care.

Community, School, and Vocational Re-entry

Many factors affect the burned child's transition back into society and school. Some of these are the child's age, developmental level, ability to adjust, severity of disfigurement, family support, and peer acceptance. Interventions that include family members and classmates prior to the return to home and school allow a positive adjustment. A plan for school re-entry should be developed as early as possible and could include the following steps:

With parental permission, a member of the team collaborates with the child's school to develop a program that can be incorporated into the child's daily activities as their condition permits.

Parents or guardians are encouraged to actively participate as advocates for their child. This goal is achieved through consistent efforts to include parents in the planning for treatment, discharge, and school re-entry. It is necessary, however, to remain aware of the emotional demand that this places on the parents. The team should support the parents and encourage mutual communication with the school regarding their child's progress.

Plans should be individualized for each child and family. The interdisciplinary team should discuss which member will contact the school and what actions should be taken (e.g., discussion with the teachers, a presentation to the class). The developmental level of the child and class and the degree of injury will influence the plan.

Each child is approached with the expectation of returning to school after discharge. It should be consistently conveyed by each team member that the burn injury is only a temporary setback to what the child was involved in before. With time, and perhaps some adaptation, the child will be able to resume previous activities.

Continued availability of the team for consultation with the school is important. A liaison at the school to communicate any difficulties back to the team should be identified, and a means for therapists and educators to periodically discuss the child's progress and concerns should be developed.

Follow-Up Care

Long-term follow-up is necessary to ensure maximum function and minimal cosmetic defect over the growth periods that occur in children. Changes in treatment regimen and pressure garments may be indicated. Skin integrity and progress of scars should be evaluated carefully. Indications for reconstructive surgery should be monitored. Family members should be reminded to bring all appliances with them to each appointment so the devices can be evaluated and possibly adjusted. Monitoring of the child's motor and functional development should be conducted in an ongoing manner.

SUMMARY

Burn injuries in children are traumatic. Physically, children have immature systems that do not tolerate the insult well; psychologically, children have not attained the skills necessary to assist in understanding and coping with the treatment and outcome. Rehabilitation of a child with burns requires a cohesive team approach that involves the child and the family at every step. It is important to recognize the child's level of development and ability and evaluate the family's supportive network, both physically and emotionally, when providing care. The development of knowledge and skill of the child and family is integral in achieving a successful outcome.

REFERENCES

Dutcher, K., & Johnson, C. (1994). Neuromuscular and musculoskeletal complications. In R.L. Richard & M.J. Staley (Eds.). *Burn care and rehabilitation: principles and practice*, pp. 576–602. Philadelphia: FA Davis.

Fratianne, R.B., & Brandt, C.P. (1994). Medical management. In K.J. Tarnowski (Ed.). *Behavioral aspects of pediatric burns*, pp. 23–53. New York: Plenum.

Graves, T. A., Cioffi, W.G., McManus, W.E., Mason, A.D., & Pruitt, B.A. (1988). Resuscitation of infants and children with massive thermal injury. *Journal of Trauma, 28*, 1656–1659.

Lund, C.C., & Browder, N.C. (1944). The estimation of areas of burns. *Surgical Gynecology and Obstetrics, 79*, 352.

Schweich, P.J. (1994). Emergency medicine. In F.A. Oski (Ed.). *Principles and practice of pediatrics* (2nd ed.), pp. 808–832. Philadelphia: JB Lippincott.

Tarnowski, K. (1994). Overview. In K.J. Tarnowski (Ed.). *Behavioral aspects of pediatric burns*, p. 9. New York: Plenum.

Waymack, J., & Herndon, D. (1992). Nutritional support of the burned patient. *World Journal of Surgery, 16*, 80–86.

ADDITIONAL RESOURCES

Blakeney, P. (1994). School reintegration. In K.J. Tarnowski (Ed.). *Behavioral aspects of pediatric burns*, pp. 217–241. New York: Plenum.

Kaslow, N.J., Koon-Scott, K., & Dingle, A.D. (1994). Family considerations and interventions. In K.J. Tarnowski (Ed.). *Behavioral aspects of pediatric burns*, pp. 193–215. New York: Plenum.

Walters, C. (1987). *Splinting the burn patient.* Laurel, MD: RAMSCO.

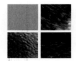

Chapter 22

Traumatic Injuries

Patricia A. Edwards

Traumatic injuries to the head and spinal cord continue to be a major cause of death and disability in the pediatric population. Advances in trauma care have increased the survival rate for children with these injuries, and although many children and adolescents who survive traumatic injuries have few or no long-term problems, those with significant deficits may require lifelong services. It is essential for the pediatric rehabilitation nurse to have an in-depth understanding of these two conditions and their varying degrees of severity to assess the needs of these children and adolescents and their families and plan for appropriate care and services. Spinal cord and traumatic brain injuries are discussed in this chapter, with an emphasis on the nursing process and functional outcomes.

SPINAL CORD INJURY

Spinal cord injury (SCI) is an acute traumatic lesion of the spinal cord and roots. When such injury occurs in children from newborns through 15 years of age it is referred to as pediatric SCI. Of the estimated new cases of SCI that occur in the United States annually, nearly 10% (300 to 500 per year) affect children aged 1 to 15 years. These injuries are caused by accidents (41.5%), sports (27%), violence (20.5%), falls (9%) and other causes (2%). Complete and incomplete paraplegia, or loss of function in the legs, accounts for 44% of these injuries, and tetraplegia (previously known as quadriplegia), or loss of function in the arms and legs, accounts for 56%. The most common time to sustain an SCI is adolescence

and early adulthood, and boys are more frequently injured than girls. Table 22–1 lists the demographic information associated with SCI. Although the incidence of SCI injuries to children is low, the severity of their injuries is consistently high. Nursing management is critical both for a successful transition to rehabilitation and return to home, school, and community and for maintaining function, preventing complications, and promoting adjustment during the rehabilitation phase and beyond (National Spinal Cord Injury Association [NSCIA], 1996; Southard & Massagli, 1994; Spoltore & O'Brien, 1995).

Pathophysiology

The amount and type of force at the time of the accident is a determining factor in the extent of injury to the spinal cord and the resultant damage. Those mechanisms of injury commonly seen are the hyperflexion and rotation occurring in a motor vehicle accident, which cause a fracture dislocation, and the longitudinal trauma after a fall, which results in a compression fracture. A knife wound or bullet may also cause damage to the spinal cord (Hanak, 1992).

The immediate effect of the trauma is disruption of neural transmission at and below the injured area of the spinal cord. This destructive process results in edema, bleeding, inflammation, and ischemia. Over the first hours following injury, these physiologic reactions induce secondary injury to the spinal cord and ultimately result in loss of function. Treatment during the first 48 to 72 hours post-

Table 22–1 SPINAL CORD INJURY DEMOGRAPHICS

Male more frequent than female
Pediatric—newborn to age 15 years
Causes: accidents (motor vehicle), violence, sports, falls
Types: complete and incomplete
Pediatric cases account for 10% of new cases in the United States (300–500 cases/year)
Most common age group: adolescent/young adult (15–25 years)
Results in paraplegia (44%) and tetraplegia (56%)

Data from National Spinal Cord Injury Association (NSCIA). (1996). *Fact sheet 14: resources for pediatric spinal cord injury.* Silver Spring, MD: NSCIA; Southard, T., & Massagli, T. (1994). Spinal cord injury. In S. Campbell (Ed.). *Physical therapy for children,* pp. 525–547. Philadelphia: WB Saunders; and Spoltore, T., & O'Brien, A. (1995). Rehabilitation of the spinal cord injured patient. *Orthopedic Nursing,* 14(3), 7–14.

injury is aimed at counteracting these effects and reducing the secondary damage. Alignment of the vertebrae following the injury is important to maintain blood flow. Surgery may be performed to remove pressure on the cord, and steroids may be administered to decrease inflammation (Southard & Massagli, 1994; National Institute of Neurological Disorders and Stroke [NINDS], 1996; UW Rehabilitation Medicine, 1995).

The location and severity of the injury determine the amount of motor and sensory function loss. The American Spinal Injury Association (ASIA) developed a standardized method of communicating functional classifications. The ASIA Impairment Scale is described in Table 22–2.

The ASIA Impairment Scale uses the findings from the neurologic examination to categorize the injury. These categories allow researchers to identify the outcomes of various types of injuries and degrees of spinal cord damage. Figure 22–1 provides specific evalua-

tion information on the motor and sensory areas. Additional information on the components of the examination can be found in *International Standards for Neurological and Functional Classification of Spinal Cord Injury, Revised* (1996) available from ASIA.

The term "tetraplegia" is currently preferred to "quadriplegia" and is used when the injury occurs in the cervical region (between C1 and T1) and results in paralysis of all four extremities. Function is impaired in the arms, trunk, pelvic area, and legs. Paraplegia, or paralysis of the lower extremities, results when the injury is in the thoracic, lumbar, or sacral region. Function is maintained in the arms, but involvement of other areas depends on the level of the injury. With either tetraplegia or paraplegia, other problems such as muscle deterioration, lack of bowel and bladder control, and the development of contracture deformities may result.

A standard measure of the impact of SCI on self-care activities that provides a functional assessment is the Functional Independence Measure (FIM) or its pediatric counterpart, the WeeFIM, described in Chapter 11. The WeeFIM is widely used as an initial evaluation tool and to measure progress in some of the areas affected by SCI: self-care, sphincter control, and mobility.

Systemic Effects and Related Complications

The pediatric rehabilitation nurse must be cognizant of the potential systemic effects and complications that occur in children and adolescents with spinal cord injuries. These include autonomic dysreflexia, heterotropic ossification, and spasticity; other complications are listed in Table 22–3.

Autonomic dysreflexia is a life-threatening complication characterized by hypertension, reflex bradycardia, and diaphoresis. It is usu-

Table 22–2 ASIA IMPAIRMENT SCALE

A = Complete	No motor or sensory function is preserved in the sacral segments S4–S5
B = Incomplete	Sensory but not motor function is preserved below the neurologic level and includes the sacral segments S4–S5
C = Incomplete	Motor function is preserved below the neurologic level, and more than half of key muscles below the neurologic level have a muscle grade <3
D = Incomplete	Motor function is preserved below the neurologic level, and at least half of key muscles below the neurologic level have a muscle grade ≥3
E = Normal	Motor and sensory function is normal

From American Spinal Injury Association (ASIA). (1996). International standards for neurological and functional classification of spinal cord injury. Atlanta: ASIA.

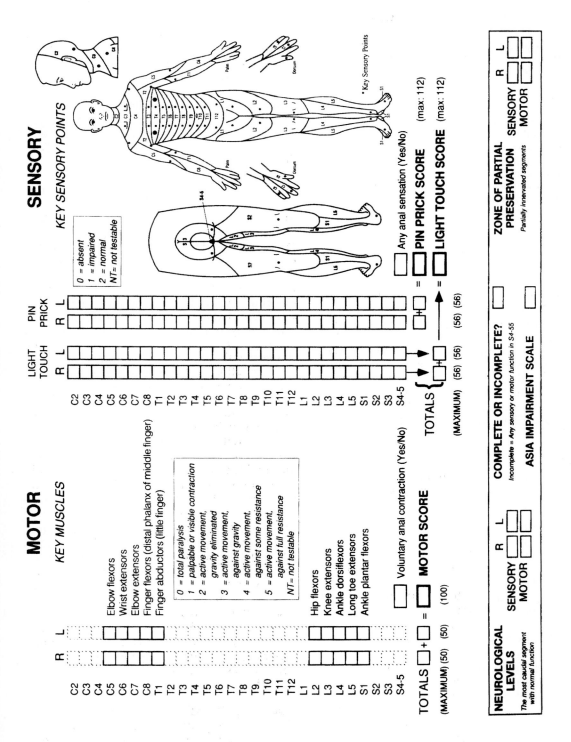

Figure 22-1 Standard neurological classification of spinal cord injury. (From the American Spinal Injury Association.)

Table 22-3 SPINAL CORD INJURY SYSTEMIC EFFECTS AND COMPLICATIONS

Skin breakdown
Heterotropic ossification
Postural hypotension
Chronic pain
Neurogenic bowel and bladder
Reduced pulmonary function
Hypercalcemia
Spine deformities
Temperature regulation
Venous stasis and edema of the lower extremities
Autonomic dysreflexia
Spasticity and contractures
Osteopenia
Sexual dysfunction

ally seen in individuals with an injury at T6 or higher and is the result of increased autonomic activity caused by a noxious stimulus, often a distended bladder or bowel. This leads to an uncontrolled rise in blood pressure and decrease in pulse. Signs and symptoms include hypertension with pounding headache, flushing and blotching of the skin, and cold sweating above the level of the injury. Immediate treatment measures include

---

Teaching Topic: Autonomic Dysreflexia Signs, Symptoms, and Treatment

Important Areas:

Place the child or adolescent in a sitting position.
Determine the precipitating stimulus and remove it.
　Unplug a catheter or catheterize to empty a distended bladder.
　Remove a fecal impaction.
　Remove skin stimuli (e.g., heat, cold, pressure, pain).
Administer medications (anti-hypertensive agents) if the stimulus cannot be removed.
Provide emotional support and measures to decrease anxiety.
Discuss signs and symptoms and prevention activities.
Demonstrate how to measure blood pressure and the meaning of the result.
Identify emergency referrals.

---

having the child or adolescent sit up to reduce blood pressure by postural means and removing the source of stimulation. Treatment with anti-hypertensive agents may be needed. Education of the child and family is essential and should include the signs and symptoms with specific interventions as outlined in Teaching Topic: Autonomic Dysreflexia Signs, Symptoms, and Treatment (Spoltore & O'Brien, 1995; Hanak, 1992; Tepperman, 1989).

Heterotropic ossification occurs when areas that do not normally produce bone, namely soft tissue, form new bone. Initial indications might be redness, swelling, warmth, and gradual loss of joint motion, or it may be asymptomatic. Heterotropic ossification commonly affects the hips, knees, elbows, and shoulders. Treatment is very important because this condition can have an impact on the child or adolescent's ability to perform activities of daily living. Heterotropic ossification may require increasing the frequency of range of motion exercises and position changes, splinting, a surgical intervention, or a combination of these measures (Spoltore & O'Brien, 1995; Tepperman, 1989).

Spasticity is a fairly common systemic problem among children and adolescents with SCI. It is a condition of excessive reflex activity, with involuntary movements and clonus and increased muscle tone. Often those with incomplete injuries and some voluntary movement have more significant problems because the reflex nerves below the level of injury develop new connections and the reflex response is strengthened. Spasms evolve over a period of time and have both positive and negative effects. Spasms offer some benefits, such as maintaining bone density and preventing pressure sores by increasing muscle mass. However, they often interfere with movement, for example, jumping extensor spasms that straighten the leg. When spasms begin to interfere with the rehabilitation process, contributing factors should be determined and interventions planned. These include

- assessing for painful stimuli below the injury level (e.g., urinary tract infection, pressure ulcer, bowel impaction, tight clothing)
- planning a regular program of stretching the muscles and performing range of motion exercises to decrease spasms
- administering medications such as baclofen, clonidine HCl, dantrolene sodium, and diazepam; these must be monitored for

signs of adverse reactions, toxicity, or both; baclofen can be applied directly by means of an implanted pump

- use of other treatments such as rhizotomy, nerve blocks, and intraspinal stimulation (Spoltore & O'Brien, 1995; UW Rehabilitation Medicine, 1994)

Spine deformity occurs in children and adolescents with SCI, and they should be evaluated frequently for scoliosis because of their potential for growth. If a brace is used, proper application and placement is important, as is skin observation and care.

The child or adolescent with SCI needs assistance in maintaining his or her sexual identity. The pediatric rehabilitation nurse can be supportive by minimizing the number of embarrassing procedures; encouraging the maintenance of physical appearance; acknowledging concerns and the expression of feelings; and facilitating the exploration of methods of sexual expression. This may be accomplished by age-appropriate education to increase biologic knowledge and acceptance of viewing and touching their body (Hanak, 1992; Spoltore & O'Brien, 1995).

Ozer (1988) proposed a description of a life cycle of the person with SCI, which includes three unequal phases of changing problems that are important for the pediatric rehabilitation nurse to understand in planning for care. During the first phase, which lasts for hours to days after injury, the health care team is concerned with maintaining life and minimizing damage. The goal is to prevent further impairment, and this phase is completed at medical stabilization. The risk of death is greatest at this phase (approximately 4%). The second phase, which lasts from weeks to months after injury, is a time of restoration and minimizing the disability despite the continuation of impairment. The traditional rehabilitation team is actively involved with the individual and family in the treatment program. In the third phase, which lasts for years after injury, continuing care is provided to minimize disability by maximizing health and enabling the individual to function independently in the community.

Transition From Acute Care to Rehabilitation

As the condition stabilizes, the child or adolescent and his or her family develop trust in the acute care staff. If arrangements are being made for a transfer to rehabilitation, which

is a dramatically different environment, it is essential that the nursing staff in both areas attempt to facilitate the process. Rehabilitation requires a totally different focus for everyone's efforts, and it will be beneficial for the child and family to be introduced to rehabilitation concepts. Anxiety can be alleviated prior to transfer by allowing the child and family the opportunity to interact with and meet the rehabilitation nursing staff and therapists and to see the new setting. This will reduce fears and form the foundation for the beginning of a new trusting relationship (Swarczinski & Graham, 1990).

Application of the Nursing Process

The pediatric rehabilitation nurse, as the coordinator of care for the child and family, interacts in a variety of settings with other nurses and health professionals. The critical thinking skills inherent in the nursing process are essential in the provision of quality care that meets the needs of the child and family and obtains desired outcomes. Many nursing diagnostic statements and collaborative problems are applicable to the complex care of children with traumatic SCI. Age, developmental level, and level of injury and associated problems greatly affect the priorities in nursing assessment.

Nursing Assessment

A health history and nursing and functional assessment, focusing on information about the injury and associated problems; a systems review including current problems and preexisting conditions; a list of medications and known allergies; and a personal history focusing on diet, sleep patterns, exercise, and psycho-social status are important initial elements in determining the needs and problems of the child and family. Significant areas to incorporate into the assessment are listed in Table 22–4.

Nursing Diagnoses and Plan

After a thorough, individualized assessment of the child and family, a list of problems should be developed and nursing diagnoses and a plan of care identified. The main problems identified depend on the age of the child and the level and severity of the injury, and the problems identified are specific to the nurse's clinical practice setting (e.g., rehabilitation unit, school, home). If the nursing diagnosis of "High risk for impaired skin integ-

Table 22–4 NURSING ASSESSMENT AREAS: SPINAL CORD INJURY

Skin
Cardiovascular function
Bowel function
Psychologic status
Musculoskeletal deficits
Respiratory function
Bladder function
Nutrition
Neuromotor function
Pain

rity" is identified, the plan of care, as outlined in Table 22–5, can be initiated after it is specifically tailored to the age and abilities of the child and family.

Rehabilitation nursing standards, such as the one developed by Miller (1996) for maintaining skin integrity, should be in place in each clinical practice setting. This standard includes additional information useful in maintaining and restoring the integrity of the skin as well as protocols for the treatment of skin breakdown and pressure sores. The standard also provides a consistent format for assessment and documentation, a teaching tool for new staff, and a quality monitor for

determining prevalence of skin breakdown and timeliness of instituting treatment. Other nursing diagnoses that must be considered and their associated interventions are shown in Table 22–6.

In all areas, education of the child and family is a key element, and there should be constant reinforcement by all involved health care professionals. The signs and symptoms of infection and the importance of prevention must be discussed and reinforced. The use of intermittent catheterization for individuals who sustained an SCI is common and is often a means of introducing bacteria into the bladder, causing an infection. A study was conducted (Charbonneau-Smith, 1993) to compare the straight, intermittent catheterization technique with the no-touch method. Results showed a decrease in the urinary tract infection rate for hospitalized patients, both in number of infections and length of time infected, with the no-touch method. Another study (Moore et al., 1993) compared the infection rates of subjects who used sterile, single-use catheters and those who cleaned and reused catheters for intermittent self-catheterization in the home setting. Results showed that the single-use catheters did not reduce the infection rate and supported the current practice of re-using catheters.

Table 22–5 NURSING PLAN OF CARE

Nursing Diagnosis: High Risk for Impaired Skin Integrity

| **Related to:** | Lack of sensation | Immobility |
| | Circulatory impairment | Altered nutrition |

Goals	Nursing Interventions/Teaching
Identify individual risk factors	Determine factors that will impair skin integrity and teach elements of early detection of skin changes and pressure ulcer prevention
	Understand the child/adolescent/family interpretation of the importance of measures to maintain skin integrity
Demonstrate behaviors to minimize risk	Provide for optimum nutrition with supplements high in protein as needed
	Teach hygiene, safety, skin care, and skin inspection techniques (e.g., use of a mirror to inspect certain areas, safety factors for use of equipment and appliances)
	Reinforce elements of pressure ulcer prevention (e.g., schedule for skin inspection, repositioning schedule, proper fit of clothing, using push-ups or backward tilt if in a wheelchair)
	Use appropriate devices such as water or egg-crate mattress, sheepskin, or special wheelchair pads

Expected Outcomes

Behaviors to prevent skin breakdown are demonstrated
Skin integrity is maintained

Table 22–6   NURSING DIAGNOSES WITH INTERVENTIONS

Nursing Diagnoses	Interventions
High risk for ineffective airway clearance	Deep breathing and coughing Postural drainage and percussion Incentive spirometry Encourage fluid intake
High risk for infection Respiratory	Stress proper handwashing Meticulous respiratory care Chest physiotherapy Deep breathing and positioning
Urinary	Perineal care Catheter care
Altered patterns of urinary elimination	Toileting routines Intermittent catheterization Adequate fluids
Constipation	Establish bowel program Stool softeners Balanced diet and adequate fluids Exercise and activity program
High risk for altered family processes	Promote and support family cohesiveness Encourage expressions of feelings Identify coping behaviors Encourage family participation in care and therapy

The child or adolescent with SCI may experience pain, which will negatively affect the rehabilitation process and the performance of daily activities. The type, severity, and location of the pain, as well as the child's or adolescent's response to it, should be assessed and appropriate action taken. A study conducted by Quigley and Veit (1996) used the McGill-Melzack Pain Questionnaire (MMPQ) as an interdisciplinary pain assessment. They found that it provided a systemic assessment to specify and quantify the types of clinical pain associated with SCI and could also be used to determine the response to pain management.

Psycho-social Impact

Adolescence is a difficult time of psychological development while physical changes, new demands and responses from others, and higher levels of thinking and reasoning skills are expected. The adolescent who sustains an SCI encounters additional problems—medical, psychological, and developmental—and struggles to restore a balance among all these factors.

The primary psychological features that occur with SCI are sudden and massive change with loss of control; dependency in a new environment; fear and pain, which interfere with judgment and tolerance; effects of medications that impair function and cognition; and separation from normal means of coping with stress or change. The reaction stages depend on the adolescent's level of physical, emotional, and cognitive development. Reactions often include anger, as the injury may be seen as punishment, and the adolescent may express hostility and show signs of depression and noncompliance. In many studies, immobility and hospitalization have been associated with periods of paranoia, panic, depression, disorientation, and temporary diminution of cognitive function. Special attention must be paid to the elements of sensory deprivation and appropriate actions taken to facilitate expression of feelings and concerns.

It is important to remember that some issues and problems will slow or impede the child or adolescent's progress. Inadequate social support systems and lack of variety in behavioral skills to assist in coping can negatively affect outcomes and slow the reintegration process. The issues of sexuality and the wide range of changes in function and expression must be dealt with and resolved to the greatest degree possible. Pre-existing issues with alcohol and drug abuse must also be addressed and included in the therapeutic regimen. Sensitive support and adequate treatment, as well as time to adjust and prove themselves, will allow adolescents to successfully resolve their physical and emotional issues and re-enter society with a healthy body image that precipitates a realistic outlook on life and its opportunities. The following was written by Dean Joyce (1997), who has C6 quadriplegia:

> When you enter the world you will be given a body, do not compare it to others, nor think it should be different, instead, realize it is the most beautiful gift you have, and the only thing that you truly own. Your true self is your mind, it controls what you think of your body, do not let your body control what you think in your mind. . . . Only then would you be handicapped.

The care that the pediatric rehabilitation nurse provides to the child or adolescent with an SCI is ongoing and must follow a well-developed, coordinated plan that provides education and psychological support. Care must also incorporate health promotion activities to decrease complications, improve function, and positively affect lifestyle. These include exercise and fitness activities, which have physical and emotional benefits including stress reduction and enhanced self-esteem (Edwards, 1996). Additional information about health promotion activities is provided in Chapter 14.

Future Implications

Pediatric rehabilitation nurses must play a key role in participating in research projects. Because fewer of these types of injuries occur in children, few centers see enough pediatric patients to do clinical trials. In some instances, results of studies done on adults can be applied to children (Massagli, 1996). One study sought to distinguish differences between adults and children with SCI and concluded that the only areas of difference were in level of injury (higher in children) and post-injury scoliosis (Apple, 1995).

Clinical and rehabilitation research being conducted through the Miami Project focuses on understanding the response of the nervous system to injury, therapies to maximize physical capabilities, and the effect of exercise on improving muscle function (University of Miami, 1996). Future directions for spasticity research include the possibility of preventing the development of spasticity, discovering whether there is a critical period after injury during which spasticity can be suppressed, and investigating whether limiting spasticity

enhances recovery after SCI (UW Rehabilitation Medicine, 1994).

TRAUMATIC BRAIN INJURY

Injury to the brain, caused by trauma to the head, is an important cause of disability in children and adolescents and presents the pediatric rehabilitation nurse and the interdisciplinary team with a tremendous challenge to identify and manage a variety of physical, psycho-social and cognitive deficits. The injury may not always be visible, but the physical, emotional, and intellectual changes may be long lasting and place an enormous burden on the family (Family Caregiver Alliance [FCA], 1996).

Incidence figures vary, but it is estimated that as many as 200,000 children and adolescents in the United States are hospitalized each year with head injuries, and 15,000 of these require prolonged hospitalization. Adolescents and young adults 15 to 24 years of age are most frequently injured, and males are twice as likely to be injured as females. These childhood injuries are caused by motor vehicle and motorcycle accidents, either to a driver, passenger, or pedestrian; by falls (especially in infants); or by violence (assaults and gunshot wounds). Massagli and Jaffe (1994) used the Glasgow Coma Scale (GCS) to evaluate injury severity and found that 5% of children have a severe traumatic brain injury (TBI) with a GCS score of 3 to 8, and 7% have a moderate TBI with a GCS score of 9 to 12. Table 22–7 lists the demographic information associated with TBI.

Pathophysiology

Damage to the brain following trauma results from two mechanisms: primary injury, caused by the initial impact of the trauma, and secondary injury. Primary injuries may be either focal (e.g., a contusion in the area where the brain comes in contact with the skull) or diffuse (e.g., acceleration-deceleration forces leading to shearing of the layers of the brain tissue and tearing of nerve fibers with associated pressure changes). Secondary injury results from the edema and increased intracranial pressure, which affects blood flow to the area and results in hypoxia and acidosis. Systemic factors such as blood loss, hypotension, and elevated temperature may also contribute to secondary injury. Immediate coma following the injury is usually the result of primary damage.

Table 22-7   TRAUMATIC BRAIN INJURY DEMOGRAPHICS

- Male-to-female ratio of 2:1
- Higher incidence in older children
- Causes: motor vehicle accident as driver, passenger, or pedestrian; bike or motorcycle accident; falls; violence
- 100,000–250,000 new cases/year
- Classified as mild, moderate, or severe
- 80% considered mild or minor
- High-risk group: alcohol or drug ingestion; previous head injury; psychiatric illness; cognitive delays, including poor judgment
- Types: closed or blunt; open or penetrating

Data from DiScala, C., Osberg, J., Gans, B., Chin, L., & Grant, C. (1991). Children with traumatic head injury: morbidity and post acute treatment. *Archives of Physical Medicine and Rehabilitation, 72*(8), 662–666; Family Caregiver Alliance. (1996). *Selected head injury statistics;* [On-line]. Available: www.caregiver.org.text Hanak, M. (1992). *Rehabilitation nursing for the neurological patient.* New York: Springer; and Henry, P., Hauber, R., & Rice, M. (1992). Factors associated with closed head injury in a pediatric population. *Journal of Neuroscience Nursing, 24*(6), 311–316.

Disability Rating Scales

Level of coma is often monitored using a criterion-based behavioral scale. Two frequently used measures are the Glasgow Coma Scale (GCS) and the Rancho Los Amigos Scale. Both of these tools assess the child's ability to respond to various stimuli ranging from a painful stimulus to a complex verbal command. The GCS, found in Table 22–8, is one of the gross classification tools used to evaluate the severity of brain injury and relates consciousness to motor response, verbal response, and eye opening. The levels of responses indicate the degree of nervous system impairment as follows:

Eye opening—eyes may open spontaneously, only on verbal request, or only with painful stimulation
Best verbal response—speaks normally and is oriented to time and place, is disoriented and uses inappropriate words, or makes incomprehensible sounds or no sounds
Best motor response—able to move about on command, has various responses to painful stimulus, or no response

Each category of the GCS is rated using "1" as the lowest possible score. This allows for classification of brain injuries as mild (score of 13 to 15), moderate (score of 9 to 12), or severe (score of 8 or less). The score is obtained by adding the eye opening, verbal response, and motor response scores to achieve a total score.

To avoid the difficulty of using different terms to describe the same children or adolescents, Reilly and colleagues (1987) recommend using the Rancho Los Amigos Scale of Cognitive Functioning and adapting it for use with the pediatric population. This descriptive scale has eight levels of functioning rang-

Table 22-8   GLASGOW COMA SCALE

Eyes	Open	Spontaneously	4
		Responds to verbal command	3
		Responds to pain	2
		No response	1
Best motor response	To verbal command	Obeys	6
	To painful stimulus	Localizes pain	5
		Flexion—withdrawal	4
		Flexion—abnormal (decerebrate rigidity)	3
		Extension (decerebrate rigidity)	2
		No response	1
Best verbal response		Oriented and converses	5
		Disoriented and converses	4
		Inappropriate words	3
		Incomprehensible sounds	2
		No response	1
Total			3–15

ing from level I (no response) through level VIII (purposeful appropriate). The levels and their characteristics are shown in Table 22–9.

The Functional Independence Measure (FIM) and the Functional Independence Measure for Children (WeeFIM) described in Chapter 11 are tools for measuring functional skills, and they provide an index of outcome measurement in the rehabilitation of children and adolescents with TBI. One study (DiScala et al., 1992) to evaluate the relationship between clinical judgment and functional status using the FIM reported that the measure effectively categorized children according to the extent of their disability.

The Disability Rating Scale proposed by Rappaport (1982) is another method of evaluating the level of disability as it reflects changes in the functional, cognitive, and psycho-social domains. This scale monitors a range of recovery from initial injury to community reintegration and is a more sensitive index of change than the GCS (Fleming & Maas, 1994).

Systemic Effects and Related Complications

The pediatric rehabilitation nurse must be aware of the potential complications that can occur following TBI, especially in the areas of neurologic, cognitive, and behavioral function shown in Table 22–10. Neurologic complications may include hydrocephalus resulting from ventricular obstruction, post-traumatic epilepsy, seizures, diabetes insipidus or inappropriate anti-diuretic hormone (ADH) secretion, and elevated intracranial pressure (Hanak, 1992).

Cognitive dysfunction affects many areas of daily activity and may result in increased distractibility, decreased concentration and short-term memory, inability to think and reason effectively and change tasks, and impaired visual motor skills. Behavioral problems can be both acute and chronic, and the site of the injury is a determining factor in the severity of the problem. After coma, confusion, agitation, low tolerance for stimulation, and emotional problems may exist. Chronic behaviors include emotional lability, disinhibition, and lack of insight, and depression may also occur. Conditions that existed prior to the injury and subsequent adjustment difficulties can exacerbate these problems (Massagli & Jaffe, 1994; Slifer et al., 1993).

Medical problems and complications must be anticipated, recognized accurately, and properly managed. The child or adolescent

Table 22–9 RANCHO SCALE LEVELS AND BEHAVIORS

Level I	No response	Deep sleep; no reaction to stimuli
Level II	Generalized response	Signs of arousal; inconsistent, nonpurposeful reaction; response to deep pain
Level III	Localized response	Response fairly consistent to pain but inconsistent to pleasant stimuli; inconsistently follows simple commands
Level IV	Confused, agitated	Increased activity and aggressive behaviors; disoriented and incoherent; no selective attention or memory; undifferentiated response to people
Level V	Inappropriate, non-agitated	Attentive and responds to simple commands; distractible with poor judgment; best response is to body needs and familiar people; automatic verbalization
Level VI	Appropriate, confused	Consistently follows commands; needs external direction; behavior control and response limited to immediate situation
Level VII	Automatic, appropriate	Can perform daily routines; judgment and memory remain impaired; requires minimal safety and supervision; responds to systematic, directive training
Level VIII	Purposeful, appropriate	Alert and oriented; recalls and integrates past and recent events; demonstrates new learning; may still have residual problems

Table 22–10   TRAUMATIC BRAIN INJURY COMPLICATIONS

Neurologic	Cognitive	Behavioral
Hydrocephalus	Decreased attention and concentration	Confusion
Epilepsy/seizures	Increased distractibility	Agitation
Diabetes insipidus	Short-term memory impairment	Emotional lability
Increased intracranial pressure	Impaired visual motor skills	Impulsiveness and disinhibition

who has sustained a TBI is at risk for altered nutrition because of feeding and swallowing disorders, initial intestinal stasis, and peripheral alimentation. The team should thoroughly evaluate nutrition and feeding-swallowing to make recommendations about food delivery method and techniques, consistency and texture of food, and positioning of the child or adolescent during feeding.

Fever may represent an infection, and the source must be determined and treatment instituted promptly because a central nervous system infection can be life threatening. Other causes of fever include urinary tract infections, pulmonary problems (e.g., aspiration, pneumonia, atelectasis), middle ear infections, and bacteremia.

Conductive hearing loss and visual and vestibular disturbances may also occur following TBI. These conditions warrant a thorough assessment and treatment as indicated by the problem. Many children and adolescents have skeletal injuries accompanying TBI. A comprehensive evaluation should be done to detect fractures or dislocations that may involve the spine, pelvis, long bones, and shoulder or clavicle (Jaffe & Hays, 1986).

Factors Influencing Outcome

Two factors that seem to be most significant in predicting outcome are the extent and severity of the injury and the rate of improvement experienced immediately after the injury. Other factors include age (the brain of a young child may have more plasticity), presence of associated injuries and complications, site of injury, and individual characteristics of the child or adolescent. Young children may be at a disadvantage, as their knowledge base and past experiences are limited and the injury can affect new learning. Physical improvement cannot be the only indicator, because complex cognitive problems, which may not be as obvious, must be considered (Hanak, 1992; Middleton et al., 1992; Hall, Johnson, & Middleton, 1990).

Studies of brain injury in children found that the GCS, especially the motor component, performed in the first few days after injury, was a better outcome predictor than initial clinical status (Michaud et al., 1992). This study also determined that severity of injury to the brain and extra-cranial injuries, especially to the chest, related significantly to the quality of life after survival. Patterns of change over a 3-year period were examined to determine the association between severity of injury and recovery patterns. Children with severe injuries had significant deficits initially but showed improvement at 1 year post-injury, after which change slowed. The most significant deficits at 1 and 3 years post-injury were in adaptive problem solving and performance intelligence quotient (IQ), but there were no significant deficits in the areas of independent living skills and psycho-motor performance (Jaffe et al., 1995).

Transition to Rehabilitation

Discharge from the intensive care unit should be the beginning of a comprehensive management plan for the provision of rehabilitation services to the child or adolescent and family. In the acute care hospital, the following elements of the rehabilitation process should be initiated:

- comprehensive examination of all systems, including collection of baseline neurologic information
- stabilization of function and prevention of further injury
- prevention of complications
- protocols for consultation with rehabilitation professionals and transfer to inpatient pediatric rehabilitation programs, to home care, and for follow-up.

As with the child or adolescent with SCI, if arrangements are being made for a transfer to a rehabilitation facility, it is essential that nursing staff in both areas attempt to facilitate the process. Anxiety can be alleviated prior to transfer by allowing the child and family the opportunity to interact with and meet the rehabilitation nursing staff and therapists and to see the setting. This should also be done if the child is being discharged to home.

Application of the Nursing Process

The pediatric rehabilitation nurse, as the coordinator of care for the child and family, interacts in a variety of settings with other nurses and health professionals. The critical thinking skills inherent in the nursing process are essential in the provision of quality care that meets the needs of the child and family and obtains desired outcomes. Many nursing diagnostic statements and collaborative problems are applicable to the complex care of children with TBI. Age, developmental level, and level of injury and associated problems greatly affect the priorities in nursing assessment.

Nursing Assessment

A health history should incorporate information about functioning and performance prior to the injury, the mechanism and cause of injury, and its clinical course. These important data, along with the standard history information, guide the assessment areas and assist in identifying problems and formulating

goals. Significant areas to incorporate in the assessment are:

Neurologic status—level of consciousness, cranial nerves, sensation and movement, potential seizure activity
Cardio-respiratory function—vital signs, orthostatic hypotension, adequacy of circulation and oxygenation
Elimination—bowel patterns and urinary function
Vision and Hearing—evaluation
Nutrition and fluid intake—including swallowing
Growth patterns—height and weight, developmental parameters
Mobility—range of motion of joints, general strength and muscle tone, spasticity
Behavior and cognitive function—ability to follow commands, presence of confusion

Nursing Diagnoses and Plan

When the pediatric rehabilitation nurse has the information derived from a thorough history and nursing assessment, a list of nursing diagnoses can be identified and a plan of care developed to address the problems of the child or adolescent and family. The main problems identified depend on the age of the

Table 22–11   NURSING PLAN OF CARE

Nursing Diagnosis: High Risk for Injury

Related to:	Altered mobility	Behavioral dysfunction
	Cognitive deficits	Sensory deficits

Goals	Nursing Interventions and Teaching
Identify risk factors in the environment	Evaluate developmental and competence level, behavior, and decision-making ability
Identify interventions to minimize or eliminate risk factors and promote safety	Evaluate knowledge of safety needs and injury prevention
	Modify environment to enhance safety
	Provide information regarding injury and the deficits that increase risk of injury
	Provide an organized, consistent environment: orient to time, place, and person; identify caregivers
	Assist to learn and follow program schedule
	Familiarize with environment and safety devices in use
	Demonstrate safe use of adaptive devices and techniques
	Evaluate home for environmental hazards and unsafe situations
	Provide information on community resources
	Teach about effects of medications and adverse interactions, especially with alcohol

Expected Outcomes

Behaviors to reduce risk factors and protect self are demonstrated
Be free from injury

Table 22–12   SETTING SPECIFIC NURSING DIAGNOSES AND INTERVENTIONS

Nursing Diagnosis	Goals	Interventions
Inpatient Pediatric Rehabilitation		
Activity intolerance	Measurable increase in activity tolerance	Promote comfort measures Increase activity levels gradually Plan care with rest periods
Ineffective airway clearance	Airway patent and lungs remain clear	Encourage deep breathing and coughing Postural drainage and percussion Humidification and respiratory therapy
Home		
Family coping, ineffective	Verbalize understanding and interact appropriately	Encourage open communication Help family to understand behaviors Involve child/adolescent and family in plan Refer to appropriate resources
Altered family processes	Express feelings appropriately and demonstrate involvement in problem solving	Encourage expression of feelings Stress importance of open family dialogue Provide information as necessary Identify coping behaviors
School		
Impaired verbal communication	Employ effective communication to convey needs	Determine appropriateness of communication Validate meaning of non-verbal communication Plan alternate means of communication Keep communication simple
Impaired physical mobility	Use techniques and equipment correctly to facilitate mobility	Program of exercises Positioning Use of splints, walker

child, the severity of the injury, and associated complications and problems specific to the setting in which the plan is being implemented. If the nursing diagnosis of "High risk for injury" is identified, the plan outlined in Table 22–11 can be initiated after it is specifically tailored to the age and abilities of the child and family.

Other nursing diagnoses with specific goals that must be considered and the resulting interventions depend on the setting in which the pediatric rehabilitation nurse is working and the cognitive level and individual problems of the child or adolescent and family. Table 22–12 lists examples of these nursing diagnoses, goals, and interventions for various settings.

Nursing diagnoses that must be considered in all settings for the child or adolescent with TBI include self-care deficits, activity intoler-

ance, impaired skin integrity, altered bowel and bladder elimination, altered nutritional status, sexual dysfunction, body image and self-esteem disturbance, and anxiety. If the child has seizures as a result of the TBI, appropriate precautions and management are essential. These are outlined in Teaching Topic: Seizure Precautions and Management.

FAMILY INVOLVEMENT

Hastening a child or adolescent's recovery requires a team effort, with numerous professionals specializing in pediatrics and rehabilitation and the family as key team members. At each of the Rancho levels, there are important nursing interventions to include in the plan of care. At level I, there should be normal conversation, familiar objects, and the

---

Teaching Topic: Seizure Precautions and Management

Important Areas:

Remain calm and stay with the child.
Speak softly.
Reassure.

Protect the child from injury.
Do not restrain or restrict movement.
Move harmful objects away.
Assist the child to lie down.
Place soft material under the child's head.
Loosen restrictive clothing.

Provide time for recovery.
Turn child to the side-lying position.
Give nothing to eat or drink.

Reassure and provide support.
Answer questions.

Call for emergency help if:
Breathing does not resume; begin mouth-to-mouth resuscitation
Seizure lasts more than 5 minutes
Seizures continue without return to consciousness between seizures
There are serious injuries
It is the child's first seizure

Safety considerations:
Helmets
Chairs with arms
Evaluate environment, especially sleeping area
Activities of daily living performed with supervision

---

presence of family members. The child or adolescent should be dressed in his or her own clothes and participate in activities when medically stable. Providing family members with information and encouragement is essential to the recovery process. This care is continued at level II, but rest is provided and stimulation in the environment is minimized. All team members should use simple commands and observe and document the child's or adolescent's response.

At level III, all previous care is continued with as much consistency as possible in the daily schedule by caregivers. The disorientation and confusion occurring at level IV makes this one of the most difficult periods for the team and family. It is important to identify and remove noxious stimuli and

heighten environmental safety awareness. The child or adolescent needs continued reorientation, and the family should be reassured that this is part of the recovery process. From level V onward, the child or adolescent should be encouraged to participate in his or her own care and attend to the tasks that need to be mastered. Positive reinforcement of correct behaviors assists in learning, but appropriate limits on behavior should also be set. Safety awareness continues to be a priority, and identification of specific deficits and problems is essential as the discharge plan is formulated. Participation of family members in therapies, mealtimes, recreational activities, and eventually in home visits makes the transition easier for all involved in care (Reilly et al., 1987).

CASE STUDY

David is a 10-year-old boy who sustained a brain injury and a fractured femur 4 months ago when he was hit by a car while riding his bicycle home from school. He was not wearing a helmet at the time and was unconscious at the scene and on admission to the hospital. A GCS score of 7 in the emergency department placed him at the severe level of brain injury. David was stabilized and transferred to the pediatric intensive care unit, and after 1 week he was moved to a pediatric nursing unit. At this point, he was evaluated to be at Rancho level III. Improvement was shown over the course of a few weeks, and he was transferred to a pediatric rehabilitation facility for intensive physical and cognitive therapy. He showed continual progress and was discharged to home at Rancho level VI–VII. David still had weakness, especially on the right side, and cognitive and behavioral deficits. He continued to be seen for outpatient therapy until he returned to school.

The nurse in the school setting must work with the therapists to develop and implement an individualized program that includes exercises to deal with continued motor deficits. Any medications that are used must be monitored and David's response observed. The program should also include strategies to deal with perceptual deficits, and written as well as verbal cues may be needed to assist with visual-spatial problems. The teachers and classroom aides must understand how to work with David to maintain his optimal level of function. David, to be successful in performing activities of daily living, will continue to need help in a number of areas: sequencing the steps of a task, mobilizing to perform the task, perceiving what he has accomplished, and executing the activity correctly. The plan must also include strategies for modulating behavior problems such as impulsivity, with positive reinforcement provided for appropriate activities.

Future Implications

Recovery after TBI can be a very long and complex process. The pediatric rehabilitation nurse working with children and adolescents with TBI must understand both the rationale for the rehabilitation intervention strategies and the effects of the recovery process on the brain. The importance of a comprehensive rehabilitation program, including the cooperation of all members of the health care team and family, is essential for initial and follow-up care. The nurse's participation in ongoing research will help to expand the knowledge base relative to pediatric head trauma; improve understanding of the physical, cognitive, and behavioral sequelae; and enable the pediatric rehabilitation nurse to better meet the needs of these children or adolescents and their families.

The pediatric rehabilitation nurse can be instrumental in helping children and adolescents who have trauma to the spinal cord or brain return to home, school, and community even if they are different in some ways than they were before. As scientific research and technologic advances have produced improvements in emergency medicine and initial diagnosis and intervention, more individuals with SCI and TBI are surviving, and additional research will be essential to help these individuals reach their optimal level of function. Studies to find more effective ways to repair damaged nervous system tissue, improve rehabilitation techniques, and prevent consequences of injuries must be initiated.

Developing a community-centered preventive education program regarding SCI and TBI is another role for the pediatric rehabilitation nurse. This could include anticipatory guidance for parents, preventive education programs, public and community awareness of safety measures for children, and education in the schools.

REFERENCES

Spinal Cord Injury

American Spinal Injury Association (ASIA). (1996). International standards for neurological and functional classification of spinal cord injury. Atlanta: ASIA Standards.

Apple, D. (1995). Spinal cord injury in youth. *Clinical Pediatrics*, 34(2), 90–95.

Charbonneau-Smith, R. (1993). No-touch catheterization and infection rates in a select spinal cord injured population. *Rehabilitation Nursing*, 18(5), 296–299.

Edwards, P. (1996). Health promotion through fitness for adolescents and young adults following spinal cord injury. *SCI Nursing*, 13(3), 69–73.

Hanak, M. (1992). *Rehabilitation nursing for the neurological patient*. New York: Springer.

Joyce, D. (1997). Personal communication [On-line]. E-mail: c67quad@aol.com

Massagli, T. (1996). Personal communication [On-line]. E-mail: massagli@u.washington.edu

Miller, L. (1996). Maintaining skin integrity: setting the standard in a rehabilitation facility. *Rehabilitation Nursing*, 20(5), 273–277.

Moore, K., Kelm, M., Sinclair, O., & Cadrain, G. (1993). Bacteriuria in intermittent catheterization users: the effect of sterile versus clean reused catheters. *Rehabilitation Nursing*, 18(5), 306–309.

National Institute of Neurological Disorders and Stroke (NINDS). (1996). *Spinal cord injury— research highlights* [On-line]. Available: www.nih.gov/ninds

National Spinal Cord Injury Association (NSCIA). (1996). *Fact sheet 14: resources for pediatric spinal cord injury*. Silver Spring, MD: NSCIA.

Ozer, M. (1988). *The management of persons with spinal cord injury*. New York: Demos.

Quigley, P., & Veit, N. (1996). Interdisciplinary pain assessment of SCI patients. *SCI Nursing*, 13(3), 62–68.

Southard, T., & Massagli, T. (1994). Spinal cord injury. In S. Campbell (Ed.). *Physical therapy for children*, pp. 525–547. Philadelphia: WB Saunders.

Spoltore, T., & O'Brien, A. (1995). Rehabilitation of the spinal cord injured patient. *Orthopedic Nursing*, 14(3), 7–14.

Swarczinski, C., & Graham, P. (1990). From ICU to rehabilitation: a checklist to ease the transition for the spinal cord injured. *Journal of Neuroscience Nursing*, 22(2), 89–91.

Tepperman, P. (1989). Primary care after SCI. *Postgraduate Medicine*, 86(5), 211–218.

University of Miami. (1996). *Clinical and rehabilitation research: The Miami Project to Cure Paralysis* [On-line]. Available: http://199.227.117.2/miaproj/curepar3.htm

UW Rehabilitation Medicine. (1994). Spasticity, SCI Forum, SCI update, November 1, 1994 [On-line]. Available: weber.u.washington.edu

UW Rehabilitation Medicine. (1995). Recovery research, SCI Forum, March 7, 1995 [On-line]. Available: weber.u.washington.edu

Traumatic Brain Injury

DiScala, C., Grant, C., Brooke, M., & Gans, B. (1992). Functional outcome in children with traumatic brain injury. *American Journal of Physical Medicine and Rehabilitation, 71*(3), 145–148.

Family Caregiver Alliance. (1996). *Selected head injury statistics* [On-line]. Available: www.caregiver.org.text

Fleming, J., & Maas, F. (1994). Prognosis of rehabilitation outcome in head injury using the disability rating scale. *Archives of Physical Medicine and Rehabilitation, 75*(2), 156–163.

Hall, D., Johnson, S., & Middleton, J. (1990). Rehabilitation of head injured children. *Archives of Disease in Childhood, 65,* 553–556.

Hanak, M. (1992). *Rehabilitation nursing for the neurological patient.* New York: Springer.

Jaffe, K., & Hays, R. (1986), Pediatric head injury: rehabilitative medical management. *Journal of Head Trauma and Rehabilitation, 1*(4), 30–40.

Jaffe, K., Polissai, N., Fay, G., & Liao, S. (1995). Recovery trends over three years following pediatric traumatic brain injury. *Archives of Physical Medicine and Rehabilitation, 76*(1), 17–26.

Massagli, T., & Jaffe, K. (1994). Pediatric traumatic brain injury: prognosis and rehabilitation. *Pediatric Annals, 23*(1), 29–36.

Michaud, L., Rivara, F., Grady, S., & Reay, D. (1992). Predictors of survival and severity of disability after severe brain injury in children. *Neurosurgery, 31*(2), 254–264.

Middleton, J., Jones, M., Moffat, V., Wintle, L., & Russell, P. (1992). Rehabilitation after acute neurological trauma. In G. McCarthy (Ed.). *Physical disability in childhood.* New York: Churchill Livingstone.

Rappaport, M., Hall, K., Hopkins, K., Belleza, T., & Cope, D. (1982). Disability rating scale for severe head trauma: coma to community. *Archives of Physical Medicine and Rehabilitation, 63,* 35–37.

Reilly, A., Lutz, M., Spiegler, B., & Lynn, P. (1987). Head trauma in children: the stages to cognitive recovery. *Maternal Child Nursing, 12*(6), 405, 407, 409, 412.

Sifer, K., Cataldo, M. Babbitt, R., Kane, A., Harrison, K., & Cataldo, M. (1993). Behavior analysis and intervention during hospitalization for brain trauma rehabilitation. *Archives of Physical Medicine and Rehabilitation, 74*(8), 810–817.

ADDITIONAL RESOURCES

DiScala, C., Osberg, J., Gans, B., Chin, L., & Grant, C. (1991). Children with traumatic head injury: morbidity and post acute treatment. *Archives of Physical Medicine and Rehabilitation, 72*(8), 662–666.

Henry, P., Hauber, R., & Rice, M. (1992). Factors associated with closed head injury in a pediatric population. *Journal of Neuroscience Nursing, 24*(6), 311–316.

Molnar, G., Easton, J., Badell, A., Binder, H., Dykstra, D., Mathews, D., Noll, S., & Perrin, J. (1989). Pediatric rehabilitation. 2. Brain damage causing disability. *Archives of Physical Medicine and Rehabilitation, 70*(5), 166–167.

RESOURCES

American Spinal Injury Association
345 East Superior Street, Room 1436
Chicago, IL 60611
312-908-1242
http://www.asia-spinalinjury.org

Family Caregiver Alliance
425 Bush Street, Suite 500
San Francisco, CA 94108
415-434-3388
fax: 415-434-3508
http://www.caregiver.org
E-mail: info@caregiver.org

In Touch with Kids Program (ITWK)
National Spinal Cord Injury Association
8300 Colesville Road
Silver Spring, MD 20910
301-588-6959
fax: 301-588-9414
http://www.erols.com/nscia

The Miami Project to Cure Paralysis
University of Miami School of Medicine
1-800-STANDUP (automated information line)
305-243-6001
fax: 305-243-6017
http://miamiproject.miami.edu
E-mail: webmaster@miamiproj.med.miami.edu

National Head Injury Foundation
1776 Massachusetts Avenue NW, Suite 100
Washington, DC 20036
800-444-6443

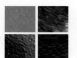

Part IV

Further Dimensions

Chapter 23

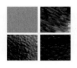

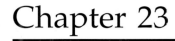

Pediatric Rehabilitation Nursing Research

Patricia A. Edwards

Research is an important component of pediatric rehabilitation nursing at all levels of practice. Related activities in which nurses are involved range from applying research findings in clinical practice to conducting research based on clinical problems. Nurses in advanced practice roles encourage research use among nursing staff and work with other team members to conduct clinical research in specific areas.

Pediatric rehabilitation nurses practice in a variety of settings and are uniquely positioned to identify research questions in their day-to-day contact with children and their families. In the past, nursing actions were based on intuition, tradition, and beliefs, but increased nursing research and dissemination has led to research-based practice. It has become very important to move away from practices that are based on tradition or expert opinion. "Using scientific inquiry to evaluate and validate nursing interventions can improve our efforts to ensure quality nursing care and optimal patient outcomes" (Prichard et al., 1994, p. 307). Nurses have many opportunities to launch investigations based on actual or potential nursing problems and to use research as a basis for clinical decision making and the development of standards.

As you read this chapter, think about the nursing-related problems in your practice that might be the basis of a research study and begin to formulate research questions. Get together with colleagues and discuss your ideas to gain support and valuable input. Brainstorm to identify broad subjects that cover everyone's interest, then narrow con-

cepts down to specific topics. Choose one and begin a literature search. A review of the literature and critiques of articles and other information obtained begin the foundation for a research study. This chapter contains an overview of the research process and the steps that should be taken as the nurse conducts research. Research priorities for rehabilitation nursing are included, with the suggestions for researchable topics and issues related specifically to pediatric rehabilitation nursing.

NURSING RESEARCHER ROLE

In the role description for Pediatric Rehabilitation Nursing (Association of Rehabilitation Nurses [ARN] Pediatric Special Interest Group, 1992), one of the main components of the practice is participation in research. Through this critical analysis of clinical practice, the pediatric rehabilitation nurse contributes to the field as well as his or her own professional growth. Inter- and intra-disciplinary research is essential for "the continuing development of knowledge and skills in the practice of nursing and rehabilitation" (ARN Pediatric Special Interest Group, 1992, p. 5).

The Advanced Practice Nurse in pediatric rehabilitation "uses research to discover, examine and evaluate knowledge, theories and creative approaches to health care" (ARN, 1996, p. 28). This includes the identification of significant issues and questions in clinical practice, critical evaluation of current practice in relation to research findings, and dissemination of findings through education and consultation. The Pediatric Rehabilitation Nurse may participate in research activities in any or all of the following ways depending on his or her education and level of expertise and practice:

- identify clinical problems and research questions
- participate in data collection
- share research activities
- conduct research
- critique research

At one rehabilitation hospital, the Nursing Research committee is composed of unit-based nurses as well as educators and an experienced researcher. The group identified a research question that dealt with intravenous therapy and changing of sites, critiqued the literature, developed a small study that was piloted by the nurses on two units, and used the results as the basis of an application for funding. Staff nurses participated in all aspects of the study and shared the information with others on the nursing units. Table 23–1 shows a comparison of the research role expectations as found in *Standards and Scope of Rehabilitation Nursing Practice* (ARN, 1994) and *Scope and Standards of Advanced Clinical Practice in Rehabilitation Nursing* (ARN, 1996).

As rehabilitation nurses at all levels move into new practice settings and roles and are involved in new and innovative models of care, their practice must incorporate the consistent integration of theoretical and practical research-based knowledge. Depending on the research skills of the nurse, this can include participating in collaborative projects or independent research. Inter-disciplinary research is very important because it allows the nurse to participate as part of a team and be identified as a knowledgeable and active member. Critical research competencies for pediatric rehabilitation nurses in advanced practice include interpreting research for others, using research in their practice, critically evaluating all aspects of practice, and conducting research.

> Advanced practice nurses should be able to use a variety of measures and methods to evaluate the effectiveness of nursing practice. Studies that document the effectiveness of specific advanced practice nursing interventions and identify outcome measures that are sensitive to nursing interventions are essential to validate the practice and obtain reimbursement for nurse managed care. (Steifbergen, 1996, p. 70)

CRITIQUING RESEARCH REPORTS

"If nursing practice is to be based on a solid foundation of scientific knowledge, the worth of studies appearing in the literature must be critically appraised" (Polit & Hungler, 1993, p. 380). A research critique is a careful appraisal of several aspects and dimensions of a piece of research. Each report includes the strengths and limitations, substantive and theoretical aspects, methodology, presentation, and style of the research. The reader must evaluate the importance of the study in terms of the significance of the problem, the appropriateness of the theoretical framework, and the application of the findings to clinical nursing practice. When reading an article about a research study, use the questions in Table 23–2 to guide the critical analysis and examine the research's relevance to actual nursing practice.

OVERVIEW OF THE RESEARCH PROCESS

Pediatric rehabilitation nurses practice in a variety of settings with children or adolescents and their families and are uniquely positioned to identify actual and potential problems and formulate researchable questions. The initial idea for a research study may begin with an intuitive feeling about a particular problem or it may develop after discussion and exploration with nursing colleagues and other members of the rehabilitation team. The nurse may wish to begin a research study but be unclear about the resources needed as well as his or her own strengths and weaknesses.

Table 23–1 COMPARISON OF RESEARCH ROLES

Pediatric Rehabilitation Nurse	Advanced Practice Pediatric Rehabilitation Nurse
Uses interventions based on research	Critically evaluates practice in light of research
Uses findings to develop guidelines for care	Identifies research questions
Participates in research committee or program	Disseminates research findings
Participates in research activities	Accountable for providing care based on research

Table 23-2 ARTICLE CRITIQUE

What is the underlying purpose of the study and the problem being examined?

Does the literature review describe the findings of key studies, weakness in existing studies, and important gaps in the literature?

Does the research report describe a theoretical or conceptual framework for the study?

What are the major strengths and limitations of the research design?

Are the target population and sample selection procedures described?

Who collected the data and under what conditions?

Does the report contain any evidence of the reliability of the data or the validity of the measures?

Do the statistics sufficiently describe the major characteristics of the data set?

Were the results of any statistical tests significant?

How relevant is the research to the actual practice of nursing?

How to Begin

The pediatric rehabilitation nurse who is working independently may need to begin by reading and critiquing articles in the professional journals, joining or forming a discussion group to stimulate ideas and explore opportunities in various practice areas, or establishing a relationship with a seasoned nurse researcher. Such a person can be identified through a variety of resources, both formal professional and informal nonprofessional, as shown in Table 23–3. "Write and

define your ideas. Be prepared with information before you approach the researcher with whom you are seeking a relationship" (Rempusheski, 1992, p. 107).

In pediatric rehabilitation clinical settings, more formal mechanisms may be available, such as nursing research committees, monthly presentations, research groups, and links with educational institutions. These groups are designed to stimulate interest in and promote awareness of research. When a research group is formed, a broad topic of interest to all members is identified and then narrowed to one that is more amenable to study and for which an adequate sample is available. This group may need to divide into smaller sections that are more practice based for discussion of actual projects.

Inter-disciplinary collaboration can also facilitate the development of questions and meet mutual research needs. In clinical practice settings where time and resources are limited, this pooling of talents distributes the workload. The pediatric rehabilitation nurse, who may lack some researcher attributes, can benefit from the knowledge and expertise of individuals from many disciplines, and from these collaborative efforts, even stronger programs can evolve.

Mentoring and Expert Consultants

The novice nurse researcher can benefit greatly from a relationship with a seasoned investigator who can act as a mentor. "Mentoring refers to guiding by example so that

Table 23-3 WHERE TO FIND A RESEARCHER

Sources	Forums	Situations	Settings
Formal/Professional			
Published directories Journals Conference proceedings Abstracts Newsletters Organizations, societies	Panels Conferences, seminars, workshops, meetings (local, regional, national, international)	Lectures (community or academic) Committee meetings	College or university Clinical sites: hospital, home health agency, nursing home Industry or business Research centers or institutes
Informal/Nonprofessional			
Media: newspaper or magazine articles Friends, relatives, neighbors, colleagues	Community or political hearings	Social gatherings Tours or holiday trips	Health club or gym Church Shopping mall, department store, or grocery store Jet or airport

Rempusheski, V. (1992). A researcher as resource, mentor, and preceptor. *Applied Nursing Research*, 5(2), 105–107. Copyright WB Saunders.

the novice can learn while taking part in some of the activities. Conducting the literature search, collecting data and helping to analyze data are other areas in which the less experienced person can perform" (Derstine & Edwards, 1991, p. 8). Look for an individual who is respected, preferably in the same specialty, and discuss with him or her the goals to be achieved and the research focus. A mentor can provide a source for networking, resources to assist the new nurse researcher, and research opportunities. Guidance with technical methodology and the process for entry into a setting to implement a study are also opportunities that can be provided by a mentor.

Expert consultants with knowledge of specific subject matter, statistics, or data analysis can be useful to the individual or the research group. These consultants can offer assistance in refining the survey tool and managing data. The consultant should have a role, that of expert advisor, and should not be involved in planning or conducting the research.

STEPS IN THE RESEARCH PROCESS

Conceptualizing, planning, and conducting research should be a systematic process that follows the following steps:

1. Intellectual conceptualization
2. Research plan and design
3. Data collection
4. Analysis and interpretation
5. Dissemination

These steps are outlined further in Table 23–4.

Step 1: Intellectual Conceptualization

Formulating and delimiting the problem is often the most difficult step, because beginning researchers are not knowledgeable about what constitutes a problem. Time spent deciding on the subject is very important to ensure that it is of interest to the people who will be involved in the study. Problems can be identified in the nursing literature and related theories as well as in clinical practice. It is wise to proceed from broad topic areas of interest to specific questions that can be studied. Some topics specific to pediatric rehabilitation nursing are found in Table 23–5. Nurse researchers ideally consider the following dimensions:

Substantive—Is this research question of theoretical or clinical significance?

Table 23–4 STEPS IN THE RESEARCH PROCESS

Step 1: Intellectual Conceptualization
Define the problem
Review relevant literature
Identify a theoretical framework
Develop hypothesis/researchable problem

Step 2: Research Plan/Design
Select a research approach
Specify the subjects
Determine procedures and interventions
Develop a sampling plan

Step 3: Data Collection
Gather data
Code data
Prepare computer program

Step 4: Analysis/Interpretation
Determine reliability and validity
Analyze data
Discern patterns/relationships
Interpret results
Examine implications of findings

Step 5: Dissemination
Prepare research report
Communicate findings
Plan for use of findings

Methodologic—How can this question best be studied?
Practical—Are adequate resources available to conduct a study?
Ethical—Can this question be studied in a manner consistent with guidelines for the protection of subjects? (Polit & Hungler, 1993, p. 37)

Literature relevant to the problem should be reviewed so that the study is an extension of previous research, builds on existing work, and provides a base for new knowledge. A literature review also provides a conceptual context and may assist the researcher in formulating and refining the problem under investigation. As the literature is reviewed, efforts should be made to identify an appropriate theoretical framework that relates to the problem to be addressed.

Theory is the ultimate aim of science in that it transcends the specifics of a particular time, place and group of people and aims to identify regularities in the relationships among variables. When research is performed within the context of a theoretical framework, it is more likely that its findings will have broad significance and utility. (Polit & Hungler, 1993, p. 37)

The problem for study can be refined in

Table 23–5   RESEARCH TOPICS BASED ON REHABILITATION NURSING FOUNDATION PRIORITIES

Health Promotion and Primary and Secondary Prevention to Facilitate Management of Self-Care and Independence for Persons With or at Risk for Chronic Illness and/or Disability
Will limiting spasticity enhance recovery after spinal cord injury?
Does management of constipation from infancy influence later continence in children with neurogenic bowel?
How does the cultural environment of the child and family affect health and wellness behaviors?
How does the provision of family support influence health and wellness behaviors?
Does teaching health promotion increase appropriate behaviors by adolescents with a disability or chronic illness?
What are the health and wellness behaviors practiced by parents of children with disabilities?

Interventions and Symptom Management for Persons With Disability to Maximize Function
Does expanding applications of the use of intrathecal baclofen for adolescents with spinal cord injury enhance their quality of life?
Does the use of intrathecal baclofen for adolescents with cerebral palsy improve self-care skills?
Which strategies are most effective for promoting wellness in the child with a neurologic disability?
What is the most cost-effective method for treating skin breakdown in children with disabilities?
Should the rehabilitation process be modified for adolescents with violence-induced disability?
Does use of assistance dogs improve quality of life for school-aged children with severe disabilities?
What is the impact of parent/child interventions on acquisition of autonomy skills in children with a disability or chronic illness?
Which interventions are most effective in managing adverse behavior in adolescents with brain injury?

Community Context of Care for Persons at Risk or With a Chronic Illness and/or Disability and Their Quality of Life
What effects do bladder management techniques have on quality of life and child development?
What are the educational needs of the home health care nurse relative to the rehabilitative care of children with disabilities and/or chronic conditions?
Does delegation of care by school nurses to non-licensed paraprofessionals result in increased health risk for children with disabilities in the schools?
Does participation in adaptive sports programs improve quality of life for children with disabilities?
Can the child or adolescent with a disability transfer newly learned skills to the home, school, and community environments?

Rehabilitation Nurse–Sensitive Outcomes and Costs in the Continuum of Care and the Interdisciplinary Setting
What common measures of outcomes should be used to compare findings across service settings and populations?
How does capitation affect the rehabilitation nursing care of children with disabilities in the community?
Which nursing interventions are the most effective in improving the functional outcomes of children with disabilities?
Which nursing interventions in the community are the most cost effective?
Is there a difference between comprehensive community-based and facility-based rehabilitation program outcomes?

Rehabilitation Practice and Roles in the Changing Health Care System
How are changing health-care priorities affecting the practice of pediatric rehabilitation nurses?
Is the use of case management in the community for the child with a disability or chronic condition and the family having a positive effect on outcomes?
What is the role of the independent pediatric rehabilitation nurse consultant in the changing health care system?
What will be the role of the pediatric rehabilitation nurse in interdisciplinary practice in the twenty-first century?

the form of a researchable question or hypothesis to guide the development of the research plan. The researcher's expectations about outcomes and the relationships that are expected as a result of the study are the basis for the hypothesis statement. This is a more formalized focus that predicts how the phenomena being investigated are related. Conversely, a simple question such as "Does management of constipation from infancy influence later continence in children with neurogenic bowel?" can be used as the focus of research.

Step 2: Research Plan and Design

After conceptualization, the researcher develops an overall plan for finding answers to the research questions or testing the research hypothesis. Decisions are made regarding methods to be used and the plan for the actual collection of data. The research design selected specifies the approaches that will be used and the types of comparisons that will be made. The design may be "experimental research (in which the researcher actively introduces some form of intervention)" or "non-experimental research (in which the researcher collects data without making any changes or introducing any treatments)" (Polit & Hungler, 1993, p. 38).

Specifying the population and determining the setting in which the study will take place are important parts of this research planning and design. Only a small portion of the population, referred to as the sample, are used as subjects. A method to collect the data is specified, outlining how the variables will be observed or measured; this may be through biophysiologic measurements, self-reports, or observational techniques. A plan is developed for selecting and recruiting the sample; this plan includes eligibility criteria and takes into account the representativeness, size, and elements of the sample that are specific to the study.

All aspects of the research plan are reviewed before actual implementation. A pilot study, which is a trial run of a major study, may be advisable to obtain information for assessing feasibility, improving design, or making revisions in the plan. As mentioned previously, a pilot study of the intravenous therapy research example was done to refine the data collection tool and provide additional information in seeking funding for the larger study.

Step 3: Data Collection

The collection of the research data proceeds according to the established plan, which specifies procedures for where, when, and how the data should be gathered. This can take place in a variety of settings: where subjects live, attend school, work, and participate in community activities; controlled laboratory settings; or hospital outpatient settings, depending on the problem and the population under consideration.

The data collected must be prepared for analysis through some preliminary steps. One is known as coding, or the process of transforming verbal data into categories or numeric form. A second step involves transferring the data from the written form to a computer program so that it can be analyzed by the researcher.

Step 4: Analysis and Interpretation

Various types of analysis and interpretation can occur during this step in the process. Analysis for validity (i.e., the degree to which an instrument measures what it is supposed to measure) and reliability (i.e., the degree of consistency of the measurement) of the instrument is useful in the interpretation of results. Various tests, such as descriptive statistics, t-tests (testing the statistical significance of a difference between the means of two groups), analysis of variance (ANOVA), and multi-variate analysis of variance (MANOVA), are used so that patterns and relationships can be discerned. ANOVA tests the significance of the difference between means, and MANOVA is an extension of this test to more than one dependent variable. The results must then be organized and interpreted in a systematic fashion, the implications of the findings examined within the broader context, and a determination made about the generalizability of the results.

Step 5: Dissemination

The results of a research study must be communicated to others and disseminated as widely as possible. This is an important part of the researcher's job, and the last step should not be considered completed until dissemination takes place and a plan is formulated for use of the results in the real world. The research report should include stated implications of the results for nursing practice and describe what the results mean for the care of children and their families. This information can be shared with others, especially the staff at the institution or agency that participated in the study. Also look at ways to apply the results to practice in different settings.

> Answer the call for abstracts for conferences and present your findings at local, state or national programs. It can be done in the form of an oral presentation of a paper or in a poster session. Obtain the publication guidelines from a number of journals and select those that best fit your topic. Submit your research for publication and enjoy seeing the results of your efforts in print. (Derstine & Edwards, 1991, p. 9)

These activities add to the body of knowledge, stimulate ideas for further investigation, generate interest and enthusiasm for the research process, and enhance the practice of nursing.

INTEGRATING RESEARCH AND PRACTICE

A conceptual framework for evaluating staff nurse activity in relation to nursing research was proposed by Killeen (1992) and is composed of four levels: valuing, understanding, practicing, and integrating. This framework can be used by educators and specialists endeavoring to implement a research utilization program. Initial activities involve presenting research literature at meetings where policies, procedures, and standards that affect nursing practice are discussed to foster awareness and commitment to research. Once the value of research-based practice is seen, it is important to involve staff in critiquing the research literature and determining its applicability to a particular setting. One tool to help evaluate research articles is presented in Table 23–2. After skills have been acquired, opportunities must be provided for practice and for integrating the new way of thinking into everyday activities. When practice problems or questions are identified, a process should be in place that bridges identification and resolution.

> The ultimate goal is to create a new mindset so that whenever a problem in practice is uncovered or whenever a staff nurse wonders 'Why am I doing this?' the question that immediately follows is 'What does the nursing research tell us?' then 'Can I apply data here?' and if so practice change occurs. (Guillett, 1995, p. 171)

According to Gift (1994), involving the nursing staff who are providing direct care in a research study provides the following benefits:

- opportunity to try an intervention before it is implemented in practice
- seeing the apparent advantages and pitfalls of the new routine or procedure
- having the opportunity to observe responses rather than reading a research report
- face-to-face communication helps the team develop into a social system with shared values
- time and process required allow staff to adjust to the innovation and observe its benefits
- outcomes are obvious and, if the procedure is well-liked and perceived to be beneficial, it is highly likely it will be adopted in practice (p. 306)

CURRENT RESEARCH TRENDS

In 1994 the Pediatric Special Interest Group of the Association of Rehabilitation Nurses surveyed its members to obtain demographic information and ascertain involvement in research activities. Thirty percent of the members ($n = 115$) responded to the survey, and of that group, 13% reported that they were currently participating in research. The broad areas of research included traumatic brain injury follow-up and outcomes, spinal cord injury causes and developmental outcomes, and community- and home-based care, as well as some more specific topics such as children's pain profile, caregiver burden, therapeutic play, and use of the baclofen pump (Edwards, 1995).

In 1994, the Rehabilitation Nursing Foundation (RNF) implemented a process to systematically identify rehabilitation nursing knowledge and its gaps and to prioritize the components of rehabilitation nursing that should be studied to achieve optimal outcomes of care. The initial stage of the process gathered information from a wide range of organization members and examined existing research-oriented organizational activities. The final stage "used experts to establish the final priorities using a technology-supported consensus process" (Gordon, Sawin, & Basta, 1996, p. 60). The five areas of research priority identified during this process are:

1. Health promotion and primary and secondary prevention to facilitate management of self-care and independence for

persons with or at risk for chronic illness or disability

2. Interventions and symptom management for persons with disability to maximize function

3. Community context of care for persons at risk for or with a chronic illness or disability and their quality of life

4. Rehabilitation nurse–sensitive outcomes and costs in the continuum of care and the interdisciplinary setting

5. Rehabilitation practice and roles in the changing health care system

Table 23–5 lists these research priorities and adds some questions for investigation derived from the literature specific to pediatric rehabilitation nursing. Many additional researchable questions can be formulated by nurses in professional practice in all pediatric rehabilitation settings.

FUNDING FOR RESEARCH

Financial support is often a major consideration that has an impact on the nurse's ability to propose and conduct research. The time and effort of the researchers and the resources of the organizations and agencies must be included in determining the cost of conducting the research. Whenever possible, funding should be sought to support the research endeavor.

At the federal level, various agencies that fund research studies exist, including the National Institute for Nursing Research. Request all the information available from the potential funding agency and target the grant specifically to the purpose and goals of the agency. Read the application over carefully and follow the step-by-step instructions for writing and submitting the proposal; these may also be the criteria that will be used to determine funding. It may also be helpful to meet with key people at the agency, either in person or by phone. Consultants with expertise in the research subject or methodology and statistical analysis can assist with both the application process and the data analysis. Having an experienced, doctorally prepared nurse researcher involved in the study may also be necessary. Do not be discouraged if the study is not approved and funded the first time it is submitted; many applications are submitted several times before funding. Use the reviewers' comments to strengthen the application for the next submission. Do not be dismayed by the amounts of money

that may be offered. Often a grant of $1000 to $3000 U.S. is enough to get started, and the nurse can continue from that point.

When seeking private funding, it is wise to begin with institutions or agencies that will support and benefit from the research. There may be funds and in-kind support available for a pilot study as well as the entire project. Because many organizations and agencies have personnel to support grant applications and funding, it is important to check to see if these resources are available to assist with the nursing research proposal. Professional and local organizations and community groups can also be sources for funding, especially if the research results have particular relevance for them. Grant funding is available through the Rehabilitation Nursing Foundation and other nursing and specialty organizations such as the American Nurses Foundation, Association of Spinal Cord Injury Nurses, and Sigma Theta Tau. It is also possible to obtain information about foundations and corporations through directories and computer searches. It is often possible to request a copy of the agency's annual report, a list of the grants awarded in the past, and guidelines and deadlines for submission of grant proposals (Derstine & Edwards, 1991). Follow the agency's guidelines, which may be as simple as a letter of intent describing the project or as complex as a proposal that is as detailed as those submitted to government agencies.

SUBMITTING TO AN INSTITUTIONAL REVIEW BOARD

Most hospitals, universities and other institutions where research is conducted have established formal committees and protocols for reviewing research plans and proposed research procedures. These committees are sometimes called human subjects committees or research advisory panels. If the institution receives federal funds that help to pay the costs of the research, it is likely that the committee will be an Institutional Review Board (IRB). (Polit & Hungler, 1993, p. 365)

According to federal regulations, an IRB must have five or more members, including one non-researcher and one person who has no affiliation with the institution. The IRB cannot be composed solely of one gender and must have members from more than one profession to safeguard against the possibility of bias.

IRBs are the institution's conscience, and they are very concerned with human rights and dignity. "The principles of patient autonomy and rights of privacy, confidentiality, anonymity, self-determination and safety are critical components of their philosophical statements" (Munhall & Boyd, 1993, p. 410). When preparing to submit to an IRB, obtain the institution's guidelines and follow the outlined process as precisely as possible. This may be time consuming, but it will help expedite the review process and ensure that all the information is communicated clearly and completely. The wording of the proposal should be specific and written clearly, and the value of the research to the goals of the organization should be suggested. If written approval is needed from specific people within the organization, it should be acquired and the forms included with the proposal. If you are expected to present your proposal to the IRB, consider it a valuable chance to discuss your research study. Anticipate the questions that might be asked and have additional details and support information available for the IRB to examine and review.

ETHICS AND NURSING RESEARCH

In recent years the increase in research involving human subjects has evoked concern regarding the protection of the rights of those who participate in the studies. "Ethical concerns are especially prominent in the field of nursing because the line of demarcation between what constitutes the expected practice of nursing and the collection of research information has become less distinct as research by nurses increases" (Polit & Hungler, 1993, p. 353). When human subjects are involved in research, care must be taken to ensure that their rights are protected and that fundamental ethical principles are upheld. One of these principles contains two dimensions: freedom from harm and freedom from exploitation. When conducting research, the risks and benefits incurred during the study must be carefully assessed. The risk-benefit ratio should consider whether the risk to the human subjects is commensurate with the benefit to the nursing profession and society and in terms of the scientific knowledge gained from the study.

Another ethical principle, the right to self-determination and full disclosure, respects the dignity of the human subjects. Potential subjects must be fully informed about the purpose of the research, the expectations of participants, and the costs and benefits of the research so they can make thoughtful decisions about their participation. "Informed

consent means that the subjects have adequate information regarding the research; are capable of comprehending the information; and have the power of free choice, enabling them to consent voluntarily to participate in the research or decline participation" (Polit & Hungler, 1993, p. 360).

The rights of special populations also need to be considered and require the researcher to have heightened sensitivity. Children and people with physical disabilities are considered especially vulnerable, and nurse researchers must keep the ethical principles foremost in their minds and respect the subjects' right to privacy and fair treatment as studies are proposed and conducted. These potential human subjects may not be capable of giving informed consent or may be at risk of unintended effects because of their disability or chronic condition. Although parents or guardians provide consent for minors, children should be informed in a way that is appropriate given their age and cognitive level. When possible, they should be involved in the consent process.

SUMMARY

As we move forward into a new era of health care initiatives, pediatric rehabilitation nurses are discovering new roles and innovative partnerships. During this exciting period, knowledge discovery must continue to be foremost in nurses' minds as they commit to conducting research and to using these discoveries to improve the health of children and their families, to teach better, and to administer more effectively. Nurses are in a position to demonstrate and reinforce the value of research by sharing findings with the rehabilitation team and providing assistance in applying findings to clinical practice. "Intelligence, energy and interest are enough for a good start; fuel the fire with participation and dissemination so the research flame burns bright in nursing's future" (Derstine & Edwards, 1994, p. 213).

REFERENCES

Association of Rehabilitation Nurses. (1994). *Standards and scope of rehabilitation nursing practice.* Skokie, IL: Association of Rehabilitation Nurses.
Association of Rehabilitation Nurses. (1996). *Scope and standards of advanced clinical practice in rehabilitation nursing.* Glenview, IL: Association of Rehabilitation Nurses.
Association of Rehabilitation Nurses Pediatric Spe-

cial Interest Group. (1992). *Pediatric rehabilitation nursing role description*. Skokie, IL: Association of Rehabilitation Nurses.

Derstine, J., & Edwards, P. (1991). Make research an integral part of your practice. *Rehability, 4*(2), 8–9.

Derstine, J., & Edwards, P. (1994). Using available resources to implement research. *Gastroenterology Nursing,* (4), 210–214.

Edwards, P. (1995). Pediatric Special Interest Group survey results. *ARN News,* 11(1), 4–5.

Gift, A. (1994). Nursing research utilization. *Clinical Nurse Specialist,* 8(6), 306.

Guillett, S. (1995) The role of staff development in creating a research-based practice environment. *Journal of Nursing Staff Development,* 11(3), 170–172.

Gordon, D., Sawin, K., & Basta, S. (1996). Developing research priorities for rehabilitation nursing. *Rehabilitation Nursing Research,* 5(2), 60–66.

Killeen, M. (1992). Organizational guidelines for RN research behaviors. Michigan Nurse, 65(11), 6–7.

Munhall, P., & Boyd, C. (1993). *Nursing research: a qualitative perspective* (2nd ed.). New York: National League for Nursing Press.

Polit, D., & Hungler, B. (1993). *Essentials of nursing research: methods, appraisal and utilization* (3rd ed.). Philadelphia: JB Lippincott.

Prichard, L., Norville, R., Oakes, L., Gattusa, J., & Howard, V. (1994). The natural connection: the CNS and bedside nursing research. *Clinical Nurse Specialist,* 8(6), 307–310.

Rempusheski, V. (1992). A researcher as resource, mentor and preceptor. *Applied Nursing Research,* 5(2), 105–107.

Steifbergen, A. (1996) Advanced practice nursing and research. *Rehabilitation Nursing Research,* 5(3), 70.

ADDITIONAL RESOURCES

Dickenson-Hazard, N. (1994). Executive officer's message. *Reflections,* Fall, 2.

Hockenberry-Eaton, M. (1992) Nursing research—moving forward through networking, collaboration and mentorship. *Journal of Pediatric Oncology Nursing,* 9(3), 132–135.

Sibley, P. (1991). Mentoring: implications for the new research investigator. *SCI Nursing,* 8(2), 53–54.

Sidoni, S. (1991). Mentoring the novice nurse researcher. *Journal of Pediatric Nursing,* 6(1), 57–59.

Wells, N., & Baggs, J. (1994). A survey of practicing nurses' research interests and activities. *Clinical Nurse Specialist,* 8(3), 145–151.

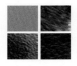

Chapter 24

Advanced Nursing Practice

Susanne R. Hays and *Patricia A. Edwards*

At a time when market forces are downsizing hospitals and eliminating professional nurse positions and patient acuity with the essential need for sophisticated nursing judgment is very high, patients are being discharged earlier in their recovery. In increasing numbers these patients are under-served in the community because of basic health care access problems and lack of professionals with the knowledge and skills to provide the necessary services. In this uncertain climate of health care reform, Advanced Practice Nurses (APN) can be an important part of the solution (Cukr, 1996). All these issues must be viewed in terms of the changing health care environment, the development of new practice sites, and the changing populations of both clients and the health care work force.

This chapter describes the evolution of advanced practice from the role of nurse-clinician, through the roles of clinical specialist and nurse practitioner, to the current scope of advanced clinical practice specific to pediatric rehabilitation nursing. Other current models are included and specific examples given of the APN as entrepreneur and consultant.

ADVANCED PRACTICE NURSE

Role Evolution

In 1943, Frances Reiter suggested the role of nurse-clinician, which included three clinical practice aspects: "(1) clinical competence in the dimensions of depth of understanding, range of function, and breadth of services; (2) clinical expertise for coordination of and responsibility for continuity of care; and (3)

professional maturity in collaboration with the medical profession" (Lynch, 1996, p. 1). At the same time, the National League for Nursing Education recommended the development of a curriculum to educate advanced clinical nurses at the master's level. A shift began to occur in nursing preparation, from the functional role to one which involved knowledge and competency in all clinical nursing areas.

In the 1960s, the first Nurse Practitioner (NP) program was developed with an emphasis on health promotion and disease prevention for children. Recently the term "advanced nursing practice" has been applied to a number of roles in nursing, most notably the Clinical Nurse Specialist (CNS) and the Nurse Practitioner (NP), and there has been an impetus to combine these into a single practitioner. The Advanced Practice Nurse (APN) would have a broad perspective of the care delivery system as well as the community in which care is provided (Davies & Hughes, 1995). In 1992, the National Council of State Boards of Nursing and the American Nurses Association recommended merging the roles of CNS and NP into that of APN. It was anticipated that this would create the following benefits: "generate control in the practice of nursing; simplify the concept of the role for consumers and practice sites; and engender greater political visibility" (Lynch, 1996, p. 2).

From their inception, the CNS and NP roles had very different perspectives and goals. The CNS role was originally designed to assist in preparing staff nurses for clinical practice quality using staff development approaches. The CNS brought specialty nursing knowledge and expertise to the patient's bedside and used skills in consultation, patient education, system analysis, and research to enhance care and improve outcomes (Cukr, 1996; Lynch, 1996). The NP role was focused on direct primary health care for patients outside of the hospital setting to increase access to health care services and promote community-based continuity of care. Today NP care includes accurate and timely problem identification, differential diagnosis, and the development of diagnostic, therapeutic, and educational plans in collaboration and consultation with other health care providers (Cukr, 1996).

Models

Five models of advanced nursing practice are described by Williams and Valdivieso (1994):

Additive Model—one role is added to another: CNS + NP = APN
Dual Pathways Model—CNS and NP preparation are separate but equal ways for nurses to achieve advanced practice
Overlapping Roles Model—both unique and shared areas of practice with both core and specialty content
Subsumed Role Model—NP skills are integrated in CNS program, or vice versa
Blended Role Model—roles and competencies of NP and CNS blend and boundaries are blurred

Characteristics and Competencies

Certain characteristics were identified by Davies and Hughes (1995) as necessary for the advanced practice nursing role: "risk taking, vision, flexibility, articulateness, inquisitiveness and ability to lead" (p. 157). Areas of competence essential for the APN were "clinical expertise, critical thinking and analysis, clinical judgment and decision making, leadership and management, communication, problem solving, collaboration, education and research and program development" (Davies & Hughes, 1995, p. 157).

Roles

Nursing roles at the advanced practice level that currently exist to provide care for children or to provide rehabilitation nursing care are: Pediatric Nurse Practitioner (American Nurses Credentialing Center, 1996); Clinical Specialist, which has recently been described as Advanced Clinical Practice in Rehabilitation Nursing (Association of Rehabilitation Nurses [ARN], 1996); Primary Care NP in family and child nursing (Brown, 1996); APN in care of children with special health and developmental needs; CNS as Case Manager of the chronically ill child (Smith, 1994); Nurse Practitioners/Clinical Managers for children with complex chronic illness (Medicaid Working Group, 1993); and CNS role as Family-Centered Nurse Coordinator—Early Childhood Intervention (Lund, 1994). Complete information about these roles and their characteristics, functions and educational preparation can be found in the references cited for each.

ADVANCED PRACTICE IN PEDIATRIC REHABILITATION NURSING

In light of these evolving roles and the trend to merge the NP and CNS roles, the following is proposed as a description of an Advanced Practice Pediatric Rehabilitation Nurse (APPRN) that includes the scope of practice, standards, and educational preparation for this new role.

Advanced Practice Nurses in pediatric rehabilitation share key characteristics and a common core of knowledge with other advanced clinical practice nurses. These include: increased complexity in clinical decision making, greater skill in managing environments, diagnosing and prescribing, and practice autonomy.

Role

Advanced Practice Pediatric Rehabilitation Nurses have an in-depth knowledge base and the requisite skills to provide care to children or adolescents and their families who are affected by disability or a chronic condition. The scope of practice "is distinguished by the level of autonomy of their practice, the dominance of nurse-initiated treatment regimens, the complexity of cases or situations they manage, and the leadership they provide within the interdisciplinary team" (ARN, 1996, p. 9). The preparation necessary for this level of practice is acquired in a graduate nursing program that integrates the role of the APN both in pediatrics, with an emphasis on developmental disabilities, and in rehabilitation.

The domains of APPRN include patient care management, coordination, consultation and education, quality improvement and research, and administration and management. "Common to all of these domains is the ability to provide leadership, work effectively with interdisciplinary teams, and integrate various components in different ways at different times, as the situation demands" (ARN, 1996, p. 6).

Standards

The Standards of Care for the APPRN are those described in the *Scope and Standards of Advanced Clinical Practice in Rehabilitation Nursing* (ARN, 1996), but the client receiving the care is a child or adolescent with a disability or chronic condition and his or her family. Six standards describe the elements of the nursing process: assessment, diagnosis, outcome identification, planning, implementation, and evaluation. Included within the standard on implementation are the specific areas of case management and coordination of care, consultation, health promotion, health maintenance and health teaching, prescriptive authority, and referral.

The APPRN also adheres to the Standards of Professional Performance, which include the following:

- developing criteria for and evaluating quality and effectiveness of care
- evaluating practice in relation to standards and regulations and providing competent care
- acquiring current knowledge and maintaining skills in the practice area
- serving as a leader, team member, and role model
- integrating ethical principles in practice
- using research in critically evaluating practice and providing evidence-based care

Education

A program of study at the graduate level provides a foundation in the clinical expertise needed for nurses planning to provide pediatric and rehabilitative care to children and adolescents with disabilities and chronic conditions and their families. Courses include nursing theory, moral and ethical issues, research, health assessment, and management of acute illnesses as well as specific disabilities and chronic conditions. Specific topics and areas of study are shown in Table 24–1.

The clinical component should provide supervised clinical activities and precepted ex-

Table 24–1 EDUCATIONAL PROGRAM CONTENT

Theories from Physical, Behavioral, and Social Sciences

Anatomy
Pathophysiology
Epidemiology
Nursing science
Medical science
Nutrition
Family systems
Growth and development

Professionalism in Advanced Practice Nursing

Advanced practice nursing role
Standards
Legal parameters
Credentialing
Peer review
Prescriptive authority
Research participation and utilization
Quality assessment and risk management

Decision Making and Clinical Management Process

Data-gathering techniques
Developmental assessment
Health promotion and management
Consultation and referral
Ethical considerations
Cultural sensitivity and diversity
Team functioning
Management of acute problems, chronic conditions, and disabilities

Health Policy and Organizational Issues

Access to care
Delivery systems
Case management and managed care
Organizational management
Health care economics
Advocacy
Practice management

periences that include research utilization, assessment and management, and technical decision-making skills needed for optimal functioning as an APPRN. Nurses functioning in this role could have a tremendous impact on the provision of community-based, family-centered care to children with disabilities and chronic conditions and their families.

ADVANCED PRACTICE NURSE AS ENTREPRENEUR

An entrepreneur is defined in Webster's dictionary (1958) as "one who assumes the risk and management of business." The characteristics of an entrepreneur as presented by Calmelat (1993) include: financially able to live without a steady income for at least 1 year; highly developed clinical and organizational skills; access to capital for start-up if necessary; commitment from spouse and children; and positive working relationship with a physician who is willing to work as a consultant or collaborator. It is believed that finding a niche, having the ability to recognize it, and having the knowledge, skills, resources, creativity, and commitment to yourself and others are also much needed characteristics for entrepreneurship.

Nurses going into business for themselves have been described in many ways: crazy, following an impossible dream, stupid, and high on energy and short on brains, as well as creative, innovative, powerful, highly skilled, and respected in their communities. Actually, at one moment or another, all these definitions may apply. But many nurses are saying "So what? Nothing ventured, nothing gained." A nurse who asks a seasoned entrepreneur about their business and then starts wondering about starting one is told that if he or she wants a challenge in developing autonomy, go ahead, but make sure there is lots of support, resilience, and commitment to the vision.

Nurses, who are predominantly female, have had the misfortune of being thought of as being in a second-rate profession and one that only fills the gaps between high school and marriage with children, and from the time when children leave home until retirement. In other words, it has been thought that nurses are not really committed to the profession of nursing, just using skills and education for a second paycheck. These perceptions are obviously not true, for as managed care sweeps the nation, the APN is being placed in mid-level management and providing primary care, not only in the community but also in the hospital.

Starting the Business

When starting out, first review the state's Nurse Practice Act regarding the rules and regulations and any restrictions that would affect the nursing business. It is possible that the first activity necessary might be getting the Nurse Practice Act changed through legislation to allow a nurse in an independent nursing practice; however, this is already legal in most states.

To start the business, the nurse may take classes in small business, access a mentor or other nurses who are already in business to provide support, seek advice from the local small business association, or go to the library. Information about types of businesses, legal issues, tax issues, developing a marketing plan, and developing a financial plan are all readily available.

The next tasks are to identify the kind of service to be provided or the type of business, decide on the type of company (e.g., sole proprietorship, partnership, incorporation), and select a name for the business. Two professionals that should be hired initially to assist in the start-up are an accountant or bookkeeper and an attorney with experience in small business law in your state. Additionally, it is important to open a separate bank account for the business and obtain malpractice insurance that covers a nurse in private practice.

Other professionals who could be of service and would be valuable resources are bankers and advertising specialists, including those who can assist with development and production of materials for the public (e.g., newspaper releases, cards, brochures, pamphlets that describe the business).

Models of Independent Nursing Practice

Many types of independent nursing practice are possible. There are nurse-owned, free-standing clinics and birthing centers; nurses in private practice providing primary and specialty care; nurse inventors; nurse-owned businesses providing case management resources; agencies for training and education of nurses and other health care providers; and nurses providing legal consultation and acting as expert witness in their area of specialty. Basically, the sky is the limit when it comes to nurses being entrepreneurs, as long as the laws are clear and the public is being protected.

One example is the nursing center model. The National League for Nursing (NLN) states that a Community Nursing Center is one in which the primary management position is held by a nurse, the nursing staff are responsible and accountable for professional practice and the care received by clients, and the nurses are the primary care providers for the center's clients. It is both a setting where clients visit and a concept that shapes the broader services provided by nurses in various practice arrangements in the home, community, hospital, nursing home, or any site across the health care continuum.

The types of Community Nursing Centers that currently exist include:

- community outreach—freestanding community public health centers
- an institution based as part of a hospital, university, or corporation
- wellness, health promotion, and health maintenance services providing screening, education, counseling, and triage
- private, independent nursing practice (Lockhart, 1995)

A study by Watson (1996) profiled the structure and function of nursing centers and the differences based on academic versus non-academic settings. The factors examined included:

- funding and fees
- organizational structure
- time elements
- demographics
- services
- qualifications and categories of staff
- functions of staff
- research endeavors
- major barriers
- major sources of support (p. 74)

One notable difference was the amount of time they had been in operation, with only 16% of the academic centers reporting more than 10 years versus 50% of the non-academic centers.

Nurses in advanced practice considering starting a nursing center should be sure to use an inter-disciplinary approach and include the community in all the planning stages. The timing is right to consider filling the gap in U.S. health care, and APNs must educate the public and legislators about the cost-effective, health promotion services they can provide, especially to children and adolescents with disabilities and chronic conditions and their families.

The following is one nurse entrepreneur's description of her personal experiences.

PERSONAL EXPERIENCE

Susanne R. Hays, MS, RN, CRRN, CCM

As a nurse specialist in pediatric rehabilitation, I left a position I had held for many years with a large pediatric rehabilitation unit in Southern California. I came to New Mexico because that is where I wanted to live. Originally, I had a job at a university working with other professionals on a developmental disabilities evaluation team that was funded by many grants. As funding got tighter and I spent more time writing grants, I became more and more aware that I missed the ongoing contact with children with disabilities or chronic illness and their families. I also became aware that families in my care were seeking resources to assist them with their children's feeding, growth, and toilet-training needs. This seemed to be an unfilled niche, and I had skills and knowledge to provide intervention and teaching in those areas. The next question was, who would pay me to do what I really wanted to do in nursing? I went to the only home health agency in the community and sought a contract like the one obtained by a speech therapist who also had a contract with the agency. Those at the agency were visionary enough to finally say "Yes." That was 1983, and to this day I still get reimbursed through that agency for seeing children who have Medicaid.

As I started to develop my sole proprietorship, I continued to work at my other job for 4 days a week. Since I was single, I felt I needed to keep my salary and benefits. As I gradually got various contracts, I cut back my other job to 50% to keep my benefits. Finally, because of the medico-legal work that I was doing and my client caseload, I was able to quit my job at the university. I have now been in full-time private practice for 8 years, and I continue to see new possibilities for my business. I am here to tell you that it has not always been easy, but it sure has been interesting and rewarding.

Possible Barriers

Nurses can be their own worst enemies when it comes to removing internal barriers and making a decision to become an entrepreneur. For too long, many nurses have believed that they are not capable of being independent and do not deserve to be in business, and therefore they sit back, taking orders from a doctor and not realizing their own potential.

Realistically, there may be many barriers when it comes to reimbursement for services. Medicare, Medicaid, Federal Employee Health Benefit Programs (FEHBP), Civilian Health and Medical Program of the Uniformed Services (CHAMPUS), private health insurance programs, and managed care programs each have their own rules for reimbursement regarding fees, services, and the providers they will reimburse for services. Many clients are also willing to pay out-of-pocket for specialty nursing services that fill their particular needs and are not covered by their health care insurance.

CASE STUDY

A nurse saw the need for her advanced practice skills in the area of management of feeding problems while doing teaching rounds with staff nurses on a pediatric unit. The particular situation involved an infant who had been born with a unilateral cleft of the lip and palate and no other defects. He was 3 months old and weighed only 0.5 kg above his birth weight. He had been admitted because of poor growth and was being evaluated for failure to thrive. His mother was very stressed and felt she had not been able to nourish her infant adequately.

After assessment, the APN made a specific modification to the nipple being used to feed the infant, taught his mother how to use the new feeding system, and recommended that his slightly red tympanic membranes be treated with medication. Within a week, he had gained 1 pound.

After doing some investigating, the nurse learned that there was no specific protocol for teaching families how to feed infants born with cleft lips and palates and no consistent plan for nursing follow-up in the community. The agency for which the APN was currently working did not feel that using those specific skills fit into her job description and was not willing to allow her to expand her role to meet the need. She decided to present a proposal to Children's Medical Services (CMS), the agency responsible for payment of services for children born with defects. This proposal included information gathered from the specific situation seen on the pediatric unit and included costs of medical care and hospitalization. It also included the cost of using the APN to provide nursing intervention for the infant as a newborn, thus preventing the need for payment of services related to complications when no specific feeding program was established.

CMS could see this as a cost-saving project and also realized that providing intervention for the newborn supported one of their program goals, which was prevention of further complications for children with congenital defects. CMS was very interested in working out payment for such services and requested that the APN obtain a Medicaid provider number. This could have been a hurdle for the nurse, because in her state Medicaid gave provider numbers only to NPs and she was a nurse specialist. Instead of feeling defeated, the nurse decided to try contracting with a home health agency for payment and also to start working with a group of nurse specialists to get the Medicaid rules changed in her state as well as getting the title of APN included in the nurse practice act.

The home health agency was very agreeable and a contract was worked out for payment. The changes in legislation to permit all nurses in advanced practice access to payment through Medicaid as well as other managed care payment resources is currently being presented to the state legislature.

ADVANCED PRACTICE NURSE AS CONSULTANT

In the *Advanced Practice Standards of Care*, a subset of the section on "Implementation" deals with consultation and states that "the APN in rehabilitation provides consultation to influence the plan of care for clients, enhance the abilities of others, and effect change in the system." (ARN, 1996, p. 17). In this context, consultation occurs when a nurse with appropriate expertise assists in resolving problems, either directly or through others. For example, when a child with a severe disability is being discharged from the hospital, an APPRN may consult with the nurses who will provide care in the home and school to assist in the formulation of a plan and instruct in techniques and procedures essential to the well being of the child or adolescent and family.

Models

Parent partnership models (Robards, 1994) provide another method for professional consultation. These range from the expert model, in which professionals with expertise assess and treat, to the emerging model of empowerment, in which the parents have control, responsibility, and power and their strengths are recognized. The type of consultation provided in each of these models will change as the nurse's emphasis is switched from being an expert to participating with the family and the child in the overall assessment and planning for services.

Another model for the APN is that of management consultant. This type of consultation, instead of being clinical practice–and child and family—focused, includes services of an individual or group to increase the effectiveness of an organization. In many aspects, consulting is an intellectual entrepreneurship, requiring the consultant to have a high achievement orientation and an ability and willingness to assume personal risk. The type of consultation provided may be "expert," in which the consultant identifies and solves problems without involving staff, or "process," in which organization members are an integral part of the activity and the consultant is the advisor. In both types of consultation, there is no magic cure for the problems, and the consultant has no direct authority but rather is dependent on members of the organization (Berger, Ray, & Togno-Armanasco, 1993). Key qualities for success in management consulting include the ability to communicate compellingly in both oral and written form, be sensitive to human interaction and organizational process, integrate information to produce clear and coherent insights into complex issues, and sustain high levels of physical and mental energy.

Client-Consultant Relationship

An important issue is the client-consultant relationship, "a partnership created when the client's investment in the consultant's unique combination of abilities equals the consultant's investment in the client's unique combination of opportunities. To achieve mutual satisfaction the client and consultant must develop a relationship based on respect and trust" (Berger, Ray, & Togno-Armanasco, 1993, p. 65). The consultation, which takes place over time, involves identification of need by the organization, selection of a consultant and the scope of activity, implementation, and evaluation and termination. Throughout the process, maintaining communication is essential to the success of the consultation. Continual feedback and an open exchange of information must occur during each of the phases, and at the termination of the contract there is a review of the accomplishments and recommendations for further change.

The following is a nurse consultant's description of her personal experiences.

PERSONAL EXPERIENCE

Patricia A. Edwards, EdD, RN, CNAA

Successful administrative consultation is a rewarding and challenging task. Over a period of years, I have provided both internal consultation as an "expert" staff member and external consultation as a nurse with advanced practice in administration to an outside agency. For me, the key to professional consulting success was in the three "C"s: concern, competency, and candor. It is always important to have a successful, trusting relationship with the client. Three areas must be considered when asked to consult: the initial contact and consulting environment, contractual issues, and process and procedures.

1. Initial Contact and Consulting Environment

When a call from a client comes in, listen to his or her individual needs. Set up a meeting to get to know each other. Pre-plan the initial meeting by getting information about the institution and the background of the individuals involved in the consultation. Allow a minimum of 2 hours for discussion of background of the problem and the organization's needs and readiness for change and intervention. Ask the organization to cover your expenses. During that initial meeting:

AFFIRM the factual situation and any background information or hidden issues. Examine values and assumptions about people and work.
PROBE: delineate difficulties, problems, and dissatisfactions with current situation.
UNCOVER implications, effects, and consequences of change.
DETERMINE the value, need, and importance of the activity.

2. Contractual Considerations

Have a written contract for the services that you will provide that establishes specific deliverables and the time commitment. Be sure you have covered the organization's explicit needs and concerns and summarized the anticipated benefits. Do not pre-price your services or demonstrate your capability too soon, and never assume that the initially stated problem is *"the* problem." When pricing your services, be aware of the hourly rate of comparable consultants and consider the value of the service to the client.

3. Process and Procedures

Problem definition and data collection are similar to the problem-solving process. Strategies include surveys with follow-up feedback sessions, focus groups, force field analysis, one-on-one or group interviews, brainstorming sessions, and nominal group sessions. Problem identification requires appropriate allocation of tasks, sufficient time for a thorough examination of the issues, and established time frames for completion.

After the data have been gathered and a tentative organizational diagnosis made, goals are established and a course of action is determined, as is a specific ongoing evaluation plan. Action is taken, and the plan is implemented. A continuous feedback loop should be established to provide all participants with information about what is or is not working to allow revision of the action plan and mobilization or reorganization of available resources. The consultation is complete when the goals and the terms of the contract have been met. Formal closure of the process should occur at a final meeting to discuss the consultation process and accomplishments. A formal evaluation and a written report on the process should be provided to the management team.

In my consulting experiences, I have enjoyed the interactions and the stimulation of organizational problem solving. I have also learned a great deal through research, opportunities to be inspired both personally and intellectually, and planning strategic and creative solutions to address complex issues.

PROFESSIONAL LIABILITY

The advanced practice role brings greater accountability and responsibility as well as risk and professional liability as nurses practice in settings that involve more independent judgment. The best protection is a safe, effective practice according to professional standards of care. However, other risk-management strategies include having adequate liability insurance and formulation of specific contracts to cover services provided by the APN. When considering purchase of a liability policy, consider the practice role and setting as well as the components of the policy and the adequacy of the scope of professional actions covered. When developing contracts, it may

be helpful to seek legal counsel so that the document delineates responsibilities and outcomes and protects against possible negative situations (Scott & Beare, 1993).

SUMMARY

It is exciting, creative, and challenging for a nurse to be in advanced practice while the health care system is being reformed. The shift in "both the population in need of care and the motivation of the new workers within the caregiving community creates an opportunity for nurses to develop workplace 2000 into a person-oriented, caring environment" (Donley, 1995, p. 87). The leadership of APNs as specialists in pediatric rehabilitation, entrepreneurs, and consultants may be a key component in the provision of quality care to children and adolescents with disabilities or chronic conditions and their families and in enhancing health care outcomes.

REFERENCES

American Nurses Credentialing Center (ANCC). (1996). *Certification guidelines*. Washington, DC: ANCC.

Association of Rehabilitation Nurses (ARN). (1996). *Scope and standards of advanced clinical practice in rehabilitation nursing*. Glenview, IL: ARN.

Berger, M., Ray, L., & Togno-Armanasco, V. (1993). The effective use of consultants. *Journal of Nursing Administration*, 23(7/8), 65–69.

Brown, M. (1996). Primary care nurse practitioners: don't blend the colors in the rainbow of advanced practice nursing. *Online Journal of Issues in Nursing*, On-line], Aug. 1, pp.1–10. Available: http://www.nursingworld.org/ojin/tpc1 E6.htm

Calmelat, A. (1993). Tips for starting your own nurse practitioner practice. *Nurse Practitioner*, 18(4), 58–68.

Cukr, P. (1996). Viva la difference! The nation needs both types of advanced practice nurses: clinical nurse specialists and nurse practitioners. *Online Journal of Issues in Nursing* [On-line], June 15, pp. 1–8. Available: http://www.nursingworld.org/ojin/tpc1 E4.htm

Davies, B., & Hughes, A.M. (1995). Clarification of advanced nursing practice: characteristics and competencies. *Clinical Nurse Specialist*, 9(3), 156–160.

Donley, R. (1995). Advanced practice nursing after health care reform. *Nursing Economics*, 13(2), 84–88.

Lockhart, C. (1995). Community nursing centers: an analysis of status and needs. In B. Murphy (Ed.). *Nursing centers: the time is now*. New York: National League for Nursing Press.

Lund, S. (1994). Family-centered nurse coordinator—early childhood intervention: development and implementation of the CNS role. *Clinical Nurse Specialist*, 8(2), 109–114.

Lynch, A. (1996). At the crossroads: we must blend the CNS and NP roles. *Online Journal of Issues in Nursing* (On-line), June 15, pp. 1–6. Available: www.nursingworld.org/ojin

Medicaid Working Group. (1993). *Nurse practitioners as clinical managers*. Boston: Medicaid Working Group.

Robards, M. (1994). *Running a team for disabled children and their families*. London: MacKeith Press.

Scott, L., & Beare, P. (1993). Nurse consultant and professional liability. *Clinical Nurse Specialist*, 7(6), 331–334.

Smith, L. (1994). Continuity of care through nursing case management of the chronically ill child. *Clinical Nurse Specialist*, 8(2), 65–68.

Watson, L. (1996). A national profile of nursing centers. *Nurse Practitioner*, 21(3), 72, 74, 79–80.

Webster's new collegiate dictionary, p. 275. (1958). Springfield, MA: G&C Merriam.

Williams, C., & Valdivieso, G. (1994). Advanced practice models: a comparison of clinical nurse specialist and nurse practitioner activities. *Clinical Nurse Specialist*, 8(6), 311–318.

ADDITIONAL RESOURCES

Association of Rehabilitation Nurses (ARN) Pediatric Special Interest Group. (1992). *Pediatric rehabilitation nursing role description*. Skokie, IL: ARN.

Blouin, A., & Brent, N. (1995). The nurse entrepreneur: legal aspects of owning a business. *Journal of Nursing Administration*, 25(6), 13–14.

Considine, R., Hughes, V., & Bloniarz, B. (1994). The development of CNS consultation forms. *Clinical Nurse Specialist*, 8(3), 168–172.

Crofts, A. (1994). Entrepreneurship: the realities of today. *Journal of Nurse Midwifery*, 39(1), 39–42.

Dougherty, A. (1990). *Consultation practice and perspectives*. Pacific Grove, CA: Brooks/Cole.

Hamric, A., Spross, J., & Hanson, C. (1996). *Advanced nursing practice: an integrative approach*. Philadelphia: WB Saunders.

Jackson, P. (1992). The primary care provider and children with chronic conditions. In P. Jackson & J. Vessey (Eds.). *Primary care of the child with a chronic condition*. Boston: Mosby–Year Book, pp. 3–11.

Mittelstadt, P. (1993). *How to get paid for your advanced practice nursing services: the reimbursement manual*. Washington, DC: American Nurses Publishing.

Rich, B., Hart, B., Barrett, A., Marks, G., & Ruderman, S. (1995). Peer consultation: a look at the process. *Clinical Nurse Specialist*, 9(3), 181–186.

Vonfrolio, L. (1993). Nurse entrepreneur . . . what are you waiting for? *Orthopedic Nursing*, 12(2), 19–22.

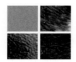

Chapter 25

Outcomes and Program Evaluation

Dalice L. Hertzberg and *Patricia A. Edwards*

Scientifically established databases should be the driving force in decisions made about health care, regardless of the service level at which the discussion is taking place. These levels include regulatory and national policy arenas, research, and most significantly, the clinical administrative level. However, this is often not the case, as reliable and valid measurement systems based on outcomes of client care are not applied as guidelines for clinical practice.

OUTCOMES

Various groups use outcome measurements to determine whether health care dollars are being spent wisely and that the care being delivered results in positive patient outcomes. These groups include the service provider, the payor (usually an insurance carrier), accrediting bodies, and other health professional and consumer groups.

Initially, outcomes were a method of providing scientific legitimacy to rehabilitation interventions, but in the evolving health care system, outcomes are increasingly being used to attract payors and justify payment. For more traditional rehabilitation service providers, superior outcomes will help to justify higher costs. Overall client outcomes traditionally have been focused more on global rehabilitation services, medical care, and therapies than on nursing. Well-established and valid nursing outcome data will help to legitimize the claims of the rehabilitation nurse for increased autonomy within rehabilitation provider systems (DeJong & Sutton, 1996).

In this chapter, key outcome and program evaluation issues are explored, as well as specific data-gathering techniques and instruments. Pediatric rehabilitation nurses are key professionals in identifying quality indicators and determining nurse-sensitive outcomes for children and adolescents with disabilities or chronic conditions and their families.

Key Issues

One of the key outcome issues is length of stay, which affects cost. Another important factor is the duration of the rehabilitation program being considered. Most outcome measures focus on functional outcome. The longer the period beyond the original injury, the less change will occur in the client's functional status, and functional outcomes will be more difficult to measure. As time passes, social roles and community integration and functioning become more important than short-term functional changes. Longer-term considerations such as community integration will become more important to a consumer-driven health care system. This trend may lead to more generic outcomes, such as those addressing quality of life, over specific functional measures, such as the distance ambulated or range of motion.

Additionally, outcome data will have to be adjusted to meet the needs of the groups of buyers of health care plans with a heterogeneous makeup These rehabilitation outcomes feed into the system that is used to score entire health plans for use when consumers make decisions regarding which plan to purchase. Full public disclosure of outcomes and case-mix data from rehabilitation providers will occur in the more competitive environment. Case-mix indexes are used to adjust risk across facilities. However, methodologies that can be applied across rehabilitation settings and across different modalities have not yet been developed (DeJong & Sutton, 1996).

Purposes for Measuring Outcomes

When developing or considering the use of a system for measuring outcomes, the purpose or purposes for the measurements must be taken into account. Areas for consideration when determining purposes are "clinical practice; utilization review; case management; program evaluation; [and] quality management" (Cole et al., 1995, p. 161). The Joint Commission on Accreditation of Healthcare Organizations (JCAHO, 1988) has indicated some possible reasons for outcome measurement:

Results are of importance to practitioners, clients, and payors.
Information about the performance of a process that leads to an outcome is brought to organizational attention. This allows priorities to be set for improvement of processes.
Organizations can then examine the effect of implementing these changes on the process.

This is especially true for outcomes that are the result of specific processes. Correct selection of outcome measurements creates a framework for the evaluation of care and identification of clinical practice improvements (Schaffer & Srp, 1996).

Definitions

Cope and Sundance (1996) define outcomes in three ways:

Global outcomes are the end results of all interventions and treatments expressed in the most general form. This term defines the objective recovery achieved as well as the subjective perceptions of the quality of life.
Outcome levels are specific categories of patient problems or conditions that are usual in rehabilitation and recovery.
Client-specific outcomes are the individual goals achieved as a result of recovery and clinical interventions that are specific to the patient and the condition.

Cope and Sundance (1996) state that once the desired outcome is conceptualized, the interventions and sequence of interventions needed to bring about that outcome can be "reverse-engineered." To achieve the process of outcome identification and to determine longitudinal outcomes, experience with a large number of clients over long periods of time is necessary. Nurses must keep in mind that outcome measurements will be dependent on their definitions and the quality of the data that are being gathered.

ICIDH Framework and Attributes

Cole and colleagues (1995) recommend using the International Classification for Impairment Disability and Handicap (ICIDH) framework for looking at outcomes. The terms used in the classification—impairment, disability, and handicap—are defined in Chapter 7. Each of the three domains is unique, and the handicap results from the interaction of impairment and disability, the physical and social environment, and economic and other resources available.

> The impairment outcomes are often the components of a particular function and each discipline has specific impairments it usually addresses in treatment. Disability outcomes usually involve the whole person and are more often functional outcomes. These are more often of primary concern to clients. Outcomes related to handicap frequently involve the individual's ability to interact with others and with the environment and are also important to the client. (Cole et al., 1995, p. 163)

When the attributes that reflect the overall treatment goals are considered in selecting outcome measures, important areas of practice are included. For example, the outcome attributes for the neurologic area might be:

Sensorimotor—trunk control, voluntary and involuntary movements, strength and coordination, range of motion, tone and fitness
Physical disabilities—mobility and locomotion, self-care, gross and fine motor function, caregiver burden
Handicaps—productive role participation, cope with disability, control over life, satisfied with quality of life, community integration (Cole et al., 1995)

Levels

Different levels of outcomes must be developed, from those with a low level of abstraction to those with a high level of abstraction. Outcomes with a low level of abstraction are those with very specific concrete descriptors, such as range of joint motion. More abstract outcomes might be less individually oriented and more group oriented or they might be more subjective, such as those addressing quality of life indicators. It is significant that outcome measures be quantifiable and psychometrically sound (Maas, Johnson, & Moorhead, 1996).

Levels of outcomes progress from physiologic instability, through physiologic maintenance, through community reintegration, to productive activity. The levels represent the basic areas of function of human beings (Cope & Sundance, 1996). Most outcome measures are designed for adults and do not take into account the changes in roles and abilities brought about by development or the level of caregiving by others typically required for children without disabilities. Most measures of functional ability do not take caregiving into account, either; the only exception is the Pediatric Evaluation of Disability Inventory (PEDI), described in Chapter 11, which includes a caregiving scale. Other measures of function that have been used to identify the nursing role in functional outcomes, such as Bobath principles, are also inappropriate for use with children (Duchene, 1996).

Adjustment for Severity

The severity of the client's condition at admission has a significant impact on outcomes, and levels of function vary widely among individuals. For example:

> . . . the strength gain expected in an individual who is debilitated by prolonged lack of normal activity will be very different from an individual who has a loss of strength due to a short period of interrupted training. As a result, comparison of simple gain scores (the score at discharge minus the score at admission) is a controversial issue. (Cole et al., 1995, p. 164)

Therefore, consideration must also be given to factors that influence outcome variability to improve the accuracy of goal setting and the determination of expected outcome. Examples of these factors include:

- severity of various impairments
- severity of various disabilities
- age
- co-morbidity or complications (e.g., incontinence)
- client attitudes, beliefs, and expectations

- social factors
- caregiver support
- financial resources
- occupation
- duration and intensity of physical therapy and other health care services (Cole et al., 1995, p. 165)

Risk adjustment systems must be developed for nursing indicators so that comparisons of quality measures and costs and staffing predictions can be made. There are many commercially available systems that fall into one of three categories of focus: mortality, resource-use, or other measures. These systems do not include nurse-specific measures such as maintaining skin integrity and nosocomial infection rates.

In an objective comparison of systems (ANA, 1995), it was found that these systems are of questionable value, do not include many nurse-specific measures, and do not provide a comprehensive system for quality assessment. It was recommended that appropriate systems using nursing quality indicators be developed, and it was suggested that existing acuity systems used in nursing might be the base upon which to build. Nursing acuity systems can be used in two ways: "1) by providing data on patient acuity and 2) by providing algorithms relating patient acuity to nurse staffing requirements" (ANA, 1995, p. B-12). Figure 25–1 displays the use of acuity systems in risk adjustment development.

Outcomes of Interest to Nursing

All outcomes should be of interest and concern to nursing, but those most consistent with nursing's practice and theory base must be identified if nursing is to prove the effectiveness and quality of nursing care provided to clients. In evaluating nursing's effectiveness, some areas of particular interest are functional status, satisfaction with care, and cost of care. Categories of outcomes found in a review of nursing literature by Harris and Warren (1995) included:

- physiologic outcome indicators
- psycho-social measures
- functional status
- behavioral
- knowledge
- symptom control
- home maintenance
- well-being
- goal attainment
- patient satisfaction

Figure 25–1 Use of the nursing acuity systems in risk adjustment development. (From American Nurses Association. (1995). *Nursing Care Report Card for Acute Care.* Washington, D.C.: ANA.)

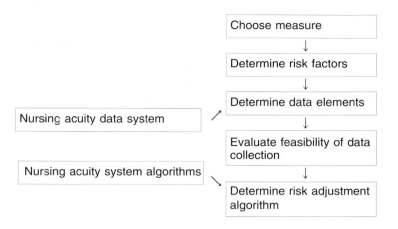

- safety
- frequency of service
- cost
- re-hospitalization
- resolution of nursing diagnosis (p. 82)

Nurse-Sensitive Patient Outcomes

Global rehabilitation client outcomes may or may not be nursing sensitive; that is, they may or may not recognize the contribution of nursing care to the overall level of function at the point of final measurement. Nursing-sensitive outcomes must recognize that they are influenced by nursing and encompass all aspects of nursing practice. Most global client outcomes are more likely to be the result of interventions from several health care disciplines (Maas, Johnson, & Moorhead, 1996). Nursing-sensitive outcome indicators are defined as "variable patient or family caregiver states, behaviors or perceptions at a low level of abstraction that are responsive to nursing intervention and used for determining a patient outcome" (Maas, Johnson, & Moorhead, 1996, p. 296). The traditional use of the term patient may be too limiting, because families and others are often involved in care and benefit from nursing interventions. Based on their research, Maas, Johnson, and Moorhead (1996) developed criteria for evaluating evidence of nursing sensitivity in outcomes (Table 25–1).

Most nursing-sensitive outcomes are related to the resolution of nursing diagnoses. However, these measures are limited to outcome levels rated low in abstraction and do not take into account client satisfaction or more global abstract outcomes such as quality of life. Additionally, nursing diagnosis is not yet well recognized among other disciplines that may be involved in the care of the child

or adolescent with a disability or chronic condition.

Nursing as a discipline must seize the opportunity to fully participate in outcome identification and evaluation. This requires knowledge of client assessments, specific assessment tools, and the data needs of both outcome evaluation and research. Advanced Practice Nurses especially are uniquely positioned to participate in the identification of methods and tools and make recommendations for documenting assessments and evaluations of individual responses to nursing care (Harris & Warren, 1995).

PROGRAM EVALUATION

As mentioned previously, one of the purposes for measuring outcomes is program evalua-

Table 25–1 CRITERIA FOR EVALUATING EVIDENCE OF NURSING SENSITIVITY IN OUTCOMES

The nursing intervention produced a positive outcome

The nursing intervention influenced a positive outcome

The nursing intervention is implemented with the intent to produce or influence the client outcome

The nursing intervention produced improvement or maintenance of the outcome or prevented deterioration or occurrence of a negative outcome

The failure to provide a nursing intervention resulted in failure to achieve a positive outcome or prevent a negative outcome

The nursing intervention occurred before observation of the outcome

The interventions that produced or influenced the outcomes are within the nursing scope of practice

tion. The evaluation may focus on structure, process, or outcome as the effectiveness and efficiency of the program is evaluated. An important outcome of rehabilitation programs is the measurement of the patient's functional performance, which involves global outcome measurement at the start of the program and at discharge and follow-up. The evaluation is often done by the interdisciplinary team, who can also use it to assist in future program planning and to determine expected change for future clients (Cole et al., 1995).

Program evaluation is concerned with both quality of service and the overall result of service, or outcome. Program evaluation begins during the initial phase of the client's contact with the program and continues until discharge from the program, whether it is an inpatient, outpatient, or continuous program. Collection of data about the client's progress, client satisfaction, and ongoing evaluation of quality, as well as a system for determining the validity of the outcome data, are all parts of the process. Most hospitals, centers, and clinics develop their own program evaluation systems in lieu of using commercially available systems. Some problems with commercially available systems are that they do not address participant satisfaction, and they do not directly address the pediatric population (Duchene, 1996).

Program evaluation information can be used in any or all of the following areas:

- program planning
- efficiency improvement
- quality improvement
- risk management
- cost analysis
- operational decision making
- trending and forecasting
- marketing (Glass, 1989)

Gray and Swope (1989) suggested combining the process of program evaluation with quality improvement efforts. At one hospital, this resulted in a cost-savings opportunity as well as an excellent system to measure outcomes.

Quality Indicators

Nursing quality indicators can be divided into three areas:

- outcome indicators
- process of care indicators
- structure of care indicators

Specific measures have been identified for each category (Table 25–2). It should be recog-

nized that, in addition to nursing, a variety of other factors may influence these measures. For example, the behavior of the other professionals caring for the child or adolescent and family, as well as excellent nursing care, influence the nosocomial infection rate. Additional explanations of each of the measures and their relations to nursing care can be found in the *Nursing Care Report Card for Acute Care* (ANA, 1995).

Data Gathering

The Uniform Data Set for Medical Rehabilitation (UDSMR) provides a method for uniform assessment of the severity of the client's disability and the outcomes of medical rehabilitative care. The effectiveness and efficiency of medical rehabilitation services can be analyzed using the Functional Independence Measure (FIM), which is the functional assessment component of the UDSMR; its pediatric equivalent, the WeeFIM; and other data. Program evaluation models based on the UDSMR and the FIM are useful for measuring resource cost of disability. The FIM and WeeFIM are described in detail in Chapter 11. The UDSMR is a valid and reliable measure of level of disability and functional gain during inpatient rehabilitation and after discharge. This tool provides quantitative information on individual program effectiveness and efficiency and allows comparisons with regional facilities of the same type. Other commercially available program evaluation systems used by rehabilitation facilities include the Level of Rehabilitation Scale (LORS-II) and the Patient Evaluation and Conference System (PECS). These tools are described further in Chapter 11.

Outcome-Based Critical Pathways

"Critical pathways are patient care processes—in other words, a mapped out route of care" (Schaffer & Srp, 1996, p. 11). Critical pathways are an outcome-driven system that specifies responsibilities, time frames for completing activities, and expected outcomes. In providing rehabilitation services in both the hospital and the community, the use of outcome-based critical pathways can be beneficial in the provision of care, foster continuity and efficiency, predict costs, and allow the agency to control delivery of care.

When clinical and financial outcomes are clearly defined, patients and caregivers know what to expect; third party payors know what

Table 25–2 NURSING QUALITY INDICATORS

Patient-Focused Outcome Indicators

Mortality rate
Length of stay
Adverse incidents
  Adverse incident rate (total)
  Medication error rate
  Patient injury rate
Complications
  Total complication rate
  Decubitus ulcer rate
  Nosocomial infection rate (total)
  Nosocomial urinary tract infection rate
  Nosocomial pneumonia rate
  Nosocomial surgical wound infection rate
Patient/family satisfaction with nursing care
  Patient willingness to recommend hospital to others/use hospital again
Patient adherence to discharge plan
  Readmission rates
  Emergency department visits post-discharge
  Unscheduled physician visits post-discharge
  Patient knowledge of disease/condition and care requirements

Process of Care Indicators

Nurse satisfaction
Assessment and implementation of patient care requirements
  Assessment of patient care requirements
  Development of a nursing care plan
  Accurate and timely execution of therapeutic interventions and procedures
  Documentation of nursing diagnoses, therapeutic objectives, and care given
Pain management
Maintenance of skin integrity
Patient education
Discharge planning
Assurance of patient safety
  Overall assurance of patient safety
  Appropriate use of restraints (all)
  Appropriate use of pharmaceutical restraints
  Appropriate use of physical restraints
Responsiveness to unplanned patient care needs

Structure of Care Indicators—Nurse Staffing Patterns

Ratio of total nursing staff to patients
  RN patient ratio
  LPN patient ratio
  Unlicensed workers–patient ratio
Ratio of RNs to total nursing staff
  Mix of RNs, LPNs, and unlicensed workers
RN staff qualifications
  RN staff experience
  RN staff education (i.e., MSNs, BSNs)
Total nursing care hours provided per patient (case mix, acuity adjusted)
  RN hours per patient
  LPN hours per patient
  Unlicensed worker hours per patient
Staff continuity
  Use of agency nurses
  Use of float nurses
  Unsafe assignment rate
  Nursing staff turnover rates
  Full time–part time ratio
RN overtime
Nursing staff injury rate

From American Nurses Association. (1995). *Nursing care report card for acute care.* Washington, DC: American Nurses Publishing.

they are paying for, and agency staff are in a better position to advocate for patients and negotiate services. (VanDyck, Maturen, & Gahn, 1996, p. 37)

Additionally, the resource use and cost data that can be generated from the critical pathways are useful in projecting staffing needs. Defining the outcomes also makes it possible to clearly describe the interventions needed to achieve these outcomes. In home care, critical pathways help decrease variability in the care and number of visits and in the services provided by diverse clinicians (VanDyck, Maturen, & Gahn, 1996).

Schaffer and Srp (1996) described other key elements in measuring outcomes—for example, disease management and patient education—and recommended incorporating several other practices to create an overview of the complete picture of care. These elements include:

Problem reporting—allows the clinician to record all client problems

Customer satisfaction surveys—allows the client to communicate to the provider how satisfied he or she is with the care received

Clinical outcomes—allow the clinician to analyze the events of the condition to verify if certain elements (critical pathway, care provided, use of resources, the client himself or herself) affected the care outcome in any way

Quality-of-life surveys—allow the client to comment on the extent to which changes in functioning or well-being met his or her needs or expectations (Schaffer & Srp, 1996, p. 12)

SUMMARY

Delineation of client outcomes will be a crucial part of rehabilitation services in the near future. Outcomes that show the most efficient, cost-effective method of providing services will aid insurance companies in determining which programs receive referrals and payment. Outcomes measurement will be crucial to the developing consumer-driven health care system that is emerging.

There is a great need for a common language among health care providers with regard to client outcomes in general and pediatric rehabilitation outcomes in particular. Outcome language must address not only individual client outcomes but those of the family and other important caregivers as a unit (Maas, Johnson, & Moorhead, 1996) Long-term outcomes must be considered and are

even more crucial with children, where long-term may represent 20 or 30 years and a considerably different developmental level with differing roles and expectations is present. More abstract concepts must also be considered, such as those related to quality of life and overall life satisfaction. Pediatric rehabilitation nurses have a challenge ahead: to work with rehabilitation colleagues to develop comprehensive, discipline-sensitive outcomes that address child or adolescent and family goals and dreams in both the short and long term.

REFERENCES

American Nurses Association. (1995). *Nursing care report card for acute care.* Washington, DC: American Nurses Publishing.

Cole, B., Finch, E., Gowland, C., & Mayo, N. (1995). *Physical rehabilitation outcome measures.* Philadelphia: Williams & Wilkins.

Cope, N., & Sundance, P. (1996). Conceptualizing clinical outcomes. In P. Landrum, N. Schmidt, & A. McLean (Eds.). *Outcome-oriented rehabilitation principles: strategies and tools for effective program management.* Gaithersburg, MD: Aspen, pp. 43–56.

DeJong, G., & Sutton, J. (1996). Rehab 2000: the evolution of medical rehabilitation in American health care. In P. Landrum, N. Schmidt, & A. McLean (Eds.). *Outcome-oriented rehabilitation principles, strategies and tools for effective program management.* Gaithersburg, MD: Aspen, pp. 3–42.

Duchene, P. (1996). Total quality management and outcome evaluation. In S. Hoeman (Ed.). *Rehabilitation nursing: process and application* (2nd ed.). St. Louis: CV Mosby, pp. 87–100.

Glass, R. (1989). Program evaluation. In B. England, R. Glass, & C. Patterson (Eds.). *Quality rehabilitation results-oriented patient care,* pp. 19–37. Chicago: American Hospital Publishing.

Gray, C., & Swope, M. (1989). Integrated program evaluation and quality assurance processes. In B. England, R. Glass, & C. Patterson (Eds.). *Quality rehabilitation results-oriented patient care,* pp. 53–59. Chicago: American Hospital Publishing.

Harris, M., & Warren, J. (1995). Patient outcomes: assessment issues for the CNS. *Clinical Nurse Specialist,* 9(2), 82–86.

Maas, M., Johnson, M., & Moorhead, S. (1996). Classifying nursing-sensitive patient outcomes. *Image: Journal of Nursing Scholarship,* 28(4), 295–301.

Schaffer, C., & Srp, F. (1996). Outcome-driven home care: quality, savings and results. *Caring,* June, 11–12.

VanDyck, L., Maturen, V., & Gahn, G. (1996). Outcome-based critical pathways: quality management. *Caring,* June, 30–37.

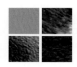

Chapter 26

Current Trends and Future Directions

Dalice L. Hertzberg, Susanne R. Hays,
Patricia A. Edwards, and *Nancy M. Youngblood*

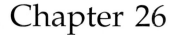

As the twenty-first century approaches, predictions are inevitable about what life will be like during the next 100 years. Life is already so fast-paced it seems difficult to predict what events will take place even within the next decade. In this chapter, selected issues and future trends in the field of pediatric rehabilitation nursing are described and related to the care of children with disabilities or chronic conditions and their families.

CHANGING DEMOGRAPHICS

Depending on the definition of the terms "disability" and "chronic illness," estimates of the prevalence of these conditions in children in the United States vary from 2% to 32% (Ireys & Katz, 1997). There are a limited number of major chronic diseases causing disability in adults, and each of these occurs with a relatively high frequency. These include stroke-related conditions, cardiovascular disorders, musculoskeletal conditions, cancer, and hearing and vision limitations. In children a different picture emerges, that of many different chronic conditions (more than 200), each with limited prevalence. In addition to prevalence rates based on diagnosis and activity limitation, specific subgroups of children are defined by their reliance on medical technologies or services. Estimates of these populations is important because the technologies and services used are often quite costly and require specialized skills to administer. For example, there was a maximum of 100,000 children dependent on medical tech-

nology in the United States in 1987 (Office of Technology Assessment, 1987).

Several factors unique to children influence patterns of disability and service use across the developmental stages (Ireys & Katz, 1997). One of these factors, the age of the child, influences the intensity, cost, and focus of services needed. For example, a very-low-birth-weight premature infant requires intensive and costly medical services in the first few years of life. As the child becomes older and more medically stable, interventions focus on learning and development of independence and are much less intensive. Adolescents with disabilities require transition services that will enable them to be more successful in the world of work and to move into adult health care systems unaccustomed to serving individuals with what were previously considered "pediatric" conditions such as cystic fibrosis or muscular dystrophy. Pediatric services, both health and educational, use age-based criteria. These needed services are often lost when the individual reaches adulthood, and there is no corresponding system to serve adults with disabilities.

Gender-linked disorders are common in children and young adults due to the large number of conditions that are genetically based. This phenomenon influences prevalence rates of certain conditions and in turn affects the intensity of services available (Ireys & Katz, 1997).

Race and poverty also have a great influence on prevalence of disability and chronic conditions in children. Some conditions, such as sickle cell anemia, occur primarily in one racial group. Other conditions predominate in a racial group, such as the prevalence of spina bifida in families of English-Irish descent. According to Ireys and Katz (1997),

> From a national perspective, white children are more likely to have at least one chronic condition than African-American or Hispanic children. However, the latter two groups, more than white children, experience more limitation in their usual activities and more days of restricted activity as a result of a chronic condition. Thus, absolute prevalence differences among races appear to result from higher prevalence of comparatively mild conditions (e.g. respiratory conditions, skin allergies) among white children. Minority children may experience more severe consequences of their conditions although these differences may result in part from heightened exposure to social and economic impoverishment and associated deficits in access to health care services. (p. 6)

However, more information is needed about the relationships of genetic and racial factors to disability and chronic illness.

Trends in prevalence and distribution of conditions reflect changes in birth rate, incidence, survival, and classification or diagnostic practices. Although the birth rate has been increasing since 1975, it is expected to remain relatively stable for the next 10 years. Incidence rates of conditions will probably not change substantially, with the possible exception of pediatric human immunodeficiency virus (HIV) infection, which will most likely increase. Survival rates of children with disabilities and chronic conditions continue to show increases, but at a slower rate. Increased prevalence estimates will probably reflect improved reporting and screening as well as changes in survey techniques (Ireys & Katz, 1997).

Although actual prevalence of disability and chronic illness in children will most likely not show a major increase in the next decade, new trends in service delivery are evolving. These trends include more children living with severe medical conditions; more children with complex medical conditions living and being cared for in the home; a greater trend toward inclusion of children with disabilities and their families in mainstream activities in communities; and an increased interest in prevention of secondary disability in children with disabilities and chronic conditions. These trends suggest that families and advocates will become more involved in policy, programs, and education of health care providers (Ireys & Katz, 1997).

Adequacy of insurance coverage will continue to be an issue, with health care inadequate or inaccessible to many poor or working poor families of children with disabilities. Managed care systems will change the picture of health care service delivery and the nature and quantity of services provided. Although many public integrated programs are available for children with disabilities, duplication of programs with complex and often conflicting rules and eligibility requirements can create barriers to service (Ireys & Katz, 1997).

Some new populations of children with major chronic conditions are emerging, including children with HIV, very-low-birthweight infants, and children with fetal alcohol syndrome and pre-natal drug effects. These subgroups represent relatively small numbers of children but account for a disproportionately high number of services and supports, including new or redesigned services for their special needs. Earlier identification of children with serious conditions leading to disability, such as pre-natal and post-natal treatment of conditions such as bronchopulmonary dysplasia or cystic fibrosis, may lead to changes in prevalence or in the level and sites of service provision (Ireys & Katz, 1997).

Prevention efforts have the potential to reduce the numbers of children born with congenital disabilities and to decrease the occurrence of trauma. However, to be effective, these strategies must be accessible to underserved and high-risk populations such as families living in poverty, families living in the United States who do not speak English, and families who, for a variety of reasons, are unable to access supportive services.

At present, the systems of services and supports that provides for the health care, education, and vocational and life training of children and young adults with disabilities and chronic conditions is woefully inadequate. Newspapers are filled with stories of children and families who "fall through the cracks" of health and welfare safety nets. Placement out of the natural home of the child continues to be an issue for many children with disabilities and chronic conditions when the birth family is unable to provide adequately for the child's needs. Many children with disabilities and chronic conditions who enter the foster care system remain in that system for far too long, with little consistency or permanence in their lives. Educational systems are overwhelmed with the numbers of children who fall outside the norm of behavior, educational achievement, and need for comprehensive health and related services within the school system. The preparation and availability of resources for teachers on the front lines, to aid them in teaching children with diverse academic, health, and behavioral issues is in question. Services and supports for adults who have grown up with childhood disabilities and chronic conditions are lacking, from knowledgeable and accessible health care services to community-based work and living arrangements. In many states, these adults remain on waiting lists for assisted living support for years before services are finally obtained, if they are obtained at all.

In this era of shrinking resources, pediatric rehabilitation nurses must join with families, individuals with disabilities, and others to influence public policy on national, state, and local levels to advocate for the needs and basic civil rights of children and adults with disabilities. New and innovative methods of funding and of allocating resources to benefit all people in this country must be found, or all people, with and without disabilities and chronic health conditions, will lose.

HEALTH CARE REFORM: CHILD HEALTH

In previous chapters, the differences between adult and pediatric rehabilitation were outlined and the need was stressed for nursing care that addresses the special health concerns of the child or adolescent with a disability or chronic condition and their family. These differences must be linked to both access to health insurance and the provision of appropriate health care services. Jameson and Wehr (1995) advocate for the creation by Congress of a standard of care for children that would protect their health interests. This would include access to appropriate services for children and adolescents with disabilities and chronic conditions with guarantees that they will not be compromised by cost-containment efforts at various levels. This has not yet happened, but Congress is beginning to focus on children's issues. For example, legislation was introduced in the following areas:

- expanding the quality of child care
- increasing access to early intervention programs
- expanding health coverage for uninsured children

Additionally, proposals such as the "Early Learning Act" and the "Children's National Security Act" have been drafted (Healy, 1997). At a summit meeting convened at the White House by President Clinton (Healy, 1997), the importance of the first 3 years of life was discussed, focusing attention on how important they are to long-term physical and mental development. There is increasing evidence that early intervention programs save money in the long run because of their impact on violence, substance abuse, and teen pregnancy. Pediatric rehabilitation nurses must remain knowledgeable about legislative initiatives and advocate for children and adolescents with disabilities or chronic conditions and their families.

REHABILITATION INTEGRATION IN THE COMMUNITY

The changing health care system and methods of financing are challenging rehabilitation professionals to conceptualize and propose new models of care delivery. These models need to be community-based rehabilitation systems that offer a continuum of services in disability prevention and treatment that promote community living and independence. Sandstrom, Hoppe, and Smutko (1996) proposed the Community Integration Rehabilitation Model: "a coordinated care delivery system emphasizing prevention and wellness at the community level" (p. 48). This model has two components:

1. Institution-based rehabilitation (IBR), which includes acute and sub-acute medical rehabilitation and long-term skilled nursing care
2. Community-based rehabilitation continuum (CBRC), which includes outpatient services (nursing and therapy), home health, day services, and community education and advocacy groups.

Implementing this model will require a redefinition of comprehensive rehabilitation as well as a rethinking of resource utilization, forging partnerships between institutions and the community and focusing on expanding opportunities for independent living.

An interdisciplinary care continuum model was proposed by Broughton & Lutner (1995) to "offer a unique service that is needed to achieve such goals as disease prevention, optimal health promotion, rehabilitation and a continuum of care" (p. 321). This model is aimed at the child and family in the community and involves an interdisciplinary team composed of the following professionals:

- advanced practice nurses as care coordinators
- therapists (e.g., physical, occupational, speech-language)
- physicians
- social workers and psychologists
- clergy
- teachers
- case managers

These team members have unique knowledge and skills to provide culturally sensitive services encompassing health promotion, disease prevention, and rehabilitation.

ROLE OF TECHNOLOGY

Assistive technology enables children and young adults with disabilities and chronic conditions to lead more useful and successful lives, to communicate and learn more effectively, and to develop and maintain independence. In 1990, the U.S. Census Bureau's National Health Interview Survey on Assistive Devices revealed that more than 13.1 million people in the United States used assistive technology. Since 1969, the number of individuals using assistive technology devices and services has more than doubled and continues to increase (U.S. Census Bureau, 1990). Three key factors in this increase have been identified: improvement in medical care resulting in greater rates of survival and longer lives for individuals with disabilities, advances in microelectronics and the availability of microcomputers, and the passage of legislation that mandated the consideration of assistive technology for children and adults with disabilities, much of which occurs in conjunction with the educational system and work settings.

Many barriers to the use of assistive technology devices and services remain. These barriers include the lack of educational opportunities for families of children with disabilities, professionals, and school personnel regarding access to and use of assistive technology devices and services; a lack of understanding of the benefits of assistive technology devices and services; and a lack of funding to provide needed technology and services for families, agencies, and institutions.

Children and young adults with disabilities and chronic conditions who use assistive technology devices for communication face many challenges when attempting to actively communicate with health care providers. Many health care providers are unfamiliar with such devices and their use. Often, physicians are required to write prescriptions for assistive technology devices and services even though they have received little if any training in the proper use of these devices. Few managed care systems recognize the benefits and cost savings of assistive technology devices and services. Professionals in the field of assistive technology, such as speech-language pathologists and occupational therapists, have not provided information to these agencies in a manner in which the information can be used and applied within the system. Families are also at a disadvantage because they are unable to communicate their needs within the managed care systems in a way that can be heard. Research into efficacy and cost savings provided by assistive technology devices is needed, as well as advocacy on the part of pediatric rehabilitation nurses and other health and rehabilitation personnel to promote knowledge and use of assistive technology for children and young adults with disabilities and chronic conditions.

Computer technology has also been used to help children with disabilities to learn in interactive, fun, non-threatening, and accessible ways. Children who are unable to access a keyboard can use a variety of methods, including voice, joysticks, or pressure-sensitive pads stimulated by finger, hand, forehead pointer, tongue, or sip-and-puff stick. Nurses working with children with disabilities and chronic conditions can learn how to use these adaptive programs to teach children and to design rehabilitation interventions.

Assistive technology holds the promise of improved functioning and greatly enhanced independence for children and young adults with disabilities, facilitating full participation in all aspects of life. Fewer dollars within the health care system may threaten this promise while ever-expanding technologic advances make assistive technology more portable, more easy to use, and more applicable to the needs of children and young adults with disabilities. Research, advocacy, and efforts to change policies and systems will be increasingly necessary to ensure the accessibility of assistive technology devices and services to children and young adults with disabilities and their families. Additional information about assistive technology is provided in Chapter 14.

COMPUTERS AND EDUCATIONAL TECHNOLOGY

Computers are more and more becoming a part of every home as well as an indispensable tool in hospitals, clinics, private offices, and other health and rehabilitation settings. No longer relegated solely to the realm of word processing, financial spreadsheets, and laboratory data, computers are increasingly used as a primary information and communication resource for nurses, individuals with disabilities, children, and families. Nursing informatics, which addresses information science and technology, represents a new discipline for nurses (Turley, 1996).

Technologic advances over the past 25 years have resulted in faster, more powerful computers linked within businesses or agencies in a networked system (intranet or ethernet), as well as computers linked through fiberoptic telephone lines worldwide (the Internet or World Wide Web). These worldwide systems, initially developed for the purpose of national defense and then taken over by universities to be used for the exchange of knowledge and research, are now available to anyone with a computer, a modem, and a telephone line. For nursing, the applications of computer technology are endless.

The electronic transfer of computer mail (E-mail), data, images, sounds, and video are available with the point and click of a mouse. Computer technology is the basis for telemedicine, which allows physicians or other health care providers to "link up" with other centers or clinics and perform real-time consultations, attend interactive lectures, and have face-to-face meetings with patients or other providers hundreds or thousands of miles away. Telemedicine is in its infancy and is currently very expensive, but it promises to be a useful method of providing education and direct health care.

Uses of computers and computer technology for nurses include the more traditional applications such as word processing, desktop publishing, and formulation and maintenance of databases and forms for uses such as patient acuity, charting, and statistical analysis. Wider applications are now possible and include nursing education through Internet resources; communication with individual nurses, companies, and organizations via the Internet or E-mail; electronic consultation; electronic patient and family teaching; virtual reality technology for education, such as the

Visible Human Project at the University of Colorado Health Sciences Center, as well as to enhance clinical decision making; and computer-based programs that analyze patient data and make prognostications about risk, treatment options, and nursing interventions (Turley, 1996).

Educational Applications of Computers

The educational applications of computers are endless. Books, including nursing textbooks and resource books such as medication references, are available on disk, CD-ROM, and on the Internet. Problem-solving programs and continuing education (CE) courses are also available in these media. Most colleges not only have computers with Internet access available to students, but many now require students to bring their own computers to school and demonstrate competency in computer use. Clinical problem-solving methods such as problem-based learning (PBL) are available through the Internet on the home pages of individuals and university health science centers. These electronic programs provide a text-based description of the clinical situation with all of the visual aids (e.g., radiographs, laboratory reports, video presentations of the patient) in a step-wise manner that the learner can access from home or office, with the resource person's E-mail address for questions and comments. One Web Site, "Pediatric Nursing Practice Management Problems" offers clinical case studies for nurses that are primarily text-based (Kilmon, 1996). Few of these types of programs are as yet available for nurses, and none are available as yet for nurses working with children with disabilities or chronic conditions; however, the application is clear. Other computer-based educational programs are available for purchase, usually on a CD-ROM, which combine print, audio, and video with an interactive program.

Most schools of nursing use distance learning, where a lecture or patient presentation can be sent over telephone or cable television circuits to other communities and groups of students, often many at once. Workshops and seminars can be broadcast from one central site to many other sites all across the country and even the world. Using telephone link-ups, these participants can ask questions and interact with the presenter and other participants. This type of technology makes the best use of experts in a field, such as that of pediatric rehabilitation, and enables participants to share their expertise with many others.

E-mail discussion groups composed of class cohorts can facilitate discussion among students and faculty, even when they are located in different cities, states, or countries.

The Internet and computer technology is still in its infancy. Computers represent a vast new resource of unique applications for nurses, the potential of which as yet remains largely untapped. In the future, nurses will travel the "information superhighway" to provide innovative services to children with disabilities and chronic conditions and their families as easily as nurses today walk down the halls of a hospital. See Tables 26–1, 26–2, and 26–3 for a glossary of computer-related resource terms, Web Sites, home pages, and LISTSERVs of interest to pediatric rehabilitation nurses.

THE IMPACT OF GENETIC RESEARCH ON CHILDREN AND FAMILIES

The Human Genome Project has brought about tremendous advances in the under-standing of genetic influences on humans. The genetic aspects of many inherited diseases are becoming much better understood, as are the genetic contributions to many personal characteristics such as mood and behavior. Identification of the exact gene and area of the gene that causes inherited disease is now possible for a number of conditions and will be possible for more in the near future. This research will lead to more accurate and earlier diagnostic tests, as well as to new therapies and new strategies for disease prevention based on individual as well as population risks.

Genome research has also led to advances in gene therapy, which is the use of genetic information to replace, correct, or supplement malfunctioning genes. Gene therapies for inherited diseases such as cystic fibrosis and adenosine deaminase deficiency are currently under investigation (Williams & Lessick, 1996). Therapies for Duchenne's muscular dystrophy are also being investigated but have as yet shown little promise.

Table 26–1 GLOSSARY OF COMPUTER-RELATED RESOURCE TERMS

Bulletin Boards: Computer system, separate from the World Wide Web, that users can send messages to, and read messages from, on a large variety of topics. There are no membership requirements; anyone can post a message or read messages. Usenet is one of the largest. Also called **newsgroups.**

Downloading: Transferring a file by copying it from another computer or from the Internet.

E-mail: Electronic mail is written communication between individuals via computers within a network or a system of networks: May operate with or without the Internet.

FTP: File transfer protocol is the method used to copy file and executable programs between computers on the Internet.

Home Page or Web Page: A site on the World Wide Web that contains a directory of its contents as well as directories of related information.

HTML: Hypertext markup language is the language used to format the information contained in individual sites in the World Wide Web.

HTTP: Hypertext transfer protocol is the primary method for transferring data throughout the World Wide Web.

Internet: Computer "network of networks" where millions of computers all around the world are linked

Listserv: Electronic discussion lists on various topics. Listservs are limited to members who must subscribe using their E-mail address, and messages are sent only to members.

Nursing Informatics: The combination of nursing science, cognitive science, computer science, and information science designed to enhance nursing knowledge and functions.

Uploading: Transferring a file by making a copy from a user's computer to another computer on a network or on the Internet.

URL: Uniform resource locator is a combination of letters, numbers, and symbols that makes up the address of a particular web site or home page. The URL usually starts out with the letters http://www

World Wide Web: A computer database available on the Internet that includes text, sounds, video, and a variety of other information formats.

From Yerks, A. (1996). The Internet and pediatric nursing: guide to the information superhighway. *Pediatric Nursing,* 22(1), 11–15, 26–27. Levine, J., Baroudi, C., & Young, M. (1995). *The Internet for dummies* (3rd ed.). Foster City, CA: IDG Books Worldwide.

Table 26–2 INTERESTING WEB SITES AND HOME PAGES

Nursing

Peter Ramme "Idea Nurse": Computer consultant, political action, nurses, and the Internet
http://ideanurse.com/index1.html

NurseNet: General nursing links, nurses, and the Internet
http://www.ualberta.ca/~irnorris/nursenet/nn.html

Developmental Disability Community Nurses Coalition: Nursing organization and links
http://ourworld.compuserve.com/homepages/A Hodas/

Child Health and Disability Sites

Pediatric Points of Interest: Links to numerous pediatric health and medical sites
http://www.med.ihu.edu/peds/neonatology/poi.html

Rare Genetic Diseases in Children: Genetic and disability resources
http://moror2.med.nyu.edu/murphy01/homenew.htm

Virtual Children's Hospital: Multiple resources on child health and disease, including tutorials
http://www.med.thu.edu/peds/neonatology/poi.html

The American Academy of Pediatrics: Information and guidelines for child health and disability
http://www.aap.org

The Family Village: A global community of disability-related resources
http://www.familyvillage.wisc.edu.8000/

Internet Resources for Special Children: Links to many child disability sites
http://www.irsc.org/

However, advances in detection of inherited conditions have a down side as well. Individuals identified as carriers or pre-symptomatic bearers of a disease-causing gene may face discrimination from insurance carriers, employers, and others and may face difficult life decisions (Cook-Deegan, 1994; Lapham, Kozma, & Weiss, 1996). Those forms of cancer that have a strong genetic component for which the genes are identified and do not cause disease until adulthood are one example. As a result of advanced carrier detection methods, it is now possible to identify children who carry the gene for some forms of neuromuscular disease that do not manifest until adulthood. This knowledge of imminent disease can affect an individual's life choices with regard to marriage, having children, forming close relationships, and employment. The question arises regarding whether or not it is ethical to inform families when their child carries a gene for a disabling condition or even whether or not it is essential to carry out such a test. These decisions are a matter of individual choice on the part of family members.

Table 26–3 LISTSERVS OF INTEREST TO PEDIATRIC REHABILITATION NURSES

The Family Village: Health and disability-related mailing lists; more than 75 categories, including those for parents, children, and adults with disabilities or chronic conditions and health care professionals
http://www.familyvillage.wisc.edu/master.html

Martha Dewey Bergren's Home Page: Sign up for "School-RN" school nurse discussion list
http://www.usinternet.com/users/bergren/

Children With Special Health Care Needs Discussion List: "CHCSN-L"
To subscribe send message to:
listserv@nervn.nerdc.ufl.edu
Leave subject line blank
In message type: subscribe cshcn-l Yourfirstname Yourlastname

Parents of Children with Disabilities List: "Our Kids"
To subscribe send message to:
listserv@maelstrom.stjohns.edu
Leave subject line blank
In message type: subscribe our-kids Yourfirstname Yourlastname

Parents of Children With Spina Bifida Discussion List: "SB-Parents"
To subscribe send message to:
listserv@waisman.wisc.edu
Leave subject line blank
In message type: subscribe sb-parents Yourfirstname Yourlastname

Health and Developmental Disabilities Discussion List: "DD-Health"
To subscribe send message to:
listserver@relay.doit.wisc.edu
Leave subject line blank
In message type: subscribe ddhealth Yourfirstname Yourlastname

---

From Yerks, A. (1996). The Internet and pediatric nursing: guide to the information superhighway. *Pediatric Nursing,* 22(1), 11–15, 26–27.

Diagnosis of an inherited disease in a family member can cause strife and discord within the family. Family members may blame others for carrying or passing on the disease. A parent whose child is identified with an inherited disorder may not want any other family members to be notified even if a sibling of the parent is pregnant and there is a risk of the unborn child inheriting the condition. Counseling families and individuals on a long-term basis and forming therapeutic relationships with them is an important intervention for pediatric rehabilitation nurses.

Discrimination by insurance companies is another risk. There have been instances in which families who have a relative identified with a genetic disorder had a difficult time obtaining health insurance coverage or lost coverage. Families who are affected by fragile X syndrome have experienced moderate to extreme worry about losing insurance (Wingrove et al., 1996). Although confidentiality is maintained as well as possible, the increasing ease of information transfer using computerized records makes it easier for insurance companies to obtain this type of information. Several states, such as Washington, have enacted laws against genetic discrimination by insurance carriers. Five states have laws barring discrimination against individuals who are carriers of sickle cell trait. Seven other states provide some legal protection to people with inherited conditions (Lapham, Kozma, & Weiss, 1996).

A 1996 survey of people who have inherited diseases in their families found that 15% of people were asked about genetic disease on a job application, and 13% were denied or let go from a job (Lapham, Kozma, & Weiss, 1996). As a result, people surveyed were less likely to reveal genetic information to insurance companies or potential or actual employers and were likely to refuse testing for a genetic condition.

Another important implication of genetic research for children and families pertains to the benefits obtained from participating in research. Ethical practices require that parents be fully informed about their options when considering participation in a genetic research protocol. Options include voluntary participation, the right to refuse testing or release of any information that is generated by testing or research, and the right to withdraw from the study at any time without any change in care, non-investigational treatment, or support (Baumiller et al., 1996).

Families also need to be fully informed about the benefits of the research study to themselves and to their child. Many times the benefits of genetic research are long term rather than immediate, and no clear benefit to the child or family may result. Parents should also be aware that in contributing a genetic sample for research, future applications of the samples may also exist, and that there may be commercial interests in derivatives from biologic specimens. Families should also have the opportunity to refuse any future or potential use of blood or tissue samples supplied by their child (Baumiller et al., 1996).

Children who are developmentally able to give consent to genetic testing should be asked. Younger children or those who are not developmentally able to understand the implications of testing may be asked to give assent or may be given an abbreviated explanation of the study.

Although genetic research promises the hope of prevention, treatment, and even cure for genetic conditions in children, the risks of discrimination on the basis of diagnosis with a genetic condition may be far-reaching and could affect distant family members as well as parents and siblings. Nurses working with children who have been diagnosed with a genetic condition and their families must be aware of and sensitive to the risks of loss of confidentiality and discrimination. Pediatric rehabilitation nurses can advocate for children and families by providing access to local resources and information about insurance and other social issues. Adherence to the ethical principles surrounding genetic testing, research, and informed consent is imperative.

ALTERNATIVE OR COMPLEMENTARY THERAPY

The term "alternative" is used to describe any medical intervention not generally taught or accepted by U.S. medical schools and not usually reimbursable by third-party payors (Eisenberg et al., 1993). The term "complementary" is used widely in Europe to describe medical intervention that is used in combination with allopathic medicine or treatment (Cleaveland & Biester, 1995).

According to the Office of Alternative Medicine (OAM) at the National Institutes of Health, alternative therapies include acupuncture, acupressure, antioxidant therapies, bioelectromagnetic therapies, biofeedback, chiropractic, guided imagery, herbal medicines, hypnosis, massage, macrobiotic nutrition, intercessory prayer, therapeutic touch, tai chi, and yoga, among other nontraditional modalities (McDowell, 1994).

According to Eisenberg and colleagues (1993), unconventional medicine is used predominately by persons with chronic, non–life-threatening medical conditions. Reports in the literature suggest that for children with chronic illnesses such as juvenile arthritis, chronic diarrhea, cancer, cystic fibrosis, and asthma, alternative therapies, complementary therapies, or both have been used with varying levels of success.

Information in the media regarding alternative and complementary therapies has increased significantly. The public is becoming more widely educated, and attitudes are changing as a result. In some cultures, such as some Native American groups, alternative therapy has always been common but was not well known or understood by others outside those communities. Families turned to alternative and complementary therapies because they hoped to get more personalized attention, were dissatisfied with conventional medicine, feared the side effects of drugs, or their child had a chronic problem and they were encouraged to explore alternatives (Spigelblatt et al., 1994).

Krieger (1979) was one of the nursing pioneers in integrating alternative therapy in the form of therapeutic touch into clinical practice, education, and research. Many nurses are learning about alternative therapies and their use in prevention of recurrence of some acute illnesses, relief of some symptoms in both acute and chronic illnesses, and promotion of a sense of well-being when the disease progress cannot be stopped (Cleaveland & Biester, 1995).

The pediatric rehabilitation nurse, whether in the hospital or in the community, may be the first person a concerned family turns to for information about and use of alternative and complementary therapies and medicine for their child. The nurse must be informed, be involved with consumer and legislative efforts to integrate safe alternative therapies into health care, establish collaborative relationships with non-nurse providers of alternative and complementary care, and empower the families who are seeking answers.

AGING WITH A DISABILITY

Now more than ever before, adults who had pediatric onset of a disability are being seen by health care providers. Whereas in the past such persons would probably have died before reaching adulthood, today they are naturally growing older because of advances in all aspects of care, advances in technology and research, and legislative acts that protected their rights to live in the community and participate in community life. Most however, have not had the benefit of habilitation and rehabilitation to assist them in learning to live in the community, much less to care for themselves and have healthy relationships. Neither have they had much encouragement to live in their own home, marry, or have children if those were their goals.

Many of these adults have continued to live with their families until there was a crisis, usually a situation in which the parents could no longer physically or emotionally provide care or one or both parents died. These individuals then lived out their years in institutions, shut away from society at large. Their care was provided by residential staff, and they were not expected to be independent. Today, however, these systems are changing, and many institutions are closing or closed, making another model of care in the community a necessity.

There continue to be many barriers to adults with pediatric onset of disabilities living in the community: adequate health care by staff who understand them as adults and yet have an understanding of their past and current needs; housing; insufficient trained, consistent support staff; lack of vocational training and placements for employment; and too few multi-disciplinary teams who have an understanding of how to support the individual in learning the skills to support successful community living.

Many adults with developmental disabilities also have secondary disabilities; these are principally mobility limitations, but often mental disorders are present as well. One study indicates that 20% to 35% of adults with developmental disabilities living in the community also have mental disorders (Landsberg, Fletcher, & Maxwell, 1987). This group of persons with a combination of developmental, psychiatric, and mental health disorders are greatly under-served in the community, making community placement difficult. Their needs are very complex and require not only increased daily staff to provide therapeutic programs but also a multi-disciplinary team to support them while they learn to live successfully in the community. Ideally, the team should have experience and training in both developmental disabilities and mental health, because these clients' needs are complex. The team core should include a community psychiatrist, a behavioral counselor, a psychiatric nurse specialist, vocational staff, and case managers. Many of these adults with developmental and secondary disabilities also have other medical conditions and substance abuse problems and have been involved with the local police. These issues all add to the complexity of their care needs. In the past, these individuals were cared for by mental health staff with little attention given to their developmental disability needs, or they were cared for by the developmental disability staff with little concentrated effort to manage their mental health concerns. Some communities have used a highly specialized team of professionals to provide consultation, including annual evaluations and ongoing consultation management, to provide support to the local team working with these individuals.

Barriers still exist, even for adults who had the benefit of a family's and community's vision that as children they would eventually become adults. Social stigmas regarding disabled adults having relationships, bearing children, and becoming productive citizens remain. Health care is also a problem for this population. How many obstetric and gynecology offices have examination facilities for a woman in a wheelchair? How many are prepared to support her during pregnancy and afterwards? How many community systems are ready and able to support a physically and mentally challenged family in raising their child?

The challenge for the rehabilitation team, today and for the future, is to continue working toward a higher level of community access and integration for the adult with pediatric-onset disability. This includes working with the child with a disability or chronic illness and their family to achieve full community inclusion and access.

FUTURE DIRECTIONS FOR NURSING EDUCATION AND PRACTICE

Pediatric rehabilitation nurses are being affected by the major system changes currently underway in health care and must begin exploring ways to position themselves for the future. As mentioned in previous chapters, the focus of care is shifting to the community, and this is creating new opportunities for the nurse working with children with disabilities or chronic conditions and their families. This shift in emphasis will require the nurse to update knowledge and skills, especially in the areas of primary and preventive care and case management. Opportunities will develop that allow nurses to expand their practice into collaborative arrangements and manage care across a variety of settings. Employment may be sought in a variety of settings, including schools, day care centers, public health centers, and nursing homes, or the nurse may wish to explore the possibility of starting a business.

At the ARISTA II conference (Sigma Theta Tau Leadership Institute, 1996), recommendations were formulated that identified five strategic action areas that would position nursing as a member of the team plotting the future of both nursing and health care. The following are strategic areas for action and some of their component parts.

Public communication—create and disseminate a clear description of the role of nursing; establish information networks; educate nurses in public communication; publicize collaborations with various constituencies; target a range of audiences.

Policy formulation—be a presence at the decision-making table; find opportunities for nurses to be involved in policy formulation; develop coalitions to set reform agendas; identify partnerships.

Education—implement standard entry level for practice; disseminate "best practices" in nursing education; develop curricula with a broader, more sophisticated role for nursing as the context.

Leadership development—enhance ability to manage change; raise awareness of economic realities and value of nursing; acknowledge and reward innovation and leadership.

Research, models and partnerships—focus agenda on health promotion, systems, and outcomes; participate in interdisciplinary research; facilitate knowledge exchange; disseminate information on models of excellence.

Based on the knowledge that nurses have the ability to generate solutions to health care issues and are highly regarded and trusted by the public, the following conclusions emerged:

It will be important that nurses align themselves with the needs of the populations as well as the needs of the system. Nurses must join with communities in determining how best to improve health and care and in defining the role that nurses will play within an ideally structured health care system.

Nursing needs to create partnerships with individuals and families in providing direct care; with communities in promoting health and preventing disease in a community-based and designed system; and with their colleagues in developing and managing health care systems that are both cost-efficient as well as humane and holistic. (ARISTA, 1996, p. 11)

More nurses will be needed in advanced practice roles, and those with a background in pediatric rehabilitation should position themselves as cost-effective alternatives for physicians in the delivery of some basic services. Pediatric rehabilitation nurses considering graduate education would find a program that combines pediatrics and rehabilitation with community-based practice as an excellent curriculum for advanced practice and ultimately for certification in the advanced practice role.

Academic centers and nursing faculty must examine undergraduate and graduate curricula and re-focus course work and clinical experiences to emphasize prevention and early intervention as well as the management of disabilities and complex chronic conditions. Skills in case management, delegation, supervision, and financial planning should also be essential components of nursing education.

Berger and colleagues (1996) proposed a number of advanced practice roles in the changing system of health care to promote optimal use of nurses' knowledge and ability. These roles "are designed to position health-care facilities to meet the demands of serving patients with increasingly complex health care needs while meeting cost-containment goals" (Berger et al., 1996, p. 255). The proposed roles are:

Case manager—responsible for overseeing the overall plan and providing leadership in producing cost effective outcomes

Clinical educator—coordinates educational activities within a clinical practice area including ensuring staff competency

Clinical researcher—plans and monitors nursing care outcomes and designs research activities to examine difficult clinical problems

Clinical consultant—acts as a resource to the staff, both clinical and management, in project work, research, staff development, and care initiatives

Nurse practitioner—provides health promotion and disease prevention, as well as diagnostic and management services, to individuals, families, and groups

Corporate/community nurse practitioner—provides health care at the work site or at a location in the community for a specific group

Patient care manager—manages human and financial resources for one or more patient areas

Graduate education is necessary for all these roles, and the nurse must also demonstrate core competencies that have been identified for the role. For example, the core competencies identified for the case manager role are:

- advanced assessment
- outcomes management
- educational strategies
- pharmacology
- health promotion (Berger et al., 1996)

Nursing education must include core content in communication, research, quality management, health policy, information technology, and diversity. These roles are designed to maximize the contribution of nurses and can serve as a model for the organization in planning integrated services that promote optimal care and cost savings.

SUMMARY

The pediatric rehabilitation nurse is challenged as never before to move forward and face head-on the changes that are occurring in health care. Meeting these challenges involves community-based action and focusing on the needs of children and families where they live, go to school, and work. Nurses must assume leadership roles in creating new care models that improve outcomes for both the child and his or her family and the community. "As the most trusted of all health care providers, nurses now have the unparalleled opportunity to achieve their long-standing vision of holistic, continuous, integrated and cost-effective health care" (ARISTA, 1996, p. 7). Now is the time, and nurses are the individuals who must envision the future and go out and lead others toward a restructured health care system that is accessible, child- and family-centered, community-based, and outcome-oriented. It is your responsibility to be ever mindful of the current trends in health care and take a leadership role in charting a course for the future of pediatric rehabilitation nursing.

REFERENCES

Baumiller, R., Cunningham, G., Fisher, N., Fox, L., Henderson, M., Lebel, R., McGrath, G., Pelias, M., Porter, I., Seydel, F., & Willson, N. (1996). Code of ethical principles for genetics professionals: an explanation. *American Journal of Medical Genetics*, 65, 179–183.

Berger, A., Eilers, J., Pattria, L., Rolf-Fixley, M., Pfeifer, B., Rogge, J., Wheeler, L., Bergstrom, N., & Heck, C. (1996). Advanced practice roles for nurses in tomorrow's healthcare systems. *Clinical Nurse Specialist*, 10(5), 250–255.

Broughton, B., & Lutner, N. (1995) Chronic childhood illness: a nursing health promotion model for rehabilitation in the community. *Rehabilitation Nursing*, 20(6), 318–322.

Sigma Theta Tau Leadership Insitute. (1996). *Nursing leadership in the 21st century, a report of ARISTA II healthy people: leaders in partnership*. Indianapolis, IN: Center Nursing Press.

Cleaveland, M., & Biester, D. (1995). Alternative and complementary therapies: considerations for nursing practice. *Journal of Pediatric Nursing*, 10(2), 121–123.

Cook-Deegan, R. (1994). Private parts. *The Sciences*, March-April, 18–23.

Eisenberg, D., Kessler, R., Foster, C., Norlock, F., Calkins, D., & Delbanco, T. (1993). Unconventional medicine in the United States. *New England Journal of Medicine*, 328, 246–252.

Healy, M. (1997). Babies on board in politicians' latest bills. *The Seattle Times*, Monday, June 2 [On-line]. Available: http://www.seattletimes.com/extra/browse/html97/altchil

Ireys, H., & Katz, S. (1997). The demography of disability and chronic illness among children. In H. Wallace, J. MacQueen, R. Biehl, & J. Blackman (Eds.). *Mosby's resource guide to children with disabilities and chronic illness*. St. Louis: CV Mosby.

Jameson, E., & Wehr, E. (1995). *Drafting national health care reform legislation to protect the health interests of children* [abstract] [On-line]. Available: http://nncf.unl.edu/health.pedstand.html

Kilmon, C. (1996). Computerized approaches to teaching nurse practitioner students. *Pediatric Nursing*, 22(1), 16–28.

Krieger, D. (1979). *The therapeutic touch: how to use your hands to heal*. Englewood Cliffs, NJ: Prentice-Hall.

Landsberg, G., Fletcher, R., & Maxwell, T. (1987). Developing a comprehensive community care system for the mentally ill/mentally retarded. *Community Mental Health Journal*, 23, 131–134.

Lapham, E., Kozma, C., & Weiss, J. (1996). Genetic discrimination: perspectives of consumers. *Science*, 274(5287), 621–624.

McDowell, B. (1994). The National Institutes of Health Office of Alternative Medicine: evaluating research outcomes. *Alternative and Complementary Therapies*, 1(1), 17–25.

Office of Technology Assessment. (1987). Technology-dependent children: hospital versus home care—a technical memorandum. Washington, DC: U.S. Government Printing Office.

Sandstrom, R., Hoppe, K., & Smutko, N. (1996). Comprehensive medical rehabilitation in the 1990s: the community integration rehabilitation model. *Health Care Supervisor*, 15(2), 44–54.

Spigelblatt, L. Laine-Ammara, G., Pless, B., & Guyver, A. (1994). The use of alternative medicine for children. *Pediatrics*, 94(6), 811–814.

Turley, J. (1996). Toward an model for nursing informatics. *Image: Journal of Nursing Scholarship*, 28(4), 309–313.

U.S. Census Bureau. (1990). *National health interview survey on assistive services, (NHIS-AD)*. Washington, DC: U.S. Government Printing Office.

Williams, J., & Lessick, M. (1996). Genome research: implications for children. *Pediatric Nursing*, 22(1), 40–46.

Wingrove, K., Norris, J., Barton, P., & Hagerman, R. (1996). Experiences and attitudes concerning genetic testing and insurance in a Colorado population: a survey of families diagnosed with fragile X syndrome. *American Journal of Medical Genetics*, 64, 378–381.

ADDITIONAL RESOURCES

Cavalcanti, R.S. & de Freitas, G.G. (1992). Alternative medicine in a patient with juvenile chronic arthritis [letter]. *Journal of Rheumatology*, 19(11), 1827–1828.

Cleeg, J.A., & Standen, P.J. (1991). Friendship among adults who have developmental disabilities. *American Journal on Mental Retardation*, 95(6), 663–671.

Dossey, B.M., Keegan, L., Guzzetta, C. E., & Kolkmeier, L. G. (1995). *Holistic nursing: a handbook for prcctice* (2nd ed.). Gaithersburg, MD: Aspen.

Eisenberg, D.M. Kessler, R.C., Foster, C., Norlock, F.E., Calkins, D.R., & Delbanco, T.L. (1993). Unconventional medicine in the United States. *New England Journal of Medicine*, 328, 246–252.

Engebretson, J. (1996). Comparison of nurses and alternative healers. *Image: Journal of Nursing Scholarship*, 23(2),

Engebretson, J., & Wardell, D. (1996). A contemporary view of alternative healing modalities. *Nurse Practitioner*, 12(9), 51–55 (1993).

Felsenthal, G. Garrison, S., & Steinberg, F. (Eds.). (1994). *Rehab litation of the aging and elderly patient*. Baltimore: Williams & Wilkins.

France, N.E. (1993). The child's perception of the human energy field. *Journal of Holistic Nursing*, 11(4), 319–331.

Graves, J., & Corcoran, S. (1989) The study of nursing informatics. *Image: Journal of Nursing Scholarship*, 21, 227–231.

Hallum, A. (1995). Disability and the transition to adulthood: issues for the disabled child, the family, and the pediatrician. *Current Problems in Pediatrics*, January, 12–50.

Hubble, M., & Middleton, M. (1995). A nurse's role in complementary medicine. *Complementary Therapies in Medicine*, 3(3), 171–178.

Kenyon, J.N. (1993). Hyperactivity: a consideration of the alternatives. *Complementary Therapies in Medicine*, 1(2), 78–80.

Kilmon, C. (1996). Computerized approaches to teaching nurse practitioner students. *Pediatric Nursing*, 22(1), 16–18.

Kramer, N.A. (1990). Comparison of therapeutic touch and casual touch in stress reduction of hospitalized children. *Pediatric Nursing*, 16(5), 43–45.

Levine, J., Baroudi, C., & Young, M. (1995). *The Internet for dummies* (3rd ed.). Foster City, CA: IDG Books Worldwide.

Neal, L. (1997). There is a need for more nurses in home care practice. *Rehabilitation Nursing*, 22(3), 153.

Nelson, M.R., & Alexander, M.A. (1994). Pediatric-onset disabilities. In G. Felsenthal, S. Garrison, & F. Steinberg (Eds.). *Rehabilitation of the aging and elderly patient*, p. 407. Baltimore: Williams & Wilkins.

Robbins, J. (1996). *Reclaiming our health: exploding the medical myth and embracing the source of true health*. Tiburon, CA: H.J. Kramer.

Sawyer, M.G., Gannoni, A. F., Toogood, I. R., & Rice, M. (1994). The use of alternative therapies for children with cancer. *Medical Journal of Australia*, 160(6), 320–322.

Southwood, T.R., Malleson, P. N., Roberts-Thomson, P. J., & Mahy, M. (1990). Unconventional remedies used for patients with juvenile arthritis. *Pediatrics*, 85, 150–154.

Spigelblatt, L.S. (1995). Alternative medicine: should it be used by children? *Current Problems in Pediatrics*, 25(7), 180–188.

Stern, R.C., Danda, E. R., & Doershuk, C. F. (1992). Use of nonmedical treatment by cystic fibrosis patients. *Pediatric Nursing*, 19(1), 71–75.

Torrey, W.C. (1993). Psychiatric care of adults with developmental disabilities and mental illness in the community. *Community Mental Health Journal*, 29(5), 461–476.

Ullman, D. (1992). *Homeopathic medicine for children and infants*. New York: G.P. Putnam's Sons.

Watson, J. (1995). Nursing's care-healing paradigm as exemplar for alternative medicine? *Alternative Therapies*, 1(3), 64–69.

Yerks, A. (1996). The Internet and pediatric nursing: guide to the information superhighway. *Pediatric Nursing*, 22(1), 11–15, 26–27.

Zagorsky, E.S. (1993). Caring for families who follow alternative health care practices. *Pediatric Nursing*, 19(1), 71–74.

Zand, J., Walton, R., & Rountree, B. (1995). *Smart medicine for a healthier child*. Garden City, NY: Avery.

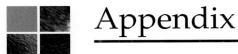

Appendix

Components of Pediatric Rehabilitation Nursing Practice

Dalice L. Hertzberg, Susanne R. Hays, Patricia A. Edwards, and *Nancy M. Youngblood*

Using Appropriate Theory and Content

The pediatric rehabilitation nurse uses appropriate theory and specialized content from the biophysical, psychosocial, behavioral, and developmental sciences as the basis for decision making in rehabilitation nursing practice.

The nursing process provides the systematic approach through which relevant decision making can occur. Related theories and bodies of knowledge include growth and development, biological processes, hierarchy of needs, learning, crisis, family, group dynamics, change and leadership, and pharmacokinetics.

Maintaining Professional Practice Standards

The pediatric rehabilitation nurse maintains professional practice standards by providing nursing interventions that meet individual needs and are consistent with the total rehabilitation program.

Nursing care is designed to restore and maintain health, support adaptive capabilities, and promote independence. The nurse assumes the challenge of helping children, adolescents, and families in making the transition from the hospital to the community and of helping the young client to function in the community. Because of the complex needs of

children and adolescents, pediatric rehabilitation nurses have a leadership role as family educators, counselors, and discharge planners.

Approaching Crises Systematically

The pediatric rehabilitation nurse uses a systematic process to assist children and adolescents and their families in dealing with recurrent actual or potential crises and the impact of these events.

The nurse establishes goals in collaboration with the child or adolescent, the family, and the members of the interdisciplinary team. The plans of care then are implemented through direct intervention or delegation. Systematic evaluation facilitates the child's or adolescent's progress toward his or her maximal level of function, especially as it changes during the various stages of development.

Collaborating With All Members of the Team in the Plan of Care

The pediatric rehabilitation nurse collaborates with other professionals, the child or adolescent, and the family in assessing, planning, implementing, and evaluating an individual interdisciplinary plan of care.

Nursing practice demands sharing and planning with other disciplines to facilitate optimum development. Knowledge of the scope and practice of fellow members of the rehabilitation team is essential to collegial relationships. The team develops an interdisciplinary plan that reflects the expertise of each

Adapted from *Pediatric rehabilitation nursing role description.* (1992). Skokie, IL: Association of Rehabilitation Nurses.

discipline as well as coordination among disciplines.

Participating in Research

The pediatric rehabilitation nurse contributes to nursing and the field of pediatric rehabilitation through participation in research.

As a professional, the pediatric rehabilitation nurse has a responsibility for the continuing development of knowledge and skills in the practice of nursing and rehabilitation. Intra-disciplinary and inter-disciplinary research is essential to this process.

Pursuing Professional Development

The pediatric rehabilitation nurse assumes responsibility for his or her continuing professional development.

Ongoing professional growth and development is an essential component of pediatric rehabilitation nursing because the field is constantly growing and developing, and the nurse must possess diverse knowledge and skills to meet the complex needs of children, adolescents, and families.

Providing Health Education

The pediatric rehabilitation nurse provides health education for professionals and consumers regarding the health needs of children with disabilities and their families.

Nursing service to the pediatric rehabilitation population requires specialized knowledge and skills beyond a baccalaureate education, and nurses must have the necessary expertise to provide advanced nursing care to children and adolescents with disabilities and their families. This expertise includes the ability to observe, conceptualize, and analyze complex health problems; educate others regarding relevant theories and concepts; serve as a role model; evaluate the effectiveness of interventions; and adapt to changing needs and changing environments.

Pediatric Evaluation of Disability Inventory

Stephen M. Haley, Ph.D., P.T., Wendy J. Coster, Ph.D., OTR/L, Larry H. Ludlow, Ph.D.,
Jane T. Haltiwanger, M.A., Ed.M., Peter J. Andrellos, Ph.D.

SCORE FORM

ABOUT THE CHILD

ID# _____

Name _____

Sex M ☐ F ☐ Ethnic group or race _____

Age   Year   Month   Day

Interview Date   _____   _____   _____

Birth Date   _____   _____   _____

Chronological age _____   _____   _____

Diagnosis (if any) _____

ICD-9 code(s) _____ _____ _____
                          primary   additional

CURRENT STATUS OF CHILD

☐ hospital inpatient   ☐ lives at home

　☐ acute care   ☐ lives in residential facility

　☐ rehabilitation

other (specify) _____

School or other facility _____

Grade placement _____

ABOUT THE RESPONDENT (Parent or Guardian)

Name _____

Sex M ☐ F ☐

Relationship to child _____

Type of work (be specific) _____

Years of education _____

ABOUT THE INTERVIEWER

Name _____

Position _____

Facility _____

ABOUT THE ASSESSMENT

Referred by _____

Reason for the assessment

_____

_____

_____

Notes _____

_____

GENERAL DIRECTIONS

Below are the general guidelines for scoring. All the items have specific descriptions. Consult the Manual for individual item scoring criteria.

PART I Functional Skills:
197 discrete items of functional skills

Self-care, Mobility, Social Function

0 = unable, or limited in capability, to perform item in most situations

1 = capable of performing item in most situations, or item has been previously mastered and functional skills have progressed beyond this level

PART II Caregiver Assistance:
20 complex functional activities

Self-care, Mobility, Social Function

5 = Independent
4 = Supervise/Prompt/Monitor
3 = Minimal Assistance
2 = Moderate Assistance
1 = Maximal Assistance
0 = Total Assistance

PART III Modifications:
20 complex functional activities.

Self-care, Mobility, Social Function

N = No Modifications
C = Child-oriented (non-specialized) Modifications
R = Rehabilitation Equipment
E = Extensive Modifications

PLEASE BE SURE YOU HAVE ANSWERED ALL ITEMS.

PEDI Research Group, c/o Stephen M. Haley, Department of Rehabilitation Medicine, New England Medical Center Hospital, # 75K/R, 750 Washington St, Boston, MA 02111-1901 • Phone (617) 956-5031, Fax (617) 956-5353 **VERSION 1.0**

Part I: Functional Skills

SELF-CARE DOMAIN Place a check corresponding to each item:
Item scores: 0 = unable; 1 = capable

UNABLE / CAPABLE

A. Food Textures
0 1

1. Eats pureed/blended/strained foods
2. Eats ground/lumpy foods
3. Eats cut up/chunky/diced foods
4. Eats all textures of table food

B. Use of Utensils
0 1

5. Finger feeds
6. Scoops with a spoon and brings to mouth
7. Uses a spoon well
8. Uses a fork well
9. Uses a knife to butter bread, cut soft foods

C. Use of Drinking Containers
0 1

10. Holds bottle or spout cup
11. Lifts cup to drink, but cup may tip
12. Lifts open cup securely with two hands
13. Lifts open cup securely with one hand
14. Pours liquid from carton or pitcher

D. Toothbrushing
0 1

15. Opens mouth for teeth to be brushed
16. Holds toothbrush
17. Brushes teeth; but not a thorough job
18. Thoroughly brushes teeth
19. Prepares toothbrush with toothpaste

E. Hairbrushing
0 1

20. Holds head in position while hair is combed
21. Brings brush or comb to hair
22. Brushes or combs hair
23. Manages tangles and parts hair

F. Nose Care
0 1

24. Allows nose to be wiped
25. Blows nose into held tissue
26. Wipes nose using tissue on request
27. Wipes nose using tissue without request
28. Blows and wipes nose without request

G. Handwashing
0 1

29. Holds hands out to be washed
30. Rubs hands together to clean
31. Turns water on and off, obtains soap
32. Washes hands thoroughly
33. Dries hands thoroughly

H. Washing Body & Face
0 1

34. Tries to wash parts of body
35. Washes body thoroughly, not including face
36. Obtains soap (and soaps washcloth, if used)
37. Dries body thoroughly
38. Washes and dries face thoroughly

I. Pullover/Front-Opening Garments
0 1

39. Assists, such as pushing arms through shirt
40. Removes T-shirt, dress or sweater
    (pullover garment without fasteners)
41. Puts on T-shirt, dress or sweater
42. Puts on and removes front-opening shirt,
    not including fasteners
43. Puts on and removes front-opening shirt,
    including fasteners

J. Fasteners
0 1

44. Tries to assist with fasteners
45. Zips and unzips, doesn't separate or hook zipper
46. Snaps and unsnaps
47. Buttons and unbuttons
48. Zips and unzips, separates and hooks zipper

K. Pants
0 1

49. Assists, such as pushing legs through pants
50. Removes pants with elastic waist
51. Puts on pants with elastic waist
52. Removes pants, including unfastening
53. Puts on pants, including fastening

L. Shoes/Socks
0 1

54. Removes socks and unfastened shoes
55. Puts on unfastened shoes
56. Puts on socks
57. Puts shoes on correct feet; manages velcro fasteners
58. Ties shoelaces

M. Toileting Tasks (clothes, toilet management, and wiping only)
0 1

59. Assists with clothing management
60. Tries to wipe self after toileting
61. Manages toilet seat, gets toilet paper and flushes toilet
62. Manages clothes before and after toileting
63. Wipes self thoroughly after bowel movements

N. Management of Bladder (Score = 1 if child has previously mastered skill)
0 1

64. Indicates when wet in diapers or training pants
65. Occasionally indicates need to urinate (daytime)
66. Consistently indicates need to urinate with time to get to toilet (daytime)
67. Takes self into bathroom to urinate (daytime)
68. Consistently stays dry day and night

O. Management of Bowel (Score = 1 if child has previously mastered skill)
0 1

69. Indicates need to be changed
70. Occasionally indicates need to use toilet (daytime)
71. Consistently indicates need to use toilet with time to get to toilet (daytime)
72. Distinguishes between need for urination and bowel movements
73. Takes self into bathroom for bowel movements, has no bowel accidents

SELF-CARE DOMAIN SUM	

PLEASE BE SURE YOU HAVE ANSWERED ALL ITEMS.

Comments

MOBILITY DOMAIN

Place a check corresponding to each item:
Item scores: 0 = unable; 1 = capable

A. Toilet Transfers

	UNABLE 0	CAPABLE 1
1. Sits if supported by equipment or caregiver		
2. Sits unsupported on toilet or potty chair		
3. Gets on and off low toilet or potty		
4. Gets on and off adult-sized toilet		
5. Gets on and off toilet, not needing own arms		

B. Chair/Wheelchair Transfers

	0	1
6. Sits if supported by equipment or caregiver		
7. Sits unsupported on chair or bench		
8. Gets on and off low chair or furniture		
9. Gets in and out of adult-sized chair/wheelchair		
10. Gets in and out of chair, not needing own arms		

C. Car Transfers

	0	1
11. Moves in car; scoots on seat or gets in and out of car seat	▨	▨
12. Gets in and out of car with little assistance or instruction	▨	
13. Gets in and out of car with no assistance or instruction	▨	
14. Manages seat belt or chair restraint		
15. Gets in and out of car and opens and closes car door		

D. Bed Mobility/Transfers

	0	1
16. Raises to sitting position in bed or crib		
17. Comes to sit at edge of bed; lies down from sitting at edge of bed	▨	
18. Gets in and out of own bed		
19. Gets in and out of own bed, not needing own arms		

E. Tub Transfers

	0	1
20. Sits if supported by equipment or caregiver in a tub or sink	▨	
21. Sits unsupported and moves in tub		
22. Climbs or scoots in and out of tub		
23. Sits down and stands up from inside tub		
24. Steps/transfers into and out of an adult-sized tub		

F. Indoor Locomotion Methods (Score = 1 if mastered)

	0	1
25. Rolls, scoots, crawls, or creeps on floor		
26. Walks, but holds onto furniture, walls, caregivers or uses devices for support	▨	
27. Walks without support		

G. Indoor Locomotion: Distance/Speed (Score = 1 if mastered)

	0	1
28. Moves within a room but with difficulty (falls; slow for age)	▨	
29. Moves within a room with no difficulty		
30. Moves between rooms but with difficulty (falls; slow for age)	▨	
31. Moves between rooms with no difficulty		
32. Moves indoors 50 feet; opens and closes inside and outside doors		

H. Indoor Locomotion: Pulls/Carries Objects

	0	1
33. Changes physical location purposefully		
34. Moves objects along floor		
35. Carries objects small enough to be held in one hand		
36. Carries objects large enough to require two hands		
37. Carries fragile or spillable objects		

PEDI — 3

I. Outdoor Locomotion: Methods

	UNABLE 0	CAPABLE 1
38. Walks, but holds onto objects, caregiver, or devices for support	▨	
39. Walks without support		

J. Outdoor Locomotion: Distance/Speed (Score = 1 if mastered)

	0	1
40. Moves 10-50 feet (1-5 car lengths)		
41. Moves 50-100 feet (5-10 car lengths)		
42. Moves 100-150 feet (35-50 yards)		
43. Moves 150 feet and longer, but with difficulty (stumbles; slow for age)	▨	
44. Moves 150 feet and longer with no difficulty		

K. Outdoor Locomotion: Surfaces

	0	1
45. Level surfaces (smooth sidewalks, driveways)		
46. Slightly uneven surfaces (cracked pavement)		
47. Rough, uneven surfaces (lawns, gravel driveway)		
48. Up and down incline or ramps		
49. Up and down curbs		

L. Upstairs (Score = 1 if child has previously mastered skill)

	0	1
50. Scoots or crawls up partial flight (1-11 steps)		
51. Scoots or crawls up full flight (12-15 steps)		
52. Walks up partial flight		
53. Walks up full flight, but with difficulty (slow for age)		▨
54. Walks up entire flight with no difficulty		

M. Downstairs (Score = 1 if child has previously mastered skill)

	0	1
55. Scoots or crawls down partial flight (1-11 steps)		
56. Scoots or crawls down full flight (12-15 steps)		
57. Walks down partial flight		
58. Walks down full flight, but with difficulty (slow for age)		▨
59. Walks down full flight with no difficulty		

MOBILITY DOMAIN SUM

PLEASE BE SURE YOU HAVE ANSWERED ALL ITEMS.

SOCIAL FUNCTION DOMAIN

Place a check corresponding to each item: Item scores: 0 = unable; 1 = capable

A. Comprehension Word Meanings

	0	1
1. Orients to sound		
2. Responds to "no"; recognizes own name or that of familiar people		▨
3. Understands 10 words		
4. Understands when you talk about relationships among people and/or things that are visible		
5. Understands when you talk about time and sequence of events		

B. Comprehension of Sentence Complexity

	0	1
6. Understands short sentences about familiar objects and people		▨
7. Understands 1-step commands with words that describe people or things		
8. Understands directions that describe where something is		
9. Understands 2-step commands, using if/then, before/after, first/second, etc.		
10. Understands two sentences that are about the same subject but have a different form		

	UNABLE	CAPABLE
C. Functional Use of Communication	0	1

11. Names things
12. Uses specific words or gestures to direct or request action by another person
13. Seeks information by asking questions
14. Describes an object or action
15. Tells about own feelings or thoughts

		0	1
D. Complexity of Expressive Communication		0	1

16. Uses gestures with clear meaning
17. Uses single word with meaning
18. Uses two words together with meaning
19. Uses 4-5 word sentences
20. Connects two or more thoughts to tell a simple story

	0	1
E. Problem-resolution	0	1

21. Tries to show you the problem or communicate what is needed to help the problem
22. If upset because of a problem, child must be helped immediately or behavior deteriorates
23. If upset because of a problem, child can seek help and wait if it is delayed a short time
24. In ordinary situations, child can describe the problem and his/her feelings with some detail (usually does not act out)
25. Faced with an ordinary problem, child can join adult in working out a solution

	0	1
F. Social Interactive Play (Adults)	0	1

26. Shows awareness and interest in others
27. Initiates a familiar play routine
28. Takes turn in simple play when cued for turn
29. Attempts to imitate adult's previous action during a play activity
30. During play child may suggest new or different steps, or respond to adult suggestion with another idea

	0	1
G. Peer Interactions: (Child of similar age)	0	1

31. Notices presence of other children, may vocalize and gesture toward peers
32. Interacts with other children in simple and brief episodes
33. Tries to work out simple plans for a play activity with another child
34. Plans and carries out cooperative activity with other children; play is sustained and complex
35. Plays activities or games that have rules

	0	1
H. Play with Objects	0	1

36. Manipulates toys, objects or body with intent
37. Uses real or substituted objects in simple pretend sequences
38. Puts together materials to make something
39. Makes up extended pretend play routines involving things the child knows about
40. Makes up elaborate pretend sequences from imagination

Comments

	UNABLE	CAPABLE
I. Self-Information	0	1

41. Can state first name
42. Can state first and last name
43. Provides names and descriptive information about family members
44. Can state full home address; if in hospital, name of hospital and room number
45. Can direct an adult to help child return home or back to the hospital room

	0	1
J. Time Orientation	0	1

46. Has a general awareness of time of mealtimes and routines during the day
47. Has some awareness of sequence of familiar events in a week
48. Has very simple time concepts
49. Associates a specific time with actions/events
50. Regularly checks clock or asks for the time in order to keep track of schedule

	0	1
K. Household Chores	0	1

51. Beginning to help care for own belongings if given constant direction and guidance
52. Beginning to help with simple household chores if given constant direction and guidance
53. Occasionally initiates simple routines to care for own belongings; may require physical help or reminders to complete
54. Occasionally initiates simple household chores; may require physical help or reminders to complete
55. Consistently initiates and carries out at least one household task involving several steps and decisions; may require physical help

	0	1
L. Self-Protection	0	1

56. Shows appropriate caution around stairs
57. Shows appropriate caution around hot or sharp objects
58. When crossing the street with an adult present, child does not need prompting about safety rules
59. Knows not to accept rides, food or money from strangers
60. Crosses busy street safely without an adult

	0	1
M. Community Function	0	1

61. Child may play safely at home without being watched constantly
62. Goes about familiar environment outside of home with only periodic monitoring for safety
63. Follows guidelines/expectations of school and community setting
64. Explores and functions in familiar community settings without supervision
65. Makes transaction in neighborhood store without assistance

SOCIAL FUNCTION DOMAIN SUM	

PLEASE BE SURE YOU HAVE ANSWERED ALL ITEMS.

Parts II and III: Caregiver Assistance and Modification

Circle the appropriate score for Caregiver Assistance and Modification for each item.

	Caregiver Assistance Scale						Modification Scale			
	Independent	Supervision	Minimal	Moderate	Maximal	Total	None	Child	Rehab	Extensive
SELF-CARE DOMAIN	5	4	3	2	1	0	N	C	R	E
A. **Eating**: eating and drinking regular meal; do not include cutting steak, opening containers or serving food from serving dishes	5	4	3	2	1	0	N	C	R	E
B. **Grooming**: brushing teeth, brushing or combing hair and caring for nose	5	4	3	2	1	0	N	C	R	E
C. **Bathing**: washing and drying face and hands, taking a bath or shower; do not include getting in and out of a tub or shower, water preparation, or washing back or hair	5	4	3	2	1	0	N	C	R	E
D. **Dressing Upper Body**: all indoor clothes, not including back fasteners; include help putting on or taking off splint or artificial limb; do not include getting clothes from closet or drawers	5	4	3	2	1	0	N	C	R	E
E. **Dressing Lower Body**: all indoor clothes; include putting on or taking off brace or artificial limb; do not include getting clothes from closet or drawers	5	4	3	2	1	0	N	C	R	E
F. **Toileting**: clothes, toilet management or external device use, and hygiene; do not include toilet transfers, monitoring schedule, or cleaning up after accidents	5	4	3	2	1	0	N	C	R	E
G. **Bladder Management**: control of bladder day and night. clean-up after accidents, monitoring schedule	5	4	3	2	1	0	N	C	R	E
H. **Bowel Management**: control of bowel day and night, clean-up after accidents, monitoring schedule	5	4	3	2	1	0	N	C	R	E
Self-Care Totals **SELF-CARE SUM**										

Self-Care Modification Frequencies

MOBILITY DOMAIN										
A. **Chair/Toilet Transfers**: child's wheelchair, adult-sized chair, adult-sized toilet	5	4	3	2	1	0	N	C	R	E
B. **Car Transfers**: mobility within car/van, seat belt use, transfers, and opening and closing doors	5	4	3	2	1	0	N	C	R	E
C. **Bed Mobility/Transfers**: getting in and out and changing positions in child's own bed	5	4	3	2	1	0	N	C	R	E
D. **Tub Transfers**: getting in and out of adult-sized tub	5	4	3	2	1	0	N	C	R	E
E. **Indoor Locomotion**: 50 feet (3-4 rooms); do not include opening doors or carrying objects	5	4	3	2	1	0	N	C	R	E
F. **Outdoor Locomotion**: 150 feet (15 car lengths) on level surfaces; focus on physical ability to move outdoors (do not consider compliance or safety issues such as crossing streets)	5	4	3	2	1	0	N	C	R	E
G. **Stairs**: climb and descend a full flight of stairs (12-15 steps)	5	4	3	2	1	0	N	C	R	E
Mobility Totals **MOBILITY SUM**										

Mobility Modification Frequencies

SOCIAL FUNCTION DOMAIN										
A. **Functional Comprehension**: understanding of requests and instructions	5	4	3	2	1	0	N	C	R	E
B. **Functional Expression**: ability to provide information about own activities and make own needs known; include clarity of articulation	5	4	3	2	1	0	N	C	R	E
C. **Joint Problem Solving**: include communication of problem and working with caregiver or other adult to find a solution; include only ordinary problems occurring during daily activities; (for example, lost toy; conflict over clothing choices.)	5	4	3	2	1	0	N	C	R	E
D. **Peer Play**: ability to plan and carry out joint activities with a familiar peer	5	4	3	2	1	0	N	C	R	E
E. **Safety**: caution in routine daily safety situations, including stairs, sharp or hot objects and traffic	5	4	3	2	1	0	N	C	R	E
Social Function Totals **SOCIAL FUNCTION SUM**										

Social Function Modification Frequencies

Pediatric Evaluation of Disability Inventory

Name _____   Test Date _____   Age _____

ID# _____   Respondent/Interviewer _____

SCORE SUMMARY

Composite Scores

DOMAIN		RAW SCORE	NORMATIVE STANDARD SCORE	STANDARD ERROR	SCALED SCORE	STANDARD ERROR	FIT SCORE*
Self-Care	Functional Skills						
Mobility	Functional Skills						
Social Function	Functional Skills						
Self-Care	Caregiver Assistance						
Mobility	Caregiver Assistance						
Social Function	Caregiver Assistance						

*Obtainable only through use of software program

MODIFICATION FREQUENCIES

SELF-CARE (8 ITEMS)				MOBILITY (7 ITEMS)				SOCIAL FUNCTION (5 ITEMS)			
None	Child	Rehab	Extensive	None	Child	Rehab	Extensive	None	Child	Rehab	Extensive

Score Profile

DOMAIN		NORMATIVE STANDARD SCORES	SCALED SCORES
Self-Care	Functional Skills	10 30 50 70 90	0 50 100
Mobility	Functional Skills	10 30 50 70 90	0 50 100
Social Function	Functional Skills	10 30 50 70 90	0 50 100
Self-Care	Caregiver Assistance	10 30 50 70 90	0 50 100
Mobility	Caregiver Assistance	10 30 50 70 90	0 50 100
Social Function	Caregiver Assistance	10 30 50 70 90	0 50 100

± 2 standard errors

VERSION 1.0

Values

The New England SERVE Regional Task Force on Quality Assurance began its work by reviewing and defining core beliefs and values regarding health care for children with specialized needs. These values formed the philosophical base for the development of the standards contained in *Enhancing Quality*. The following values adopted by the Task Force focus on the rights of the child and his or her family to have access to and receive appropriate care.

All care for children with special health care needs shall be:

Community-based Services delivered at a local level or as close to the child's home as possible; the major responsibility for planning, designing, and implementing the services rests within the community as defined by the family.

Comprehensive The inclusion of a broad range of health, educational, social, and related services in delivering care.

Continuous Care that is maintained without interruption despite changes in the child's health care delivery site, caregivers, or method of payment.

Coordinated Care that is planned and implemented so as to form a cohesive therapeutic program.

Adapted from Epstein, S., Taylor, A., Halberg, A., Gardner, J., Walker, D., & Crocker, A. (1989). *Enhancing quality: standards and indicators of quality care for children with special health care needs*. Boston: New England SERVE.

Developmentally-oriented Care that is based on the individual's functional level and chronological age. Functional level includes physical, cognitive, psycho-social, and communications development.

Documented All aspects of care (assessment, problem-identification, ongoing interventions, and outcomes) are periodically recorded in a system that is easily accessible to the family, providers, and authorized monitors and evaluators of health care.

Efficacious Care that is based on acceptable scientific evidence and practices, achieving the anticipated outcomes in health status.

Family-centered Care that recognizes and respects the pivotal role of the family in the lives of children. It supports families in their natural caregiving roles, promotes normal patterns of living, and ensures family collaboration and choice in the provision of services to the child.

Geographically-available Care that is accessible to all children regardless of place of residence.

Individualized Care that reflects the unique physical, developmental, emotional, social, educational, and cultural needs of the individual within the context of the family.

Integrated Care that includes a system for communication and advocacy in order to ensure that the individual and his or her family participate fully in all aspects of society.

Interdisciplinary A process of communication and interaction among persons who bring a variety of diagnostic, therapeutic, and habilitative skills and knowledge to bear on the development and implementation of a health care plan.

Non-discriminatory Care that is available to all individuals and their families regardless of race or ethnic identity, primary language, religion, gender, sexual orientation, marital status, medical condition, or method of payment.

Payment-assured The cost of health services provided to the child are paid for while protecting the financial integrity of the family.

Safe Care that is free from unnecessary risk by ensuring use of adequate facilities, staff, procedures and equipment.

Neutropenia: A Parents' Guide

Michael Comeau

■

As part of your child's therapy, the complete blood count (CBC), or "counts," will be checked on a regular basis. Counts consist of the white blood cell count (WBC), the hematocrit (Hct), and the platelet count. It is important to know what each type of cell does. White blood cells are the infection-fighting cells of the blood. The hematocrit measures the amount of red blood cells, which carry oxygen to the organs and tissues. Platelets are necessary for proper blood clotting.

One of the major side effects of chemotherapy is its effect on the WBC. Chemotherapy lowers the WBC. White blood cells are the body's main defense against infection, and they fight infection in several ways. The CBC tells us the WBC, HCT, and platelet count. A differential count is a breakdown of the different types of white blood cells. When looking at the differential count, the most important factors are the number of polymorphonuclear cells, or polys, and the number of bands. Polys may also be called segmented neutrophils, or segs. Other white blood cells also will be listed, such as monocytes (monos), eosinophils (eos), and lymphocytes

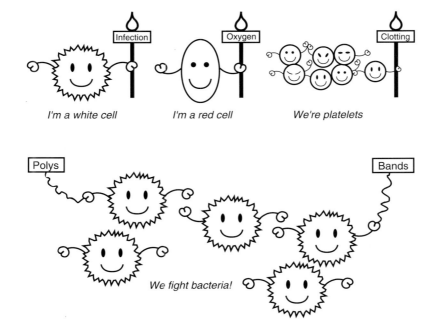

I'm a white cell   I'm a red cell   We're platelets

Polys   Bands

We fight bacteria!

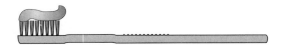

(lymphs), but for our purposes, it is the polys and the bands that are most important.

The polys and the bands are types of white blood cells that fight infection caused by bacteria. The body uses polys to destroy and remove bacteria that could be harmful. When there are few polys, the body is at greater risk for infection and may not show some of the symptoms that normally would occur in someone who had plenty of polys and bands. Normal symptoms of infection such as redness or swelling may not occur; therefore, particular attention must be paid to the skin and any cuts or scratches. It is also important that areas that normally have bacteria, such as the mouth or rectal area, be kept clean. It is important to never take a temperature rectally or give any medication rectally unless ordered by your doctor.

One way that you can determine whether your child is at greater risk for infection is by determination of the absolute neutrophil count (ANC). The ANC is the percentage of bacteria-fighting white cells (polys and bands) in relation to the total WBC. Technically, an ANC <1000 cells/mm³ is considered neutropenia, and an ANC <500 cells/mm³ must be treated very seriously.

$$ANC = WBC \times 1000 \, (\% \text{ polys} + \% \text{ bands})$$

Example

J.R. has a WBC of 3.0; the differential consists of 20 polys and 5 bands. What is his ANC?

$$WBC \times 1000 = 3.0 \times 1000 = 3000$$

$$\text{polys} + \text{bands} = 20 + 5 = 25$$

Expressed as a percentage, $25 \div 100 = .25$

$$25\% \text{ of } 3000 = .25 \times 3000 = 750$$

Therefore, J.R's ANC is 750 cells/mm³

The ANC is an important number for two reasons the ANC determines when chemotherapy can be given, and the ANC determines when your child is neutropenic and more at risk for infection. Most people need practice in figuring out the ANC; your primary nurse is available to assist you as needed. Your primary nurse will also be available to review with you the ANC as well as the normal laboratory values for the Hct and platelet count.

If you need to call the doctor or have questions for your primary nurse, please call the clinic.

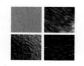

Index

Note: Page numbers in *italics* refer to illustrations; page numbers followed by t refer to tables.

ISBN 0-7216-5425-8

90038